Theranostics Approaches to Gastric Cancer

Theranostics Approaches to Gastric Cancer

Editor: Donald Maxmilian

AMERICAN
MEDICAL PUBLISHERS
www.americanmedicalpublishers.com

AMERICAN
MEDICAL PUBLISHERS
www.americanmedicalpublishers.com

Cataloging-in-Publication Data

Theranostics approaches to gastric cancer / edited by Donald Maxmilian.
p. cm.
Includes bibliographical references and index.
ISBN 979-8-88740-505-6
1. Stomach--Cancer. 2. Stomach--Cancer--Diagnosis. 3. Stomach--Cancer--Treatment.
4. Stomach--Diseases. I. Maxmilian, Donald.
RC280.S8 T44 2023
616.994 33--dc23

American Medical Publishers,
41 Flatbush Avenue,
1st Floor, New York,
NY 11217, USA

ISBN 979-8-88740-505-6 (Hardback)

Contents

Preface

The term theranostics is derived from the combination of two words, namely, therapeutics and diagnostics. It is a practical aspect of personalized medicine. It involves using a combination of one radioactive drug to identify (diagnose) and a second radioactive drug to provide therapy in order to treat a tumor. Gastric cancer, also known as stomach cancer, develops due to the formation of malignant cancer cells in the lining of the stomach. The factors such as age, diet, and stomach diseases result in the development of gastric cancer. Some of the common symptoms of this cancer include unexplained weight loss, severe abdominal pain, nausea and vomiting, difficulty in swallowing, etc. It can be diagnosed with the help of imaging tests such as CT or CAT scans, PET scans, MRI, or upper gastrointestinal endoscopy. Theranostics includes molecular targeting and nanotechnologies which are increasingly finding many applications in the treatment of gastric cancer. In this book, the various advancements in the field of theranostics as well as their application for the treatment of gastric cancer have been looked at in detail. For all readers who are interested in this area of study, the case studies included herein will serve as an excellent guide to develop a comprehensive understanding.

After months of intensive research and writing, this book is the end result of all who devoted their time and efforts in the initiation and progress of this book. It will surely be a source of reference in enhancing the required knowledge of the new developments in the area. During the course of developing this book, certain measures such as accuracy, authenticity and research focused analytical studies were given preference in order to produce a comprehensive book in the area of study.

This book would not have been possible without the efforts of the authors and the publisher. I extend my sincere thanks to them. Secondly, I express my gratitude to my family and well-wishers. And most importantly, I thank my students for constantly expressing their willingness and curiosity in enhancing their knowledge in the field, which encourages me to take up further research projects for the advancement of the area.

Editor

1

Comparison of Early Oral Feeding with Traditional Oral Feeding After Total Gastrectomy for Gastric Cancer: A Propensity Score Matching Analysis

Juan Wang[1†], *Min Yang*[2†], *Quan Wang*[1†] *and Gang Ji*[1*]

[1] *Department of Digestive Surgery, Xi Jing Hospital, The Fourth Military Medical University, Xi'an, China,* [2] *Emergency Department, Huangpu Branch of the Ninth People's Hospital Affiliated to the Medical College of Shanghai Jiaotong University, Shanghai, China*

***Correspondence:**
Gang Ji
jigangfmmu@163.com

† *These authors have contributed equally to this work*

Background: The present study aimed to compare the feasibility and safety of early oral feeding (EOF) with traditional oral feeding (TOF) after radical total gastrectomy for gastric cancer.

Methods: This retrospective study included consecutive patients who underwent total gastrectomy from April 2016 and November 2018. These patients were divided into two groups, according to their postoperative feeding protocol: EOF group (n = 314) and TOF group (n = 433). Propensity score matching was used to balance the potential confounders, and 276 patients were selected from each group. The EOF group received oral diet on postoperative day one, while the TOF group were started on oral feeding after the passage of flatus.

Results: No significant differences were found in the postoperative complications ($P = 0.426$) and tolerance to oral feeding ($P > 0.056$) between the two groups. The changes in perioperative nutritional markers were also similar between the two groups ($P > 0.05$). The time to first passage of flatus or defecation (47.19 ± 12.00 h vs. 58.19 ± 9.89 h, $P < 0.0001$) and length of postoperative hospital stay (6.84 ± 2.31 days vs. 7.72 ± 2.86 days, $P < 0.0001$) were significantly lower in the EOF group compared to the TOF group.

Conclusion: EOF may be safe and feasible after radical total gastrectomy with faster recovery and no increased risk of postoperative complications.

Keywords: early oral feeding, traditional oral feeding, total gastrectomy, gastric cancer, propensity score matching

INTRODUCTION

Gastric cancer is the third most common cause of cancer-related death, and has the fifth highest incidence of cancer worldwide (1). Most of these patients require multimodality treatment including endoscopic resection, surgical resection, chemotherapy, immunotherapy, and radiation therapy. The stomach is also the most common site for gastrointestinal lymphoma (2). However, the treatment for both these diseases are completely different. For early stage gastric adenocarcinoma, complete endoscopic, or surgical resection is the only curative treatment as recommended by the NCCN guidelines (3). Chemotherapy and immunotherapy are used in the neoadjuvant and adjuvant settings to take care of the micro-metastases and cannot achieve complete pathological response. Hence, they are not the preferred first line therapies. Unlike adenocarcinoma, gastric lymphoma shows very good response to chemotherapy, and Helicobacter pylori eradication therapy. Hence, chemotherapy is the first-line treatment for gastric lymphoma (4).

Traditionally, oral feeding is delayed after gastric surgery, until the passage of flatus, or appearance of audible bowel sounds or bowel movements due to the theoretical concerns of increased risk of anastomosis leakage (5). The rationale of nil by mouth was to allow the anastomosis to heal before being stressed by food (6). However, recent studies have questioned this traditional concept of fasting until passage of flatus after gastric surgery (7–9).

Contrary to the widespread belief, various studies have confirmed the safety and feasibility of early oral feeding (EOF) (6, 7, 10–13). A randomized clinical trial performed by Hur et al. demonstrated that EOF was feasible, and could result in shorter hospitalization and improvements in the quality of life of 54 patients receiving open gastrectomy (7). A case-control study and pilot study revealed that EOF after gastrectomy is feasible, with no increase in morbidity (8, 14). A meta-analysis of patients who underwent distal gastrectomy also revealed that EOF is safe and feasible (15). Another systematic review and meta-analysis conducted by Liu et al. revealed that EOF after gastrectomy did not increase the incidence of postoperative complications or readmissions, and significantly reduced the length of hospital stay (15). Furthermore, a recent meta-analysis of six randomized controlled trials (RCTs) of gastric cancer surgery (15) and the combined meta-analysis of 15 RCTs and other studies of open upper gastrointestinal surgery (16) revealed that EOF could reduce the length of hospital stay and bowel recovery time without increasing postoperative complications in gastrectomy patients. Moreover, early oral nutrition is one of the most important elements of the enhanced recovery after surgery (ERAS) strategy after gastrointestinal surgery (7, 8).

Although a number of studies have reported the outcomes of EOF after gastric surgery, most of these studies have focused on EOF after distal gastrectomy. Hence, the outcomes of early oral nutrition after total gastrectomy for gastric cancer is scarce and limited. In recent years, gastric cancer surgery has developed from open surgery, laparoscopic-assisted surgery, to total laparoscopic surgery. However, due to the high position of the gastroesophageal junction and small operating space, it remains difficult to laparoscopically perform a complete total gastrectomy. At present, in China, pure laparoscopic total gastrectomy is only performed in few high-volume centers, and its safety and long-term survival effects have not been confirmed by large-scale clinical studies. Therefore, in the present study, a single center retrospective cohort study was conducted using propensity score matching, in order to compare EOF with traditional oral feeding (TOF) following total gastrectomy (for both open and laparoscopic surgery) in gastric cancer patients. The propensity score matching analysis was used to for the confounding factors by forming a matched cohort, taking in to consideration various variables (17).

PATIENTS AND METHODS

Study Design and Propensity Score Matching

In the present study, the data of patients who underwent radical total gastrectomy for gastric carcinoma between April 2016 and November 2018 at the Department of Gastrointestinal Surgery of Xijing Hospital Affiliated to the Fourth Military Medical University were retrospectively analyzed (**Figure 1**). According to the time when oral nutrition was initiated, these patients were divided into two groups: EOF group and TOF group. Propensity score matching was performed using the logistic regression model to generate a propensity score for balancing the baseline characteristics and potential confounders between these two groups. Specifically, the tendency score was used to synthesize all the observed variable information and balance the variables in order to reduce bias. In the present study, patients were matched one-to-one by propensity score (random selection from severe nearest-neighbor individual propensity score match of which difference between the standard and the matching value <0.001, calculated and matched with logistic regression, a caliper of 0.2 without replacement) using the covariates of age, gender, body mass index (BMI), NRS2002 score (18), American Society of Anesthesiologists (ASA) score, tumor differentiation, clinical stage, and surgical approach as the confounding variables for propensity score matching. The propensity scoring function of the SPSS 22.0 software was used to perform the variable matching. The confounding factors were balanced in the two groups after the propensity score matching. McNemar's Test was used for sensitivity analysis (19). Then, the matched and adjusted cohort data were analyzed, and the results were obtained.

NRS2002 was first introduced by Kondrup (18), and has three components: impaired nutritional status (0–3 points), severity of disease (0–3 points), and age (0–1 points). Patients with NRS 2002 <3 and ≥3 (original scale) were classified as "no nutritional risk" and "nutritional risk," respectively.

Selection Criteria

The present study included patients with histologically proven gastric adenocarcinoma by preoperative gastroscopy biopsy or postoperative pathology, who received radical total gastrectomy with R0 resection margins.

The exclusion criteria were as follows: (1) patients with severe cardiovascular disease, respiratory disease, hepatopathy, renal impairment, and abnormal nutritional status; (2) patients with metastatic disease or another type of cancer; (3) patients with a history of neoadjuvant chemo/radiotherapy; (4) patients who underwent emergency operation due to gastric perforation or bleeding; (5) patients with serious complications such as major bleeding occurring within 24 h after surgery, which may affect the oral feeding; (6) patients with combined resection of other organs (except for the gallbladder) or thoracotomy; (7) patients with a preoperative NRS2002 score >3 points or BMI <17 kg/m^2; (8) patients who were admitted to the intensive care unit (ICU) after surgery.

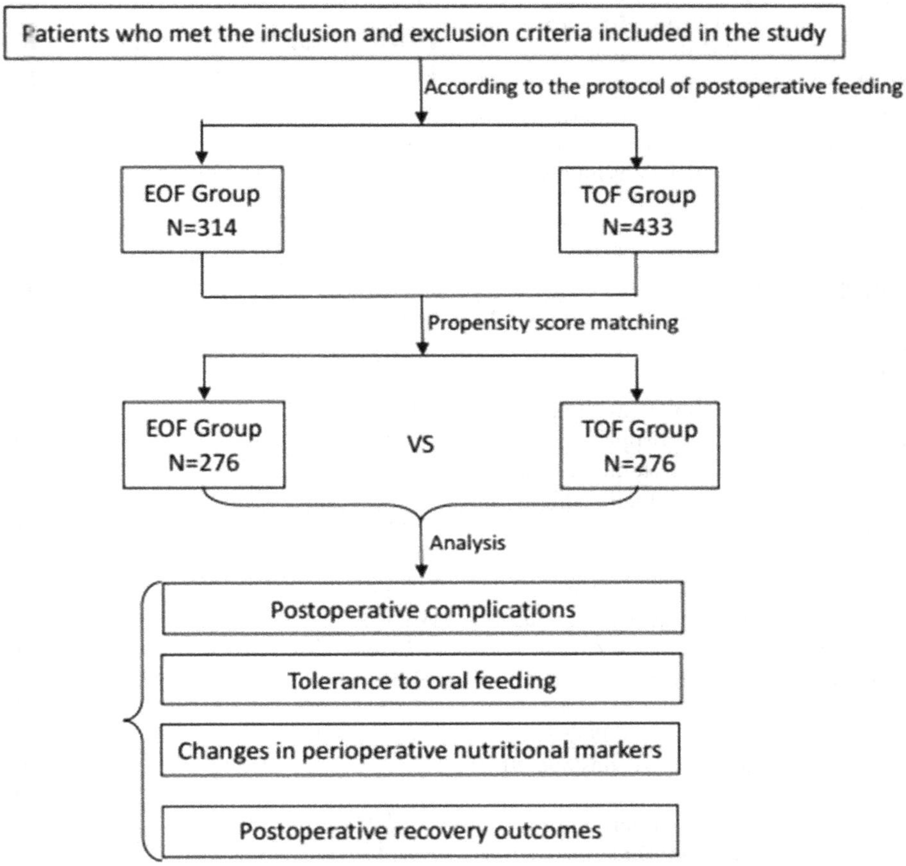

FIGURE 1 | Flow chart depicting the patient selection, propensity score matching, and postoperative variables used for analysis (EOF, early oral feeding; TOF, traditional oral feeding).

An informed consent was obtained from all patients. The Institutional Review Board of the Air force Military Medical University approved the present study.

Postoperative Feeding

For patients in the EOF group, oral feeding was initiated by giving water on the first postoperative day. These patients were started on a clear liquid diet on the second postoperative day, which contained glucose, sodium chloride water, and enteral nutrient solution. From the third postoperative day up to the day of discharge, patients were instructed to eat a liquid diet, and when they passed the flatus or bowel sounds appeared, soft diet was gradually given. The daily calorie requirements were met by supplementing with parenteral nutrition (1,200–1,400 kcal, 20–25 mL/kg/d). For patients who developed intractable nausea, vomiting, or distension, the diet was stopped, and a nasogastric tube was inserted.

For patients in the TOF group, oral feeding was started by giving water when the bowel sounds were audible, or with the passage of flatus. Prior to that, patients were maintained nil-by-mouth, and the daily calorie requirements were provided by parenteral nutrition. A clear liquid diet was given on the next day, and a soft diet was gradually given when the liquid diet was well-tolerated. The diet was stopped and a nasogastric tube was inserted when patients complained of intractable nausea, vomiting, or abdominal distension.

Perioperative Treatment

Before surgery, preoperative bowel preparation was avoided. Both groups received similar prophylactic antibiotics before the skin incision. General anesthesia with similar anesthetic drugs was administered to all patients. All surgeries were performed by experienced surgeons. Total gastrectomy with a Roux-en-Y esophagojejunostomy reconstruction and D2 lymph node dissection was performed for all patients, as described in the Japanese gastric cancer treatment guidelines (20). All anastomoses were strengthened by a 3–0 silk thread. A nasogastric tube and urinary catheter were routinely inserted in the operating room, and was removed on the morning of postoperative day (POD) 1. An abdominal drain was also routinely placed. Postoperative pain was managed by non-steroidal anti-inflammatory drugs (NSAIDs), but no epidural analgesia was given. All the patients were encouraged to start active ambulation from POD1. Patients in both the groups were discharged using the same criteria. The criteria for discharge were as follows: (1) no pyrexia; (2) passage of flatus and feces in the postoperative period; (3) removal of the abdominal drain; (4) no obvious symptoms such as nausea, vomiting and abdominal distention; (5) tolerance of oral feeding for at least 24 h. When the patients were suspected to have anastomotic complications, such as anastomotic leakage or ileus, oral intake was immediately stopped, and the appropriate treatment was given.

Data Collection and Definitions

Data regarding the demographic and clinicopathologic characteristics of the patients were retrieved from the medical records. The following data was collected: age, gender, NRS2002 score, ASA score, BMI, histologic differentiation, pathological stage, surgical approach (laparoscopic surgery or open surgery), complications (including anastomotic leakage, duodenal stump leakage, pancreatic fistula, abdominal bleeding, abdominal infection, pulmonary infection, wound infection, wound dehiscence, and ileus), the prevalence and grade of all postoperative complications (revised Clavien-Dindo classification) (21), reoperation, re-hospitalization, 30-day mortality, oral feeding tolerance (including postoperative nausea or vomiting, and abdominal distention), changes in nutritional markers (preoperative and postoperative serum albumin and serum prealbumin level on POD1 and POD3), time to first passage of flatus or feces, and length of postoperative hospital stay.

The pathological stage was performed according to the seventh edition of the American Joint Committee on Cancer TNM classification of gastric carcinoma. Complications were detected using the clinical symptoms, or the laboratory and imaging tests. The anastomotic leakage was radiologically (extravasation of the contrast medium at the anastomotic site) or clinically (abdominal pain, fever, and discharge of gastrointestinal content through a drain) confirmed. Postoperative morbidity and mortality were defined as complications or deaths within 30 days after surgery.

Follow-Up

After discharge from the hospital, patients were followed up in the Outpatient Department or by telephone. Blood or imaging studies (X-radiography, CT scan, or angiography) were performed according to the clinical symptoms.

Statistical Analysis

Data were expressed as mean ± standard deviation (SD), or number and percentage. The categorical variables were compared using chi-square test, and Student *t*-test was used to compare continuous variables. The difference in changes in postoperative nutritional markers was analyzed by two-way repeated-measures ANOVA. Two-sided *P*-values <0.05 were considered to be statistically significant. The statistical analysis was performed using the IBM® SPSS® Statistics Version 22.0 (Corp, Armonk, NY, USA).

RESULTS

Patient Characteristics Before and After Propensity Score Matching

A total of 747 patients were included in the present study. Among these patients, 314 patients (42.03%) were treated with EOF, while the remaining 433 patients (57.97%) received TOF. The clinicopathological characteristics of these patients are presented in **Table 1**. Before the propensity score matching, there were significant differences in gender ($P = 0.022$), histological differentiation ($P < 0.0001$), and surgical approach ($P < 0.0001$) between the EOF and TOF groups (**Table 1**). However, there were no statistically significant differences in age, NRS2002 score, ASA score, BMI and pathological stage between the two groups (**Table 1**). After the propensity score matching, 276 patients were selected from each group, and the baseline characteristics were well-balanced between the two matched groups (**Table 1**).

Postoperative Complications

Table 2 presents the incidence of each complication in the two groups. In the two matched groups, 43 (15.58%) and 50 (18.12%) patients developed postoperative complications in the EOF and TOF groups, respectively. Although the incidence of postoperative complications was higher in the TOF group, the difference was not statistically significant ($P > 0.050$, **Table 2**). Serious complications (Clavien-Dindo grade >III) developed in 27.91% (12/43) and 36.00% (18/50) of patients in the EOF and TOF groups, respectively. Reoperation were performed in 11 (3.99%) patients in EOF group and 17 (6.16%) patients in TOF group, and the re-hospitalization rate was 0.36% both in the EOF and TOF groups. The reoperation rate ($P = 0.245$), re-hospitalization rate ($P = 1.000$), and serious complications (Clavien-Dindo grade >III) rate ($P = 0.405$) were not statistically different between the two groups. No 30 day-mortality occurred in either of the groups.

Tolerance to Oral Feeding

After the propensity score matching, 15 (5.43%) and nine (3.26%) patients had nausea or vomiting in the EOF and TOF groups, respectively ($P = 0.210$). Furthermore, 20 patients (7.25%) in the EOF group and 10 patients (3.62%) in the TOF group had abdominal distention ($P = 0.060$). The tolerance of oral feeding in the EOF and TOF groups was 88.41 and 93.12%, respectively ($P = 0.056$, **Table 3**).

Changes in Perioperative Nutritional Markers

In the present study, serum albumin levels and serum prealbumin were used as the nutritional markers. There was no statistical difference between these nutritional markers in the EOF and TOF groups, before and after the surgery (**Table 4**). The two-way repeated-measures ANOVA analysis revealed that the changes in serum albumin levels from the day before surgery to POD3 was similar between these two groups ($P = 0.638$).

Serum pre-albumin, which has a short half-life and is more sensitive to changes in nutritional status, was also tested, and no statistical difference was found between the two groups, before

TABLE 1 | Patient demographics and baseline clinicopathological characteristics before and after propensity score matching.

Characteristics	Before matching		χ^2	P1 value	After matching		χ^2	P2 value
	EOF group	TOF group			EOF group	TOF group		
Age (years)			0.343	0.558			0.000	1.000
≤60	162	214			140	140		
>60	152	219			136	136		
Gender			5.246	0.022			0.011	0.915
Male	244	365			222	221		
Female	70	68			54	55		
NRS2002 Score			0.727	0.394			0.034	0.854
1	216	285			190	192		
2	98	148			86	84		
ASA score			5.079	0.079			2.225	0.329
I	79	86			71	63		
II	182	250			153	170		
III	53	97			52	43		
BMI			0.014	0.907			0.282	0.595
≤25	252	346			218	223		
>25	62	87			58	53		
Tumor differentiation			23.860	<0.001			5.455	0.065
I	52	107			52	41		
II	168	258			149	176		
III	94	68			75	59		
Pathological stage			0.155	0.694			0.212	0.645
I+II	103	148			88	83		
III	211	285			188	193		
Surgical approach			15.56	<0.001			0.000	1.000
Laparoscopic surgery	166	166			142	142		
Open surgery	148	267			134	134		

EOF, early oral feeding; TOF, traditional oral feeding; P1, represents the variable comparison of baseline clinicopathological characteristics before matching; P2, represents the variable comparison of baseline clinicopathological characteristics after matching.

and after surgery (before surgery: $t = 0.155$, $P = 0.877$; POD1: $t = 0.188$, $P = 0.851$; POD3: $t = 1.620$, $P = 0.106$). The two-way repeated-measures ANOVA analysis also revealed that the changes in serum prealbumin levels from the day before surgery to POD3 was similar between the two groups ($P = 0.285$).

Postoperative Recovery Outcomes

There was a significant decrease in the time to first passage of flatus or feces in the EOF group, when compared to the TOF group (47.19 ± 12.00 h vs. 58.19 ± 9.89 h, $P < 0.0001$; **Table 5**). Furthermore, the length of postoperative hospital stay also significantly decreased in the EOF group (6.84 ± 2.31 days vs. 7.72 ± 2.86 days, $P < 0.0001$; **Table 5**).

Sensitivity Analysis for Propensity Score Matching

Since the propensity score only balances the matched variables between the two groups and does not eliminate potential confounding factors, sensitivity analyses were performed to determine the impact of potential confounding factors that fail to match between the two groups. In the sensitivity analysis, the calculations for gamma values ranged between 1.0 (i.e., no hidden bias) and 6.0, stepping by 0.5. The sensitivity analysis tips over significance at the two-tailed $\alpha = 0.05$ level somewhere between gamma = 5.0 and gamma = 5.5. A gamma threshold was 5.472 for overall postoperative complications and the tolerance of oral feeding. This suggests that an unobserved covariate would be need to produce more than a 5-fold increase in the odds of overall postoperative complications and the tolerance of oral feeding (**Supplementary Tables 1, 2**).

DISCUSSION

In China, there is high incidence of gastric cancer. Approximately 40% of new cases of gastric cancer diagnosed every year, worldwide occur in China (1). Various newer therapies, including targeted therapy and immunotherapy, have been developed to improve the survival outcomes of gastric cancer (22). However, the best treatment option for gastric cancer continues to be surgery despite its associated morbidities and the risk of postoperative mortality. Various advancements in the surgical techniques such as minimally invasive surgeries

TABLE 2 | Comparison of postoperative complications between the EOF and TOF groups after propensity score matching.

Complications	EOF group (n = 276)	TOF group (n = 276)	χ^2	*P*-value
All postoperative complications	43 (15.58%)	50 (18.12%)	0.634	0.426
Clavien-dindo grade >III	12/43 (27.91%)	18/50 (36.00%)		
Anastomosis leakage	7 (2.54%)	8 (2.90%)	0.069	0.793
Duodenal stump leakage	3 (1.09%)	6 (2.17%)	1.017	0.313
Pancreatic fistula	0	0		
Abdominal bleeding	2 (0.72%)	4 (1.45%)	0.674	0.412
Abdominal infection	5 (1.81%)	9 (3.26%)	1.173	0.279
Pulmonary infection	23 (8.33%)	27 (9.78%)	0.352	0.553
Wound infection	5 (1.81%)	4 (1.45%)	0.113	0.737
Wound dehiscence	2 (0.72%)	6 (2.17%)	2.029	0.154
Ileus	6 (2.17%)	6 (2.17%)	0.000	1.000
Reoperation	11 (3.99%)	17 (6.16%)	1.354	0.245
Rehospitalization	1 (0.36%)	1 (0.36%)	0.000	1.000
30-day mortality rate	0	0		

TABLE 3 | Comparison of tolerance to oral feeding between the EOF and TOF groups after propensity score matching.

Symptoms	EOF group (n = 276)	TOF group (n = 276)	χ^2	*P*-value
Nausea or vomiting	15 (5.43%)	9 (3.26%)	1.568	0.210
Abdominal distention	20 (7.25%)	10 (3.62%)	3.525	0.060
Tolerance of oral feeding	244 (88.41%)	257 (93.12%)	3.651	0.056

and perioperative care, have led to substantial improvements in postoperative outcomes. Various studies have shown laparoscopic gastrectomy to be associated with lesser blood loss, reduced postoperative pain, faster recovery, and reduced hospital stay (23–25). A key aspect of perioperative care that has been found to improve short-term outcomes includes the adaptation of the ERAS strategy.

Traditionally, oral feeding is started after the appearance of bowel movements, or passage of flatus or defecation after gastric surgery (26). Early oral intake has been considered dangerous due to the fear of anastomotic leakage caused by the increased intraluminal pressure of the postoperative atonic intestine and poor tolerability of patients (6). This concern is particularly evident after total gastrectomy, because the esophageal-jejunal anastomosis is considered to be more prone to develop anastomotic leakage. However, EOF is an important component of ERAS strategy. In the present study, it was found that EOF after radical total gastrectomy for gastric cancer significantly enhanced the recovery of bowel function ($P < 0.0001$) and decreased the length of hospital stay ($P < 0.0001$) without increasing the risk of postoperative complications and mortality. Although a lower occurrence of postoperative complications was observed in the EOF group, the difference was not statistically significant ($P > 0.05$), which implies that EOF is a safe option after radical total gastrectomy. It was also found that there were no

TABLE 4 | Comparison of perioperative nutritional markers between the EOF and TOF groups after propensity score matching.

Nutritional markers	EOF group	TOF group	*t*-value	*P*-value
Serum preoperative albumin (g/L)	39.27 ± 2.34	39.20 ± 2.24	0.391	0.696
Serum preoperative prealbumin (g/L)	30.89 ± 2.96	30.86 ± 3.06	0.155	0.877
Serum albumin on POD1 (g/L)	34.33 ± 2.35	34.03 ± 2.84	1.355	0.176
Serum prealbumin on POD1 (g/L)	38.51 ± 2.21	28.54 ± 2.32	0.188	0.851
Serum albumin on POD3 (g/L)	31.80 ± 3.17	31.78 ± 2.24	0.080	0.937
Serum prealbumin on POD3 (g/L)	30.08 ± 3.64	30.57 ± 3.45	1.620	0.106

TABLE 5 | Comparison of postoperative outcomes between the EOF and TOF groups after propensity score matching.

Outcomes	EOF group	TOF group	*t*-value	*P*-value
Time to first passage of flatus or defecation (hr)	47.19 ± 12.00	58.19 ± 9.89	11.750	<0.0001
Length of postoperative hospital stay (d)	6.84 ± 2.31	7.72 ± 2.86	3.984	<0.0001

significant differences in serum albumin and prealbumin levels before and after surgery in EOF and TOF groups. Hence, it was considered that EOF not only provides nutritional support, but also accelerates the recovery of gastrointestinal function through food stimulation, thereby reducing surgical complications.

In recent years, various studies have shown that EOF after surgery for gastric cancer is feasible and safe (8, 10, 14, 15, 27, 28). Fukuzawa et al. revealed that EOF can promote anastomotic healing (27). A meta-analysis reported by Willcutts et al. (16) analyzed eight RCTs and seven non-RCTs to compare EOF with TOF, and demonstrated that the mean postoperative hospital stay was significantly shorter in the EOF group, with no significant difference in postoperative complications. Liu et al. (15) reported another meta-analysis of six RCTs on EOF after gastrectomy, and demonstrated that postoperative complications and tolerability of oral feeding were not significantly different, and that EOF was associated with a significantly earlier onset of flatulence and defecation, and shorter postoperative hospital stay. However, in the above-mentioned studies, oral feeding was started on postoperative day two or three, while in the present study, oral intake was started in the EOF group on the first postoperative day.

Tolerability of patients is another important factor that should be considered when adopting EOF. Most patients tolerate immediate postoperative feeding without developing major complications, as reported in several studies (26, 29, 30). In the present study, although the rate of intolerance in the EOF group was higher than that in the conventional feeding group, the difference was not statistically significant. This indicates that EOF remains feasible.

Many studies have demonstrated that EOF is safe, and provides nutritional and immunological benefits with better protein kinetics and preservation of the immune system over TOF (31–33). Furthermore, starting EOF can accelerate wound healing and increase anastomotic strength (34). Animal studies conducted using a rat model revealed that starvation after intestinal anastomosis leads to poor quality of healing, and demonstrated that EOF can increase wound healing and strength in esophageal anastomoses (27, 35, 36).

Studies on early oral nutrition after total gastrectomy are limited. Some early RCTs (7, 37) and retrospective studies (14, 38) have reported the outcomes of EOF after total gastrectomy. Kamei et al. revealed that patients who underwent total gastrectomy for gastric cancer were randomized to receive oral enteral nutrition beginning on post-operative day three (39). However, the present results revealed that the mean time to the first passage of flatus or defecation was 58.19 ± 9.89 h, which means that bowel movements starts by third postoperative day three. Hence, oral feeding initiated on POD3 cannot be regarded as EOF. In a RCT and retrospective study that compared early oral nutrition and conventional diet after total gastrectomy, patients who received EOF exhibited no increase in morbidity and anastomosis-related complications, when compared with patients receiving a conventional diet (40). Jang et al. (41) also reported a retrospective study that used propensity score matching to compare EOF with conventional oral feeding after total gastrectomy in gastric carcinoma patients. However, that study was limited by the fact that the patients in the two groups were treated in different time periods, causing the results to be likely in?uenced by the advances in operative skills and perioperative management with time.

At present, surgery is the only curative treatment for gastric cancer. Although, distal gastrectomy is the most common surgery for gastric cancer, total gastrectomy is performed in selected cases with advanced gastric cancer in order to achieve R0 resection. The long-term survival of gastric cancer continues to remain poor despite R0 resection especially for advanced stages of the disease. Hence, multimodality treatment is very important for improving long-term survival. Apart from surgery, other therapies used to treat gastric cancer includes chemotherapy, radiation therapy, immunotherapy and targeted therapy. Since surgery alone is insufficient for most patients with cT2 or higher tumors perioperative chemotherapy (category 1; preferred) or preoperative chemoradiation (category 2B) are recommended (42–45). Chemoradiation or systemic therapy are the recommended treatment options for medically fit patients whose locoregional cancer is found to be surgically unresectable (46, 47). Postoperative chemoradiation is recommended for all patients following an R1 or R2 resection. Postoperative chemoradiation is also recommended following an R0 resection in selected patients having pT2N0 tumors with high-risk features (poorly differentiated tumor, lymphovascular invasion, neural invasion, age <50 years, and patients who did not undergo D2 lymph node dissection) (48) and for patients with pT3-pT4, any N or any pT, N+ tumors who received less than a D2 dissection (category 1). Patients with pT3-pT4, any N or any pT, N+ tumors who have undergone primary D2 lymph node dissection should receive postoperative chemotherapy (category 1) (49, 50). Recently, biological therapies such as ramucirumab, trastuzumab have been found to improve overall survival in patients with advanced gastric cancer (51). In locally advanced or unresectable cases of gastric cancer, neoadjuvant therapy has been found to be effective in downstaging the tumor (52). In patients showing favorable response to neoadjuvant therapy, subtotal or distal gastrectomy with lymph node dissection can be performed thereby avoiding the morbidities associated with total gastrectomy. Malignant gastric lymphoma refers to a malignant tumor originating from the submucosal lymphoid tissue of the stomach, and may also be a part of systemic malignant lymphoma. Gastric lymphoma is highly sensitive to chemotherapy and can achieve good survival in most patients. Surgery is considered in patients with local complications such as bleeding, obstruction, etc. In addition, the surgical strategy for gastric cancer and gastric lymphoma is different. In gastric adenocarcinoma, due to high incidence of lymph node metastasis, D2-lymph node dissection is performed along with gastrectomy. While, in gastric lymphoma lymph node dissection is not required. Moreover, the first-line chemotherapy for gastric cancer is tegafur, gimeracil, and oteracil potassium (S-1) with oxaliplatin, while the chemotherapy for lymphoma is mostly CHOP (cyclophosphamide + doxorubicin + vincristine + prednisone).

There were some limitations of the present study. First, the present study was retrospective in nature. Retrospective studies have their own biases, which may not be correctable even with propensity score matching. Although propensity score matching can balance the confounding factors between the two groups, the one-on-one matching itself will result in a decrease in the sample size of the pairing and decrease the statistical efficiency to some extent. Furthermore, only observed confounders could be included in the construction of the propensity scores which does not represent all confounding factors. Some other potential confounders not included in this study may affect oral feeding after surgery, for example, anesthetics. The use of opioid analgesics may cause nausea and vomiting in some patients after surgery. This will affect the patient's early oral intake. In addition, the amount of oral intake in the early postoperative period is also a potential confounding factor. The difference in early oral intake of different patients will have certain effects on the tolerance of enteral nutrition and nutritional indicators. Therefore, we intend to include these factors in our future research. Second, this was a single-center study. A single hospital-based design might limit the generalizability of this study. Third, the sample size of this study was relatively small. For safety evaluation, future studies with larger sample size are required.

CONCLUSION

The present study reveals that EOF may be safe and feasible after radical total gastrectomy, with faster postoperative recovery and no increased risk of postoperative complications. Future prospective multicenter studies are required to validate the findings of the present study. A wider clinical use of the ERAS strategy can help in significantly reducing hospital cost and improving the postoperative outcomes of patients with gastric cancer.

ETHICS STATEMENT

All the procedures performed in this study that involved humans were in accordance with the ethical standards of the Research Ethics Committee of the Fourth Military Medical University.

AUTHOR CONTRIBUTIONS

GJ and JW conceived and designed the study. JW wrote the paper. MY participated in the statistical analysis. QW reviewed and edited the manuscript. All authors read and approved the manuscript and agree to be accountable for all aspects of the research in ensuring that the accuracy or integrity of any part of the work are appropriately investigated and resolved.

REFERENCES

1. Bray F, Ferlay J, Soerjomataram I, Siegel RL, Torre LA, Jemal A. Global cancer statistics 2018: GLOBOCAN estimates of incidence and mortality worldwide for 36 cancers in 185 countries. *CA Cancer J Clin.* (2018) 68:394–424. doi: 10.3322/caac.21492
2. Khuroo MS, Khwaja SF, Rather A, Hassan Z, Reshi R, Khuroo NS. Clinicopathological profile of gastrointestinal lymphomas in Kashmir. *Ind J Med Paediatr Oncol.* (2016) 37:251–5. doi: 10.4103/0971-5851.195736
3. Ajani JA, D'Amico TA, Almhanna K, Bentrem DJ, Chao J, Das P, et al. NCCN clinical practice guidelines in oncology, gastric cancer, Version 3.2016. *J Natl Compr Canc Netw.* (2016) 14:1286–312. doi: 10.6004/jnccn.2016.0137
4. Yoon SS, Hochberg EP. Chemotherapy is an effective first line treatment for early stage gastric mucosa-associated lymphoid tissue lymphoma. *Cancer Treat Rev.* (2006) 32:139–43. doi: 10.1016/j.ctrv.2006.01.006
5. Bisgaard T, Kehlet H. Early oral feeding after elective abdominal surgery: what are the issues? *Nutrition.* (2002) 18:944–8. doi: 10.1016/S0899-9007(02)00990-5
6. Bowling TE. Does disorder of gastrointestinal motility affect food intake in the post-surgical patient? *Proc Nutr Soc.* (1994) 53:151–7. doi: 10.1079/PNS19940018
7. Hur H, Kim SG, Shim JH, Song KY, Kim W, Park CH, et al. Effect of early oral feeding after gastric cancer surgery: a result of randomized clinical trial. *Surgery.* (2011) 149:561–8. doi: 10.1016/j.surg.2010.10.003
8. Hur H, Si Y, Kang WK, Kim W, Jeon HM. Effects of early oral feeding on surgical outcomes and recovery after curative surgery for gastric cancer: pilot study results. *World J Surg.* (2009) 33:1454–8. doi: 10.1007/s00268-009-0009-3
9. Osland EJ, Memon MA. Early postoperative feeding in resectional gastrointestinal surgical cancer patients. *World J Gastrointest Oncol.* (2010) 2:187–91. doi: 10.4251/wjgo.v2.i4.187
10. Fanaie SA, Ziaee SA. Safety of early oral feeding after gastrointestinal anastomosis: a randomized clinical trial. *Indian J Surg.* (2005) 67:185–8. Available online at: http://hdl.handle.net/1807/6325
11. Lassen K, Kjaeve J, Fetveit T, Trano G, Sigurdsson HK, Horn A, et al. Allowing normal food at will after major upper gastrointestinal surgery does not increase morbidity: a randomized multicenter trial. *Ann Surg.* (2008) 247:721–9. doi: 10.1097/SLA.0b013e31815cca68
12. Lewis SJ, Andersen HK, Thomas S. Early enteral nutrition within 24 h of intestinal surgery versus later commencement of feeding: a systematic review and meta-analysis. *J Gastrointest Surg.* (2009) 13:569–75. doi: 10.1007/s11605-008-0592-x
13. Osland E, Yunus RM, Khan S, Memon MA. Early versus traditional postoperative feeding in patients undergoing resectional gastrointestinal surgery: a meta-analysis. *JPEN J Parenter Enteral Nutr.* (2011) 35:473–87. doi: 10.1177/0148607110385698
14. Suehiro T, Matsumata T, Shikada Y, Sugimachi K. Accelerated rehabilitation with early postoperative oral feeding following gastrectomy. *Hepatogastroenterology.* (2004) 51:1852–5.
15. Liu X, Wang D, Zheng L, Mou T, Liu H, Li G. Is early oral feeding after gastric cancer surgery feasible? A systematic review and meta-analysis of randomized controlled trials. *PLoS ONE.* (2014) 9:e112062. doi: 10.1371/journal.pone.0112062
16. Willcutts KF, Chung MC, Erenberg CL, Finn KL, Schirmer BD, Byham-Gray LD. Early oral feeding as compared with traditional timing of oral feeding after upper gastrointestinal surgery: a systematic review and meta-analysis. *Ann Surg.* (2016) 264:54–63. doi: 10.1097/SLA.0000000000001644
17. Austin PC. An introduction to propensity score methods for reducing the effects of confounding in observational studies. *Multivariate Behav Res.* (2011) 46:399–424. doi: 10.1080/00273171.2011.568786
18. Kondrup J. Nutritional risk screening (NRS 2002): a new method based on an analysis of controlled clinical trials. *Clin Nutrition.* (2003) 22:321–36. doi: 10.1016/S0261-5614(02)00214-5
19. Love TE. *Spreadsheet-Based Sensitivity Analysis Calculations for Matched Samples.* Center for Health Care Research & Policy, Case Western Reserve University (2008). Available online at: http://www.chrp.org/propensity
20. Japanese Gastric Cancer Association. Japanese gastric cancer treatment guidelines 2010 (ver. 3). *Gastric Cancer.* (2011) 14:113–23. doi: 10.1007/s10120-011-0042-4
21. Katayama H, Kurokawa Y, Nakamura K, Ito H, Kanemitsu Y, Masuda N, et al. Extended Clavien–Dindo classifcation of surgical complications: Japan Clinical Oncology Group postoperative complications criteria. *Surg Today.* (2016) 46:668–85. doi: 10.1007/s00595-015-1236-x
22. Wang F, Wei XL, Wang FH, Xu N, Shen L, Dai GH, et al. Safety, efficacy and tumor mutational burden as a biomarker of overall survival benefit in chemo-refractory gastric cancer treated with toripalimab, a PD1 antibody in phase Ib/II clinical trial NCT02915432. *Ann Oncol.* (2019) 30:1479–86. doi: 10.1093/annonc/mdz197
23. Reyes CD, Weber KJ, Gagner M, Divino CM. Laparoscopic vs open gastrectomy. A retrospective review. *Surg Endosc.* (2001) 15:928–31. doi: 10.1007/s004640080185
24. Jiang L, Yang KH, Guan QL, Cao N, Chen Y, Zhao P, et al. Laparoscopy-assisted gastrectomy versus open gastrectomy for resectable gastric cancer: an update meta-analysis based on randomized controlled trials. *Surg Endosc.* (2013) 27:2466–80. doi: 10.1007/s00464-012-2758-6
25. Wang W, Li Z, Tang J, Wang M, Wang B, Xu Z. Laparoscopic versus open total gastrectomy with D2 dissection for gastric cancer: a meta-analysis. *J Cancer Res Clin Oncol.* (2013) 139:1721–34. doi: 10.1007/s00432-013-1462-9
26. Han-Geurts IJ, Jeekel J, Tilanus HW, Brouwer KJ. Randomized clinical trial of patient-controlled versus fixed regimen feeding after elective abdominal surgery. *Br J Surg.* (2001) 88:1578–82. doi: 10.1046/j.0007-1323.2001.01934.x
27. Fukuzawa J, Terashima H, Ohkohchi N. Early postoperative oral feeding accelerates upper gastrointestinal anastomotic healing in the rat model. *World J Surg.* (2007) 31:1234–9. doi: 10.1007/s00268-007-9003-9
28. Velez JP, Lince LF, Restrepo JI. Early enteral nutrition in gastrointestinal surgery: a pilot study. *Nutrition.* (1997) 13:442–5. doi: 10.1016/S0899-9007(97)91283-1
29. Heslin MJ, Latkany L, Leung D, Brooks AD, Hochwald SN, Pisters PW, et al. A prospective, randomized trial of early enteral feeding after resection of upper gastrointestinal malignancy. *Ann Surg.* (1997) 226:567–80. doi: 10.1097/00000658-199710000-00016

30. Carr CS, Ling KD, Boulos P, Singer M. Randomized trial of safety and efficacy of immediate postoperative enteral feeding in patients undergoing gastrointestinal resection. *BMJ.* (1996) 312:8698–71. doi: 10.1136/bmj.312.7035.869
31. Aiko S, Yoshizumi Y, Sugiura Y, Matsuyama T, Naito Y, Matsuzaki J, et al. Beneficial effects of immediate enteral nutrition after esophageal cancer surgery. *Surg Today.* (2001) 31:971–8. doi: 10.1007/s005950170005
32. Harrison LE, Hochwald SN, Heslin MJ, Berman R, Burt M, Brennan MF. Early postoperative enteral nutrition improves peripheral protein kinetics in upper gastrointestinal cancer patients undergoing complete resection: a randomized trial. *J Parenter Enteral Nutr.* (1997) 21:202–7. doi: 10.1177/0148607197021004202
33. Hochwald SN, Harrison LE, Heslin MJ, Burt ME, Brennan MF. Early postoperative enteral feeding improves whole body protein kinetics in upper gastrointestinal cancer patients. *Am J Surg.* (1997) 174:325–30. doi: 10.1016/S0002-9610(97)00095-0
34. Schroeder D, Gillanders L, Mahr K, Hill GL. Effects of immediate postoperative enteral nutrition on body composition, muscle function, and wound healing. *J Parenter Enteral Nutr.* (1991) 15:376–83. doi: 10.1177/0148607191015004376
35. Tadano S, Terashima H, Fukuzawa J, Matsuo R, Ikeda O, Ohkohchi N. Early postoperative oral intake accelerates upper gastrointestinal anastomotic healing in the rat model. *J Surg Res.* (2011) 169:202–8. doi: 10.1016/j.jss.2010.01.004
36. Yurtçu M, Toy H, Arbag H, Caglayan O. The effects of early and late feeding on healing of esophageal anastomoses: an experimental study. *Int J Pediatr Otorhinolaryngol.* (2011) 75:1289–91. doi: 10.1016/j.ijporl.2011.07.013
37. Mahmoodzadeh H, Shoar S, Sirati F, Khorgami Z. Early initiation of oral feeding following upper gastrointestinal tumor surgery: a randomized controlled trial. *Surg Today.* (2015) 45:203–8. doi: 10.1007/s00595-014-0937-x
38. Jeong O, Ryu SY, Jung MR, Choi WW, Park YK. The safety and feasibility of early postoperative oral nutrition on the frst postoperative day after gastrectomy for gastric carcinoma. *Gastric Cancer.* (2014) 17:324–31. doi: 10.1007/s10120-013-0275-5
39. Kamei H, Hachisuka T, Nakao M, Takagi K. Quick recovery of serum diamine oxidase activity in patients undergoing total gastrectomy by oral enteral nutrition. *Am J Surg.* (2005) 189:38–43. doi: 10.1016/j.amjsurg.2004.03.015
40. Sierzega M, Choruz R, Pietruszka S, Kulig P, Kolodziejczyk P, Kulig J. Feasibility and outcomes of early oral feeding after total gastrectomy for cancer. *J Gastrointest Surg.* (2015) 19:473–9. doi: 10.1007/s11605-014-2720-0
41. Jang A, Jeong O. Early postoperative oral feeding after total gastrectomy in gastric carcinoma patients: a retrospective before-after study using propensity score matching. *J Parenter Enteral Nutr.* (2019) 43:649–57. doi: 10.1002/jpen.1438
42. Ajani JA, Winter K, Okawara GS, Donohue JH, Pisters PW, Crane CH, et al. Phase II trial of preoperative chemoradiation in patients with localized gastric adenocarcinoma (RTOG 9904): quality of combined modality therapy and pathologic response. *J Clin Oncol.* (2006) 24:3953–8. doi: 10.1200/JCO.2006.06.4840
43. Al-Batran SE, Homann N, Pauligk C, Goetze TO, Meiler J, Kasper S, et al. Perioperative chemotherapy with fluorouracil plus leucovorin, oxaliplatin, and docetaxel versus fluorouracil or capecitabine plus cisplatin and epirubicin for locally advanced, resectable gastric or gastro-oesophageal junction adenocarcinoma (FLOT4): a randomised, phase 2/3 trial. *Lancet.* (2019) 393:1948–57. doi: 10.1016/S0140-6736(18)32557-1
44. Ychou M, Boige V, Pignon J-P, Conroy T, Bouché O, Lebreton G, et al. Perioperative chemotherapy compared with surgery alone for resectable gastroesophageal adenocarcinoma: an FNCLCC and FFCD multicenter phase III trial. *J Clin Oncol.* (2011) 29:1715–21. doi: 10.1200/JCO.2010.33.0597
45. Stahl M, Walz MK, Stuschke M, Lehmann N, Meyer HJ, Riera-Knorrenschild J, et al. Phase III comparison of preoperative chemotherapy compared with chemoradiotherapy in patients with locally advanced adenocarcinoma of the esophagogastric junction. *J Clin Oncol.* (2009) 27:851–6. doi: 10.1200/JCO.2008.17.0506
46. Moertel CG, Childs DS, Reitemeier RJ, Colby MY Jr, Holbrook MA. Combined 5-fluorouracil and supervoltage radiation therapy of locally unresectable gastrointestinal cancer. *Lancet.* (1969) 2:865–7. doi: 10.1016/S0140-6736(69)92326-5
47. The Gastrointestinal Tumor Study Group. (1990). The concept of locally advanced gastric cancer. Effect of treatment on outcome. *Cancer.* 66:2324–30. doi: 10.1002/1097-0142(19901201)66:11<2324::aid-cncr2820661112>3.0.co;2-c
48. Du C, Zhou Y, Huang K, Zhao G, Fu H, Shi Y. Defining a high-risk subgroup of pathological T2N0 gastric cancer by prognostic risk stratification for adjuvant therapy. *J Gastrointest Surg.* (2011) 15:2153–8. doi: 10.1007/s11605-011-1684-6
49. Noh SH, Park SR, Yang HK, Chung HC, Chung IJ, Kim SW, et al. Adjuvant capecitabine plus oxaliplatin for gastric cancer after D2 gastrectomy (CLASSIC): 5-year follow-up of an open-label, randomised phase 3 trial. *Lancet Oncol.* (2014) 15:1389–96. doi: 10.1016/S1470-2045(14)70473-5
50. Bang Y-J, Kim Y-W, Yang H-K, Chung HC, Park YK, Lee KH, et al. Adjuvant capecitabine and oxaliplatin for gastric cancer after D2 gastrectomy (CLASSIC): a phase 3 open-label, randomised controlled trial. *Lancet.* (2012) 379:315–21. doi: 10.1016/S0140-6736(11)61873-4
51. Yazici O, Sendur MA, Ozdemir N, Aksoy S. Targeted therapies in gastric cancer and future perspectives. *World J Gastroenterol.* (2016) 22:471–89. doi: 10.3748/wjg.v22.i2.471
52. Newman E, Marcus SG, Potmesil M, Sewak S, Yee H, Sorich J, et al. Neoadjuvant chemotherapy with CPT-11 and cisplatin downstages locally advanced gastric cancer. *J Gastrointest Surg.* (2002) 6:212–23. doi: 10.1016/S1091-255X(01)00054-3

2

Association Between Liquid Biopsy and Prognosis of Gastric Cancer Patients

Yunhe Gao[1,2†], Hongqing Xi[1†], Bo Wei[1,2†], Jianxin Cui[1], Kecheng Zhang[1], Hua Li[1], Aizhen Cai[1,2], Weishen Shen[1,3], Jiyang Li[1,2], Rafael Rosell[4], Joseph Chao[5], Tianhui Chen[6], Samuel Klempner[7,8], Zhi Qiao[1†] and Lin Chen[1,2*] on behalf of Gastric Cancer Collaborative Group*

[1] Department of General Surgery, Chinese PLA General Hospital, Beijing, China, [2] General Surgery Institute, Chinese PLA General Hospital, Beijing, China, [3] Nanjing General Hospital of Nanjing Military Command, Nanjing, China, [4] Catalan Institute of Oncology, Germans Trias i Pujol Health Science Institute and Hospital, Barcelona, Spain, [5] Department of Medical Oncology and Therapeutics Research, City of Hope Comprehensive Cancer Center, Duarte, CA, United States, [6] Department of Cancer Prevention, Institute of Cancer and Basic Medicine (ICBM), Zhejiang Provincial Office for Cancer Prevention and Control, Cancer Hospital of the University of CAS, Chinese Academy of Sciences (CAS), Hangzhou, China, [7] The Angeles Clinic and Research Institute, Los Angeles, CA, United States, [8] Samuel Oschin Comprehensive Cancer Institute, Cedars-Sinai Medical Center, Los Angeles, CA, United States

***Correspondence:**
Zhi Qiao
drqiaozhi@126.com
Lin Chen
chenlin@301hospital.com.cn

† These authors have contributed equally to this work and share first authorship

Background: Reports regarding liquid biopsy and gastric cancer (GC) have emerged rapidly in recent decades, yet their prognostic value still remains controversial. This study was aimed to assess the impact of liquid biopsy, including circulating tumor cells (CTCs) and cell-free nucleic acids, on GC patients' prognosis.

Methods: PubMed, Medline, EMBASE, and ClinicalTrial.gov databases were searched for studies that report GC patient survival data stratified by CTC/circulating tumor DNA (ctDNA)/circulating miRNAs' status. The hazard ratios (HRs) and their 95% confidence intervals (CIs) for patients' overall survival (OS) and disease-free survival (DFS)/progression-free survival (PFS) were recorded or calculated depending on circulating target status.

Results: We initially identified 4,221 studies, from which 43 were eligible for further analysis, comprising 3,814 GC patients. Pooled analyses showed that detection of certain CTCs, ctDNA, and circulating miRNA was associated with poorer OS (CTCs: HR = 1.84, 95%CI 1.50–2.26, $p < 0.001$; ctDNA: HR = 1.78, 95%CI 1.36–2.34, $p < 0.001$; circulating miRNA: HR = 1.74, 95%CI 1.13–2.69, $p < 0.001$) and DFS/PFS (CTCs: HR = 3.39, 95%CI 2.21–5.20, $p < 0.001$; ctDNA: HR = 2.38, 95%CI 1.31–4.32, $p = 0.004$; circulating miRNA: HR = 3.30, 95%CI 2.39–4.55, $p < 0.001$) of GC patients, regardless of disease stage and time point at which sample is taken (at baseline or post-treatment).

Conclusions: The presence of CTCs and/or cellular components identifies a group of GC with poorer prognosis. Among circulating markers, CTCs demonstrated a stronger and more stable predictive value for late-stage disease and among Mongolian populations with GC. Less data are available for ctDNA and miRNA; however, their presence may also reflect aggressive biology and warrants further prospective study.

Keywords: liquid biopsy, circulating tumor cells, circulating tumor DNA, circulating mRNA, gastric cancer, prognosis

INTRODUCTION

Gastric cancer (GC) remains the fifth most common cancer and the third leading cause of cancer-related death worldwide (1, 2). Although some therapeutic advances have been made, its prognosis remains unfavorable owing to the aggressive tumor biology, late detection, and high disease progression/recurrence rate (3). Few clinicopathological factors are used to guide therapy or disease monitoring, and ideal peripheral blood biomarkers have been lacking. Although enhanced endoscopic techniques, such chromoendoscopy (4) and endoscopy with narrow-band imaging (NBI) (5), are considered to be the more reliable and credible methods for diagnosis of GC than conventional diagnostic tools, their applications are limited because of their invasive nature and cost-efficacy concerns (5).

Although serum-based protein biomarkers such as carcinoembryonic antigen (CEA) (6), carcinoma antigen 125 (CA-125) (7), carcinoma antigen 724 (CA-724) (8), and carcinoma antigen 19-9 have commonly been used for GC patient management, they are plagued by limited diagnostic, and prognostic capacity (9). Circulating tumor cells (CTCs) and cell-free nucleic acids (cfNAs), known as "liquid biopsies," are detectable biomarkers across tumor types and represent attractive putative targets in GC (10–13). The potential advantages of liquid biopsy have been demonstrated in the management of breast cancer, colorectal cancer, and prostate cancer (14–16), but evidence of their effectiveness in GC management is limited and controversial.

Theoretically, tumor-derived blood-based biomarker tests have multiple application in GC including detecting/monitoring response after therapies, identification of actionable tumor alterations, and patient stratification (17, 18). Currently, the diagnostic value of liquid biopsy is still under debate, and it has been questioned for its low sensitivity and yields in some series (12, 19). In contrast, the prognostic importance is increasingly supported by mounting evidence in breast (20) and colorectal (21) cancers. Although cfNAs include several cellular components, the most commonly investigated in GC research are circulating tumor deoxyribonucleic acid (ctDNA) (22) and circulating microRNA (miRNA) (23). Variability in detection methodology, genomic coverage, specimen processing, and reproducibility has not always been consistent. Moreover, the most appropriate sampling time point for accurate detection (at baseline or post-treatment), the most appropriate test population and disease stage, and even the predictive value of certain types of biomarkers have not yet been agreed (12, 24). With the continuously emerging data in GC, there is a need to conduct quantitative analysis evaluating the most commonly used liquid biopsy methods currently in GC management. Therefore, we sought to conduct a systematic review and meta-analysis to evaluate the significance of CTCs and cfNAs in predicting GC progression and recurrence in a methodologically consistent manner.

METHODS

Literature Search

MOOSE (Meta-analysis Of Observational Studies in Epidemiology) (25) and PRISMA (Preferred Reporting Items for Systematic Reviews and Meta-Analyses) (26) guidelines were applied to conduct the systematic review. The following databases were systematically searched for relevant studies published up to December 2017: PubMed, Medline, EMBASE, Web of Science, and the Cochrane Central Register of Controlled Trials. Bibliographies of all relevant papers were also checked for further eligible studies. There was no restriction on language of publication (**Table S1**).

Selection Criteria

Studies were included in the analysis if they met the following criteria: (1) they enrolled patients with pathologically confirmed gastric or gastroesophageal junction adenocarcinoma; (2) they reported GC patient survival data stratified by CTC/ctDNA/circulating miRNA status (presence/positive and absence/negative); (3) they provided sufficient data for determining or calculating a hazard ratio (HR) and 95% confidence interval (95%CI); and (4) they enrolled patients who did not overlap with patients included in other eligible studies.

Studies were excluded if (1) fewer than 20 patients were analyzed; (2) samples were not drawn from peripheral blood (e.g., from urine or bone marrow); or (3) the histology type of included GC patients was squamous carcinoma or neuroendocrine carcinoma.

Data Extraction

Two authors (HX and JC) independently reviewed the eligible studies and extracted the following information: first author name, publication year, number of patients analyzed, age, gender, tumor stage, clinical treatment, volume and timing of blood withdrawal, marker detection method, cutoff value, positive ratio, and follow-up duration, if provided. When more than one marker was assessed in studies and an HR for survival or the survival curve was provided for each marker, results for all these markers were recorded as independent data sets.

Assessment of Risk of Bias

Risk of bias for individual studies was assessed using a modified Cochrane risk of bias instrument that included evaluation options of "definitely or probably yes" or "definitely or probably no" or "unknown or unclear" (27). The items included "adequate eligibility," "the measurement equality," "controlled confounding," "adequate follow-up," "free of selective outcomes," and "other factors" (**Table S2**) (21).

Statistical Analysis

The HRs and their 95%CIs for overall survival (OS) and disease-free survival (DFS)/progression-free survival (PFS) were recorded. For studies where HRs were not provided, we approximated HRs from the Kaplan–Meier curves with the use of an HR calculation Excel spreadsheet provided by

Tierney et al. (28). All HR data extraction and calculations were performed independently by YHG and HQX, and disagreements were resolved by discussion. Survival outcomes generated using multivariate analysis models were preferentially used if available, to ensure results are as clinically relevant as possible. By convention, an HR > 1 implies a worse prognosis in the circulating marker positive/upregulated group than in the negative/downregulated group, and $p < 0.05$ indicated statistical significance.

We pooled the extracted HRs using the generic inverse variance method. We anticipated interstudy heterogeneity and so used a random-effect analysis model preferentially (29). If no obvious heterogeneity was observed ($p > 0.05$), then a fixed-effect model was applied. Analyses were conducted using Stata 12.0 (StatCorp, College Station, TX, USA).

Sensitivity Analysis, Subgroup Analysis, and Meta-Regression Analysis

The stability of pooled HRs was tested by one-way sensitivity analysis with omission of a single study. Subgroup analyses and meta-regression were performed to explore potential sources of heterogeneity, and the following clinicopathological features were stratified: sampling time (at baseline or postoperatively), number of tested targets, cutoff value, tumor–node–metastasis (TNM) stage, risk of bias level, statistical methodology employed, ethnicity, and sample size. Any subgroup comprising fewer than two studies was excluded from the analysis.

RESULTS

Baseline Study Characteristics

Forty-three studies were eligible for inclusion, comprising 3,814 patients. These included 20 studies reporting on CTCs, 10 on ctDNA, and 13 on circulating miRNAs. Considering CTCs could also be performed at the DNA or RNA (mRNA or microRNA) level, we classified enrolled studies into relevant groups according to the authors' description in their report (**Figure 1**).

The baseline characteristics and study design variables of the included studies are shown in **Table 1**. All studies were written in English. Sample sizes ranged from 27 to 277 patients (median: 73 patients). The studies were conducted in 11 countries or regions (China, Egypt, Germany, Greece, Hong Kong, Italy, Japan, Poland, Spain, Taiwan, and Thailand).

All 43 studies applied a molecular or cytological detection method analyzing venous blood [polymerase chain reaction (PCR), quantitative reverse PCR (qRT-PCR), methylation-specific PCR (MSP), quantitative MSP (qMSP), next-generation sequencing (NGS), immunofluorescence (IF), CellSearch System, or colorimetric membrane array (CMA)]. Notably, three studies applied a combination of molecular and cytological detection methods (35, 37, 39). Five studies (37, 43, 57, 71, 72) analyzed the same patient cohort but using two different targets. To account for this, both markers were included in the pooled analysis, whereas the total number of patients was only counted once. The assessment of risk of bias for individual studies showed 31 and 12 studies with a low risk of bias and a high risk of bias, respectively. HRs for OS and DFS/relapse-free survival (RFS) could be extracted from 35 to 16 studies, respectively. Publication bias analyses were carried out for the analysis of all studies in Egger's and Begg's tests on OS and DFS/RFS, but no relevant publication bias was observed (**Figure S1**).

Circulating Tumor Cells

HRs for OS were available in 17 studies, representing 1,239 patients. Two HR estimates for OS were extracted from Uen et al. for the reason mentioned in the *Methods* part (43). The pooled HR showed a significant prognostic effect of CTC detection in GC patients (HR = 1.84, 95%CI 1.50–2.26, $p < 0.001$, **Figure 2A**), with moderate heterogeneity ($I^2 = 44\%, p = 0.024$).

HRs for DFS/PFS were available in 11 studies, representing 848 patients. The pooled HR showed a significantly increased risk of disease progression or recurrence in patients with CTC positivity (HR = 3.39, 95%CI 2.21–5.20, $p < 0.001$). The heterogeneity between studies was significant ($I^2 = 63.8\%, p = 0.002$).

Sensitivity analyses conducted by omitting each single study changed this result only marginally (**Figure S2**). **Table 2** shows the results of subgroup analysis stratified by covariates of clinical importance as described in the Methods. The most popular applied markers were CellSearch-associated [a combination of cytokeratins and epithelial cell adhesion molecule (EpCAM)] cytokeratins and survivin, and a subgroup analysis based on CTC markers showed that all CTC markers were significantly associated with GC patients' OS and DFS/PFS, except for CEA (OS: HR = 1.68, 95%CI 0.76–3.71, $p = 0.20$; DFS/PFS: HR = 1.41, 95%CI 0.77–2.55, $p = 0.262$) (**Figures 2B–D**). There was a more pronounced predictive value for CellSearch in both OS and DFS/PFS prediction (OS: HR = 2.33, 95%CI 1.51–3.61; DFS/PFS: HR = 4.54, 95%CI 1.82–11.33) than other CTC detection markers. However, this observation could not be substantiated by further statistical tests of interaction.

Meta-regression identified cancer stage and patient ethnicity as variables influencing OS HR estimates for CTCs (**Table 2**, $p = 0.010$ and $p = 0.008$, respectively). The presence of CTCs is associated with a higher HR for OS in studies enrolling only late-stage patients (HR = 2.81, 95%CI 1.79–4.40, $p < 0.001$) than studies enrolling with both early- and late-stage patients (HR = 1.84, 95%CI 1.50–2.26, $p < 0.001$). Nevertheless, both results from subgroups by TNM stage indicated a significant association between CTCs presence and worse prognosis of GC patients.

Studies involving GC patients of Mongolian ethnicity had a significantly higher pooled HR (2.04, 95%CI 1.64–2.54, $p < 0.001$) than had studies involving Caucasian patients (HR = 1.34, 95%CI 1.16–1.54, $p < 0.001$). This was further supported by tests for interaction ($p = 0.008$, **Table 2**). However, these differences by disease stage and ethnicity found in a subgroup analysis of OS HRs were absent in the analysis of DFS/PFS (**Table 2**). No other variables were found to be significant, which may be because of the relatively limited number of studies reporting DFS/PFS (11 studies in total, only one of which studied a primarily Caucasian patient population).

The subgroup analysis on sampling time showed a prognostic effect of CTC detection for both time points (baseline and during/post-treatment). HRs for CTCs predicting the survival

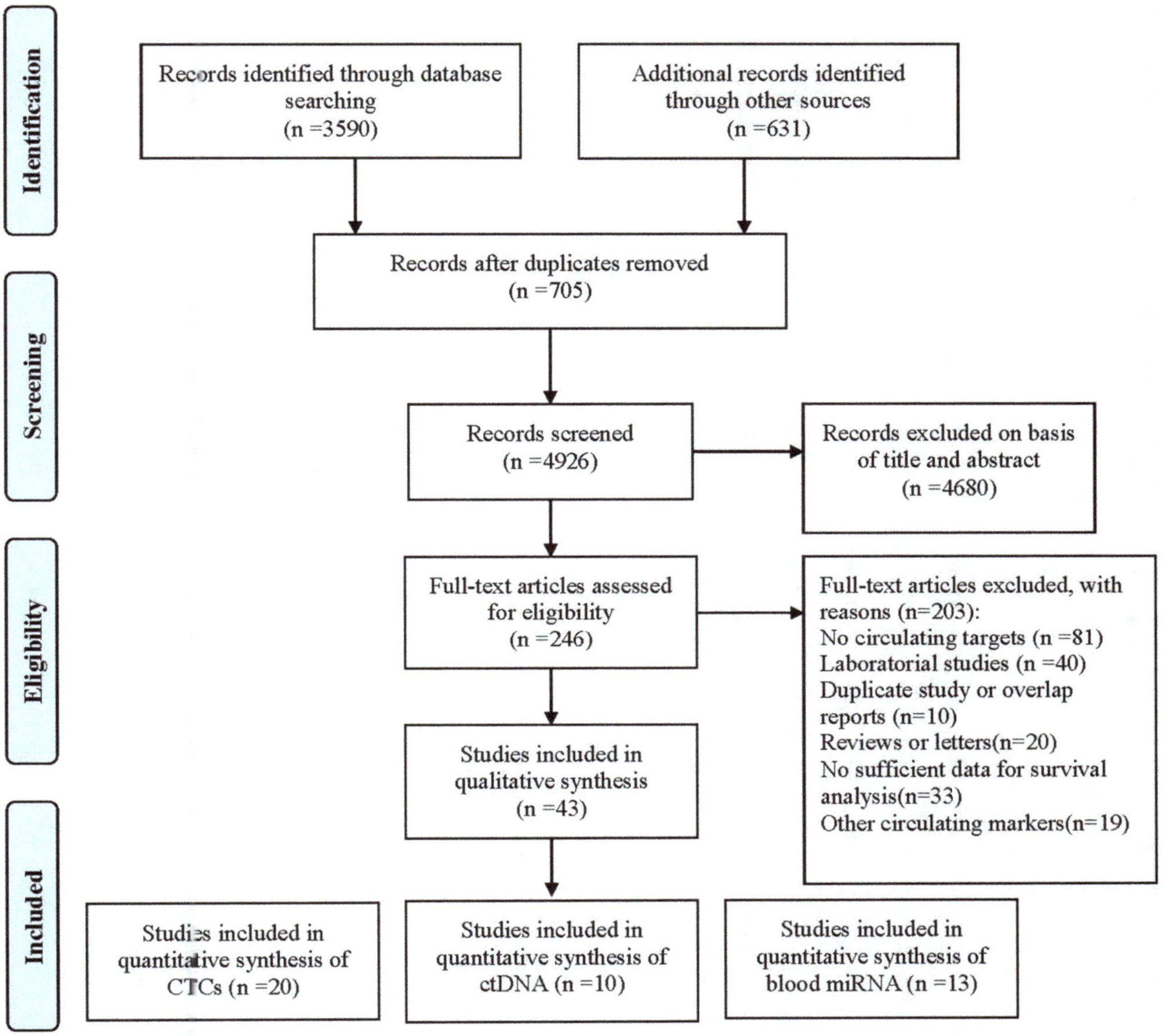

FIGURE 1 | Flowchart of enrolled studies investigating the association of liquid biopsy and gastric cancer patients' prognosis.

of GC patients where liquid biopsies were taken during/post-treatment were higher than HRs of patients where biopsies were taken at baseline. This was the case for both OS (HR = 2.30, 95%CI 1.52–3.49, $p < 0.001$ during/post-treatment; HR = 1.63, 95%CI 1.30–2.04, $p < 0.001$ at baseline) and DFS/PFS (HR = 4.04, 95%CI 1.21–13.44, $p = 0.023$ during/post-treatment; HR = 3.15, 95%CI 1.99–5.0, $p < 0.001$ at baseline). However, this difference did not reach statistical significance and could not be substantiated by further tests of interaction.

Circulating Tumor DNA

HRs for OS were reported in six studies, representing 624 patients. More than one HR for OS was extracted from three studies, because multiple detection approaches were used. The pooled HRs showed a significant prognostic effect of the detection of ctDNA in GC patients' OS (HR = 1.78, 95%CI 1.36–2.34, $p < 0.001$, **Figure 3A**), with moderate heterogeneity ($I^2 = 46.7\%$, $p = 0.059$). No ctDNA targets were assessed by more than two independent studies. Therefore, a subgroup analysis by target was not performed. A subgroup analysis by other variables revealed that ctDNA presence was significantly associated with shorter survival for all subgroups except in studies conducted primarily in Caucasian patients ($N = 2$, HR = 1.55, 95%CI 0.85–2.83, $p = 0.156$). However, this result must be interpreted with caution, given the small sample size. A Galbraith plot indicated that the study by Pimson et al. (58) might be one important source of heterogeneity (**Figure S3A**). Exclusion of Pimson et al. focusing on PCDH10 resulted in a significant

TABLE 1 | Baseline characteristics of included studies.

Target	Detection method	References	Year	Number	M/F	Age	Region	Cancer stage	Treatment	Sample volume	Sample time	Positive ratio	Follow-up	Cutoff	HR estimate	Outcomes	Bias
CIRCULATING TUMOR CELLS																	
CellSearch	CellSearch	Hiraiwa et al. (30)	2008	27	NR	68.9 ± 9.6	Japan	IV^m	NR	7.5 ml	Baseline	15/27	5.8 (1.0–15.0)	2/7.5 ml	FC	OS	Low
CellSearch	CellSearch	Matsusaka et al. (31)	2010	52	44/8	62 (24–78)	Japan	IV^m	Chemo	7.5 ml	AOT	17/52	/	4/7.5 ml	Provided (M)	PFS, OS	High
CellSearch	CellSearch	Uenosono et al. (32)	2013	148	99/49	57 (>70)	Japan	I–IV	Surgery (R0)	7.5 ml	Baseline	16/148	31.6 (4–72)	1/7.5 ml	Provided (M)	OS	Low
CellSearch	CellSearch	Li et al. (33)	2015	136	89/47	59 (25–80)	China	II–IV	Chemo	7.5 ml	Post-therapy	57/136	28.3 (median)	3/7.5 ml	Provided (M)	RFS, OS	Low
CellSearch	CellSearch	Okabe et al. (34)	2015	136	87/49	NR	Japan	II–IV	NR	7.5 ml	Baseline	25/136	26	1/7.5 ml	Provided (M)	PFS, OS	Low
Survivin	RT-PCR ELISA	Yie et al. (35)	2008	26	NR	NR	China	I–IV	Surgery (R0) + chemo	2 ml	Baseline	12/26	36	ROC	Provided (M)	RFS	High
Survivin	qRT-PCR	Bertazza et al. (36)	2009	70	39/31	68 (28–90)	Italy	I–IV	Surgery	6 ml	AOS	53/70	15 (6–119)	75th	Provided (M)	OS	Low
Survivin	RT-PCR ELISA	Cao et al. (37)	2011	98	63/35	NR	China	I–IV	Surgery	6 ml	Baseline	45/98	47.5 (36.5–56)	ROC	Provided (M)	DFS	Low
CK19	RT-PCR	Majima et al. (38)	2000	52	NR	NR	Japan	I–IV	Surgery	10 ml	Baseline	5/52	NR	HC	FC	OS	High
CK	FC+ IF	Noworolska et al. (39)	2007	57	44/13	NR	Poland	I–IV	Surgery + chemo	NR	Baseline	31/57	NR	3/slides	FC	OS	Low
CK20	RT-PCR	Illert et al. (40)	2005	70	48/22	69 (41–87)	Germany	I–IV	Surgery (R0 + R2)	9 ml	Baseline	28/70	20 (1–57)	HC	FC	OS	High
CK18/ E-cadherin	qRT-PCR	Saad et al. (41)	2010	30	16/14	NR	Egypt	I–IV	Surgery + chemo	2 ml	Baseline	15/15	NR	HC	Provided (M)	OS, RFS	Low
CK	IF	Liu et al. (42)	2017	59	35/24	59 (median)	China	III–IV	Chemo	5 ml	Baseline	36/23	NR	2/5 ml$^+$	Provided (M)	OS/DFS	Low
MUC1/C-Met	RT-PCR	Uen et al. (43)	2006	52	31/21	30 (>60)	Taiwan	I–IV	Surgery	5 ml	AOS	32/52 (C-met), 37/52 (MUC1)	NR	5/ml	FC	OS	High
hTERT/ CK19/CEA/MUC1	CMA^3	Wu et al. (44)	2006	64	41/23	60.5 (36–84)	Taiwan	I–IV	Surgery	4 ml	AOS	25/39	28 (20–33)	ROC	FC	OS/DFS	Low
CEA	RT-PCR	Ikeguchi et al. (45)	2005	59	38/21	66.3 (26–86)	Japan	I–IV	Surgery	1.5 ml	AOS	27/43	20.1 (2–31)	PC	FC	OS/DFS	High
CEA	qRT-PCR	Ishigami et al. (46)	2007	67	46/21	65 (median)	Japan	I–IV	Surgery (R0)	5 ml	AOS	33/67	37 (23–48)	PC	FC	OS	High
CEA	RT-PCR	Qiu et al. (47)	2010	123	82/41	59 (28–84)	China	I–IV	Surgery (R0) + chemo	5 ml	Baseline	45/123	37 (3.0–73.6)	PC	Provided (M)	DFS	Low
B7-H3	RT-PCR	Arigami et al. (48)	2010	95	64/31	47 (>70)	Japan	I–IV	Surgery (R0)	5 ml	Baseline	48/95	24 (1–74)	ROC	Provided (M)	OS	Low
Telomerase	IF	Ito et al. (49)	2016	65	46/19	58.8 (33–76)	Japan	I–IV	Surgery (R0 + R1)	7.5 ml	Baseline	18/47	60	ROC	Provided (M)	OS/RFS	Low

(Continued)

TABLE 1 | Continued

Target	Detection method	References	Year	Number	M/F	Age	Region	Cancer stage	Treatment	Sample volume	Sample time	Positive ratio	Follow-up	Cutoff	HR estimate	Outcomes	Bias
CIRCULATING TUMOR DNA																	
APC/E-cadherin	MSP	Leung et al. (50)	2005	60	35/25	66 (35–96)	Hong Kong	I–IV	Surgery	NR	Baseline	7/53	8 (0–40)	HC	FC	OS	High
SOX17	MSP	Ioanna et al. (51)	2013	73	51/22	56 (>60)	Greece	NR	Surgery (R0)	NR	Baseline	43/30	56 (20–111)	HC	FC	OS	Low
BCL6B	BGS	Yang et al. (52)	2013	40	33/7	NR	China	IV	NR	1 ml	Baseline	17/23	NR	HC	FC	OS	High
XAF1	MSP	Ling et al. (53)	2013	202	120/87	57 (≥60)	China	I–IV	Surgery	NR	Baseline	141/61	NR	HC	FC	DFS	Low
MINT2	qMSP	Han et al. (54)	2014	92	53/39	24 (≥60)	China	I–IV	Surgery	NR	Baseline	36/56	NR	ROC	Provided (U)	DFS	Low
P16	qMSP	Wu et al. (55)	2014	92	53/39	24 (≥60)	China	I–IV	Surgery	NR	NR	63/29	NR	HC	FC	DFS	Low
TIMP−3	MSP	Yu et al. (56)	2014	92	54/38	24 (≥60)	China	I–IV	Surgery	NR	Baseline	54/38	NR	ROC	Provided (U)	PFS	Low
APC/RASSF1A	MSP	Ioanna et al. (57)	2015	73	51/11	70.5 (28–82)	Greece	I–III	Surgery(R0)	NR	Baseline	61.50/73	56 (12–111)	HC	FC	OS	Low
PCDH10/RASSF1A	MSP	Pimson et al. (58)	2016	101	44/57	30 (≥61)	Thailand	I–IV	NR	NR	NR	95.17/101	NR	HC	FC	OS	High
ARID1A/P53/PIK3CA/PTEN/AKT2	NGS	Fang et al. (59)	2016	277	212/65	174/277	Taiwan	I–IV	Surgery	NR	Baseline	138/139	61 (2–232)	Median	FC	OS	Low
CIRCULATING microRNAs																	
MiR-200c	RT-PCR	Ayerbes et al. (60)	2012	52	42/10	65.3 (49–74)	Spain	I–IV	Surgery + chemo	10 ml	AOS	28/24	24 (6–53)	ROC	Provided (M)	OS, PFS	Low
MiR-200c	qRT-PCR	Zhang et al. (61)	2015	98	53/45	51 (≥60)	China	I–IV	Surgery	5 ml	Baseline	50/48	NR	Median	Provided (M)	OS	Low
MiR-20a-5p	RT-qPCR	Yang et al. (62)	2017	55	35/20	33 (≥60)	China	I–IV	Surgery	4 ml	Baseline	27/28	NR	Median	FC	OS	High
MiR-20a	qRT-PCR	Wang et al. (63)	2012	65	34/31	44 (>60)	China	I–IV	Surgery	2 ml	Baseline	34/31	NR	Median	Provided (M)	OS	Low
MiR-21	qRT-PCR	Komatsu et al. (64)	2013	69	43/26	40 (>65)	China	I–IV	Surgery	7 ml	Baseline	47/22	NR	HC	Provided (M)	DFS	Low
MiR-21	qRT-PCR	Song et al. (65)	2013	103	68/35	60 (27–87)	China	I–IV	Surgery	5 ml	Baseline	51/52	35.9 (24.4–53.1)	Median	Provided (U)	OS	Low
MiR-206	RT-PCR	Hou et al. (66)	2016	150	98/52	59.8 (mean)	China	I–IV	Surgery (R0)	5 ml	Baseline	75/75	38	ROC	FC	OS, DFS	Low
Mir203	qRT-PCR	Imaoka et al. (67)	2016	130	122/61	66 (≥68)	Japan	I–IV	Surgery + chemo	5 ml	NR	53/77	31.4 (1–78)	ROC	FC	OS, DFS	Low
MiR-222	qRT-PCR	Fu et al. (68)	2014	114	54/60	46 (>50)	China	I–IV	NR	<8 ml	Baseline	75/39	24 (4–60)	ROC	Provided (M)	OS, DFS	Low
MiR-27a	qRT-PCR	Huang et al. (69)	2014	82	52/30	31 (>60)	China	IV	Chemo	NR	Baseline	41/41	NR	Median	Provided (M)	OS	Low
MiR-23b	qRT-PCR	Zhuang et al. (70)	2016	138	85/53	64 (≥60)	China	I–IV	NR	5 ml	Baseline	79/79	NR	Median	Provided (M)	OS, DFS	Low
MiR-196a/b	qRT-PCR	Tsai et al. (71)	2016	98	57/41	53 (≥65)	Taiwan	I–IV	Surgery	NR	Baseline/AOS	49/49	83 (64–137)	ROC	Provided (M)	OS,	Low
MiR-192/MiR-122	qRT-PCR	Chen et al. (72)	2013	72	54/18	57 (44–62)	China	III–IV	Chemo	3–5 ml	Baseline	34, 35/72	NR	ROC	Provided (M)	OS	Low
Total	43		3814														

HC, healthy control; NC, negative control; PC, positive control; NR, not reported; FC, figure calculation; HR, hazard ratio; ROC, receiver operating characteristic curve; OS, overall survival; DFS, disease-free survival; PFS, progression-free survival; +, 5/ml KATO-III GC cell in healthy control volunteers; 3, colorimetric membrane array; MSP, methylation-specific PCR; BGS, bisulfite genomic sequence; qMSP, quantitative methylation-specific PCR; NGS, next generation sequencing; U, univariate; M, multivariate; R0, radical resection; m, metastatic cancers.

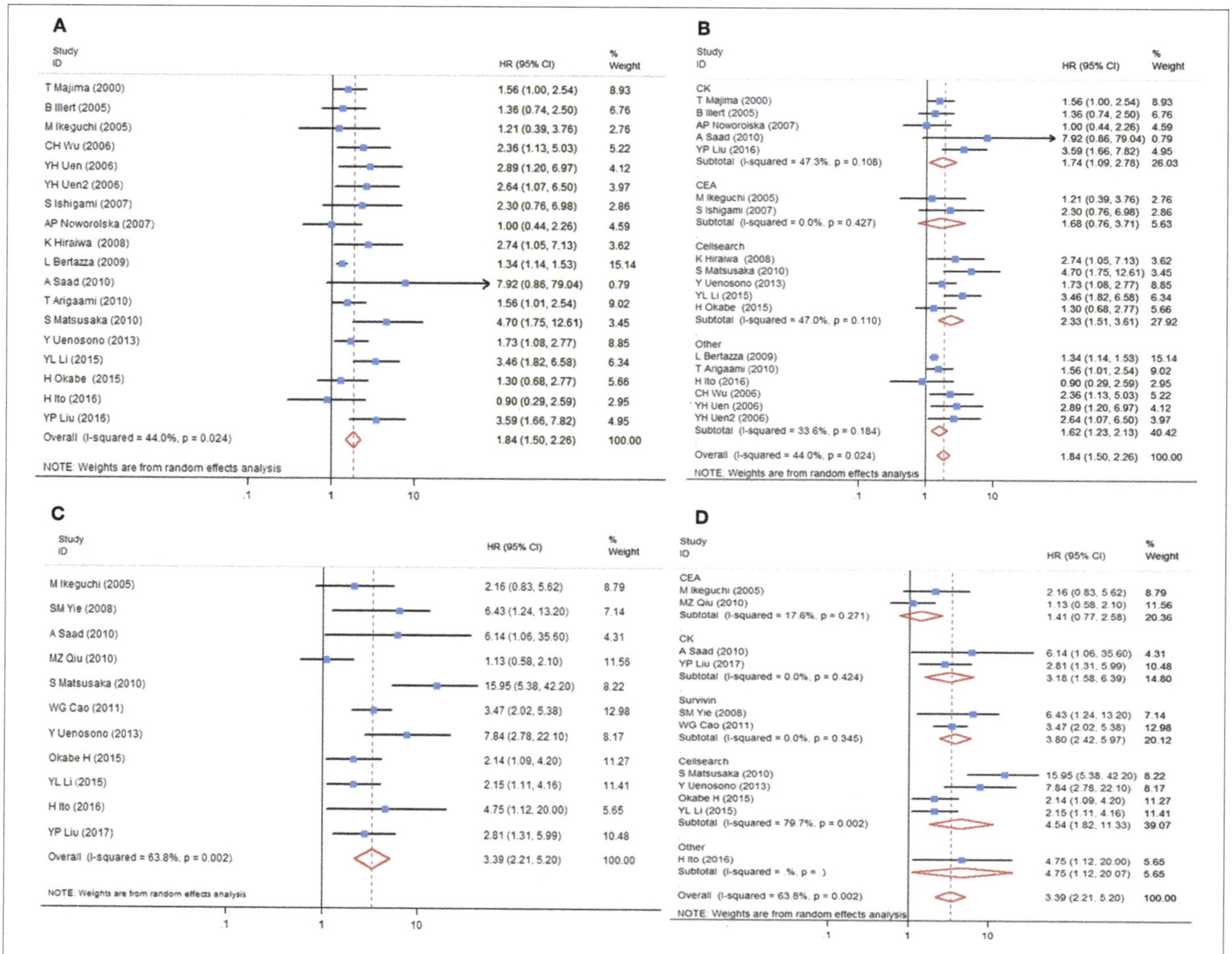

FIGURE 2 | Forest plots of HRs for OS and DFS/PFS of GC patients, by CTC status. **(A)** Overall analysis of HR for OS of GC patients. **(B)** Subgroup analysis of HR for OS of the GC patients by detection targets. **(C)** Overall analysis of HR for DFS/PFS of GC patients. **(D)** Subgroup analysis of HR for DFS/PFS of GC patients by detection targets. HRs, hazard ratios; OS, overall survival; DFS, disease-free survival; PFS, progression-free survival; GC, gastric cancer; CTC, circulating tumor cell.

decrease in heterogeneity ($I^2 = 33.2\%$, $p = 0.163$), but the association between ctDNA and OS remained significant (HR = 1.64, 95%CI 1.28–2.10, $p < 0.001$).

HRs for DFS/PFS were reported by five studies utilizing ctDNA, representing 731 patients. The pooled HR showed a significantly increased risk of disease progression or recurrence in patients with ctDNA detection (HR = 2.38, 95%CI 1.31–4.32, $p = 0.004$). Heterogeneity between studies was significant ($I^2 = 87.2\%$, $p < 0.001$). A Galbraith plot and a sensitivity analysis were performed to explore the source of heterogeneity and stability of the results. Although a sensitivity analysis showed that omission of any single study would not substantially alter the outcomes, the Galbraith plot showed that Fang et al. (59) and Ling et al. (53) were outliers and the main contributors to heterogeneity (**Figure S3B**). Excluding these two studies reduced heterogeneity somewhat ($I^2 = 56.5\%$, $p = 0.100$) and made the association between ctDNA and DFS/PFS more significant (HR = 2.19, 95%CI 1.31–3.66, $p = 0.003$, **Figure 3B**).

Circulating miRNA

HRs for OS in circulating miRNA were available in 13 studies, representing 1,157 patients, and indicated a prognostic effect of circulating miRNA detection (HR = 1.75, 95%CI 1.13–2.70, $p < 0.001$), and there was considerable heterogeneity ($I^2 = 83.3\%$, $p = 0.000$) (**Figure 4A**).

After sensitivity analyses were performed, it was found that by excluding the only two studies with an HR estimate < 1 (67, 72), the adjusted pooled HR for OS was higher (HR = 2.13, 95%CI 1.61–2.83, $p < 0.001$) whereas heterogeneity was substantially reduced ($I^2 = 53.4\%$, $p = 0.014$). In a manual review of the original work of these two studies, the authors considered the two targets, miR-203 and miR-122, as anti-tumor

TABLE 2 | Subgroup analyses and meta-regression analyses.

	CTCs								miRNA				ctDNA			
	OS				DFS				OS				OS			
	N	HR (95%CI)	I^2 (%)	P^m	*N*	HR (95%CI)	I^2 (%)	P^m	*N*	HR (95%CI)	I^2 (%)	P^m	*N*	HR (95%CI)	I^2 (%)	P^m
Sampling time																
Baseline	10	1.63 (1.30–2.04)	13.3	0.225	8	3.15 (1.99–5.0)	56.1	0.755	2	2.58 (1.55–4.31)	0	0.9	/	/	/	/
Post-op	8	2.30 (1.52–3.49)	64.4		3	4.04 (1.21–13.44)	82.4		9	2.04 (1.45–2.88)	63.9	/	/	/	/	/
Cutoff																
HC/NC	5	1.57 (1.13–2.19)	0	0.267	3	1.86 (0.84–4.13)	46.6	0.278		/	/	/	5	1.94 (1.35–2.78)	49.7	0.520
ROC	3	1.62 (1.10–2.39)	5.8		3	3.88 (2.52–5.97)	0.00		5	2.60 (1.83–3.71)	15.3	0.275	/	/	/	/
Percentiles	9	2.27 (1.60–3.22)	67.0		5	4.02 (2.00–8.10)	73.4		6	1.86 (1.26–2.75)	63.0		1	1.78 (1.36–2.34)	/	/
TNM stage																
With early stage	13	1.45 (1.28–1.63)	0.2	0.01	7	3.38 (1.91–5.99)	61.4	0.437	9	2.32 (1.67–3.23)	57.7	0.268	5	1.79 (1.28–2.49)	58.8	0.865
Advanced or late stage	5	2.81 (1.79–4.40)	38.0		4	3.49 (1.63–7.53)	75.2		2	1.53 (0.97–2.41)	0		2	1.92 (1.15–3.20)	0	/
Risk bias																
Low	11	1.84 (1.50–2.26)	52.1	0.689	6	2.87 (1.58–5.24)	60.0	0.497	2	2.34 (1.37–3.98)	0	0.27	3	1.52 (1.14–2.05)	41.	0.148
High	7	1.96 (1.36–2.82)	21.3		5	4.06 (2.15–7.68)	67.6		9	2.11 (1.51–5.94)	61.0		3	2.33 (1.56–3.50)	17.5	
Ethnicity																
Caucasian	4	1.34 (1.16–1.54)	0	0.008	1	6.14 (1.06–35.58)	/	0.600	1	2.24 (1.09–4.61)	/	/	4	1.92 (1.38–2.67)	45.3	0.465
Mongolian	14	2.04 (1.64–2.54)	20.8		10	3.31 (2.12–5.16)	66.6		10	2.13 (1.57–2.90)	57.4		2	1.55 (0.85–2.83)	54.2	
Sample size																
<100	14	1.84 (1.45–2.33)	44.5	0.955	6	4.95 (2.92–8.37)	43.0	0.075	7	2.04 (1.56–2.67)	25.3	0.14	4	1.81 (1.25–2.62)	42.3	0.975
≥100	4	1.86 (1.19–2.92)	44.0		5	2.25(1.32–3.86)	59.1		4	2.27 (1.08–4.76)	53.4)		2	1.81 (1.11–2.95)	66.2	

HR, hazard ratio; P^h, p value for inter-study heterogeneity; P^m, p value for meta-regression; HC, healthy control; NC, negative control; ROC, receiver operating characteristic curve.

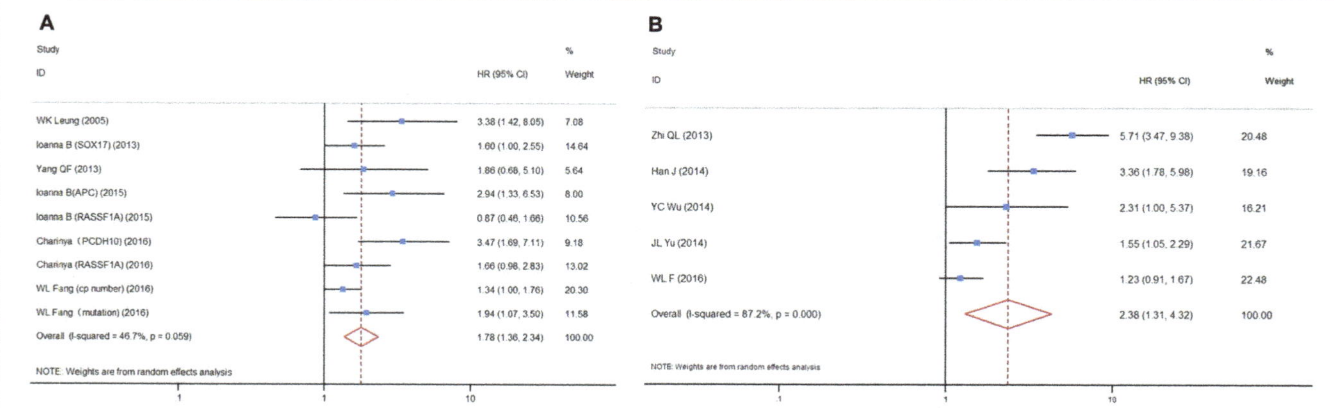

FIGURE 3 | Forest plots of HRs for **(A)** OS and **(B)** DFS/PFS of GC patients, based on detection of circulating tumor DNA status. HRs, hazard ratios; OS, overall survival; DFS, disease-free survival; PFS, progression-free survival; GC, gastric cancer.

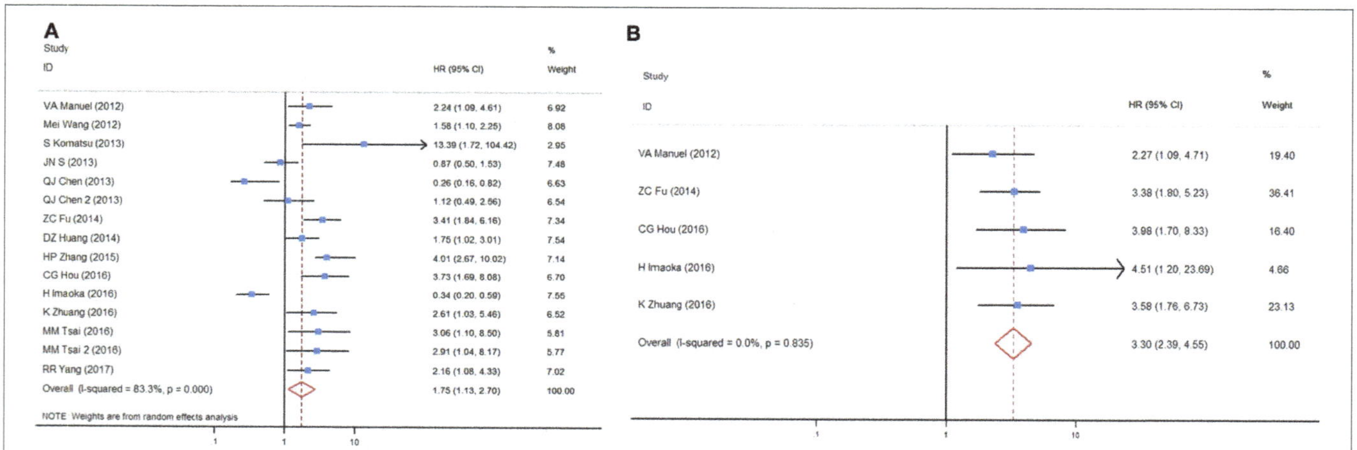

FIGURE 4 | Forest plots of HRs for **(A)** OS and **(B)** DFS/PFS of GC patients, based on detection of circulating miRNA status. HRs, hazard ratios; OS, overall survival; DFS, disease-free survival; PFS, progression-free survival; GC, gastric cancer.

microRNAs on the basis of biological function. Therefore, a subgroup analysis and a meta-regression analysis were performed after excluding these targets, and then significant associations between circulating miRNA detection and OS were found in both sample time point groups (baseline and during/post-treatment). Unlike CTC analyses, a subgroup analysis stratified by tumor stage (all stages vs. advanced stage only) and ethnicity (Caucasian vs. Mongolian) did not alter the bias and differences significantly between these subgroups.

HRs for DFS/PFS in circulating miRNA were available in five studies, representing 584 patients. The pooled HR for DFS/PFS was 3.30 (95%CI 2.39–4.55, $p < 0.001$, **Figure 4B**). Heterogeneity between HR estimates was not significant ($I^2 = 0.0\%$, $p = 0.835$).

DISCUSSIONS

Here, we report the largest meta-analysis of circulating tumor-derived biomarkers and identify prognostic value for CTCs. Our meta-analysis provides strong evidence, even after adjustment for clinical variables. With over 3,800 included GC patients, our study is the most comprehensive systematic review of the association between liquid biopsy and GC prognosis to date, substantially larger than previous studies (73, 74).

Importantly, we attempted to address biomarker detection method, study heterogeneity, and disease stage. The association between biomarker detection (CTC, ctDNA, or miRNA) was relatively stable and not influenced largely by liquid biopsy detection methods or disease stage. Even among GC patients where samples were taken post-treatment, the association remained significant, highlighting the potential clinical utility of blood-based biomarkers in GC.

Overall, we observed a stronger association between circulating marker detection and DFS than OS, suggesting an important role in prognosis and patient stratification, particularly in non-metastatic patients. We acknowledge that an optimal cutoff value for each detection method remains to be determined, and a decreased heterogeneity was observed in the receiver operating characteristic (ROC) cutoff determination subgroups, indicating more consistent results in studies that adapted ROC curves to determine patients' tumor status.

Among the detection platforms examined, several important observations warrant further discussion, and the analysis of whole CTCs can be performed at the DNA or RNA (mRNA or microRNA) and protein levels, whereas the analysis of ctDNA and microRNAs can be performed only at the genomic level. For example, one alternative to enumerating CTCs by immunocytochemistry (ICC) is to estimate their presence using RT-PCR to discover epithelial transcripts, which should not be present in normal hematopoietic cells. However, detection of CTCs often requires more cumbersome enrichment and detection methods, whereas the detection of cfNAs can be performed using blood plasma or serum, and easier methods (24). Huang et al. (73) and our previous report (75) have demonstrated the significance of CTC and ctDNA in GC patients' prognosis prediction.

Among studies examining CTCs, the CellSearch System was the most widely used method for detecting and enumerating CTCs from blood samples, using a combination of epithelial markers (EpCAM+; cytokeratin 8, 18, and/or 19; and CD45−). It is still the first and only actionable commercial test for detecting CTCs in cancer patients, including metastatic breast (14), prostate (15), and colorectal cancers (16). Our results further support its application for GC patients as a statistically significant predictor of shorter OS and DFS/PFS.

Another popular marker type in CTC detection was found to be cytokeratins (CKs). CKs have been found to have different predictive values in patients from Asian ($N = 2$, HR = 3.54, 95%CI 1.84–6.82, $p < 0.001$) and Western populations ($N = 3$, HR = 1.38, 95%CI 0.73–2.61, $p = 0.328$), which suggests that they may play a different role in different ethnicities. Moreover, CKs have tended to serve as biomarkers in a combination of their own components (e.g., CK18, CK19, and CK20) (76) or alongside other targets such as EpCAM (77, 78) to identify the epithelial cells more precisely.

Circulating tumor DNA is composed of small fragments of nucleic acid that are not associated with cells or cell fragments (79). The most widely used method of detection is methylated DNA in plasma/serum, which is usually identified by MSP or quantitative MSP (qPCR) assays (80). All included studies withdrew blood for ctDNA detection at the baseline time point, which is probably because ctDNA is rapidly cleared from circulation after surgery or other therapy because of its short half-life (80). However, a previous study reported that DNA methylation is relatively chemically stable and can be detected at a sensitivity of up to 1:1,000 molecules (81). It is therefore not surprising that most of the studies included in our review focused on epigenetic regulation of circulating markers. Only Fang et al. investigated the role of gene mutation and copy number.

Although the dysregulation of ctDNA is relatively common in gastroesophageal cancers (22), a reliably detectable prognostic ctDNAs with high specificity is yet to be identified. Our meta-analysis only covers genes and epigenetic regulators relevant to GC. Whole gene screening assays, especially for genetic mutations, are required to identify more associations (82, 83).

Beyond CTCs and ctDNA, circulating miRNAs (miRNAs) are a large group of short, non-coding RNAs, 19–25 nucleotides long, which regulate gene expression by pairing to the 3′ untranslated region (3′-UTR) of their target mRNA (84). It has been suggested that miRNAs could function as either tumor suppressor or oncogenes by regulating gene expression at transcriptional and translational levels in GC (85). Notably, although not all detected CTCs are predictors of adverse outcomes (86), the majority of them are. In contrast, certain miRNAs detected in serum/plasma may be positive predictors of GC patient survival, acting as tumor-suppresser genes, such as miR-192 and miR-203. Nevertheless, our results also support previous evidence that oncogenic circulating miRNAs are strongly significant predictors of poorer outcomes, particularly for GC recurrence, and progression (HR = 3.41, 95%CI 2.48–4.69, $p < 0.001$; $I^2 = 0.0\%$, $p = 0.670$).

In the past, it has been difficult to obtain tumor samples from GC patients without surgery, as endoscopic biopsy provides limited genetic or cellular materials in most cases. Although the optimal platform remains open to debate, the ability of ctDNA to simultaneously detect genomic alterations is attractive and might have a prognostic role. Our meta-analysis supports the use of a series of detection targets and methods for predicting GC patients' OS and DFS. Intriguingly, our data suggest that detection of certain circulating markers at any time, pre-treatment, or post-treatment, provides important prognostic information. Among the overall advanced disease population, the presence of CTCs and tumor-related nucleic acids may help identify those patients that could benefit most, or at least, from systematic therapy including chemotherapy, target therapy, or immunotherapy (87, 88). In the era of NGS and a combination of multi-analytic biomarkers (89–91), our meta-analysis provides a solid foundation and methodological reference for further study.

We acknowledge several limitations to our large meta-analysis. First, studies may tend to selectively report their positive results, leading to risk of selection and publication bias. Second, the majority of our studies enrolled patients from all disease stages, making it difficult to stratify the prognostic value of circulating biomarkers by stage. In addition, a subgroup analysis of some variables involved groups with small sample sizes, which might bias our conclusions. Although meta-regression has indicated that tumor stage and ethnicity may contribute to inter-study heterogeneity in prognostic value, large, multicenter prospective studies based on homogeneous patient populations are still required to validate our findings.

CONCLUSIONS

In conclusion, results of this meta-analysis demonstrated a significant role for liquid biopsy, including CTCs, ctDNA, and circulating miRNA, in predicting worse prognosis of patients with GC. By analyzing currently available studies, CTCs demonstrated a stronger and more stable predicative value in late-stage disease and Mongolian populations compared with early-stage disease and Caucasian populations, respectively. Careful selection of circulating markers and standard detection methods are likely to be fundamental to optimizing the accuracy of liquid biopsy in determining GC patients' prognosis. And further multicentered studies applying specific circulating biomarkers are warranted to clarify the clinical validity of liquid biopsy and its utility in GC patients.

AUTHOR CONTRIBUTIONS

YG, BW, and LC conceived the study. YG, HX, and JCu conducted the literature searches and extracted the data. AC, WS, and JL took part in the analysis and interpreted the data. YG, ZQ, and HX drafted the manuscript. RR, TC, JCh, and SK critically revised the manuscript. HL, JL, and ZQ helped in making the figures and tables. BW and KZ double-checked the extracted data.

ACKNOWLEDGMENTS

We thank Rebecca Baggaley, Ph.D., from the Department of Global Health and Development, London School of Hygiene & Tropical Medicine, for editing the English text of a draft of this manuscript.

REFERENCES

1. Bray F, Ferlay J, Soerjomataram I, Siegel RL, Torre LA, Jemal A. Global cancer statistics 2018: GLOBOCAN estimates of incidence and mortality worldwide for 36 cancers in 185 countries. *CA Cancer J Clin.* (2018) 68:394–424. doi: 10.3322/caac.21492
2. Siegel RL, Miller KD, Jemal A. Cancer statistics, 2017. *CA Cancer J Clin.* (2017) 67:7–30. doi: 10.3322/caac.21387
3. Thrumurthy SG, Chaudry MA, Hochhauser D, Mughal M. The diagnosis and management of gastric cancer. *BMJ.* (2013) 347:f6367. doi: 10.1136/bmj.f6367
4. Zhao Z, Yin Z, Wang S, Wang J, Bai B, Qiu Z, et al. Meta-analysis: the diagnostic efficacy of chromoendoscopy for early gastric cancer and premalignant gastric lesions. *J Gastroenterol Hepatol.* (2016) 31:1539–45. doi: 10.1111/jgh.13313
5. Pasechnikov V, Chukov S, Fedorov E, Kikuste I, Leja M. Gastric cancer: prevention, screening and early diagnosis. *World J Gastroenterol.* (2014) 20:13842–62. doi: 10.3748/wjg.v20.i38.13842
6. Ruibal Morell A. CEA serum levels in non-neoplastic disease. *Int J Biol Markers.* (1992) 7:160–6. doi: 10.1177/172460089200700307
7. Emoto S, Ishigami H, Yamashita H, Yamaguchi H, Kaisaki S, Kitayama J. Clinical significance of CA125 and CA72-4 in gastric cancer with peritoneal dissemination. *Gastric Cancer.* (2012) 15:154–61. doi: 10.1007/s10120-011-0091-8
8. Yang AP, Liu J, Lei HY, Zhang QW, Zhao L, Yang GH. CA72-4 combined with CEA, CA125 and CAl9-9 improves the sensitivity for the early diagnosis of gastric cancer. *Clin Chim Acta.* (2014) 437:183–6. doi: 10.1016/j.cca.2014.07.034
9. Shimada H, Noie T, Ohashi M, Oba K, Takahashi Y. Clinical significance of serum tumor markers for gastric cancer: a systematic review of literature by the Task Force of the Japanese Gastric Cancer Association. *Gastric Cancer.* (2014) 17:26–33. doi: 10.1007/s10120-013-0259-5
10. Alix-Panabières C, Pantel K. Circulating tumor cells: liquid biopsy of cancer. *Clin Chem.* (2013) 59:110–8. doi: 10.1373/clinchem.2012.194258
11. van de Stolpe A, Pantel K, Sleijfer S, Terstappen LW, den Toonder JM. Circulating tumor cell isolation and diagnostics: toward routine clinical use. *Cancer Res.* (2011) 71:5955–60. doi: 10.1158/0008-5472.CAN-11-1254
12. Crowley E, Di Nicolantonio F, Loupakis F, Bardelli A. Liquid biopsy: monitoring cancer-genetics in the blood. *Nat Rev Clin Oncol.* (2013) 10:472–84. doi: 10.1038/nrclinonc.2013.110
13. Schwarzenbach H, Hoon DS, Pantel K. Cell-free nucleic acids as biomarkers in cancer patients. *Nat Rev Cancer.* (2011) 11:426–37. doi: 10.1038/nrc3066
14. Hayes DF, Cristofanilli M, Budd GT, Ellis MJ, Stopeck A, Miller MC, et al. Circulating tumor cells at each follow-up time point during therapy of metastatic breast cancer patients predict progression-free and overall survival. *Clin Cancer Res.* (2006) 12:4218–24. doi: 10.1158/1078-0432.CCR-05-2821
15. de Bono JS, Scher HI, Montgomery RB, Parker C, Miller MC, Tissing H, et al. Circulating tumor cells predict survival benefit from treatment in metastatic castration-resistant prostate cancer. *Clin Cancer Res.* (2008) 14:6302–9. doi: 10.1158/1078-0432.CCR-08-0872
16. Cohen SJ, Punt CJ, Iannotti N, Saidman BH, Sabbath KD, Gabrail NY, et al. Relationship of circulating tumor cells to tumor response, progression-free survival, and overall survival in patients with metastatic colorectal cancer. *J Clin Oncol.* (2008) 26:3213–21. doi: 10.1007/978-1-59745-183-3
17. Kim ST, Banks KC, Pectasides E, Kim SY, Kim K, Lanman RB, et al. Impact of genomic alterations on lapatinib treatment outcome and cell-free genomic landscape during HER2 therapy in HER2-positive gastric cancer patients. *Ann Oncol.* (2018) 29:1037–48. doi: 10.1093/annonc/mdy034
18. Schrock AB, Pavlick D, Klempner SJ, Chung JH, Forcier B, Welsh A, et al. Hybrid capture-based genomic profiling of circulating tumor DNA from patients with advanced cancers of the gastrointestinal tract or anus. *Clin Cancer Res.* (2018) 24:1881–90. doi: 10.1158/1078-0432.CCR-17-3103
19. Qiu M, Wang J, Xu Y, Ding X, Li M, Jiang F, et al. Circulating tumor DNA is effective for the detection of EGFR mutation in non-small cell lung cancer: a meta-analysis. *Cancer Epidemiol Biomarkers Prev.* (2015) 24:206–12. doi: 10.1158/1055-9965.EPI-14-0895
20. Zhang L, Riethdorf S, Wu G, Wang T, Yang K, Peng G, et al. Meta-analysis of the prognostic value of circulating tumor cells in breast cancer. *Clin Cancer Res.* (2012) 18:5701–10. doi: 10.1158/1078-0432.CCR-12-1587
21. Rahbari NN, Aigner M, Thorlund K, Mollberg N, Motschall E, Jensen K, et al. Meta-analysis shows that detection of circulating tumor cells indicates poor prognosis in patients with colorectal cancer. *Gastroenterology.* (2010) 138:1714–26. doi: 10.1053/j.gastro.2010.01.008
22. Bettegowda C, Sausen M, Leary RJ, Kinde I, Wang Y, Agrawal N, et al. Detection of circulating tumor DNA in early- and late-stage human malignancies. *Sci Transl Med.* (2014) 6:224ra24. doi: 10.1126/scitranslmed.3007094
23. Huang YK, Yu JC. Circulating microRNAs and long non-coding RNAs in gastric cancer diagnosis: an update and review. *World J Gastroenterol.* (2015) 21:9863–86. doi: 10.3748/wjg.v21.i34.9863
24. Alix-Panabières C, Pantel K. Challenges in circulating tumour cell research. *Nat Rev Cancer.* (2014) 14:623–31. doi: 10.1038/nrc3820
25. Stroup DF, Berlin JA, Morton SC, Olkin I, Williamson GD, Rennie D, et al. Meta-analysis of observational studies in epidemiology: a proposal for reporting. Meta-analysis Of Observational Studies in Epidemiology (MOOSE) group. *JAMA.* (2000) 283:2008–12. doi: 10.1001/jama.283.15.2008
26. Moher D, Liberati A, Tetzlaff J, Altman DG. Preferred reporting items for systematic reviews and meta-analyses: the PRISMA statement. *BMJ.* (2009) 339:b2535. doi: 10.1136/bmj.b2535
27. Higgins JP GS. *Cochrane Handbook for Systematic Reviews of Interventions Version 5.1.0* [updated March 2011]. Cochrane Collaboration (2011).

28. Tierney JF, Stewart LA, Ghersi D, Burdett S, Sydes MR. Practical methods for incorporating summary time-to-event data into meta-analysis. *Trials.* (2007) 8:16. doi: 10.1186/1745-6215-8-16
29. DerSimonian R, Laird N. Meta-analysis in clinical trials. *Control Clin Trials.* (1986) 7:177–88. doi: 10.1016/0197-2456(86)90046-2
30. Hiraiwa K, Takeuchi H, Hasegawa H, Saikawa Y, Suda K, Ando T, et al. Clinical significance of circulating tumor cells in blood from patients with gastrointestinal cancers. *Ann Surg Oncol.* (2008) 15:3092–100. doi: 10.1245/s10434-008-0122-9
31. Matsusaka S, Chìn K, Ogura M, Suenaga M, Shinozaki E, Mishima Y, et al. Circulating tumor cells as a surrogate marker for determining response to chemotherapy in patients with advanced gastric cancer. *Cancer Sci.* (2010) 101:1067–71. doi: 10.1111/j.1349-7006.2010.01492.x
32. Uenosono Y, Arigami T, Kozono T, Yanagita S, Hagihara T, Haraguchi N, et al. Clinical significance of circulating tumor cells in peripheral blood from patients with gastric cancer. *Cancer.* (2013) 119:3984–91. doi: 10.1002/cncr.28309
33. Li Y, Gong J, Zhang Q, Lu Z, Gao J, Li Y, et al. Dynamic monitoring of circulating tumour cells to evaluate therapeutic efficacy in advanced gastric cancer. *Br J Cancer.* (2016) 114:138–45. doi: 10.1038/bjc.2015.417
34. Okabe H, Tsunoda S, Hosogi H, Hisamori S, Tanaka E, Tanaka S, et al. Circulating tumor cells as an independent predictor of survival in advanced gastric cancer. *Ann Surg Oncol.* (2015) 22:3954–61. doi: 10.1245/s10434-015-4483-6
35. Yie SM, Lou B, Ye SR, Cao M, He X, Li P, et al. Detection of survivin-expressing circulating cancer cells (CCCs) in peripheral blood of patients with gastric and colorectal cancer reveals high risks of relapse. *Ann Surg Oncol.* (2008) 15:3073–82. doi: 10.1245/s10434-008-0069-x
36. Bertazza L, Mocellin S, Marchet A, Pilati P, Gabrieli J, Scalerta R, et al. Survivin gene levels in the peripheral blood of patients with gastric cancer independently predict survival. *J Transl Med.* (2009) 7:111. doi: 10.1186/1479-5876-7-111
37. Cao W, Yang W, Li H, Lou G, Jiang J, Geng M, et al. Using detection of survivin-expressing circulating tumor cells in peripheral blood to predict tumor recurrence following curative resection of gastric cancer. *J Surg Oncol.* (2011) 103:110–5. doi: 10.1002/jso.21777
38. Majima T, Ichikura T, Takayama E, Chochi K, Mochizuki H. Detecting circulating cancer cells using reverse transcriptase-polymerase chain reaction for cytokeratin mRNA in peripheral blood from patients with gastric cancer. *Jpn J Clin Oncol.* (2000) 30:499–503. doi: 10.1093/jjco/hyd130
39. Pituch-Noworolska A, Kolodziejczyk P, Kulig J, Drabik G, Szczepanik A, Czupryna A, et al. Circulating tumour cells and survival of patients with gastric cancer. *Anticancer Res.* (2007) 27:635–40.
40. Illert B, Fein M, Otto C, Cording F, Stehle D, Thiede A, et al. Disseminated tumor cells in the blood of patients with gastric cancer are an independent predictive marker of poor prognosis. *Scand J Gastroenterol.* (2005) 40:843–9. doi: 10.1080/00365520510015557
41. Saad AA, Awed NM, Abd Elkerim NN, El-Shennawy D, Alfons MA, Elserafy ME, et al. Prognostic significance of E-cadherin expression and peripheral blood micrometastasis in gastric carcinoma patients. *Ann Surg Oncol.* (2010) 17:3059–67. doi: 10.1245/s10434-010-1151-8
42. Liu Y, Ling Y, Qi Q, Lan F, Zhu M, Zhang Y, et al. Prognostic value of circulating tumor cells in advanced gastric cancer patients receiving chemotherapy. *Mol Clin Oncol.* (2017) 6:235–42. doi: 10.3892/mco.2017.1125
43. Uen YH, Lin SR, Wu CH, Hsieh JS, Lu CY, Yu FJ, et al. Clinical significance of MUC1 and c-Met RT-PCR detection of circulating tumor cells in patients with gastric carcinoma. *Clin Chim Acta.* (2006) 367:55–61. doi: 10.1016/j.cca.2005.11.013
44. Wu CH, Lin SR, Yu FJ, Wu DC, Pan YS, Hsieh JS, et al. Development of a high-throughput membrane-array method for molecular diagnosis of circulating tumor cells in patients with gastric cancers. *Int J Cancer.* (2006) 119:373–9. doi: 10.1002/ijc.21856
45. Ikeguchi M, Kaibara N. Detection of circulating cancer cells after a gastrectomy for gastric cancer. *Surg Today.* (2005) 35:436–41. doi: 10.1007/s00595-004-2978-z
46. Ishigami S, Sakamoto A, Uenosono Y, Nakajo A, Okumura H, Matsumoto M, et al. Carcinoembryonic antigen messenger RNA expression in blood can predict relapse in gastric cancer. *J Surg Res.* (2008) 148:205–9. doi: 10.1016/j.jss.2007.08.013
47. Qiu MZ, Li ZH, Zhou ZW, Li YH, Wang ZQ, Wang FH, et al. Detection of carcinoembryonic antigen messenger RNA in blood using quantitative real-time reverse transcriptase-polymerase chain reaction to predict recurrence of gastric adenocarcinoma. *J Transl Med.* (2010) 8:107. doi: 10.1186/1479-5876-8-107
48. Arigami T, Uenosono Y, Hirata M, Yanagita S, Ishigami S, Natsugoe S. B7-H3 expression in gastric cancer: a novel molecular blood marker for detecting circulating tumor cells. *Cancer Sci.* (2011) 102:1019–24. doi: 10.1111/j.1349-7006.2011.01877.x
49. Ito H, Sato J, Tsujino Y, Yamaguchi N, Kimura S, Gohda K, et al. Long-term prognostic impact of circulating tumour cells in gastric cancer patients. *World J Gastroenterol.* (2016) 22:10232–41. doi: 10.3748/wjg.v22.i46.10232
50. Leung WK, To KF, Chu ES, Chan MW, Bai AH, Ng EK, et al. Potential diagnostic and prognostic values of detecting promoter hypermethylation in the serum of patients with gastric cancer. *Br J Cancer.* (2005) 92:2190–4. doi: 10.1038/sj.bjc.6602636
51. Balgkouranidou I, Karayiannakis A, Matthaios D, Bolanaki H, Tripsianis G, Tentes AA, et al. Assessment of SOX17 DNA methylation in cell free DNA from patients with operable gastric cancer. Association with prognostic variables and survival. *Clin Chem Lab Med.* (2013) 51:1505–10. doi: 10.1515/cclm-2012-0320
52. Yang Q, Gao J, Xu L, Zeng Z, Sung JJ, Yu J. Promoter hypermethylation of BCL6B gene is a potential plasma DNA biomarker for gastric cancer. *Biomarkers.* (2013) 18:721–5. doi: 10.3109/1354750X.2013.853839
53. Ling ZQ, Lv P, Lu XX, Yu JL, Han J, Ying LS, et al. Circulating methylated XAF1 DNA indicates poor prognosis for gastric cancer. *PLoS ONE.* (2013) 8:e67195. doi: 10.1371/journal.pone.0067195
54. Han J, Lv P, Yu JL, Wu YC, Zhu X, Hong LL, et al. Circulating methylated MINT2 promoter DNA is a potential poor prognostic factor in gastric cancer. *Dig Dis Sci.* (2014) 59:1160–8. doi: 10.1007/s10620-013-3007-0
55. Wu YC, Lv P, Han J, Yu JL, Zhu X, Hong LL, et al. Enhanced serum methylated p16 DNAs is associated with the progression of gastric cancer. *Int J Clin Exp Pathol.* (2014) 7:1553–62.
56. Yu JL, Lv P, Han J, Zhu X, Hong LL, Zhu WY, et al. Methylated TIMP-3 DNA in body fluids is an independent prognostic factor for gastric cancer. *Arch Pathol Lab Med.* (2014) 138:1466–73. doi: 10.5858/arpa.2013-0285-OA
57. Balgkouranidou I, Matthaios D, Karayiannakis A, Bolanaki H, Michailidis P, Xenidis N, et al. Prognostic role of APC and RASSF1A promoter methylation status in cell free circulating DNA of operable gastric cancer patients. *Mutat Res.* (2015) 778:46–51. doi: 10.1016/j.mrfmmm.2015.05.002
58. Pimson C, Ekalaksananan T, Pientong C, Promthet S, Putthanachote N, Suwanrungruang K, et al. Aberrant methylation of PCDH10 and RASSF1A genes in blood samples for non-invasive diagnosis and prognostic assessment of gastric cancer. *PeerJ.* (2016) 4:e2112. doi: 10.7717/peerj.2112
59. Fang WL, Lan YT, Huang KH, Liu CA, Hung YP, Lin CH, et al. Clinical significance of circulating plasma DNA in gastric cancer. *Int J Cancer.* (2016) 138:2974–83. doi: 10.1002/ijc.30018
60. Valladares-Ayerbes M, Reboredo M, Medina-Villaamil V, Iglesias-Díaz P, Lorenzo-Patiño MJ, Haz M, et al. Circulating miR-200c as a diagnostic and prognostic biomarker for gastric cancer. *J Transl Med.* (2012) 10:186. doi: 10.1186/1479-5876-10-186
61. Zhang HP, Sun FB, Li SJ. Serum miR-200c expression level as a prognostic biomarker for gastric cancer. *Genet Mol Res.* (2015) 14:15913–20. doi: 10.4238/2015.December.7.2
62. Yang R, Fu Y, Zeng Y, Xiang M, Yin Y, Li L, et al. Serum miR-20a is a promising biomarker for gastric cancer. *Biomed Rep.* (2017) 6:429–34. doi: 10.3892/br.2017.862
63. Wang M, Gu H, Wang S, Qian H, Zhu W, Zhang L, et al. Circulating miR-17-5p and miR-20a: molecular markers for gastric cancer. *Mol Med Rep.* (2012) 5:1514–20. doi: 10.3892/mmr.2012.828
64. Komatsu S, Ichikawa D, Tsujiura M, Konishi H, Takeshita H, Nagata H, et al. Prognostic impact of circulating miR-21 in the plasma of patients with gastric carcinoma. *Anticancer Res.* (2013) 33:271–6.
65. Song J, Bai Z, Zhang J, Meng H, Cai J, Deng W, et al. Serum microRNA-21 levels are related to tumor size in gastric cancer patients but cannot predict prognosis. *Oncol Lett.* (2013) 6:1733–7. doi: 10.3892/ol.2013.1626
66. Hou CG, Luo XY, Li G. Diagnostic and prognostic value of serum MicroRNA-206 in patients with gastric cancer. *Cell Physiol Biochem.* (2016) 39:1512–20. doi: 10.1159/000447854

67. Imaoka H, Toiyama Y, Okigami M, Yasuda H, Saigusa S, Ohi M, et al. Circulating microRNA-203 predicts metastases, early recurrence, and poor prognosis in human gastric cancer. *Gastric Cancer.* (2016) 19:744–53. doi: 10.1007/s10120-015-0521-0
68. Fu Z, Qian F, Yang X, Jiang H, Chen Y, Liu S. Circulating miR-222 in plasma and its potential diagnostic and prognostic value in gastric cancer. *Med Oncol.* (2014) 31:164. doi: 10.1007/s12032-014-0164-8
69. Huang D, Wang H, Liu R, Li H, Ge S, Bai M, et al. miRNA27a is a biomarker for predicting chemosensitivity and prognosis in metastatic or recurrent gastric cancer. *J Cell Biochem.* (2014) 115:549–56. doi: 10.1002/jcb.24689
70. Zhuang K, Han K, Tang H, Yin X, Zhang J, Zhang X, et al. Up-Regulation of plasma miR-23b is associated with poor prognosis of gastric cancer. *Med Sci Monit.* (2016) 22:356–61. doi: 10.12659/MSM.895428
71. Tsai MM, Wang CS, Tsai CY, Huang CG, Lee KF, Huang HW, et al. Circulating microRNA-196a/b are novel biomarkers associated with metastatic gastric cancer. *Eur J Cancer.* (2016) 64:137–48. doi: 10.1016/j.ejca.2016.05.007
72. Chen Q, Ge X, Zhang Y, Xia H, Yuan D, Tang Q, et al. Plasma miR-122 and miR-192 as potential novel biomarkers for the early detection of distant metastasis of gastric cancer. *Oncol Rep.* (2014) 31:1863–70. doi: 10.3892/or.2014.3004
73. Huang X, Gao P, Sun J, Chen X, Song Y, Zhao J, et al. Clinicopathological and prognostic significance of circulating tumor cells in patients with gastric cancer: a meta-analysis. *Int J Cancer.* (2015) 136:21–33. doi: 10.1002/ijc.28954
74. Zhang ZY, Dai ZL, Yin XW, Li SH, Li SP, Ge HY. Meta-analysis shows that circulating tumor cells including circulating microRNAs are useful to predict the survival of patients with gastric cancer. *BMC Cancer.* (2014) 14:773. doi: 10.1186/1471-2407-14-773
75. Gao Y, Zhang K, Xi H, Cai A, Wu X, Cui J, et al. Diagnostic and prognostic value of circulating tumor DNA in gastric cancer: a meta-analysis. *Oncotarget.* (2017) 8:6330–40. doi: 10.18632/oncotarget.14064
76. Oyama K, Fushida S, Kinoshita J, Okamoto K, Makino I, Nakamura K, et al. Serum cytokeratin 18 as a biomarker for gastric cancer. *Clin Exp Med.* (2013) 13:289–95. doi: 10.1007/s10238-012-0202-9
77. Zhao S, Yang H, Zhang M, Zhang D, Liu Y, Liu Y, et al. Circulating tumor cells (CTCs) detected by triple-marker EpCAM, CK19, and hMAM RT-PCR and their relation to clinical outcome in metastatic breast cancer patients. *Cell Biochem Biophys.* (2013) 65:263–73. doi: 10.1007/s12013-012-9426-2
78. Govaere O, Komuta M, Berkers J, Spee B, Janssen C, de Luca F, et al. Keratin 19: a key role player in the invasion of human hepatocellular carcinomas. *Gut.* (2014) 63:674–85. doi: 10.1136/gutjnl-2012-304351
79. Stroun M, Lyautey J, Lederrey C, Olson-Sand A, Anker P. About the possible origin and mechanism of circulating DNA apoptosis and active DNA release. *Clin Chim Acta.* (2001) 313:139–42. doi: 10.1016/S0009-8981(01)00665-9
80. Tsujiura M, Ichikawa D, Konishi H, Komatsu S, Shiozaki A, Otsuji E. Liquid biopsy of gastric cancer patients: circulating tumor cells and cell-free nucleic acids. *World J Gastroenterol.* (2014) 20:3265–86. doi: 10.3748/wjg.v20.i12.3265
81. Ye T, Chen Y, Fang J. DNA methylation biomarkers in serum for gastric cancer screening. *Mini Rev Med Chem.* (2010) 10:1034–8. doi: 10.2174/1389557511009011034
82. Dias-Santagata D, Akhavanfard S, David SS, Vernovsky K, Kuhlmann G, Boisvert SL, et al. Rapid targeted mutational analysis of human tumours: a clinical platform to guide personalized cancer medicine. *EMBO Mol Med.* (2010) 2:146–58. doi: 10.1002/emmm.201000070
83. Merker JD, Oxnard GR, Compton C, Diehn M, Hurley P, Lazar AJ, et al. Circulating tumor DNA analysis in patients with cancer: American Society of Clinical Oncology and College of American Pathologists Joint Review. *J Clin Oncol.* (2018) 36:1631–41. doi: 10.1200/JCO.2017.76.8671
84. Zhang Y, Yang P, Sun T, Li D, Xu X, Rui Y, et al. miR-126 and miR-126* repress recruitment of mesenchymal stem cells and inflammatory monocytes to inhibit breast cancer metastasis. *Nat Cell Biol.* (2013) 15:284–94. doi: 10.1038/ncb2690
85. Zhang Z, Li Z, Li Y, Zang A. MicroRNA and signaling pathways in gastric cancer. *Cancer Gene Ther.* (2014) 21:305–16. doi: 10.1038/cgt.2014.37
86. Wicha MS, Hayes DF. Circulating tumor cells: not all detected cells are bad and not all bad cells are detected. *J Clin Oncol.* (2011) 29:1508–11. doi: 10.1200/JCO.2010.34.0026
87. Liang Z, Cheng Y, Chen Y, Hu Y, Liu WP, Lu Y, et al. EGFR T790M ctDNA testing platforms and their role as companion diagnostics: correlation with clinical outcomes to EGFR-TKIs. *Cancer Lett.* (2017) 403:186–94. doi: 10.1016/j.canlet.2017.06.008
88. Diaz LA, Bardelli A. Liquid biopsies: genotyping circulating tumor DNA. *J Clin Oncol.* (2014) 32:579–86. doi: 10.1200/JCO.2012.45.2011
89. Visvanathan K, Fackler MS, Zhang Z, Lopez-Bujanda ZA, Jeter SC, Sokoll LJ, et al. Monitoring of serum DNA methylation as an early independent marker of response and survival in metastatic breast cancer: TBCRC 005 Prospective Biomarker Study. *J Clin Oncol.* (2017) 35:751–8. doi: 10.1200/JCO.2015.66.2080
90. Cohen JD, Li L, Wang Y, Thoburn C, Afsari B, Danilova L, et al. Detection and localization of surgically resectable cancers with a multi-analyte blood test. *Science.* (2018) 359:926–30. doi: 10.1126/science.aar3247
91. Qin Z, Ljubimov VA, Zhou C, Tong Y, Liang J. Cell-free circulating tumor DNA in cancer. *Chin J Cancer.* (2016) 35:36. doi: 10.1186/s40880-016-0092-4

3

How Does Combined Resection Affect the Clinical Outcomes After Laparoscopic Surgery for Serosa-Positive Gastric Cancer?: A Retrospective Cohort Study to Investigate the Short-Term Outcomes of Laparoscopic Combined Resection in Patients with T4b Gastric Cancer

Chang Min Lee [1,2*]***, San Lee*** [2]***, Danbi Lee*** [2] ***and Sungsoo Park*** [1,3]

[1] *Department of Surgery, Korea University College of Medicine, Seoul, South Korea,* [2] *Department of Surgery, Korea University Medical Center Ansan Hospital, Ansan, South Korea,* [3] *Department of Surgery, Korea University Medical Center Anam Hospital, Seoul, South Korea*

***Correspondence:**
Chang Min Lee
laparosamurai@gmail.com

Background: Only few surgeons have tried to perform laparoscopic combined resection for T4b gastric cancer. The purpose of this study was to investigate the feasibility of laparoscopic combined resection through a comparison of the clinical outcomes between cT4a and cT4b cases.

Methods: We reviewed the medical charts of patients who underwent laparoscopic gastrectomy for clinically T4 gastric cancer from May 2014 and July 2018. During this period, 62 patients with serosa-positive gastric cancer underwent laparoscopic curative surgery. The patients were divided into the following groups: patients who underwent gastrectomy and combined resection for the invaded organs (combined resection group) and those who did not undergo combined organ surgery (gastrectomy only group). Clinical outcomes were compared between the gastrectomy only and combined resection groups.

Results: Of 62 patients included in this study, 43 and 19 patients were included in the gastrectomy only and combined resection groups, respectively. The operation time was significantly longer in the combined resection group (364.6 ± 102.5 vs. 247.7 ± 66.1 min; $p < 0.001$). The incidence of grade $\geq$ III complications was comparable between the groups (26.3% vs. 11.6%; $p = 0.147$). The time from the first operation to the initiation of adjuvant chemotherapy showed no statistically significant difference between the groups (48.1 ± 45.4 days vs. 31.6 ± 9.2; $p = 0.134$).

Conclusions: Focusing on the high quality of image and new devices of laparoscopic surgery, it is necessary to re-evaluate the oncologic outcomes of combined resection for T4b gastric cancer.

Keywords: combined resection, gastric cancer, laparoscopic, T4a, T4b

INTRODUCTION

R0 resection is the mainstay to achieve the survival benefit in patients with gastric adenocarcinoma. This principle should be also considered as a significant endpoint in the treatment for locally advanced cases; therefore, the current treatment guideline suggested combined resection in T4b gastric cancer. However, regarding this issue, several representative trials showed that combined organ resection resulted in a high rate of morbidities after curative surgery for advanced gastric cancer (AGC). Cuschieri et al. reported that combined pancreatectomy and splenectomy to achieve D2 resection increased the morbidity and mortality rates after gastric cancer surgery (1). Similarly, combined organ resection might be attributed to the higher morbidity rate of patients undergoing D2 dissection than D1 dissection according to the result of a Dutch trial (2). Given that postoperative morbidity is known to be correlated with oncologic outcomes, many concerns in performing combined surgery for patients with T4b disease have existed.

However, it is remarkable that all of these data have been acquired from the clinical experiences of open surgery for gastrectomy. To date, it has been difficult to apply the minimally invasive procedures in patients with AGC. Although several trials have been planned for investigating the oncologic safety of laparoscopic surgery in patients with AGC, many concerns still exist in the minimally invasive approach for serosa-positive disease. Thus, it has taken quite a long time to apply laparoscopic combined resection in patients with T4b cases.

These reluctances to the laparoscopic approach for AGC seem to be contradictory to the known advantages of minimally invasive approaches. For decades, many trials have proved that adjuvant chemotherapy (AC) showed a significant prognostic effect in patients undergoing curative gastrectomy (3, 4). With regard to this issue, it is necessary to consider the key characteristics of laparoscopic surgery. The fast recovery resulted from the reduced wound size, which enables the patients to undergo AC in a timely period. Actually, even though we achieve R0 resection in patients with AGC, the late induction of AC may cause a poor oncologic outcome (5).

In T4b diseases that necessitate combined organ resection, laparoscopic surgery is more effective than open surgery in terms of reducing the abdominal wound size. Although it can be necessary to extend the abdominal incision for combined resection during open surgery, laparoscopic combined resection requires only the addition of no or several port incisions.

For the recent years, we accumulated the clinical experience of laparoscopic surgery for serosa-positive gastric cancer. Of these, some patients with cT4b diseases underwent laparoscopic combined resection. Therefore, in this study, we investigated the feasibility of laparoscopic combined resection through a comparison of the clinical outcomes between cT4a and cT4b cases.

METHODS

Study Design and Participants

This was a retrospective cohort study performed in a single institution. We reviewed the medical charts of patients who underwent laparoscopic gastrectomy for clinically T4 gastric cancer between May 2014 and July 2018. During this period, a total of 65 patients with serosa-positive gastric cancer underwent laparoscopic curative surgery. Of these, 62 patients were treated with AC (**Figure 1**). According to whether combined organ resection was performed, the patients were divided into the following two groups: patients who underwent gastrectomy and combined resection for the invaded organs (named the combined resection group) and those who did not undergo combined organ surgery (named the gastrectomy only group). Clinical outcomes were compared between the gastrectomy only and combined resection groups.

The approval to perform research on human subjects in this study was provided by the Institutional Review Board of Korea University Medical Center Ansan Hospital (registration number:

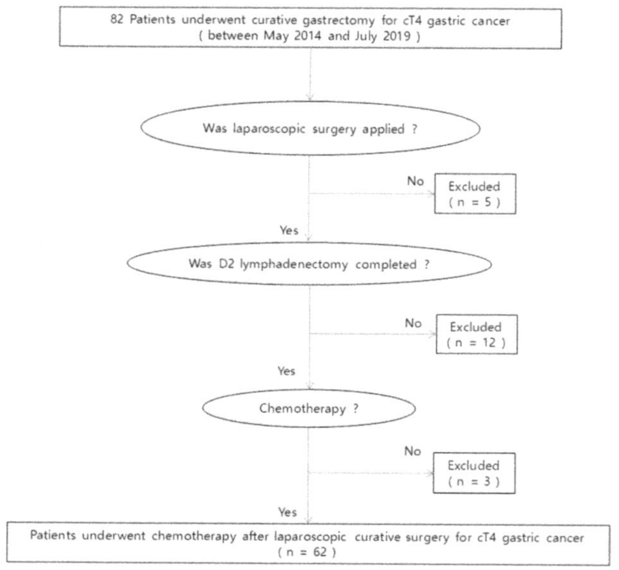

FIGURE 1 | Schematic of this study.

2019AS0205). This study adhered to the tenets of the Declaration of Helsinki.

Procedures

All surgical procedures were performed by one surgeon (CML), who had been trained in a high-volume center performing more than 500 laparoscopic gastric cancer surgeries per year.

In the operating room, the procedure was performed under general anesthesia with the patient placed on the bed with both legs abducted. The bed was adjusted to create a reverse Trendelenburg position for the patient. The operator sat on the right side of the patient, while the scopist was positioned between the patient's legs.

A 12-mm channel trocar was inserted through a transumbilical incision using the Hasson's method (6). After a pneumoperitoneum was formed with carbon dioxide at a pressure of 15 mmHg, a flexible scope was inserted through this umbilical port. Under the guidance of flexible scope, one 5-mm channel trocar was established on the right subcostal margin and the other 12-mm channel trocar on the right midclavicular line. Additionally, two 5-mm channel trocars were established on the left subcostal margin and left midclavicular line.

The falciform ligament and the left lobe of the liver were raised toward the cephalad direction by combined suture retraction (7).

Lymphadenectomy for curative distal gastrectomy was accomplished based on the criteria of the Japanese Gastric Cancer Treatment Guidelines 2010 (ver. 3) (8). We performed D2 lymphadenectomy in all of the patients who were preoperatively diagnosed with clinically T4.

After the completion of lymphadenectomy, the stomach and adjacent organs (particularly in the combined resection group) were resected. The gastrointestinal or hepatopancreaticoenteric continuity was recovered according to the following types of the resected organs: (i) in cases of Billroth II anastomosis after subtotal gastrectomy, Braun anastomosis was also performed to reduce bile reflux to the remnant stomach. All of the gastrointestinal anastomoses were performed with laparoscopic linear staplers; (ii) in cases of Roux-en-Y esophagojejunostomy after total gastrectomy, jejunojejunostomy was made at the 45-cm distal point from the esophagojejunostomy. In all of these cases, the mesentery defect was closed using non-absorbable knotless barbed sutures. All of the gastrointestinal anastomoses were performed with laparoscopic linear staplers; (iii) in cases invading the transverse colon, the involved segment was resected using laparoscopic linear staplers (**Figure 2a**). Colo-colic anastomosis was performed by overlap stapling using laparoscopic linear staplers; (iv) in cases invading the body or tail of the pancreas, distal pancreatectomy was performed using laparoscopic linear staplers (**Figure 2b**). Reinforcement sutures were performed using knotless barbed sutures; (v) in cases invading the head of the pancreas, pancreaticoduodenogastric resection was performed (**Figure 2c**). To restore the bilio-pancreatico-intestinal continuity, pancreaticojejunostomy and hepaticojejunostomy were performed by hand-sewing. Billroth II

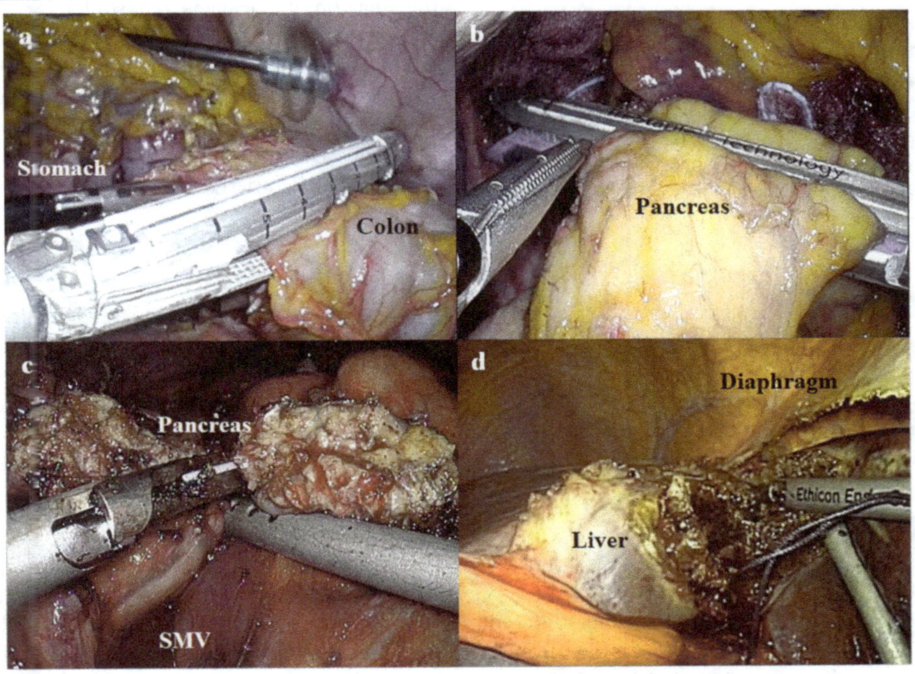

FIGURE 2 | The procedures of combined resection for advanced gastric cancer invading the adjacent organs. **(a)** Laparoscopic linear stapler is used to resect the colon invaded by advanced gastric cancer. **(b)** Distal pancreatectomy is performed using a laparoscopic linear stapler. **(c)** Pancreas is transected using an ultrasonic energy device during pancreaticoduodenectomy (SMV, superior mesenteric vein). **(d)** Ultrasonic energy device is used to resect the liver invaded by advanced gastric cancer.

anastomosis was performed for the recovery of gastrointestinal continuity; and (vi) in cases invading the liver, the resection ranges were determined according to the location and size of the involved segments. If the tumor extensively involved both segments 2 and 3, left lateral sectionectomy was performed (**Figure 2d**). If the invaded lesion was localized in segment 2 or 3, non-anatomical resection was performed.

Assessments

Demographic data, including age, sex, body mass index (BMI), and American Society of Anesthesiologists (ASA) score, were obtained from all enrolled patients. In addition, clinical outcomes, including the operation time, conversion to open surgery, reconstruction method, resected organs, postoperative hospital stay, time to the first semi-blend diet, postoperative complications, and the time from the first operation to the initiation of AC were also investigated. Postoperative complications were classified based on the Clavien-Dindo classification of surgical complications (9).

We also investigated the pathologic results, including tumor depth, and number of retrieved and metastatic lymph nodes.

As a subgroup analysis, the patients in the combined resection group were subdivided into the following three groups: patients who underwent splenectomy (named as SP group), those who underwent distal pancreatectomy and splenectomy (named as DP group), and the others (named as OT group). Clinical outcomes were compared between the SP, DP, and OT groups.

Analysis

Patients with and without undergoing combined resection were compared using chi-square test or Fisher's exact test for categorical data and Student's *t*-test or Mann–Whitney *U* test or one-way ANOVA for continuous data without normal distribution. In the two-tailed tests, a $p \leq 0.05$ was considered statistically significant. Statistical analysis was performed using SPSS 24.0 (SPSS Inc., Chicago, IL, USA).

RESULTS

Of 62 patients included in this study, 43 patients had clinically T4a disease (gastrectomy only group) and 19 had clinically T4b (combined resection group). All of the patients in the combined resection group underwent laparoscopic en bloc resection of the stomach and adjacent organs.

Demographic Data

The mean age of the patients was 62.6 ± 13.1 years, and the gastrectomy only group was significantly older (65.9 ± 13.1 vs. 55.2 ± 9.6 years; $p = 0.001$). The sex ratio was not different between two groups ($p = 0.172$). Baseline BMI was significantly higher in the gastrectomy only group (23.0 ± 3.1 vs. 21.0 ± 3.5 kg/m^2; $p = 0.031$). Most of the patients' pathologic T stages were similar to the clinical T stage before the surgery (83.9%), with the exception of 10 patients (seven with combined resection and three with gastrectomy only).

Clinical Outcomes

The clinical outcomes showed that the operation time was significantly longer in the combined resection group (247.7 ± 66.1 vs. 364.6 ± 102.5 min; $p < 0.001$). The time to the first semi-blend diet and the length of hospital stay were also significantly longer in the combined resection group (**Table 1**).

The combined resection group experienced postoperative complications more frequently (63.2%) than the gastrectomy only group (20.9%); however, the incidence of grade ≥ III was comparable between the groups (11.6% in the gastrectomy only group vs. 26.3% in the combined resection group; $p = 0.147$). In addition, the time from the first operation to the initiation of AC showed no statistically significant difference between the groups (31.6 ± 9.2 in gastrectomy only group vs. 48.1 ± 45.4 days in combined resection; $p = 0.134$) (**Table 1**). There was no complication that resulted in mortality in both groups.

Detailed Information for the Combined Resection Group

In the combined resection group, three transverse colon invasions, six pancreas invasions (one head, three body, and two tail), five liver invasions, seven spleen invasions, and one lung invasion were noted in the laparoscopic images (**Table 2**).

The postoperative complications in cases 8, 9, 10, and 19 appeared as intra-abdominal fluid collections, which were treated with the intravenous antibiotics (grade II by the Clavien-Dindo classification of surgical complications). Cases 2 and 17 also manifested the intra-abdominal fluid collection, but required the percutaneous abscess drainage (grade IIIa). Case 4 showed the anastomotic leakage of esophagojejunostomy, which was conservatively treated after endoscopic stent insertion (grade IIIa). Case 5 manifested duodenal stump leakage, which was treated with intravenous antibiotics (grade II). Case 12 was diagnosed with intractable pneumonia, which was treated in intensive care unit for more than 5 months; therefore, started AC treatment was started at 182 days postoperatively.

Subgroup Analysis for the Combined Resection Group

The subgroup analysis (performed in the combined resection group) showed a statistically significant difference between the SP, DP, and OT groups in terms of the pathologic T stage. However, the operation time, the pathologic N stage, the length of hospital stays, morbidity, severe morbidity, and the time from the first operation to the initiation of AC did not differ between the three groups (**Table 3**).

DISCUSSION

Laparoscopic surgery has been established as an effective modality for the surgical treatment of gastric cancer. Although it is still necessary to acquire the clinical evidences regarding laparoscopic combined surgery in patients with gastric cancer, the laparoscopic approach also has some advantages in terms of multi-organ resection. Most importantly, surgical trauma is minimized, because the diversity of the laparoscopic procedures

TABLE 1 | Characteristics of patients who underwent laparoscopic gastrectomy with D2 lymphadenectomy for clinical T4 gastric cancer ($n = 62$).

	Gastrectomy only group ($n = 43$)	Combined resection group ($n = 19$)	p
Age	65.9 ± 13.1	55.2 ± 9.6	0.001
Sex (Male:Female)	2.1:1	5.3:1	0.172
BMI	23.0 ± 3.1	21.0 ± 3.5	0.031
ASA score (%)			0.710
1	4 (9.3)	3 (15.8)	
2	31 (72.1)	12 (63.2)	
3	8 (18.6)	4 (21.1)	
The type of surgery (DG:TG)			<0.001
DG	31 (72.1)	4 (21.1)	
TG	12 (27.9)	15 (78.9)	
The operation time (min)	247.7 ± 66.1	364.6 ± 102.5	<0.001
Suture for intraoperative bleeding (%)	5 (11.6)	6 (31.6)	0.135
Portal vein injury	3 (7.0)	3 (15.8)	
Splenic artery injury	0	2 (10.5)	
Gastroduodenal artery injury	1 (2.3)	1 (5.3)	
Proper hepatic artery injury	1 (2.3)	0	
Pathologic T stage (%)			<0.001
pT1	0	0	
pT2	3 (7.0)	0	
pT3	0	1 (5.3)	
pT4a	40 (93.0)	6 (31.6)	
pT4b	0	12 (63.2)	
Number of retrieved lymph nodes	43.1 ± 22.2	54.4 ± 27.3	0.090
Number of metastatic lymph nodes	10.3 ± 13.4	7.5 ± 7.8	0.400
Pathologic N stage			0.601
pN0	8 (18.6)	3 (15.8)	
pN1	6 (14.0)	5 (26.3)	
pN2	9 (20.9)	5 (26.3)	
pN3a	11 (25.6)	3 (15.8)	
pN3b	9 (20.9)	2 (10.5)	
The length of hospital stays (day)	15.2 ± 5.4	36.0 ± 40.9	0.040
Morbidity (%)	9 (20.9%),	12 (63.2%)	0.001
Severe morbidity (≥grade III) (%)	5 (11.6%)	5 (26.3%)	0.147
The details of morbidity (%)			0.014
Fluid collection	4 (9.3)	8 (42.1)	
Duodenal stump leakage	2 (4.7)	1 (5.3)	
Anastomosis leakage	0	1 (5.3)	
Pneumonia	2 (4.7)	1 (5.3)	
Bleeding	1 (2.3)	0	
Afferent loop syndrome	0	1 (5.3)	
The time to adjuvant chemotherapy	31.6 ± 9.2	48.1 ± 45.4	0.134

BMI, body mass index; ASA score, score graded by the American Society of Anesthesiologists physical status classification; DG, distal gastrectomy; TG, total gastrectomy.

can be expanded by adding several (sometimes no) port wounds. This characteristic has been known to be correlated with the fast recovery; therefore, the promising outcomes are expected in laparoscopic combined resection. Although many surgeons are concerned about whether all the procedures could not be realized with the laparoscopic approach, the recent advances in laparoscopic instruments (i.e., energy devices, surgical staplers, and high-resolution laparoscopes) have facilitated us to overcome the technical difficulty of laparoscopic procedures.

Nevertheless, only few surgeons have tried to perform laparoscopic combined resection for T4b gastric cancer (10). This tendency involves the following reasons. First, when gastric cancer shows the feature of T4b disease, the adjacent organs or tissues might be deprived of their inherent structures. Such deformities make it difficult to perform a laparoscopic approach; therefore, open surgery is generally preferred to control the risk from the unusual anatomy of T4b disease (i.e., the distorted flow of the named vessels, unexpected hemorrhage due to the neovascularization around the tumor, and ambiguous boundaries between the organs).

Meanwhile, another reason is associated with the current training systems for the surgeons. Nowadays, to acquire the qualified procedures for the oncologic principles, the surgeon's training program has been subdivided in Korea. Thus, most surgeons who had been trained for gastric cancer surgery might be unfamiliar with laparoscopic resection of the colon, pancreas, and liver. To solve these problems, some surgeons adopt the multidisciplinary approach for combined resection. However, unlike concomitant resection for the double primary malignancies, combined resection for T4b gastric cancer should be very organized that the main procedures cannot be distributed to each surgeon of the multidisciplinary team. Therefore, the foregut surgeons who usually deal with AGC should take the responsibility for en bloc resection of the invaded organs, which has been usually performed in open surgery.

Regarding this issue, we have prepared the clinical practice for a foregut surgeon to perform laparoscopic en bloc resection in patients with AGC invading the adjacent organs. Before the actual practice, we had organized many times multidisciplinary conference between the surgeons with different subspecialties in our institute. Nowadays, the well-developed video recording systems could provide high-quality images showing the details of laparoscopic surgery; therefore, our multidisciplinary conference has been operated based on the discussions regarding such video records. Moreover, in Korea, there had been some annual international conferences held by the Korean Society of Endoscopic and Laparoscopic Surgeons, in which many surgeons share the expertise from each subspecial division of laparoscopic surgery. From all of these programs outside and inside our institute, we have accumulated expertise in performing surgeries of the adjacent organs surrounding the stomach.

Nevertheless, there are several technically demanding points when performing combined surgery for T4b gastric cancer. First, such an advanced tumor makes the significant desmoplastic reaction around the major vessels; therefore, it can cause unexpected bleeding during the operation. In our results, there were many hemorrhagic events, all of which were controlled by laparoscopic suture. Even though the unexpected hemorrhage can happen during laparoscopic surgery for AGC, it can be even more dangerous to control the bleeding from the unaccustomed structures beyond the perigastric vascular anatomies. However,

TABLE 2 | Clinicopathologic data of the patients who underwent laparoscopic combined resection.

Serial number	Age	Sex	BMI	ASA score	Tumor location	Tumor size (cm)*	Type of gastrectomy	Invaded organ in laparoscopic view	Procedures for invaded organs	Operation time (min)	EBL (ml)	Hospital stay (days)	Time to the first SBD (days)	Morbidity	C-D grade
1	58	Male	23.0	1	Low body	7.0	TG	Transverse colon	Segmental resection of transverse colon	282	50	13	6	None	0
2	50	Male	18.2	2	Antrum	7.0	DG	Pancreas (head)	Pancreaticoduodenectomy	650	500	34	9	Fluid collection	IIIa
3	73	Male	15.3	1	High body	6.0	TG	Liver	LLS	463	100	15	7	None	0
4	59	Male	17.6	2	From high body to distal esophagus	10.0	TG	Liver, lung	Splenectomy, LLS, wedge resection of lung	487	100	49	42	Anastomotic leakage of esophagojejunostomy	IIIa
5	40	Male	17.0	2	Antrum	4.5	DG	Liver	Wedge resection of liver	282	100	39	9	Leakage of duodenal stump	II
6	55	Male	20.0	2	High body	9	TG	Spleen	Splenectomy	358	250	20	8	None	0
7	51	Male	22.6	2	High body	6.5	TG	Spleen	Splenectomy	350	350	15	8	Afferent loop syndrome	IIIa
8	53	Male	20.4	1	High body	8	TG	Spleen	Splenectomy	402	50	43	4	Fluid collection	II
9	55	Male	23.5	2	High body	6.5	TG	Spleen	Splenectomy	273	50	22	9	Fluid collection	II
10	46	Male	22.1	2	From high body to cardia	6	TG	Pancreas (body)	DP, Splenectomy	412	450	22	8	Fluid collection	II
11	62	Male	22.0	2	Low body	4.5	DG	Liver	Wedge resection of liver	266	100	17	5	None	0
12	66	Male	26.1	3	From mid to high body	9	TG	Spleen	Splenectomy	369	300	182	10	Pneumonia	IVa
13	53	Male	24.3	2	High body	5	TG	Pancreas (body)	DP, splenectomy, segmental resection of transverse colon	397	50	16	5	None	0
14	45	Female	16.8	2	From mid to high body	12.5	TG	Spleen	Splenectomy.	340	100	11	9	None	0
15	41	Female	19.9	2	High body	6	TG	Spleen	Splenectomy	285	350	22	8	Fluid collection	II
16	71	Male	29.7	3	From cardia to distal esophagus	8	TG	Liver	Wedge resection of liver	319	100	13	6	None	0
17	69	Male	19.7	3	From high body to cardia	10	TG	Pancreas (tail), transverse colon	DP, splenectomy, segmental resection of transverse colon	391	100	22	12	Fluid collection	IIIa
18	52	Male	20.9	3	From low body to cardia	13	TG	Pancreas (body)	DP, splenectomy	293	450	52	7	Fluid collection	II
19	49	Female	29.3	2	From high body to cardia	10	TG	Pancreas (tail), transverse colon	DP, splenectomy	408	200	27	8	Fluid collection	II

BMI, body mass index; ASA score, score graded by the American Society of Anesthesiologists physical status classification; EBL, estimated blood loss; C-D grade, grade by the Clavien-Dindo classification of surgical complications; TG, total gastrectomy; DG, distal gastrectomy; LLS, left lateral sectionectomy of liver; DP, distal pancreatectomy.

**These values are expressed as the longest diameter of the tumor.*

TABLE 3 | Subgroup analysis for combined resection group.

	Splenectomy ($n = 7$)	Splenectomy and DP ($n = 3$)	Others ($n = 9$)	p
Age	52.3 ± 8.0	49.0 ± 3.0	59.4 ± 10.8	0.164
Sex (Male:Female)	2.5:1	2:1	9:0	0.198
BMI	21.3 ± 3.0	24.1 ± 4.5	19.6 ± 3.2	0.170
ASA score (%)				0.869
1	1 (14.3)	0	2 (22.2)	
2	5 (71.4)	2 (66.7)	5 (55.6)	
3	1 (14.3)	0	2 (22.2)	
The type of surgery (DG:TG)				0.060
DG	0	0	4 (44.4)	
TG	7 (100)	3 (100)	5 (55.6)	
The operation time (min)	339.6 ± 45.9	371.0 ± 67.6	381.9 ± 141.6	0.733
Suture for intraoperative bleeding (%)				0.481
Portal vein injury	1 (14.3)	1 (33.3)	1 (11.1)	
Splenic artery injury	2 (28.6)	0	0	
Gastroduodenal artery injury	0	0	1 (11.1)	
Proper hepatic artery injury	0	0	0	
Pathologic T stage (%)				0.020
pT1	0	0	0	
pT2	0	0	0	
pT3	1 (14.3)	0	0	
pT4a	5 (71.4)	0	1 (11.1)	
pT4b	1 (14.3)	3 (100)	8 (88.9)	
Number of retrieved lymph nodes	65.3 ± 33.5	49.7 ± 13.3	47.4 ± 24.7	0.434
Number of metastatic lymph nodes	6.7 ± 9.8	8.3 ± 6.4	7.8 ± 7.4	0.949
Pathologic N stage				0.690
pN0	1 (14.3)	1 (33.3)	1 (11.1)	
pN1	3 (42.9)	1 (33.3)	1 (11.1)	
pN2	1 (14.3)	0	4 (44.4)	
pN3a	1 (14.3)	1 (33.3)	1 (11.1)	
pN3b	1 (14.3)	0	1 (11.1)	
The length of hospital stays (days)	45.0 ± 61.3	33.7 ± 16.1	29.8 ± 27.6	0.777
Morbidity (%)	5 (71.4)	3 (100)	4 (44.4)	0.191
Severe morbidity (≥grade III) (%)	3 (42.9)	0	2 (22.2)	0.344
The details of morbidity (%)				0.359
Fluid collection	3 (42.9)	3 (100)	2 (22.2)	
Duodenal stump leakage	0	0	1 (11.1)	
Anastomosis leakage	0	0	1 (11.1)	
Pneumonia	1 (14.3)	0	0	
Bleeding	0	0	0	
Afferent loop syndrome	1 (14.3)	0	0	
The time to adjuvant chemotherapy	59.7 ± 70.8	35.7 ± 3.8	43.1 ± 26.0	0.698

DP, distal pancreatectomy; BMI, body mass index; ASA score, score graded by the American Society of Anesthesiologists physical status classification; DG, distal gastrectomy; TG, total gastrectomy.

the recent technologic advances have enabled us to overcome the difficulties of laparoscopic surgery for AGC. Most of all, the high-resolution view of the current laparoscopic image induces us to comprehend the distorted anatomies around the tumor (11). Such a high-quality imaging system is expected to enhance the surgeons' eyes during gastric cancer surgery; therefore, it is possible that we may reach the stage that our ancestor surgeons could not achieve. Moreover, the diverse types of the energy devices allow us to perform the meticulous dissection over the desmoplastic adhesion.

The next demanding point lies in the poor surgical view due to the heavy tumor burden. Since lymph node dissection should precede the removal of tumor-involved organs, the huge and heavier tumor causes significant obstacles to the surgical

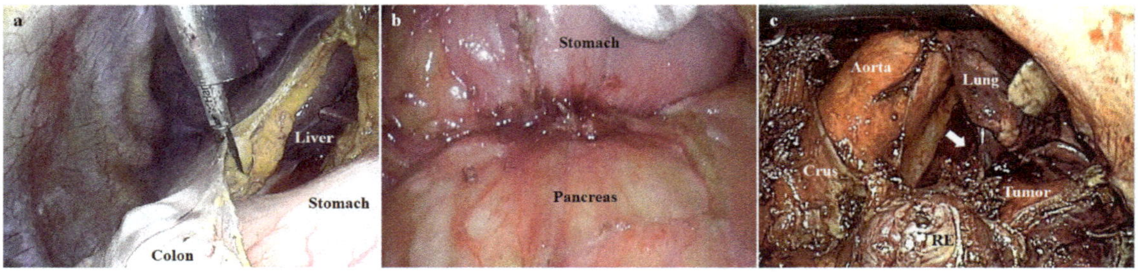

FIGURE 3 | The poor surgical views due to the heavy tumor burden. **(a)** The surgical view can be limited by the heavy stomach (due to tumor weight or impacted food contents). **(b)** The pancreatic invasion can limit the exposure of the surgical field. **(c)** The surgical view can be limited by lung invasion (indicated by the white arrow) in case of esophagogastric junction cancer (RE, resected esophagus).

view. For instance, when we elevate the stomach to expose the lymphadenectomy field, the heavy stomach (due to tumor weight or impacted food contents) can restrict the surgical view (**Figure 3a**). Sometimes, tumor invasion also limits the exposure of the surgical field (**Figure 3b**). Additionally, in case of esophagogastric junction cancer, the surgical view can be limited by the chest organ invasion that is rarely encountered during gastric cancer surgery (**Figure 3c**). In our practice, the only strategy we applied in such conditions was to find the appropriate arrangement of the counter-traction. To ameliorate the clinical outcomes, it was necessary to establish an innovative method of overcoming tumor burden during lymphadenectomy.

Finally, combined resection itself can increase the postoperative morbidity rate regardless if the approach is laparoscopic or open. This issue should be solved to take the legitimacy of laparoscopic combined surgery, since the postoperative complications can delay the initiation of AC. In other words, it is necessary to show that the poor prognosis is not caused by the "laparoscopic combined resection" itself. In this study, no statistically significant difference was found between gastrectomy only and combined resection groups in terms of the time to the initiation of AC. Even though we investigated the small number of cases, it is expected that combined resection itself was not the only factor delaying the initiation of AC, because duodenal stump leakage, postoperative ileus, and complicated fluid collection can happen after the standard surgery for gastric cancer, even in early disease. Moreover, these parameters should be carefully interpreted in our results, because we have contrived ways to proceed with AC despite the postoperative complications, which are as follows: (1) we have intraoperatively inserted percutaneous transhepatic biliary drainage (PTBD) to prepare for postoperative pancreatic fistula (POPF) in patients undergoing pancreaticoduodenectomy (12); therefore, a patient in the combined resection group (case 2, **Table 2**) started treatment with AC at 52 days postoperatively with PTBD kept; (2) although a patient in the combined resection group (case 7, **Table 2**) had afferent loop syndrome, AC was started at 21 days postoperatively with PTBD kept. He recovered later without any re-operation; (3) a sump drain was routinely inserted to prepare for POPF in patients undergoing distal pancreatectomy; therefore, a patient in the combined resection group (case 18, **Table 2**) started AC treatment at 33 days postoperatively. All of these strategies have been adopted to avoid the delay of AC.

In conclusion, it is necessary to reboot the survival outcomes regarding gastric cancer surgery. Such trials can be supported by the results of CLASS-01 studies, in which non-inferiority of laparoscopic surgery for AGC was shown (13). Although laparoscopic surgery for AGC should be verified in the various aspects, it obviously provides the new surgical view and skills for gastric cancer surgery. These items may provide us with a chance to re-evaluate the oncologic outcomes of combined resection for T4b gastric cancer. In addition, if we consider the ways to abolish the correlation between postoperative complication and chemotherapy, all of these strategies should be based on the surgeon performing AC (14).

ETHICS STATEMENT

The studies involving human participants were reviewed and approved by the Institutional Review Board of Korea University Medical Center Ansan Hospital. The patients/participants provided their written informed consent to participate in this study.

AUTHOR CONTRIBUTIONS

CL designed the main concept of this study, and write the manuscript. SL collected the data. DL interpreted the data. SP verified all the contents of the study and manuscript.

REFERENCES

1. Cuschieri A, Fayers P, Fielding J, Craven J, Bancewicz J, Joypaul V, et al. Postoperative morbidity and mortality after D1 and D2 resections for gastric cancer: preliminary results of the MRC randomised controlled surgical trial. The Surgical Cooperative Group. *Lancet.* (1996) 347:995–9. doi: 10.1016/S0140-6736(96)90144-0
2. Bonenkamp JJ, Songun I, Hermans J, Sasako M, Welvaart K, Plukker JT, et al. Randomised comparison of morbidity after D1 and D2 dissection for gastric cancer in 996 Dutch patients. *Lancet.* (1995) 345:745–8. doi: 10.1016/S0140-6736(95)90637-1
3. Paoletti X, Oba K, Burzykowski T, Michiels S, Ohashi Y, Pignon JP, et al. Benefit of adjuvant chemotherapy for resectable gastric cancer: a meta-analysis. *JAMA.* (2010) 303:1729–37. doi: 10.1001/jama.2010.534
4. Sakuramoto S, Sasako M, Yamaguchi T, Kinoshita T, Fujii M, Nashimoto A, et al. Adjuvant chemotherapy for gastric cancer with S-1, an oral fluoropyrimidine. *N Engl J Med.* (2007) 357:1810–20. doi: 10.1056/NEJMoa072252
5. Park HS, Jung M, Kim HS, Kim HI, An JY, Cheong JH, et al. Proper timing of adjuvant chemotherapy affects survival in patients with stage 2 and 3 gastric cancer. *Ann Surg Oncol.* (2015) 22:224–31. doi: 10.1245/s10434-014-3949-2
6. Hasson HM. A modified instrument and method for laparoscopy. *Am J Obstet Gynecol.* (1971) 110:886–7. doi: 10.1016/0002-9378(71)90593-X
7. Shabbir A, Lee JH, Lee MS, Park DJ, Kim HH. Combined suture retraction of the falciform ligament and the left lobe of the liver during laparoscopic total gastrectomy. *Surg Endosc.* (2010) 24:3237–40. doi: 10.1007/s00464-010-1118-7
8. Japanese Gastric Cancer Association. Japanese gastric cancer treatment guidelines 2010 (ver. 3). *Gastric Cancer.* (2011) 14:113–23. doi: 10.1007/s10120-011-0042-4
9. Clavien PA, Barkun J, de Oliveira ML, Vauthey JN, Dindo D, Schulick RD, et al. The Clavien-Dindo classification of surgical complications: five-year experience. *Ann Surg.* (2009) 250:187–96. doi: 10.1097/SLA.0b013e3181b13ca2
10. Lee CM, Rao J, Son SY, Ahn SH, Lee JH, Park DJ, et al. Laparoscopic gastrectomy for gastric cancer with simultaneous organ resection. *J Laparoendosc Adv Surg Tech A.* (2013) 23:861–5. doi: 10.1089/lap.2013.0081
11. Shinohara T, Uyama I, Kanaya S, Inaba K, Isogaki J, Horiguchi A, et al. Totally laparoscopic pancreaticoduodenectomy for locally advanced gastric cancer. *Langenbecks Arch Surg.* (2009) 394:733–7. doi: 10.1007/s00423-009-0492-x
12. Lee CM, Suh YJ, Yoon SY. Retrograde installation of percutaneous transhepatic negative-pressure biliary drainage stabilizes pancreaticojejunostomy after pancreaticoduodenectomy: a retrospective cohort study. *World J Surg Oncol.* (2019) 17:101. doi: 10.1186/s12957-019-1645-1
13. Yu J, Huang C, Sun Y, Su X, Cao H, Hu J, et al. Effect of laparoscopic vs open distal gastrectomy on 3-year disease-free survival in patients with locally advanced gastric cancer: the CLASS-01 randomized clinical trial. *JAMA.* (2019) 321:1983–92. doi: 10.1001/jama.2019.5359
14. Min JS, Lee CM, Choi SI, Seo KW, Park DJ, Baik YH, et al. Who can perform adjuvant chemotherapy treatment for gastric cancer? a multicenter retrospective overview of the current status in Korea. *J Gastric Cancer.* (2018) 18:264–73. doi: 10.5230/jgc.2018.18.e29

4

Frequency and Prognosis of Pulmonary Metastases in Newly Diagnosed Gastric Cancer

Zepang Sun[†], Hao Liu[†], Jiang Yu[†], Weicai Huang, Zhen Han, Tian Lin, Hao Chen, Mingli Zhao, Yanfeng Hu, Yuming Jiang and Guoxin Li**

Department of General Surgery, Nanfang Hospital, Southern Medical University, Guangzhou, China

Correspondence:
Yuming Jiang
jiangymbest@163.com
Guoxin Li
gzliguoxin@163.com

[†] These authors have contributed equally to this work

Purpose: The purpose of this study was to analyze the frequency and prognosis of pulmonary metastases in newly diagnosed gastric cancer using population-based data from SEER.

Methods: Patients with gastric cancer and pulmonary metastases (GCPM) at the time of diagnosis in advanced gastric cancer were identified using the Surveillance, Epidemiology and End Result (SEER) database of the National Cancer Institute from 2010 to 2014. Multivariable logistic regression was performed to identify predictors of the presence of GCPM at diagnosis. Receiver operator characteristics analysis was performed to significant predictors on multivariable logistic regression and was then assessed with Delong's test. Multivariable Cox regression was developed to identify factors associated with all-cause mortality and gastric cancer-specific mortality. Survival curves were obtained according to the Kaplan-Meier method and compared using the log-rank test.

Results: We identified 1,104 patients with gastric cancer and pulmonary metastases at the time of diagnosis, representing 6.02% of the entire cohort and 15.19% of the subset with metastatic disease to any distant site. Among the entire cohort, multivariable logistic regression identified six factors (younger, upper 1/3 of stomach, intestinal-type, T4 staging, N1 staging, and presence of more extrapulmonary metastases to liver, bone, and brain) as positive predictors of the presence of pulmonary metastases at diagnosis. The value of AUC for the multivariable logistic regression model was 0.775. Median survival among the entire cohort with GCPM was 3.0 months (interquartile range: 1.0–9.0 mo). Multivariable Cox model in SEER cohort confirmed five factors (diagnosis at previous period, black race, adverse pathology grade, absence of chemotherapy, and presence of more extrapulmonary metastases to liver, bone, and brain) as negative predictors for overall survival.

Conclusions: The findings of this study provided population-based estimates of the frequency and prognosis for GCPM at time of diagnosis. The multivariable logistic regression model had an acceptable performance to predict the presence of PM. These findings may provide preventive guidelines for the screening and treatment of PM in GC patients. Patients with high risk factors should be paid more attention before and after diagnosis.

Keywords: gastric cancer, pulmonary metastases, frequency, prognosis, SEER

INTRODUCTION

Gastric Cancer (GC) was the fourth most common malignant tumor in the world and the fifteenth in the United States (1, 2). Although the reported incidence and mortality rates had steadily decreased over the last decade, there was still an estimated 26 240 new GC patients and 10 800 deaths in United States in 2018 (2). Furthermore, about 40% of patients were presented with evidence of distant metastases (3–5). The most common site of distant metastases was the peritoneum, followed by the liver, lung, and bone (5). Pulmonary metastases (PM) were really rare discovery, which had been reported in only 0.5–16% of the GC patients with distant metastases in clinical practice (6–8), but 22–52% of patients at postmortem examination (9, 10). However, all these patients were unselected, including synchronous and asynchronous metastatic patients. PM was associated with poor survival in patients with advanced gastric cancer. The 5-year survival of gastric cancer and pulmonary metastases (GCPM) was only 2–4% (6, 7, 11). And the median survival time was 4 months for both newly diagnosed PM and those asynchronous patients (6, 7, 12).

An early detection of pulmonary metastases was necessary to alter patient management and result in significant cost savings and medical resources savings by reducing unnecessary surgery or other treatments. Chest CT was not recommended routine assessment in current gastric cancer screening guidelines. However, multiple studies revealed that CT was more superior in identifying some metastatic nodules than plain chest radiography and conventional liner tomography (CLT) (13–15). And the conventional chest radiograph was always adopted at the initial screening examination in clinical practice, which may lead to missed diagnosis. Thus, a population-based study including a large sample was particularly important to determine which patients need to receive further examination.

There were only limited data regarding pulmonary metastases from gastric cancer at present, and the majority of objects included in these researches were asynchronous metastatic patients (6–8, 11, 16, 17). The study in newly diagnosed gastric cancer with pulmonary metastases was lacking, so the proportion, predictive factors, prognostic factors, and optimal strategy for these patients were unknown. Therefore, a study based on population level about GCPM to describe epidemiologic characteristics and prognosis was urgently needed.

The purpose of this study was to use data from the Surveillance, Epidemiology and End Results (SEER) database between 2010 and 2014 to survey the incidence proportion and predictive factors of pulmonary metastases at the time of cancer diagnosis among patients with gastric cancer on a population-based level. We also wanted to characterize prognostic factors on the survival of patients at diagnosis of gastric cancer with pulmonary metastases.

MATERIALS AND METHODS

Study Population

Data was obtained from the SEER database, which was the largest publicly available cancer dataset and collected cancer data from 18 population-based cancer registries covering about 28 percent of the United States population (18). This database included information about cancer incidence as well as demographic information: age, gender, race, year at diagnosis, tumor staging, tumor size, treatment, marital status, insurance, education, family income, and so on. We used the SEERStat software version 8.3.4 published by SEER to identify eligible patients in this study, which we could get from the official network (https://seer.cancer.gov/). The SEERStat provided patients information up to 2014 based on the November 2016 submission, and it started to release metastatic information related to pulmonary metastases from 2010. Thus, we can get information about GCPM between 1 January 2010 and 31 December 2014 from SEERStat. Besides, pulmonary metastases included only the lung, but not pleura or pleural fluid in the SEER database.

Within the SEER database, we identified 36,982 patients with gastric cancer from 2010 to 2014. Patients with other cancers, <18 or more than 85 years old, with other pathological types were excluded from the analysis, leaving 18,331 patients in the final cohort for frequency analysis. Of these, 7268 patients were diagnosed with metastases to any distant site and 1,104 patients were diagnosed as GCPM. We subsequently removed patients with an unknown follow-up, leaving 1,098 patients eligible for survival analyses. The percentage of distant metastases to any site was 39.65% and pulmonary metastases were 6.02%. Data extraction flowchart was showed in **Figure 1.** The inclusion criteria were as follows: age more than 18 years old and <85 years old at time of diagnosis; gastric cancer as the only one primary cancer; with identified pulmonary metastases; confirmation of diagnosis based on pathology of a specimen, rather than based on radiography or laboratory; with active follow-up. And we excluded those patients conformed to any one of the following standards: age <18 years old or more than 85 years old at the time of diagnosis; with more than one primary

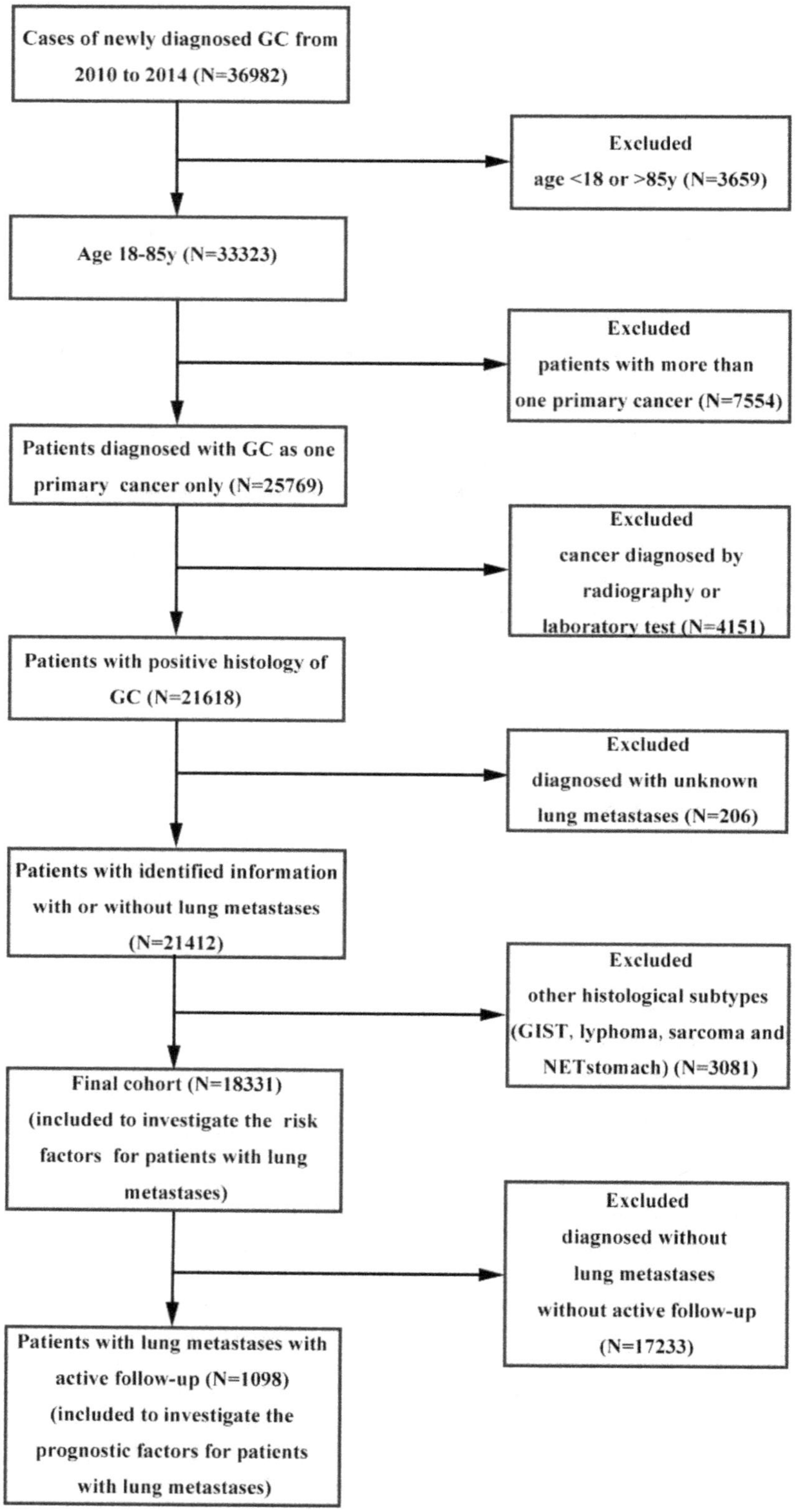

FIGURE 1 | Data extraction flowchart from the SEER database.

cancer; unknown pulmonary metastases; cancer diagnosed by radiography or laboratory; pathological type confirmed to be NET stomach, sarcoma, GIST or lymphoma; without active follow-up. 12/31/2014 was the cut-off date in this study. More details can get from SEERStat software version 8.3.4 and SEER manual 2016. The end point of this study was OS. The OS was defined from the date of diagnosis to the date of all-cause death or cancer-specific death, and patients survived to the latest follow-up identified as censoring. Toward the last follow up, there were 925 deaths and 173 censoring among patients with GCPM.

Statistical Analysis

Descriptive statistics was used to calculate the absolute number and frequency among patients with PM at the time of cancer diagnosis. Frequency was defined as the percentage of gastric cancer patients diagnosed with PM among the entire study cohort and the patients with metastatic disease to any distant site. All data were stratified by year at diagnosis, age, gender, race, original, primary site, pathology grade, Lauren classification, T staging, N staging, tumor size, treatment, number of extrapulmonary metastatic sites and other sociodemographic information, such as: marital status, residence type, insurance situation, bachelor education, median household income, and smoking status. Residence type, education level, median household income, and smoking status were defined by the county attributes from the US Census 2010–2014 American Community Survey 5-year data files, which we could get from the SEER*Stat software.

Chi-square or Fisher's test was developed for clinical characteristics of GCPM patients at the exclusion of those with unknown information. Multivariable logistic regression was used to determine predictors of the presence of pulmonary metastases at diagnosis. And only variables which demonstrated significance on both the Chi-square test and the univariate logistic regression can enter into the multivariable logistic regression. This was a population-based study, so we focused more on the entire cohorts (GC) but not subcohort (GC with metastatic disease to any distant site). Survival estimates were obtained according to the Kaplan-Meier method and compared using the log-rank test. Variables that reached significance with $P < 0.05$ were entered into the multivariable analyses using the Cox regression model to identify covariates associated with increased all-cause mortality. Besides, we used Fine and Gray's competing risk regression to assess gastric cancer-specific mortality (19). Binary-dependent receiver operator characteristics (ROC) analysis for different variables to predict the presence of PM was developed. And Delong's test was conducted to further expound the performance of multivariable logistic regression model.

All statistical analyses were performed using SPSS statistical software (version 18.0). The competing risks analysis was performed using the cmprsk package (version 2.2-7) and ROC was developed using the pROC package (version 3.2-5) in R (version 3.4.4; R Foundation). Delong's test was performed using Medcalc software. Statistical significance was set at two-sided ($P < 0.05$).

RESULTS

Frequency Analysis

A total of 18,331 patients in the U.S. were diagnosed with gastric cancer between 2010 and 2014, including 1,104 patients diagnosed with GCPM whose median age was 66 years old, consisted of 773 men (70.02%) and 331 women (29.98%). Their demographic and clinical characteristics were shown in **Table 1**. On Chi-square or Fisher's test, a significant difference was found in age, gender, race, primary site, Lauren classification, T staging, N staging, tumor size, number of extrapulmonary metastatic sites, radiotherapy, surgery, insurance situation and median household income. The proportion of younger patients (age<60 years) (40.58 vs. 36.94% $P < 0.001$), male (70.02 vs. 65.08% $P < 0.001$) and white race (74.61 vs. 69.63% $P < 0.001$) in PM group was higher compared with the no-PM group. Furthermore, presence with more upper 1/3 of stomach (67.94 vs. 49.34% $P < 0.001$), extrapulmonary metastases (63.66 vs. 17.50% $P < 0.001$) and intestinal-type tumor (72.64 vs. 64.29% $P < 0.001$) could been seen in the PM group. Besides, T4 staging (35.73 vs. 24.93% $P < 0.001$), N1 staging (49.61 vs. 30.24% $P < 0.001$) and larger tumor (>2 cm) (85.89 vs. 79.25% $P < 0.001$) were significantly associated with PM. The sociodemographic information, like insurance situation and median household income, had little value in this study. However, the no-PM group presented with higher percentage of radiotherapy (30.15 vs. 20.11% $P < 0.001$) and surgery (48.77 vs. 4.62% $P < 0.001$). Additionally, only 51 patients received gastrectomy and 7 patients received gastrectomy plus metastectomy among the cohort with GCPM. Rate of chemotherapy showed no significant difference between PM group and no-PM group. More detail information can be found in **Table S1**.

On univariable logistic regression (**Table S2**) among the entire cohort, there were nine factors that showed significance (P value < 0.05). They were age, gender, primary site, Lauren classification, T staging, N staging, tumor size, number of extrapulmonary metastatic sites to liver, bone, and brain and insurance situation. We put them on multivariable logistic regression which showed that age, primary site, Lauren classification, T staging, N staging, and number of extrapulmonary metastatic sites to liver, bone, and brain had significance among the entire cohort and primary site, Lauren classification, N staging, tumor size and number of extrapulmonary metastatic sites to liver, bone, and brain had significance among the subset with metastatic disease to any distant site.

On the multivariable logistic regression (**Table 2**) among the entire cohort, T4 (vs. T1; OR, 1.27; 95%CI, 1.02–1.57; $P = 0.03$), N1 (vs. N0; OR, 1.39; 95%CI, 1.24–1.63; $P < 0.001$), 1 extrapulmonary metastatic site (vs. 0 extrapulmonary metastatic site; OR, 4.56; 95%CI, 3.92–5.31; $P < 0.001$), 2 extrapulmonary metastatic sites (vs. 0 extrapulmonary metastatic site; OR, 13.41; 95%CI, 10.40–17.28; $P < 0.001$), 3 extrapulmonary metastatic sites (vs. 0 extrapulmonary metastatic site; OR, 21.64; 95%CI, 8.35–56.11; $P < 0.001$) were associated with significantly greater odds of having pulmonary metastases at

TABLE 1 | Clinical characteristics of patients with gastric cancer with identified pulmonary metastases at diagnosis.

Variable	Patients, no.			Proportion of pulmonary metastases, %		Survival among patients with pulmonary metastases, median (IQR), mo
	With gastric cancer (n = 18,331)	With metastatic disease (n = 7,268)	With pulmonary metastases (n = 1,104)	Among entire cohort	Among subset with metastatic disease	
YEAR AT DIAGNOSIS						
2010	3,492	1,409	221	6.33	15.68	2.0 (1.0–6.0)
2011	3,502	1,352	195	5.57	14.42	4.0 (1.0–9.0)
2012	3,751	1,469	218	5.81	14.84	3.0 (1.0–7.0)
2013	3,739	1,476	229	6.12	15.51	3.0 (1.0–11.0)
2014	3,847	1,562	241	6.26	15.43	4.0 (1.0–NA)
AGE AT DIAGNOSIS, YEARS						
18–40	773	451	63	8.15	13.97	3.0 (1.0–7.0)
41–60	6,039	2,763	385	6.38	13.93	4.0 (1.0–10.0)
61–80	9,682	3,512	581	6.00	16.54	3.0 (1.0–8.0)
80+	1,837	542	75	4.08	13.84	2.0 (0.0–7.0)
RACE						
White	12,735	5,182	820	6.44	15.82	4.0 (1.0–10.0)
Black	2,426	997	139	5.73	13.94	2.0 (1.0–7.0)
Others[a]	3,049	1,052	140	4.59	13.31	2.0 (1.0–7.0)
Unknown	121	37	5	4.13	13.51	14.0 (1–NA)
GENDER						
Male	11,984	4,743	773	6.45	16.30	3.0 (1.0–9.0)
Female	6,347	2,525	331	5.22	13.11	3.0 (1.0–8.0)
ORIGINAL						
Hispanic	3,862	1,690	216	5.59	12.78	3.0 (1.0–10.0)
Non-Hispanic	14,469	5,578	888	6.14	15.92	3.0 (1.0–9.0)
PRIMARY SITE						
Upper 1/3	7,027	2,681	553	7.87	20.63	4.0 (1.0–11.0)
Middle 1/3	1,676	694	70	4.18	10.09	3.0 (1.0–8.0)
Lower 1/3	3,808	1,186	119	3.13	10.03	3.0 (1.0–8.0)
Overlapping lesion	1,424	674	72	5.06	10.68	2.0 (1.0–5.0)
Unknown	4,396	2,033	290	6.60	14.26	2.0 (1.0–7.0)
PATHOLOGY GRADE						
I–II	4,742	1,397	269	5.67	19.26	6.0 (1.0–12.0)
III–IV	10,623	4,256	576	5.42	13.53	3.0 (1.0–7.0)
Unknown	2,966	1,615	259	8.73	16.04	2.0 (1.0–7.0)
LAUREN CLASSIFICATION						
Intestinal-type	11,878	4,621	802	6.75	17.36	3.0 (1.0–9.0)
Diffuse-type	5,552	2,241	232	4.18	10.35	3.0 (1.0–8.0)
Others[b]	901	406	70	7.77	17.24	3.0 (0.0–5.0)
TUMOR STAGING[c]						
I	3,315	0	0	NA	NA	NA
II	2,359	0	0	NA	NA	NA
III	4,351	0	0	NA	NA	NA
IV	7,268	7,268	1,104	15.19	15.19	3.0 (1.0–9.0)
Unknown	1,038	0	0	NA	NA	NA
T STAGING[c]						
T1	4,373	1,302	222	5.08	17.05	3.0 (1.0–8.0)
T2	1,650	333	35	2.12	10.51	3.0 (1.0–9.0)
T3	4,777	1,062	128	2.68	12.05	5.0 (2.0–11.0)
T4	3,672	1,642	214	5.83	13.03	2.0 (1.0–7.0)
Unknown	3,859	2,929	505	13.09	17.24	2.0 (0.0–9.0)

(Continued)

TABLE 1 | Continued

Variable	Patients, no.			Proportion of pulmonary metastases, %		Survival among patients with pulmonary metastases, median (IQR), mo
	With gastric cancer (*n* = 18,331)	With metastatic disease (*n* = 7,268)	With pulmonary metastases (*n* = 1,104)	Among entire cohort	Among subset with metastatic disease	
N STAGING[c]						
N0	7,775	2,548	362	4.66	14.21	3.0 (1.0–10.0)
N1	5,210	2572	442	8.48	17.19	4.0 (1.0–9.0)
N2	1,780	417	38	2.13	9.11	4.0 (1.0–10.0)
N3	1,893	496	49	2.59	9.88	3.0 (1.0–11.0)
Unknown	1,673	1,235	213	12.73	17.25	2.0 (1.0–6.0)
M STAGING[c]						
M0	11,063	0	0	0.00	0.00	NA
M1	7,268	7,268	1,104	15.19	15.19	3.0 (1.0–9.0)
SURGERY[d]						
Yes	8,453	883	51	0.60	5.78	4.0 (2.0–14.0)
No	9,878	6,385	1,053	10.66	16.49	3.0 (1.0–9.0)
RADIOTHERAPY						
Yes	5,416	1,251	222	4.10	17.75	5.0 (2.0–11.0)
No	12,915	6,017	882	6.83	14.66	2.0 (1.0–8.0)
CHEMOTHERAPY						
Yes	10,495	4,391	631	6.01	14.37	6.0 (3.0–13.0)
No	7,836	2,877	473	6.04	16.44	1.0 (0.0–2.0)
TUMOR SIZE, CM						
0–2	2,186	322	59	2.70	18.32	2.0 (0.0–9.0)
2–5	4,741	1,278	198	4.18	15.49	5.0 (1.0–12.0)
5+	3,742	1,226	161	4.30	13.13	3.0 (1.0–8.0)
Unknown	7,662	4,442	686	8.95	15.44	3.0 (1.0–8.0)
EXTRAPULMONARY METASTATIC SITES TO LIVER, BONE, AND BRAIN, NO.						
0	14,442	3,422	379	2.62	11.08	4.0 (1.0–13.0)
1	3,290	3,290	526	15.99	15.99	3.0 (1.0–8.0)
2	340	340	128	37.65	37.65	2.0 (1.0–8.0)
3	18	18	10	55.56	55.56	3.0 (1.0–6.0)
Unknown	241	198	61	25.31	30.81	1.0 (0.0–4.0)
INSURANCE SITUATION						
Yes	17,022	6,661	1,007	5.92	15.12	3.0 (1.0–9.0)
No	922	489	73	7.92	14.93	2.0 (1.0–7.0)
Unknown	387	118	24	6.20	20.34	2.0 (0.0–16.0)
MARITAL STATUS						
Married	10,618	4,194	627	5.91	14.95	4.0 (1.0–10.0)
Unmarried[e]	6,789	2,763	441	6.50	15.96	2.0 (1.0–7.0)
Unknown	924	311	36	3.90	11.58	3.0 (0.0–18.0)
RESIDENCE TYPE						
Rural	467	192	27	5.78	14.06	2.0 (1.0–6.0)
Urban	17,864	7,076	1,077	6.03	15.22	3.0 (1.0–9.0)
BACHELOR EDUCATION (PER 20% INCREASE)						
0–20%	5,144	1,281	173	5.50	13.51	2.0 (1.0–7.0)
20–40%	11,790	4,628	734	6.23	15.86	3.0 (1.0–9.0)
40–60%	3,397	1,359	197	5.80	14.50	4.0 (1.0–11.0)
MEDIAN HOUSEHOLD INCOME (PER $20,000 INCREASE)						
0–40,000	1,193	432	82	6.87	18.98	3.0 (1.0–8.0)
40,000–60,000	9,329	3,699	538	5.77	14.54	3.0 (1.0–8.0)

(Continued)

TABLE 1 | Continued

Variable	Patients, no.			Proportion of pulmonary metastases, %		Survival among patients with pulmonary metastases, median (IQR), mo
	With gastric cancer (n = 18,331)	With metastatic disease (n = 7,268)	With pulmonary metastases (n = 1,104)	Among entire cohort	Among subset with metastatic disease	
60,000–80,000	5,823	2,355	383	6.58	16.26	3.0 (1.0–9.0)
80,000–100,000	1,986	782	101	5.09	12.92	4.0 (1.0–14.0)
SMOKING STATUS (PER 10% INCREASE)						
0–10%	785	292	49	6.24	16.78	3.0 (1.0–7.0)
10–20%	12,201	4,829	705	5.78	14.60	3.0 (1.0–9.0)
20–30%	4,969	1,986	324	6.52	16.31	3.0 (1.0–8.0)
30–40%	376	161	26	6.91	16.15	3.0 (0.0–10.0)

CI, confidence interval, IQR, interquartile range.
[a]*Including Asian and American Indians.*
[b]*Including linitisplastica, hepatoid adenocarcinoma, adenosquamous carcinoma and so on.*
[c]*According to the eighth edition of the AJCC Cancer Staging manual.*
[d]*Including subtotal gastrectomy only, total gastrectomy only and radical surgery.*
[e]*Including divorced, separated, single (never married), and widowed.*

diagnosis. And, insurance status was not associated with a risk of pulmonary metastases at diagnosis in the multivariable model. While, age 41–60 years (vs. age 18–40 years; OR, 0.70; 95%CI, 0.52–0.94; P = 0.02), age 61–80 years (vs. age 18–40 years; OR, 0.72; 95%CI, 0.54–0.97; P = 0.03) and age 80+ years (vs. age 18–40 years; OR, 0.54; 95%CI, 0.37–0.78; P = 0.001), middle 1/3 of stomach (vs.: upper 1/3 of stomach; OR, 0.58; 95%CI, 0.44–0.76; P < 0.001), lower 1/3 of stomach (vs.: upper 1/3 of stomach; OR, 0.50; 95%CI, 0.41–0.62; P < 0.001), and overlapping lesion (vs.: upper 1/3 of stomach; OR, 0.70; 95%CI, 0.53–0.91; P = 0.01), diffused-type (vs. intestinal-type; OR, 0.83; 95%CI, 0.70–0.98; P = 0.03), T2 (vs. T1; OR, 0.58; 95%CI, 0.40–0.84; P = 0.004), T3 (vs. T1; OR, 0.65; 95%CI, 0.51–0.82; P < 0.001), N2 (vs. N0; OR, 0.64; 95%CI, 0.45–0.92; P = 0.02) were associated with marginally lower odds of pulmonary metastases at diagnosis. The multivariable logistic regression of subset with metastatic disease was also showed in **Table 2**.

In order to further expound the performance of multivariable logistic regression model, binary-dependent ROC analysis was performed for the model and different variables. The model was a combination of six significant variables (age at diagnosis, Lauren classification, primary site, T staging, N staging, and extent of extrapulmonary metastastic disease) on multivariable logistic regression. Delong's test was developed to verify the performance. The value of AUC of the model (AUC: 0.775, 95%CI: 0.760–0.790) showed better than age (AUC: 0.529, 95%CI: 0.512–0.547), Lauren classification (AUC: 0.537, 95%CI: 0.520–0.554), primary site (AUC: 0.539, 95%CI: 0.521–0.557), T staging (AUC: 0.637, 95%CI: 0.619–0.656), N staging (AUC: 0.547, 95%CI: 0.530–0.565), and extent of extrapulmonary metastastic disease (AUC: 0.745, 95%CI: 0.728–0.762) in the entire cohort. All P value was smaller than 0.001 on Delong's test. More detail was showed in **Table S4**. And the ROC curves for the entire cohort and subcohort were in **Figures S1, S2**.

Survival Analysis

Among the subset with pulmonary metastases, there were five factors that were significantly associated with overall survival on multivariable Cox regression model. **Table S3** showed univariate analysis for all-cause mortality and gastric cancer-specific mortality among GCPM. On multivariable Cox regression (**Table 3**) for all-cause mortality among patients with GCPM at diagnosis, black race (vs. white race; HR, 1.26; 95%CI, 1.03–1.54; P = 0.03), grade III-IV (vs. grade I-II; HR, 1.46; 95%CI, 1.24–1.72; P < 0.001), 1 extrapulmonary metastatic site (vs. 0 extrapulmonary metastatic site; HR, 1.40; 95%CI, 1.21–1.63; P < 0.001) and 2 extrapulmonary metastatic sites (vs. 0 extrapulmonary metastatic site; HR, 1.67; 95%CI, 1.33–2.10; P < 0.001), absence of chemotherapy (vs. chemotherapy; HR, 3.70; 95%CI, 3.18–4.30; P < 0.001) were significantly associated with an increased all-cause mortality. However, 2011 (vs. 2010; HR, 0.77; 95%CI, 0.63–0.94; P = 0.01), 2013 (vs. 2010; HR, 0.73; 95%CI, 0.59–0.88; P = 0.002), 2014 (vs. 2010; HR, 0.74; 95%CI, 0.59–0.92; P = 0.01) was significantly associated with a decreased all-cause mortality. And absence of surgery (vs. surgery; HR, 1.62; 95%CI, 1.13–2.33; P = 0.01) were significantly associated with an increased gastric cancer-specific mortality only. Gastric cancer-specific mortality among patients with GCPM at diagnosis was also presented in **Table 3**. Survival estimates of overall (**Figure 2A**) and as stratified by year at diagnosis (**Figure 2B**), race (**Figure 2C**), pathology grade (**Figure 2D**), extent of extrapulmonary metastastic disease (**Figure 2E**), and chemotherapy (**Figure 2F**) were graphically displayed in the **Figure 2**.

DISCUSSION

This study analyzed the frequency and survival of gastric cancer patients with pulmonary metastases at their initial diagnosis using data from the SEER database. We also characterized the predictive factors and prognostic factors in an attempt to better

TABLE 2 | Multivariable logistic regression for the presence of pulmonary metastases at diagnosis of gastric cancer.

Variable	Patients, no.		Among entire cohort		Among subset with metastatic disease	
	Patients (n =18,331)	With pulmonary metastases (*n* = 1,104)	OR (95% CI)	*P* Value	OR (95% CI)	*P* Value
AGE AT DIAGNOSIS, YEARS						
18–40	773	63	1 (Reference)	NA	NA	NA
41–60	6,039	385	0.70 (0.52–0.94)	0.02	NA	NA
61–80	9,382	581	0.72 (0.54–0.97)	0.03	NA	NA
80+	1,337	75	0.54 (0.37–0.78)	0.001	NA	NA
GENDER						
Female	6,347	331	1 (Reference)	NA	1 (Reference)	NA
Male	11,984	773	1.01 (0.87–1.16)	0.95	1.07 (0.92–1.24)	0.37
PRIMARY SITE						
Upper 1/3	7,027	553	1 (Reference)	NA	1 (Reference)	NA
Middle 1/3	1,676	70	0.58 (0.44–0.76)	<0.001	0.52 (0.39–0.68)	<0.001
Lower 1/3	3,808	119	0.50 (0.41–0.62)	<0.001	0.52 (0.42–0.65)	<0.001
Overlapping lesion	1,424	72	0.70 (0.53–0.91)	0.01	0.58 (0.44–0.76)	<0.001
Unknown	4,396	290	0.80 (0.68–0.95)	0.01	0.71 (0.60–0.84)	<0.001
LAUREN CLASSIFICATION						
Intestinal–type	11,878	802	1 (Reference)	NA	1 (Reference)	NA
Diffuse–type	5,552	232	0.83 (0.70–0.98)	0.03	0.70 (0.59–0.83)	<0.001
Others[a]	901	70	0.97 (0.76–1.31)	0.24	0.99 (0.75–1.31)	0.96
T STAGING[b]						
T1	4,373	222	1 (Reference)	NA	1 (Reference)	NA
T2	1,650	35	0.58 (0.40–0.84)	0.004	0.76 (0.51–1.12)	0.16
T3	4,777	128	0.65 (0.51–0.82)	<0.001	0.78 (0.61–1.00)	0.05
T4	3,672	214	1.27 (1.02–1.57)	0.03	0.96 (0.77–1.19)	0.71
Unknown	3,859	505	1.36 (1.13–1.64)	0.001	0.97 (0.81–1.17)	0.78
N STAGING[b]						
N0	7,775	362	1 (Reference)	NA	1 (Reference)	NA
N1	5,210	442	1.39 (1.24–1.63)	<0.001	1.12 (0.96–1.32)	0.15
N2	1,780	38	0.64 (0.45–0.92)	0.02	0.63 (0.44–0.92)	0.02
N3	1,893	49	0.77 (0.56–1.08)	0.13	0.79 (0.57–1.11)	0.18
Unknown	1,673	213	1.39 (1.13–1.69)	0.001	1.16 (0.95–1.41)	0.15
TUMOR SIZE, CM						
0–2	2,186	59	1 (Reference)	NA	1 (Reference)	NA
2–5	4,741	198	1.25 (0.92–1.71)	0.16	0.78 (0.56–1.09)	0.15
5+	3,742	161	1.26 (0.91–1.75)	0.16	0.73 (0.52–1.02)	0.06
Unknown	7,662	686	1.64 (1.23–2.19)	0.001	0.80 (0.59–1.09)	0.15
EXTRAPULMONARY METASTATIC SITES TO LIVER, BONE, AND BRAIN, NO.						
0	14,442	379	1 (Reference)	NA	1 (Reference)	NA
1	3,290	526	4.56 (3.92–5.31)	<0.001	1.22 (1.05–1.42)	0.01
2	340	128	13.41 (10.40–17.28)	<0.001	3.68 (2.86–4.74)	<0.001
3	18	10	21.64 (8.35–56.11)	<0.001	6.48 (2.51–16.69)	0.002
Unknown	241	61	8.02 (5.81–11.08)	<0.001	3.27 (2.35–4.54)	<0.001
INSURANCE SITUATION						
Yes	17,022	1,007	1 (Reference)	NA	NA	NA
No	922	73	1.12 (0.85–1.46)	0.42	NA	NA
Unknown	387	24	0.95 (0.61–1.48)	0.82	NA	NA

CI, confidence interval.

[a] *Including linitisplastica, hepatoid adenocarcinoma, adenosquamous carcinoma and so on.*

[b] *According to the eighth edition of the AJCC Cancer Staging manual.*

TABLE 3 | Multivariable analysis for all-cause mortality and gastric cancer-specific mortality among patients with pulmonary metastases.

Variable	Patients, no.		All-cause mortality		Gastric cancer-specific mortality	
	Patients (n = 18,331)	With pulmonary metastases (n = 1,098)	Hazard ratio (95% CI)	P value	Hazard ratio (95% CI)	P value
YEAR AT DIAGNOSIS						
2010	3,492	221	1 (Reference)	NA	1 (Reference)	NA
2011	3,502	195	0.77 (0.63–0.94)	0.01	0.91(0.75–1.11)	0.35
2012	3,751	214	0.85 (0.70–1.04)	0.12	0.89 (0.73–1.08)	0.24
2013	3,739	229	0.73 (0.59–0.88)	0.002	0.81 (0.66–0.99)	0.04
2014	3,847	239	0.74 (0.59–0.92)	0.01	0.71 (0.57–0.90)	0.004
RACE						
White	12,735	816	1 (Reference)	NA	1 (Reference)	NA
Black	2,426	138	1.26 (1.03–1.54)	0.03	0.95 (0.76–1.19)	0.67
Others[a]	3,049	139	1.14 (0.93–1.39)	0.21	1.18 (0.97–1.43)	0.10
Unknown	121	5	0.77 (0.27–2.64)	0.77	0.95 (0.32–2.87)	0.93
PRIMARY SITE						
Upper 1/3	7,027	553	1 (Reference)	NA	1 (Reference)	NA
Middle 1/3	1,676	69	1.27(0.96–1.67)	0.10	1.43(1.15–1.78)	0.001
Lower 1/3	3,808	118	1.00 (0.80–1.24)	0.97	1.08 (0.87–1.34)	0.49
Overlapping lesion	1,424	72	1.14 (0.86–1.51)	0.35	1.37 (1.04–1.80)	0.02
Unknown	4,396	286	0.97 (0.82–1.15)	0.73	0.95 (0.79–1.14)	0.59
PATHOLOGY GRADE						
I–II	4,742	269	1 (Reference)	NA	1 (Reference)	NA
III–IV	10,623	572	1.46 (1.24–1.72)	<0.001	1.35 (1.15–1.58)	<0.001
Unknown	2,966	257	1.47 (1.21–1.78)	<0.001	1.33 (1.09–1.62)	0.004
RADIOTHERAPY						
Yes	5,416	222	1 (Reference)	NA	1 (Reference)	NA
No	12,915	876	1.09 (0.92–1.30)	0.32	1.04 (0.90–1.20)	0.62
SURGERY[b]						
Yes	8,453	51	NA	NA	1 (Reference)	NA
No	9,878	1,047	NA	NA	1.62 (1.13–2.33)	0.01
CHEMOTHERAPY						
Yes	10,495	631	1 (Reference)	NA	1 (Reference)	NA
No	7,836	467	3.32 (2.87–3.84)	<0.001	2.50 (2.16–2.91)	<0.001
EXTRAPULMONARY METASTATIC SITES TO LIVER, BONE, AND BRAIN, NO.						
0	14,442	377	1 (Reference)	NA	1 (Reference)	NA
1	3,290	524	1.40 (1.21–1.63)	<0.001	1.32 (1.14–1.52)	<0.001
2	340	127	1.67 (1.33–2.10)	<0.001	1.57 (1.25–1.96)	<0.001
3	18	10	1.64 (0.97–3.11)	0.13	2.03 (1.17–3.54)	0.01
Unknown	241	60	1.44 (1.07–1.93)	0.02	1.01 (0.68–1.49)	0.97
MARITAL STATUS						
Married	10,618	626	1 (Reference)	NA	1 (Reference)	NA
Unmarried[c]	6,789	436	0.98 (0.85–1.12)	0.76	1.01 (0.88–1.17)	0.85
Unknown	924	36	0.81 (0.55–1.18)	0.27	0.77 (0.45–1.22)	0.26
RESIDENCE TYPE						
Rural	467	27	NA	NA	1 (Reference)	NA
Urban	17,864	1,071	NA	NA	0.69 (0.50–0.93)	0.01
Bachelor education (per 20% increase)	18,331	1,098	NA	NA	1.02 (0.89–1.17)	0.74
Median household income (per $20,000 increase)	18,331	1,098	NA	NA	0.89 (0.80–0.99)	0.03

CI, confidence interval.

[a]Including Asian and American Indians.

[b]Including subtotal gastrectomy only, total gastrectomy only and radical surgery.

[c]Including divorced, separated, single (never married), and widowed.

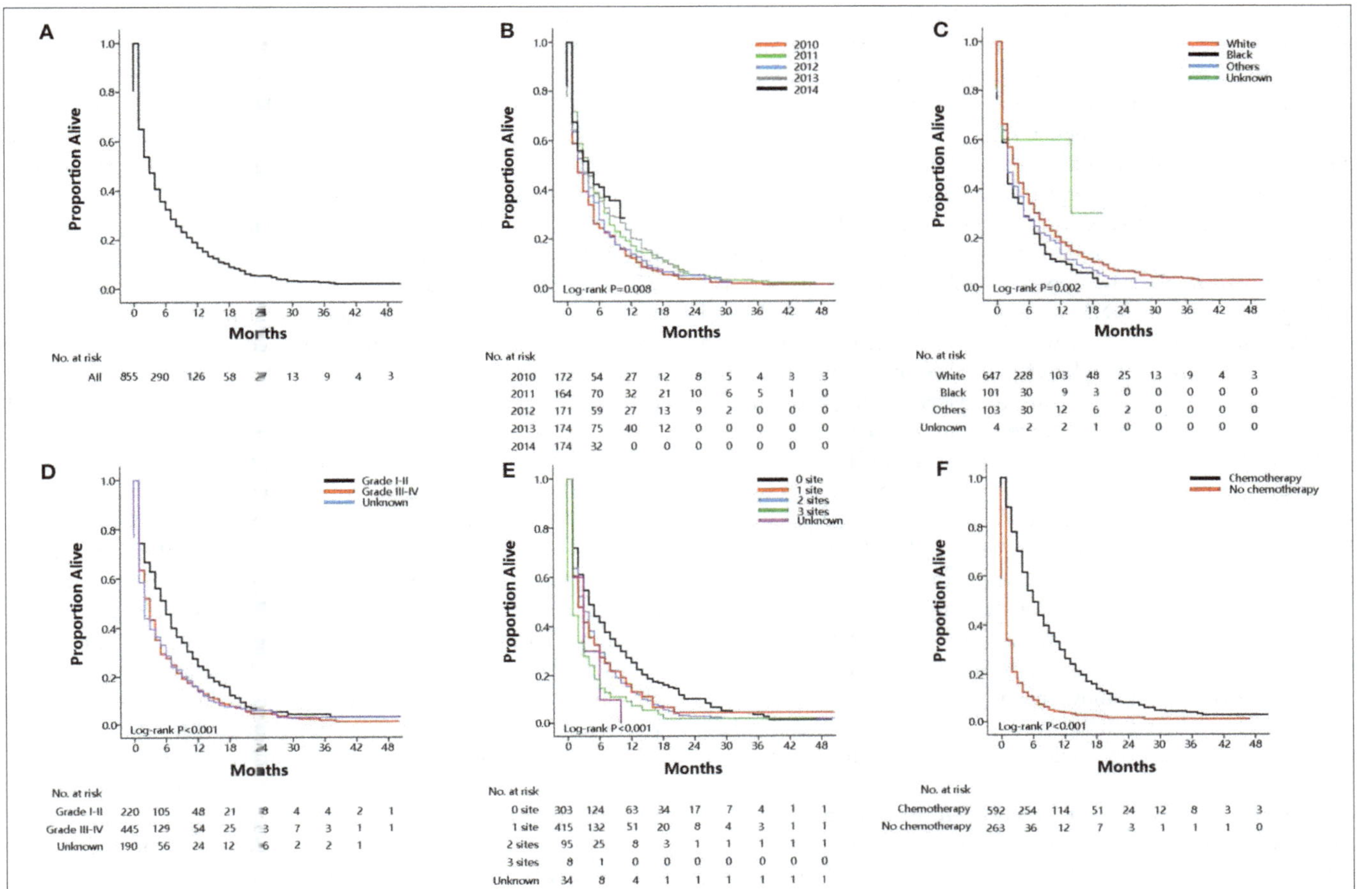

FIGURE 2 | Overall survival among patients with GCPM at diagnosis (**A** overall), stratified by year at diagnosis **(B)**, race **(C)**, pathology grade **(D)**, extent of extrapulmonary metastatic disease **(E)**, chemotherapy **(F)**.

understand the clinical impact of pulmonary metastases. To the best of our knowledge, this was the largest study including 1,104 patients with GCPM at present.

Previously published data had evaluated the incidence proportions and prognosis of GCPM roughly, and the frequency of pulmonary metastases from gastric cancer had yielded varying results, rang from 0.5 to 16% in current clinical practice (6, 7). However, the frequency of pulmonary metastases was found to be 22–52% at postmortem examination (9, 10). Most studies above were small samples from a single institution, which was unconvincing (6–10). Therefore a study based on population level to describe the frequency and prognosis of patients who presented with *de novo* pulmonary metastases was urgently needed. In this large retrospective study, we found that 6.02% of patients with gastric cancer had pulmonary metastases at diagnosis, and 15.19% of those with any metastases at diagnosis had pulmonary metastases. This result was a little different from that of previous published studies (6–10), but was in accordance with that of a previous study (12) using SEER database, which showed 5.92% of PM in all patients and 14.45% of PM in metastatic disease. Part of asymptomatic patients with lung metastases could not be found at initial diagnosis due to lack of accurate evaluation. On the other hand, most of the patients in previous studies developed pulmonary metastases in their disease course after a diagnosis of early-stage gastric cancer, so these researches contained both synchronous and asynchronous metastatic patients. And our work only focused on patients with metastatic gastric cancer at initial diagnosis, so the frequency of PM may be underestimated.

Risk factors for the presence of PM at GC diagnosis were determined using multivariate logistic regression. We found that patients had significantly greater odds of having pulmonary metastases at diagnosis when they showed the six factors as follow: younger, upper 1/3 of stomach, intestinal-type, T4 staging, N1 staging, and presence of more extrapulmonary metastases to liver, bone, and brain. Younger patients were always accompanied with more aggressive tumors which led to the common appearance of pulmonary metastases, as we guessed. An USA study by Smith found that 81% of young patients developed distant metastases compared to 50% in the elder for 15-year follow up which believed that earlier diagnosis and effective treatments were urgently needed to decrease the extreme lethality in these young patients (20). The presence of intestinal-type seemed to be associated with pulmonary metastases in this study. Huachuan et al. guessed that it might attribute to high expressions of extracellular matrix metalloproteinase inducer (EMMPRIN), which promoted tumor growth and metastasis (21). Primary tumor located at the upper 1/3 of stomach had significantly higher percentage of pulmonary metastases could be attributed to "seed-and-soil" hypothesis ("seed-and-soil" hypothesis implies organ specific tropism of circulating tumor cells) (22). Patients with T4 staging and N1 staging were easier to diagnose with pulmonary metastases, too. The finding was only seen in N1 staging because of lack of patients with N2 staging (N = 37) and N3 staging (N = 45) we guessed. And most N staging of this study was based on clinical staging which may not be accurate enough (23–25). Moreover, only T4 staging had a higher proportion of lung metastases compared with T1 staging. We thought that the same reasons existed in the variable of T staging. As we know, TNM staging was visibly associated with survival in GC. Thus, we inferred that later T staging and N staging may be associated with poor prognosis in GCPM. However, these results should be confirmed with further studies carefully. Besides, patients presented with more extrapulmonary metastatic sites were associated with a higher proportion of lung metastases. A similar result was also indicated in breast cancer (26). To say the least, our study indicated that GC patients with high risk factors above need further examination at first diagnosis, like chest CT, or PET-CT. However, it was unclear whether early detection could contribute to a more favorable survival significantly.

The multivariate logistic regression model including six significant variables had the best predictive value, with an AUC value of 0.775. And the AUC value of single predictors ranged from 0.529 to 0.745. From them, a large extent of extrapulmonary metastases hold a maximum AUC value of 0.745, and age had a minimum AUC value of 0.529. These predictors with AUC smaller than 0.6 were best to further evaluate. However, the model contains six significant variables that had an acceptable performance to predict the presence of PM in our study, which had not been reported yet.

Prognostic factors of PM at GC diagnosis were analyzed using the multivariate Cox model. We found that patients had a significantly higher risk of mortality when they showed the five factors as follows: diagnosis at previous period, black race, adverse pathology grade, absence of chemotherapy and presence of more extrapulmonary metastases to liver, bone and brain. The prognosis was better for those patients diagnosed at a later period, which may owe to those patients who receive more effective treatment with the improvement of medical conditions in recent years (2). It was worth noting that black patients had worse overall median survival which may be related to genetics and economic conditions which had not been well-explained in previous literature. And GCPM patients with adverse pathological grade and more metastatic sites predicted significantly poor survival in this study. This result had not been well-reported by published studies to the best of our knowledge. The median OS was 3.0 months from initial diagnosis of GCPM in the SEER, which was similar to the previous study (12). Chemotherapy was considered the basic treatment for advanced gastric cancer at present. The median OS of patients with and without chemotherapy was 6 and 1 months, separately, in this study. We can find a significant increase in the hazard ratio for all-cause mortality (2.87–3.84; P < 0.001) and gastric cancer-specific mortality (2.16–2.91; P < 0.001) among absence of chemotherapy vs. presence of chemotherapy. However, the role of surgery in GCPM had not been effectively identified yet. Only a few studies and case reports (8, 10, 11, 16, 17) proposed that radical surgery may improve quality of life and survival in highly selected cases with isolated pulmonary metastases, while others hold a different sound (27, 28). And our study found that surgery showed significant benefit in gastric cancer-specific mortality analysis only. The hazard ratio (1.13–2.33; P = 0.01) had a significant increase from absence of surgery to presence of surgery on a competitive risk model, while showed no significance on all-cause mortality analysis. What's more, the median OS had no significant increase from absence of surgery group (3 months) to surgery group (4 months), which may have had four reasons as follows. Firstly, most patients in published studies were confirmed pulmonary metastases after a diagnosis of early-stage gastric cancer and received metastasectomy later (6–10). Secondly, those patients in published studies were highly selected with excellent surgical conditions. Thirdly, samples in previous reports were really small with 12 patients as the largest sample (8). Finally, the GCPM patients with surgical resection were only 51 in this study, among them forty-four patients received gastrectomy and only 7 patients received radical surgery whose median survival was 6.0months (IQR:1-27mo), which needs further investigation with more patients and convincing research methods. A prospective randomized controlled trial (RCT) was not easy to conduct for patients with GCPM due to their complex characteristics, so the road may be hard and long. Besides, radiotherapy showed no significance for overall survival on multivariate Cox model in this study. In summary, chemotherapy may be the basic treatment for GCPM at present, while surgery may be available for those highly selected patients with caution. And we did not recommend routine surgery and radiotherapy at present.

Although our study was based on population-level, containing a large number of cases, we should not ignore its limitations.

Firstly, this study was a retrospective study. We could know patients with metastatic disease to bone, liver, lung and brain, but the SEER database did not provide information about other metastatic sites, like peritoneal metastases. Moreover, we only had information on synchronous metastasis to lung, lack of a relative minority compared to those patients who may develop asynchronous metastases. Secondly, information relating to comorbidities, performance status was not available in the SEER database. Thirdly, residence type, education level, and median household income were defined at a county level, not a patient level, possibly affecting the results of the logistic and Cox regressions. Fourthly, more detail information about radiotherapy, surgery and chemotherapy were not reported in the SEER database. Finally, the SEER did not record the details of pulmonary metastases.

To the best of our knowledge, this study was the first population-based analysis of patients with pulmonary metastases at initial diagnosis of gastric cancer. It provided important suggestions for clinicians to consider designing studies that evaluate the utility of screening among patients with higher risk of pulmonary metastases. The prognostic factors on GCPM were analyzed in this study too. Besides, we described the significance of different treatment on GCPM, which might provide some help to clinical practice.

CONCLUSIONS

In summary, the findings of this study based on a population level provided estimates of the frequency for GCPM at time of diagnosis. Patients present with younger, upper 1/3 of stomach, intestinal-type, T4 staging, N1 staging, and presence of more extrapulmonary metastases to liver, bone, and brain had significantly greater odds of having pulmonary metastases at diagnosis. A series of risk factors for PM in GC patients were identified, which can indicate routine screening in such patients. Furthermore, a list of prognostic factors for GCPM patients by survival estimates was found. GCPM patients present with black race, diagnosis at previous period, adverse pathology grade, presence with more extrapulmonary metastases to liver, bone and brain and absence of chemotherapy had a significantly higher risk of mortality. These finding can signify the need for individualized treatment for these patients. Chemotherapy may be the basic treatment for GCPM at present, while surgery may be available for those highly selected patients with caution. And we do not recommend routine surgery and radiotherapy at present.

ETHICS STATEMENT

The SEER was public-use data: informed consent was waived. And our study was deemed exempt from institutional review board approval by NanFang Hospital, Southern Medical University.

AUTHOR CONTRIBUTIONS

All authors listed had made a substantial contribution to the work. YJ and GL put forward the conception and designed the study. WH, TL, and ZH collected and collated the data. ZS, HL, and JY analyzed data and wrote the manuscript together. YH, HC, and MZ made contribution to proofread the article. Finally, all the authors take responsible to the final manuscript and approved it for publication.

ACKNOWLEDGMENTS

We would like to thank the staff members of the National Cancer Institute and their colleagues across the United States and at Information management Services, Inc., who have been involved with the Surveillance, Epidemiology and End Results (SEER) Program.

REFERENCES

1. Jemal A, Bray F, Center MM, Ferlay J, Ward E, Forman D. Global cancer statistics. *CA Cancer J Clin.* (2011) 61:69–90. doi: 10.3322/caac.20107
2. Siegel RL, Miller KD, Jemal A. Cancer statistics, 2018. *CA Cancer J Clin.* (2018) 68:7–30. doi: 10.3322/caac.21442
3. Bernards N, Creemers GJ, Nieuwenhuijzen GA, Bosscha K, Pruijt JF, Lemmens VE. No improvement in median survival for patients with metastatic gastric cancer despite increased use of chemotherapy. *Annals Oncol.* (2013) 24:3056–60 doi: 10.1093/annonc/mdt401
4. Irene T, Gestel YR, Van, Bert VR, Luyer MD, Koop B, Nienhuijs SW, et al. Peritoneal carcinomatosis of gastric origin: a population-based study on incidence, survival and risk factors. *Int J Cancer.* (2013) 134:622–8. doi: 10.1002/ijc.28373
5. Hundahl SA. Staging, stage migration, and patterns of spread in gastric cancer. *Semin Radiat Oncol.* (2002) 12:141–9. doi: 10.1053/srao.2002.30816
6. Kong JH, Lee J, Yi CA, Park SH, Park JO, Park YS, et al. Lung metastases in metastatic gastric cancer: pattern of lung metastases and clinical outcome. *Gastric Cancer.* (2012) 15:292–8. doi: 10.1007/s10120-011-0104-7
7. Motoki Y, Atsushi O, Narikazu B, Yoshinori M, Kuniaki S, Yasuhiro S, et al. Long-term survival and prognostic factors in patients with metastatic gastric cancers treated with chemotherapy in the Japan Clinical Oncology Group (JCOG) study. *Jpn J Clin Oncol.* (2004) 34:654–9. doi: 10.1093/jjco/hyh120
8. Kanemitsu Y, Kondo H, Katai H, Nakayama H, Asamura H, Tsuchiya R, et al. Surgical resection of pulmonary metastases from gastric cancer. *J Surg Oncol.* (2015) 69:147–50. doi: 10.1002/(SICI)1096-9098(199811)69:3<147::AID-JSO5>3.0.CO;2-H
9. D'Angelica M, Gonen M, Brennan MF, Turnbull AD, Bains M, Karpeh MS. Patterns of initial recurrence in completely resected gastric adenocarcinoma. *Ann Surg.* (2004) 240:808–16. doi: 10.1097/01.sla.0000143245.28656.15
10. Urabe M, Sakakibara T, Daibo M, Matsumura S, Mizobuchi N, Gonda H, et al. Two cases of recurrent pulmonary metastasis resected after operation for gastric cancer. *Nihon Geka Hokan.* (1996) 65:22–9.
11. Clinton DK, Mio K, Sid KR, Taylor R, Jens UM, David SS, et al. Pulmonary resection for metastatic gastric cancer. *J Thorac Oncol.* (2010) 5:1796–805. doi: 10.1097/JTO.0b013e3181ed3514
12. Qiu MZ, Shi SM, Chen ZH, Yu HE, Sheng H, Jin Y, et al. Frequency and clinicopathological features of metastasis to liver, lung, bone, and brain from gastric cancer: a SEER-based study. *Cancer Med.* (2018) 7:3662–72. doi: 10.1002/cam4.1661
13. Coppage L, Shaw C, Curtis AM. Metastatic disease to the chest in patients with extrathoracic malignancy. *J Thorac Imaging.* (1987) 2:24–30. doi: 10.1097/00005382-198710000-00006
14. Marom EM, Chasen MH. Comparison of computed and conventional whole lung tomography in detecting pulmonary nodules: a prospective radiologic-pathologic study. AJR (1978) 131:51–4. *AJR Am J Roentgenol.* (2006) 186:289–90. doi: 10.2214/AJR.05.0785
15. Chang AE, Schaner EG, Conkle DM, Flye MW, Doppman JL, Rosenberg SA. Evaluation of computed tomography in the detection of pulmonary metastases: a prospective study. *Cancer.* (2015) 43:913–63. doi: 10.1002/1097-0142(197903)43:3<913::AID-CNCR2820430319>3.0.CO;2-Q
16. Satoshi S, Toru S, Hirotoshi H, Masayuki C, Haruhisa M, Yuichi O, et al. Outcomes and prognostic factors of survival after pulmonary resection

for metastatic gastric cancer. *Eur J Cardio-Thorac Surg.* (2013) 43:E13–6. doi: 10.1093/ejcts/ezs574
17. Aurello P, Petrucciani N, Giulitti D, Campanella L, D'Angelo F, Ramacciato G. Pulmonary metastases from gastric cancer: Is there any indication for lung metastasectomy? A systematic review. *Med Oncol.* (2016) 33:9–14. doi: 10.1007/s12032-015-0718-4
18. Surveillance, Epidemiology, and End Results (SEER) Program Research Data (1973–2013), National CancerInstitute, DCCPS. *Surveillance Research Program, Surveillance Systems Branch, Released April 2016, Based on the November 2015 Submission.* Available online at: http://www.seer.cancer.gov. (accessed August 15, 2016).
19. Scrucca L, Santucci A, Aversa F. Competing risk analysis using R: an easy guide for clinicians. *Bone Marrow Transplant.* (2007) 40:381–7. doi: 10.1038/sj.bmt.1705727
20. Smith BR, Stabile BE. Extreme aggressiveness and lethality of gastric adenocarcinoma in the very young. *Arch Surg.* (2009) 144:506–10. doi: 10.1001/archsurg.2009.77
21. Huachuan Z, Hiroyuki T, Yoshihiro M, Zhengguo C, Kazuhiro N, Shigeharu M, et al. Pathobiological characteristics of intestinal and diffuse-type gastric carcinoma in Japan: an immunostaining study on the tissue microarray. *J Clin Pathol.* (2007) 60:273–7. doi: 10.1136/jcp.2006.038778
22. Kim MA, Hye Seung L, Han-Kwang Y, Woo Ho K. Clinicopathologic and protein expression differences between cardia carcinoma and noncardia carcinoma of the stomach. *Cancer.* (2010) 103:1439–46. doi: 10.1002/cncr.20966
23. Saito T, Kurokawa Y, Takiguchi S, Miyazaki Y, Takahashi T, Yamasaki M, et al. Accuracy of multidetector-row CT in diagnosing lymph node metastasis in patients with gastric cancer. *Eur Radiol.* (2015) 25:368–74. doi: 10.1007/s00330-014-3373-9
24. Hwang SW, Lee DH, Lee SH, Park YS, Hwang JH, Kim JW, et al. Preoperative staging of gastric cancer by endoscopic ultrasonography and multidetector-row computed tomography. *J Gastroenterol Hepatol.* (2010) 25:512–8. doi: 10.1111/j.1440-1746.2009.06106.x
25. Lee DH, Kim SH, Joo I, Hur BY, Han JK. Comparison between 18FFDG PET/MRI and MDCT for the assessment of preoperative staging and resectability of gastric cancer. *Euro J Radiol.* (2016) 85:1085–91. doi: 10.1016/j.ejrad.2016.03.015
26. Martin AM, Cagney DN, Catalano PJ, Warren LE, Bellon JR, Punglia RS, et al. Brain metastases in newly diagnosed breast cancer. *JAMA Oncol.* (2017) 3:1069–77. doi: 10.1001/jamaoncol.2017.0001
27. Fujitani K, Yang HK, Mizusawa J, Kim YW, Terashima M, Han SU, et al. Gastrectomy plus chemotherapy versus chemotherapy alone for advanced gastric cancer with a single non-curable factor (REGATTA): a phase 3, randomised controlled trial. *Lancet Oncol.* (2016) 17:309–18. doi: 10.1016/S1470-2045(15)00553-7
28. Müsri FY, Mutlu H, Karaagaç M, Eryilmaz MK, Gündüz S, Artaç M. Primary tumor resection and survival in patients with stage IV gastric cancer. *J Gastr Cancer.* (2016) 16:78–86. doi: 10.5230/jgc.2016.16.2.78

5

Circulating Tumor Cells in Gastrointestinal Cancers

Chaogang Yang [1,2,3†], *Fangfang Chen* [2,3,4†], *Shuyi Wang* [1,2,3] *and Bin Xiong* [1,2,3*]

[1] *Department of Gastrointestinal Surgery, Zhongnan Hospital of Wuhan University, Wuhan, China,* [2] *Hubei Key Laboratory of Tumor Biological Behaviors, Wuhan, China,* [3] *Hubei Cancer Clinical Study Center, Wuhan, China,* [4] *Department of Breast and Thyroid Surgery, Zhongnan Hospital of Wuhan University, Wuhan, China*

***Correspondence:**
Bin Xiong
binxiong1961@whu.edu.cn

† *These authors have contributed equally to this work*

Circulating tumor cells (CTCs), which are now defined as the "break away" cancer cells that derive from primary- or metastatic-tumor sites and present in the bloodstream, are considered to be the precursors of metastases. Considering the key role of CTCs in cancer progression, researchers are committed to analyze them in the past decades and many technologies have been proposed for achieving CTCs isolation and characterization with highly sensitivity and specificity until now. On this basis, clinicians gradually realize the clinical values of CTCs' detection through various clinical studies. As a "liquid biopsy," CTCs' detection and measurement can supply important information for predicting patient's survival, monitoring of response/resistance, assessment of minimal residual disease, evaluating distant metastasis, and sometimes, customizing therapy choices. Nowadays, eliminating CTCs of the blood circulation has been regarded as a promising method to prevent tumor metastasis. However, research on CTCs still faces many challenges. Herein, we present an overview to discuss the current concept of CTCs, summarize the available techniques for CTCs detection, and provide an update on the clinical significance of CTCs in gastrointestinal malignancies, especially focus on gastric and colorectal cancer.

Keywords: circulating tumor cells, gastric cancer, colorectal cancer, detection, identification, clinical application

INTRODUCTION

According to the GLOBOCAN 2018 reports, cancer is estimated to rank as the leading cause of death worldwide (1). Gastrointestinal (GI) malignancies, an important component of solid tumors, bear a heavier cancer-associated burden (2). At present, metastasis remains the main cause for GI malignancy-related deaths (3). Even for the early-stage patients who underwent curative resection, a considerable portion suffer metastatic disease within 5 years of surgery (4). This evidence implies that an occult metastatic process is parallel with primary tumor development (5) or that tumor cells with metastatic potential have entered the bloodstream from the primary tumor site during surgery and cause subsequent distant metastasis in the aforementioned patients (6). These cells are termed circulating tumor cells (CTCs), which have been proposed to be the important mediators of hematogenous metastasis of solid malignant tumors (6, 7).

CTCs, first reported by Ashworth in 1869 and further demonstrated by Engell in 1955, are now defined as the "break away" cancer cells that derive from primary or metastatic tumor sites and present in the blood circulation (8). These cells shed intermittently from the tumor site, circulate within the bloodstream, potentially seed into distant organs and finally form vital metastases (8). Therefore, research on CTCs can provide more insights into metastasis-associated progression. However, the extremely low concentration in the peripheral blood (one CTC in millions of blood cells) makes CTCs detection a technical challenge (9), which in turn greatly limits in-depth studies on the biological properties of CTCs (10). Nevertheless, given the critical role of CTCs in tumor progression, many researchers have expended much effort to explore efficiently capture CTCs (9). Consequently, a considerable amount of scientific literature has published over the past decade, occurring in parallel with technical progress that has propelled this field forward. To date, a number of technologies based on the biological or physical properties of CTCs have been developed for achieving CTCs isolation and identification (9, 11–13), which lay the technical foundation for conducting more clinical research to explore the clinical value of CTCs detection in predicting patient survival, customizing therapy choices, monitoring response/resistance, and evaluating distant metastasis in numerous types of cancer (14). Over the past few years, our group has been working on CTCs detection methods and has developed a variety of methods based on the different biophysical characteristics of CTCs (15–24); these studies have enabled us to efficiently capture CTCs in the peripheral blood and to further analyze the prognostic value of quantitative and qualitative CTCs analysis in gastrointestinal (GI) malignancies (25–27).

In this review, we aim to outline the current status of CTCs detection techniques, the clinical implications, and the limitations and opportunities in GI cancers, including gastric cancer (GC) and colorectal cancer (CRC); we then provide new insights into the applications of CTCs detection to guide clinical practice.

ISOLATION AND ENRICHMENT TECHNOLOGIES OF CTCS

Although the primary tumor or metastasis site releases tumor cells into the blood at all times, most of them are eliminated by the body's immune system, and only a few CTCs survives in the blood circulation. Therefore, the number of CTCs is sparse (~1 CTC per ml of blood) compared to the number of other cellular components in the peripheral blood (5). This situation poses a high technical challenge for us to accurately isolate CTCs from millions of blood cells, indicating that an ideal technology for CTCs separation needs to have the following characteristics: (1) the ability to isolate all heterogeneous CTCs; (2) the ability to exclude the background interference caused by normal blood cells; and (3) the ability to accurately identify all candidate CTCs. At present, it has been well-recognized that the biological and physical characteristics of CTCs are obviously different from those of other cells in the blood (8). Consequently, many capture and identification technologies based on different CTCs features are gradually being developed to pursue the ultimate goal of achieving CTCs enrichment with high specificity and sensitivity (9, 11–13). For CTC enrichment, the isolation of CTCs is usually the first step, and the characterization of CTCs (the second step) further distinguishes the CTCs from the remaining normal blood cells. As shown in **Figure 1**, we presented an overview of the technologies utilized for CTCs isolation and characterization, and these technologies are commonly used in GC and CRC.

Immunoaffinity-Based Technologies of CTCs

Immunoaffinity-based technologies, including positive or negative selection assays, achieve CTCs isolation with an antibody-immobilized inert surface combined with magnetic beads (28). Among these assays, positive selection assays frequently rely on two types of antigens, either single or a combination, that include the epithelial- or tumor-specific cell surface antigens (12). In the process of GC- and CRC-CTCs isolation, the most commonly used epithelial-specific cell surface antigens are cytokeratins (CKs) 18, 19, 20 and epithelial cell adhesion molecules (EpCAMs). CKs are intermediate filament keratins found in the cytoskeletons of epithelial cells (29). EpCAM is a human cell surface glycoprotein involved in cell-to-cell adhesion, which overexpresses in epithelial cancers and has been extensively used in proof-of-concept studies (30). Among tumor-specific cell surface antigens, carcinoembryonic antigen (CEA) has been largely utilized to isolate CRC-CTCs (31), and human epithelial growth factor receptor-2 (HER-2) was used for GC-CTCs isolation (32). Currently, several platforms, such as the CellSearch® System and AdnaTest® kit, have been developed for GC- and CRC-CTCs detection based on positive selection, and are now have achieved for commercially available (27, 33). Conversely, negative selection assays generally remove white blood cells (WBCs) from blood samples by targeting leukocyte surface-specific antigens (e.g., CD45 and CD61) that are not expressed in CTCs to achieve GC- and CRC-CTCs enrichment; the kits and techniques include the EasySep® Human CD45 Depletion Kit (34) and MACS® (35). Notably, Nagrath et al. developed the "CTC-Chip" platform by combining microfluidic technology with positive selection methods 10 years ago, and this method was able to selectively and efficiently isolate CTCs from whole blood using anti-EpCAM-coated posts with this microfluidic chip (36). Microfluidic devices are promising technologies for CTC isolation, which allow the separation of CTCs from small fluid volumes under laminar flow and eliminate the need for pre-labeling or sample processing (32). The Isoflux® System (Fluxion Biosciences Inc., South San Francisco, CA) was another classic automated EpCAM-based immunoaffinity functionalized microfluidic system that used immunomagnetic beads to facilitate the use of single or multiple capture antibodies to target cells of a specific pathology, providing near-perfect isolation efficiency (37). Although, given that there are no 100% tumor-specific antibodies, the false-positive (specificity) and false-negative (sensitivity) of CTCs isolation continue to impose shackles on immuno-magnetic detection techniques.

Among the commercially available semiautomated devices, the CellSearch® System (Veridex LLC, Raritan, NJ, USA) is the most reported immunoaffinity (EpCAM-based) method for CTCs isolation and counting, which has been approved by

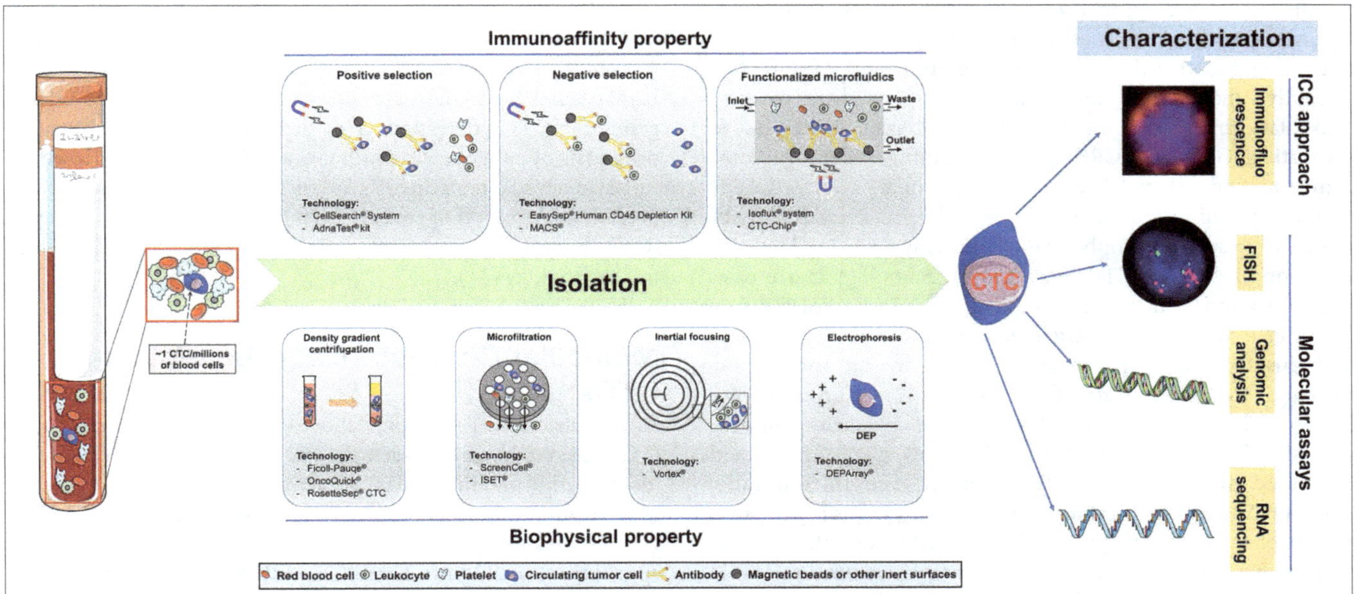

FIGURE 1 | Overview of technologies for circulating tumor cells (CTCs) capture, enrichment, and characterization. Immunoaffinity-based enrichment technologies capture CTC by positive or negative selection, typically using antibodies bound to the device surface or to magnetic beads. Positive selection is based on the specific targeting of CTCs epithelial biomarkers, whereas negative selection depletes hematopoietic cells by targeting cell-surface antigens not expressed in CTCs. Functionalized microfluidics platforms can combine the advantages of microfluidic and the characters of positive capture and negative enrichment. Biophysical methods are label-free technologies relying on cell size, shape, density, and electric charge differences between CTC and other blood constituents. Density gradient centrifugation relies in the separation of different cell populations based on their relative densities. Microfiltration consists on size-based cell separation using pores or three-dimensional geometries. Inertial focusing relies on the passive separation of cells by size, through the application of inertial forces that affect positioning within the flow channel in microfluidics devices. Electrophoresis separates cells based on their electrical signatures, using an electric field. The methods of CTCs characterization include immunocytochemistry (ICC)-based approaches and molecular assays. Of which, ICC-based approaches are consist of immunofluorescence and immunohistochemistry technology, and molecular assays are consist of fluorescent *in situ* hybridization (FISH), real-time polymerase chain reaction (RT-PCR), genomic analysis, and RNA sequencing.

the Federal Drug And Food Administration (FDA) for use in metastatic breast and colon cancer patients (38). Additionally, it has also been widely used in the capture of GC and CRC-CTCs in recent years (27, 3[illegible]). As one of the immunoaffinity assays, the major advantages of the CellSearch® System are the direct visualization and quantification of CTCs and the detection of living cells without the need for cell lysis. However, there is a non-negligible fact that CellSearch detects a relatively low number of CTCs from the peripheral blood of patients with cancer, and this low sensitivity may be because the system captures solely EpCAM-positive CTCs that are significantly reduced or absent in certain CTCs subpopulations, especially for those undergoing epithelial-to-mesenchymal transition (EMT); this characteristic is still considered a major pitfall of this device (38).

Previously, our group also reported several immunoaffinity-based technologies for CTCs detection. First, we developed a new CTCs detection platform by using an electrospun TiO2 nanofiber-deposited substrate grafted with anti-EpCAM, which achieved high efficiency in CTCs detection from the blood of GC and CRC patients (15). Meanwhile, a new CTCs capture platform based on the transparent and biocompatible TiO2 nanoparticle spin coated on a glass substrate conjugated with anti-EpCAM also was successfully used to capture GC- and CRC-CTCs (16, 17). However, preparation of the above nanostructures requires either specialized equipment or complex process control, which limits its high-throughput fabrication. Moreover, the non-transparent nature makes them incompatible with many optical imaging systems (such as immunocytochemical techniques), which also constrains further application. Therefore, our group further used a hydroxyapatite/chitosan (HA/CTS) material as a nano-substrate, which was characterized by transparency and excellent biological compatibility, and conjugated this material with anti-EpCAM to develop simple but efficient CTCs detection platforms (18, 22). More importantly, the enumeration of CTCs by these platforms in GC patients could predict the clinical response to anticancer therapy (19). Furthermore, we coated anti-CD45 and anti-EpCAM onto the surface of the above nano-substrate to develop a combined negative and positive enrichment assay, exhibiting equally high capture efficiency and excellent purity for CRC-CTCs detection (21).

Biophysical Property-Based Technologies of CTCs

Considering the bias and narrow capture spectrum presented by the aforementioned immunoaffinity-based approaches in CTCs isolation, researchers began to develop a variety of CTCs isolation technologies based on the biophysical properties of CTCs to achieve a wide-scale and high-performance capture of CTCs (39). Biophysical CTCs enrichment technologies, characterized as "label-free," isolate CTCs from the blood based on the biophysical property differences, such as density, size, deformability, and electrical charge, that present among CTCs and other blood cells for CTCs separation and capture (40). Recently, there have been commercially available reagents and platforms based on the above different principles for separating GC- and CRC-CTCs, including density gradient centrifugation (Ficoll-Pauqe®; OncoQuick®; RosetteSep® CTC), microfiltration (ScreenCell®; ISET®), inertial focusing (Vortex®), and electrophoresis (DEPArray®) (41). The most common biophysical CTCs enrichment technology is size-based microfiltration, which assumes that CTCs can be isolated from blood cells due to their larger volume and more rigid shape, and this technology has been improved by the introduction of nano to micron-sized filter pores (42). Currently, new lab-on-a-chip microfluidics devices have gradually appeared and significantly improved the GC- and CRC-CTCs yields compared with the conventional membrane microfiltration and EpCAM-based immunoaffinity assays (43, 44). Moreover, these technologies have provided improved *in situ* platforms for molecular analysis by fluorescent *in situ* hybridization (FISH) or immunofluorescence (IF) (45), as well as for the extraction of biomolecules for downstream genomic and transcriptomic sequencing (43). In addition, these platforms also provide the opportunity for CTCs release and *ex vivo* expansion, which lays an important foundation to further understand the biological characteristics of CTCs (46).

Previously, our group reported several biophysical property-based assays of CTCs detection. We fabricated a label-free wedge-shaped microfluidic chip (named CTC-Δchip) based on the size characteristics of CTCs, which exhibited high performance in capturing GC-CTCs and a great potential clinical value (24). Additionally, our group co-operated with YZY Medical Science and Technology Company (Wuhan, China) to develop a novel isolation by size of epithelial tumor cells device named CTCBIOPSY® (Wuhan YZY Medical Science and Technology Co., Ltd., Wuhan, China), which achieved CTCs isolation and identification through a polymer membrane made by biocompatible parylene and Wright's staining (23). As a one-stop ISET device, CTCBIOPSY® exhibited excellent performance in capturing patients' CTCs and has now been approved by the China Food and Drug Administration (CFDA) for clinical application in cancer management (23, 26).

Molecular (RNA-Based) Assays of CTCs (Without Prior Enrichment)

The aforementioned immunoaffinity- or biophysical property-based technologies of CTCs detection need to separate GC- and CRC-CTCs from blood cells before identification. Molecular assays, represented by RT-PCR, can directly achieve the detection and characterization of CTCs by analyzing the expression of GC and CRC-CTCs-related genes without prior CTCs enrichment (47, 48). In contrast to enrichment technologies, RT-PCR has the advantages of being rapid, well-implemented, sensitive, and cost effective (41). Previously, our group conducted a series of meta-analyses to explore the clinical role of CTCs detected by RT-PCR in GC and CRC and summarized the commonly used markers for GC-CTCs (including CK19, CK20, CEA, hTerT, c-MET, MUC1, VEGFR-1, Survivin, uPAR, B7-H3, and STCs) and CRC-CTCs (including CK19, CK20, CEA, PLS3, CD133, hTerT, EphB4, LAMγ2, and MAT) detection (25, 49). Using these cancer-related genes for CTCs detection is of great value in evaluating the prognosis of patients with both GC and CRC (25, 49). However, tumor-derived circulating RNAs (such as miRNAs and lncRNAs) present in the blood of cancer patients may affect the accuracy of RT-PCR for CTCs detection, contributing a major limitation of this technology (41).

Molecular Characterizing Technologies of CTCs

After enrichment by the above platforms, the candidate CTCs need to be further identified as "true" CTCs. Currently, the identification and molecular characterization of CTCs is achieved by (a) immunocytochemistry (ICC)-based assays, including IF and immunohistochemistry (IHC), and (b) molecular approaches, including RT-qPCR, FISH and next-generation sequencing (NGS) (41). The most commonly used assay for the identification of GC- and CRC-CTCs from contaminating cells is IF, which achieves CTCs identification by staining and visualizing related-antibody biomarkers. Such biomarkers can be specific for nuclear content, epithelial proteins (i.e., CKs), mesenchymal proteins (i.e., vimentin), and hematopoietic markers (i.e., CD45). A common immunocytological CTC definition is nucleus+/CK+/vimentin−/CD45− cell for epithelial-CTC, nucleus+/CK−/vimentin+/CD45− cell for mesenchymal-CTC, and nucleus+/CK+/vimentin+/CD45− for epithelial/mesenchymal-CTC (50). However, the detection of CTCs by classical IF, which is typically performed by pathologists through the visual observation of stained CTCs based on the above principles, is time consuming and subjective-dependent. By contrast, PCR-based molecular assays provide objective and quantifiable CTCs measurements with the advantages of automated, sensitive, relatively low-cost and amenable to quantifiable quality control. Moreover, these methods require a small amount of cells for analysis, which is also in line with the fact that the amount of CTCs is less (51). However, since the molecular characterization of CTCs by PCR assays is based on the detection of mRNA markers that are specifically expressed in CTCs but not in leukocytes, the risk of false-positive results might be increased due to the non-specific amplification of RNA (50–52).

Notably, nucleic acid-based technologies, as improvements to non-fixating enrichment procedures, allow the use of RT-PCR and qRT-PCR to amplify single or multiple gene transcripts for CTCs detection, and these technologies have provided an alternate avenue for the molecular characterization of GC- and CRC-CTCs (53–55). In particular, recent emerging single-cell sequencing techniques, including DNA and RNA sequencing, have turned the research direction toward analyzing the genetic characteristics of individual CTCs to assist in exploring tumor metastasis mechanisms, finding drug targets, monitoring therapy responses, and assessing drug resistance (54). Although, because single-cell CTC analyses are limited by the heterogeneity between

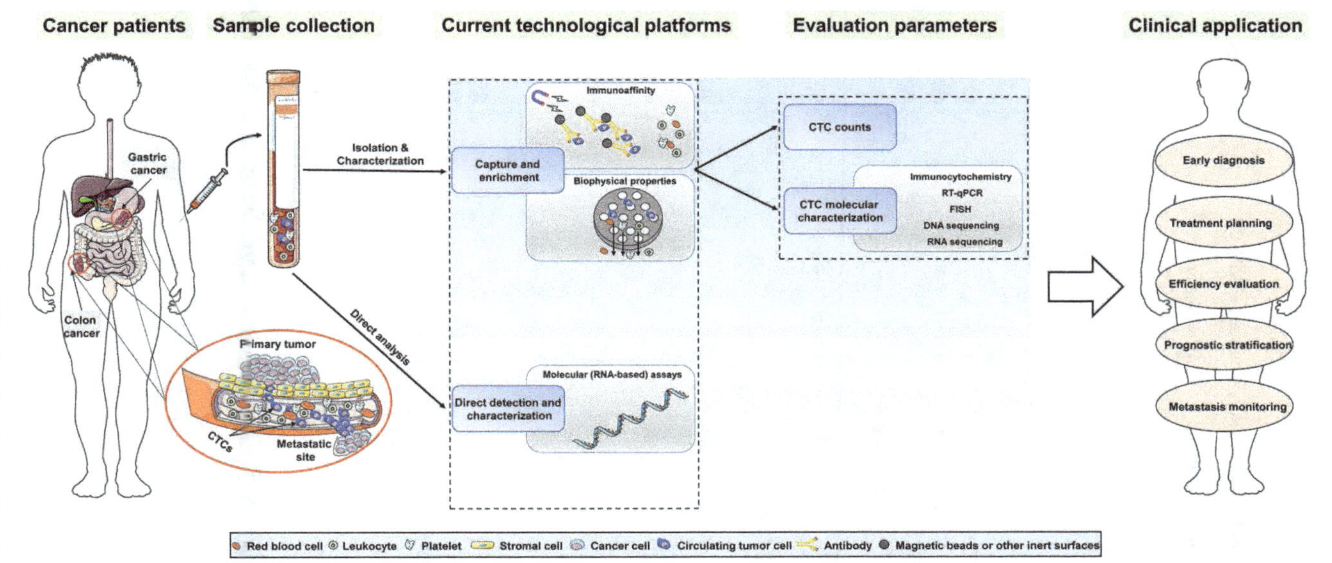

FIGURE 2 | Overview of the CTCs detection technologies and the potential clinical applications of CTCs in gastric and colorectal cancer.

cancer subtypes, the usefulness of these analyses has hindered the discovery of universal markers (54).

CLINICAL VALUE OF CTCS DETECTION IN GASTROINTESTINAL CANCER

In recent years, the clinical applications of CTCs detection via various technologies have been gradually involved in multiple aspects of GI cancers, including early diagnosis, treatment planning, efficiency evaluation, prognostic stratification, and metastasis monitoring (56) (summarized in **Figure 2**). Despite this, there is still no universally applicable "gold standard" method so far (41, 56). Therefore, the aforementioned assays must be validated in clinical trials to achieve clinical validity and utility in the future.

Prognostic Stratification

The role of CTCs in the prognostic stratification of patients with GC and CRC, as the most studied aspect of CTCs' clinical value, has been demonstrated by numerous studies (26, 57–91). For both GC and CRC, CTCs detection is considered to be significantly correlated with disease progression and patient's prognosis (56). Previously, our group conducted a prospective cohort study that recruited 138 patients with stage I–III CRC to assess the prognostic value of the change in CTCs counts before and after curative surgery. The results found that postoperative CTCs-positive but not preoperative CTCs-positive is an independent indicator of poor prognosis for CRC patients, and the patients with preoperative CTCs-positive that normalized after surgery have similar outcomes to patients with preoperative CTC-negative (26). Meanwhile, our clinical study demonstrated that combining the preoperative controlling nutritional status score and circulating tumor cell status could strongly predict the prognosis for CRC patients treated with curative resection (92), which indicated that the state of CTCs in the blood is closely related to the nutrition and immune status of the host. In addition, a series of meta-analyses conducted by our group also provided strong evidence for the prognostic significance of CTCs detection in GI malignancies, which showed that CTCs-positive predicts a poor patient prognosis and unfavorable clinicopathological factors for both GC and CRC, regardless of whether the detection method was RT-PCR, CellSearch or cytological methods (25, 27, 49, 93). In these processes, an unneglectable fact is that CTCs detection at different time points during treatment might exhibit different prognostic significance (14). The reason is that a cancer (or a minimal residual disease) evolves with time, treatment, selection pressure from surgery, chemotherapy and radiotherapy and that tumoricidal immunity could stimulate the expansion of tumor subclones, leading to a change in the number and molecular characteristics of CTCs (94). In the future, repeated CTCs detection may be necessary to capture the changing genetics attributed to anticancer therapies. In the present review, we summarized the prognostic value of CTCs detection using different methods at different time points in GC and CRC (summarized in **Table 1**). As shown in **Table 1**, although there are many CTCs detection methods, none of them are generally accepted and could be really applied to clinical practice. At the same time, the cut-off values of the same CTCs detection method are different from study to study. Therefore, it is necessary for larger clinical studies to further validate whether CTCs are used in clinical practice to guide prognostic assessment. Of course, this may still have a long way to go.

Therapeutic Implications

Currently, there is limited evidence showing that CTCs detection at baseline can predict the response to systemic therapy in

TABLE 1 | CTCs detection for prognosis of gastric and colorectal cancer.

Cancer types	Cut-off value	Technique	Patients (*n*)	HR for death (95% CI)		HR for progression/recurrence (95% CI)		References
				Before treatment	After treatment	Before treatment	After treatment	
Gastric cancer	≥2.8 CTCs	ISET	Non-metastatic GAC (88)	–	–	–	–	(57)
	≥5 CTCs	CellSearch®	Resectable GC (93)	–	–	–	–	(67)
	>17 CTCs	IsoFlux®	Stage II–IV EGC (43)	3.7 (1.2–12.4)	–	–	–	(58)
	≥1 CTCs	ISET	Stage II–IV GC (86)	2.96 (1.25–7.04)	-	3.94 (1.38–11.27)	–	(68)
	>2 CTCs	CELLection™	Stage II–IV GC (59)	3.59 (1.66–7.82)	0.77 (0.27–2.25)	2.81 (1.31–6.00)	6.58 (1.37–31.6)	(63)
	≥4 CTCs	SE-iFISH	Advanced GC (31)	–	–	–	–	(62)
	>5 CTCs	GFP fluorescence	Stage II–IV GC (65)	0.90 (0.29–2.59)	–	1.97 (0.47–8.86)	–	(59)
	≥3 CTCs	CellSearch®	Advanced EGC (106)	–	3.46 (1.82–6.58)	–	2.15 (1.11–4.16)	(61)
	≥2 CTCs	Cytometry, FISH	Advanced EGC (60)	4.30 (0.82–22.90)	–	6.70 (1.43–31.03)	–	(64)
	≥1 CTCs	CellSearch®	Advanced GC (136)	1.37 (0.68–2.77)	–	2.14 (1.09–4.20)	–	(65)
	≥5 CTCs	CellSearch®	Advanced GC (100)	2.58 (1.57–4.27)	–	2.06 (1.26–3.38)	–	(60)
	≥1 CTCs	CellSearch®	Resectable GC (148)	1.73 (1.08–2.77)	–	–	–	(66)
Colorectal cancer	≥3 CTCs	Cyttel+imFISH	Advanced CRC (121)	–	2.68 (1.19-6.03)	–	2.79 (1.01–7.71)	(69)
	≥4 CTCs	CellSearch®	Non-metastatic CRC (63)	41.03 (0.00–102.40)	–	17.6 (3.7–82.6)	–	(70)
	≥1 CTCs	ISET	Non-metastatic CRC (138)	–	–	2.17 (0.75–6.31)	2.82 (1.39–5.75)	(26)
	≥1 CTCs	Immunomagnetic selection	mCRC (77)	0.32 (0.72–2.79)	0.35 (0.12-0.99)	–	–	(71)
	≥1.92 CTCs	CEACAM5 RT-PCR	mCRC (436)	2.1 (1.3–3.2)	–	1.6 (1.1–2.5)	–	(72)
	≥6 CTCs	CanPatrol™	Stage I-IV (66)	59.7 (0.002–1.6 × 10^6)	–	7.42 (1.06–51.74)	–	(73)
	>30 CTCs	Vita-Assay™	Stage I-IV (88)	1.04 (1.01–1.06)	–	–	–	(74)
	≥2 CTCs	CellSearch®	mCRC (79)	2.51 (0.69–9.09)	–	3.28 (1.24–8.67)	–	(75)
	>30 CTCs	Negative selection	mCRC (55)	2.61 (1.39–4.93)	–	4.94 (2.60–9.39)	–	(76)

(Continued)

TABLE 1 | Continued

Cancer types	Cut-off value	Technique	Patients (*n*)	HR for death (95% CI)		HR for progression/recurrence (95% CI)		References
				Before treatment	After treatment	Before treatment	After treatment	
	NR	Multiparameter flow cytometry	mCRC (152)	6.46 (1.46–28.56)	–	–	–	(77)
	≥1 CTCs	ISET	Stage II-IV (98)	–	1.15 (0.68-1.94)	–	1.99 (1.14–3.48)	(78)
	≥1+ PCR test out of 3	CK20 RT-PCR	Resectable colon cancer (299)	1.94 (1.0–3.7)	–	1.94 (1.1–3.7)	–	(79)
	≥1 CTC	CellSearch®	Stage I-III CRC (239)	5.5 (2.3–13.6)	–	12.7 (5.2–31.1)	–	(80)
			Stage I-IV CRC (287)	5.6 (2.6–12.0)	–	7.8 (3.9–15.5)	–	
	≥1 CTC	CellSearch®	Stage III CRC (519)	–	0.96 (0.56-1.65)	–	0.97 (0.65–1.45)	(81)
	≥2 CTCs	CellSearch®	Resectable CRC LM (194)	2.48 (1.40–4.38)	–	2.32 (1.26–4.27)	–	(82)
	>0.1 ng/μL for ≥1 out of 3 gene	AdnaTest®	Metastatic RAS-BRAF wt CRC (38)	9.32 (2.63–33.1)	–	6.24 (2.54–15.3)	–	(83)
	≥1 CTC	CellSearch®	Resectable colon cancer (183)	2.88 (1.46–5.66)	–	1.96 (1.06–3.61)	–	(84)
	≥3 CTCs	CellSearch®	Metastatic KRAS wt CRC (63)	2.08 (1.16–3.73)	–	–	–	(85)
	≥1 CTC	CellSearch®	mCRC (119)	–	–	2.05 (1.29–3.28)	–	(86)
	≥3 CTCs	CellSearch®	mCRC (180)	1.54 (1.00–2.37)	–	1.47 (0.98–2.22)	–	(87)
	≥3 CTCs	CellSearch®	mCRC (64)	–	1.44 (1.14–1.82)	1.06 (0.98–1.15)	1.21 (1.09–1.34)	(88)
	All markers positive	CK19, CK20, CEA, CD133 RT-PCR	Resectable CRC (315)	3.20 (1.67–6.31)	–	3.04 (1.79–5.22)	–	(89)
	≥3 CTCs	CellSearch®	mCRC (467)	1.9	–	1.4	–	(90)
	>3 CTCs	CellSearch®	mCRC (430)	2.45 (1.77–3.39)	9.35 (5.28–16.54)	1.74 (1.33–2.26)	3.64 (2.10–6.30)	(91)

CTCs, circulating tumor cells; HR, hazard ratio; CI, confidence interval; ISET, isolation by size of epithelial tumor cells; GAC, gastric adenocarcinoma; GC, gastric cancer; EGC, esophagogastric cancer; FISH, fluorescent in situ hybridization; CRC, colorectal cancer; mCRC, metastatic CRC; RT-PCR, real-time polymerase chain reaction; CK, cytokine; CEA, carcinoembryonic antigen; wt: wild type; LM, lung metastasis; NR, not reported.

TABLE 2 | CTCs as predictive factors for cancer therapy efficacy in gastric and colorectal cancer.

Cancer types	Cut-off value	Technique	Patients (*n*)	Treatment	Conclusions	References
Gastric cancer	≥1 CTC	3D-IF-FISH method	Unresectable metastatic or recurrent GC (15)	1st-line CT + trastuzumab	ORR was 53.3% in CTCs-HER2 positive patients at first response evaluation (6 weeks) vs. 7.7% in CTCs-HER2 negative patients ($p = 0.016$)	(98)
	≥3 CTCs	CellSearch®	Advanced GC (106)	1st-line CT	ORR was 30.0% in CTCs-negative patients at first response evaluation	(61)
	≥5 CTCs	CellSearch®	Metastatic GC (100)	≥1st-line CT	Chemotherapy response (CR or PR or SD) was 76.6% in CTCs-negative patients vs. 40.0% in CTCs-positive patients ($p = 0.004$)	(60)
	≥1 of the marker genes positive	EpCAM + RT-PCR	Advanced GC (61)	1st or 2nd-line CT	100% of progressive patients were CTCs-positive at baseline vs. 73.5% of non-progressive patients ($p = 0.003$)	(96)
Colorectal cancer	2 + PCR results	RT-PCR	LARC (79)	CRT + surgery	After CRT, CTCs were detected in 54.4% of the non-responders vs. 27.2% of the responders ($p = 0.030$)	(95)
	≥1 CTC	CellSearch®	LARC (85)	CRT + surgery	pCR/downstaging/downsizing rate was 80% in baseline CTCs-negative patients vs. 40% in CTCs-positive patients ($p = 0.02$)	(97)
	≥1 out of 3 CTCs markers	AdnaTest®	Metastatic RAS-BRAF wt CRC (38)	≥1st-line CT	ORR in unfavorable and favorable CTCs-changes profiles were respectively 0% and 59% ($p < 0.0001$)	(83)
	≥3 CTCs	CellSearch®	Metastatic KRAS wt CRC (61)	3rd-line CT	ORR was not different between the high and the low CTCs groups (27.7 vs. 18.36%, $p = 0.498$)	(85)
	≥3 CTCs	CellSearch®	mCRC (180)	1st-line CT	CTCs negativity after 3 cycles of CT was associated with higher ORR (OR, 3.22; 95% CI 1.25–9.43)	(87)
	≥3 CTCs	CellSearch®	mCRC (60)	1st or 2nd-line CT	CTCs positivity at 8–12 weeks was 2% in non-PD patients vs. 43% in PD patients ($p = 0.004$)	(88)
	≥3 CTCs	CellSearch®	mCRC (307)	1st-line CT	ORR was 40% in patients with low CTCs count at 1–2 weeks vs. 11% in patients with high CTCs count ($p = 0.022$)	(90)
	≥3 CTCs	CellSearch®	mCRC (430)	1st, 2nd, or 3rd CT	CTCs positivity at 3–5 weeks was 7% in non-PD patients vs. 27% in PD patients	(91)

CTCs, circulating tumor cells; GC, gastric cancer; CRC, colorectal cancer; mCRC, metastatic CRC; LARC, localize advanced rectum cancer; IF, immunofluorescence; FISH, fluorescent in situ hybridization; EpCAM, epithelial marker epithelial cell adhesion molecule; HER2, human epidermal growth factor receptor 2; RT-PCR, real-time polymerase chain reaction; CT, chemotherapy; CRT, chemoradiotherapy; CR, complete response; PR, part response; SD, stable disease; ORR, overall response rate = complete response + partial response; OR, odds ratio.

GI cancers (60, 61, 83, 85, 87, 88, 90, 91, 95–98). However, a few studies have demonstrated the predictive value of CTCs detection during chemotherapy (summarized in **Table 2**). Li et al. conducted a single-center, prospective study to measure the level of CTCs before and at 6 weeks of chemotherapy in 136 patients with newly diagnosed advanced GC, and the results showed that the posttherapy CTCs levels may help evaluate the therapeutic response; in addition, the changes in CTCs following therapy may be useful in rapidly identifying ineffective treatments for patients with advanced GC (61). Similarly, a study including 430 patients with metastatic CRC also found that there were significantly higher disease progression rates among patients who were CTCs-positive after 3–4 weeks of chemotherapy (91). Additionally, CTCs have also been used as a vehicle to assess genotyping changes in primary tumor and metastatic lesions; this is relevant for patients for whom a targeted therapy against known resistance-causing mutations is available, such as HER2-directed treatment for GC and EGFR-directed treatment for CRC (14). Overall, although the therapeutic predictive value of CTCs is not as well-studied as their prognostic value, using CTCs detection for determining the choice of systemic treatment and monitoring the treatment effects is promising, illustrating the possibility of liquid biopsy assessments to change future cancer management.

Early Diagnosis

In the early stage of the disease, tumor cells may separate from the primary tumor and enter the bloodstream; this circumstance provides a theoretical basis for CTCs detection as a tool for early diagnosis. Over the past few years, several studies have explored the early diagnostic value of CTCs detection based on different methods in GI malignancies, and the results found that the fraction of patients positive for CTCs is generally considered too low to obtain sufficient sensitivities for true early diagnosis (66, 99–101). Therefore, screening general populations with a CTCs assessment is not logistically realistic, but may be realistic in the high-risk groups, such as those with a family history of GI cancers.

CONCLUDING REMARKS

Although the detection and measurement of CTCs is expected to become a promising tool as prognostic, predictive, and diagnostic markers for patients with GC and CRC, CTCs have yet to be realized owing to residual surmountable challenges. To achieve this goal, a CTCs detection device that is universally accepted, fast, and low-cost with low false-negative and false-positive results is first needed; simultaneously, standard procedures for CTCs detection must also be established. Then, clinical research into CTCs as a circulating marker needs to be performed, and issues and promising results should be validated in large-scale, long-term follow-up, prospective clinical trials to ensure clinical applicability. Furthermore, conducting more basic research to gain an in-depth understanding of cancer biology may provide new insights into how and when to perform CTCs detection with the best clinical use. Despite these obstacles, we still have enough reason to believe that, with advances in detection and subsequent analytical techniques, CTCs will provide abundant useful information for the diagnosis and therapy in clinical practice for patients with GI cancers in the near future.

AUTHOR CONTRIBUTIONS

BX designed the review. CY and FC drafted the manuscript and prepared the figures. SW helped to modify the manuscript. All authors read and approved the final manuscript.

ACKNOWLEDGMENTS

The authors would like to thank Wuhan YZY Medical Science and Technology Co., Ltd. for providing equipment and excellent technical support for our CTCs study.

REFERENCES

1. Bray F, Ferlay J, Soerjomataram I, Siegel RL, Torre LA, Jemal A. Global cancer statistics 2018: GLOBOCAN estimates of incidence and mortality worldwide for 36 cancers in 185 countries. *CA Cancer J Clin.* (2018) 68:394–424. doi: 10.3322/caac.21492
2. Abreu MT, Peek RM Jr. Gastrointestinal malignancy and the microbiome. *Gastroenterology.* (2014) 146:1534–46.e3. doi: 10.1053/j.gastro.2014.01.001
3. Pantel K, Brakenhoff RH. Dissecting the metastatic cascade. *Nat Rev Cancer.* (2004) 4:448–56. doi: 10.1038/nrc1370
4. Miller KD, Siegel RL, Lin CC, Mariotto AB, Kramer JL, Rowland JH, et al. Cancer treatment and survivorship statistics, 2016. *CA Cancer J Clin.* (2016) 66:271–89. doi: 10.3322/caac.21349
5. Klein CA. Parallel progression of primary tumours and metastases. *Nat Rev Cancer.* (2009) 9:302–12. doi: 10.1038/nrc2627
6. Micalizzi DS, Maheswaran S, Haber DA. A conduit to metastasis: circulating tumor cell biology. *Genes Dev.* (2017) 31:1827–40. doi: 10.1101/gad.305805.117
7. Massague J, Obenauf AC. Metastatic colonization by circulating tumour cells. *Nature.* (2016) 529:298–306. doi: 10.1038/nature17038
8. Williams SC. Circulating tumor cells. *Proc Natl Acad Sci USA.* (2013) 110:4861. doi: 10.1073/pnas.1304186110
9. Shen Z, Wu A, Chen X. Current detection technologies for circulating tumor cells. *Chem Soc Rev.* (2017) 46:2038–56. doi: 10.1039/C6CS00803H
10. Pantel K, Alix-Panabieres C. Circulating tumour cells in cancer patients: challenges and perspectives. *Trends Mol Med.* (2010) 16:398–406. doi: 10.1016/j.molmed.2010.07.001
11. Jackson JM, Witek MA, Kamande JW, Soper SA. Materials and microfluidics: enabling the efficient isolation and analysis of circulating tumour cells. *Chem Soc Rev.* (2017) 46:4245–80. doi: 10.1039/C7CS00016B

12. Esmaeilsabzali H, Beischlag TV, Cox ME, Parameswaran AM, Park EJ. Detection and isolation of circulating tumor cells: principles and methods. *Biotechnol Adv.* (2013) 31:1063–84. doi: 10.1016/j.biotechadv.2013.08.016
13. Myung JH, Park SJ, Wang AZ, Hong S. Integration of biomimicry and nanotechnology for significantly improved detection of circulating tumor cells (CTCs). *Adv Drug Deliv Rev.* (2018) 125:36–47. doi: 10.1016/j.addr.2017.12.005
14. Moon DH, Lindsay DP, Hong S, Wang AZ. Clinical indications for, and the future of, circulating tumor cells. *Adv Drug Deliv Rev.* (2018) 125:143–50. doi: 10.1016/j.addr.2018.04.002
15. Zhang N, Deng Y, Tai Q, Cheng B, Zhao L, Shen Q, et al. Electrospun TiO2 nanofiber-based cell capture assay for detecting circulating tumor cells from colorectal and gastric cancer patients. *Adv Mater.* (2012) 24:2756–60. doi: 10.1002/adma.201200155
16. Shen Q, Xu L, Zhao L, Wu D, Fan Y, Zhou Y, et al. Specific capture and release of circulating tumor cells using aptamer-modified nanosubstrates. *Adv Mater.* (2013) 25:2368–73. doi: 10.1002/adma.201300082
17. He R, Zhao L, Liu Y, Zhang N, Cheng B, He Z, et al. Biocompatible TiO2 nanoparticle-based cell immunoassay for circulating tumor cells capture and identification from cancer patients. *Biomed Microdevices.* (2013) 15:617–26. doi: 10.1007/s10544-013-9781-9
18. Cheng B, He Z, Zhao L, Fang Y, Chen Y, He R, et al. Transparent, biocompatible nanostructured surfaces for cancer cell capture and culture. *Int J Nanomed.* (2014) 9:2569–80. doi: 10.2147/IJN.S61233
19. Cheng B, Song H, Wang S, Zhang C, Wu B, Chen Y, et al. Quantification of rare cancer cells in patients with gastrointestinal cancer by nanostructured substrate. *Transl Oncol.* (2014) 7:720–5. doi: 10.1016/j.tranon.2014.10.001
20. Chen YY, Cheng BR, He ZB, Wang SY, Wang ZM, Sun M, et al. Capture and identification of heterogeneous circulating tumor cells using transparent nanomaterials and quantum dots-based multiplexed imaging. *J Cancer.* (2016) 7:69–79. doi: 10.7150/jca.12722
21. Cheng B, Wang S, Chen Y, Fang Y, Chen F, Wang Z, et al. A combined negative and positive enrichment assay for cancer cells isolation and purification. *Technol Cancer Res Treat.* (2016) 15:69–76. doi: 10.7785/tcrt.2012.500447
22. Wang S, Zhang C, Wang G, Cheng B, Wang Y, Chen F, et al. Aptamer-mediated transparent-biocompatible nanostructured surfaces for hepotocellular circulating tumor cells enrichment. *Theranostics.* (2016) 6:1877–86. doi: 10.7150/thno.15284
23. Chen F, Wang S, Fang Y, Zheng L, Zhi X, Cheng B, et al. Feasibility of a novel one-stop ISET device to capture CTCs and its clinical application. *Oncotarget.* (2017) 8:3029–41. doi: 10.18632/oncotarget.13823
24. Yang C, Zhang N, Wang S, Shi D, Zhang C, Liu K, et al. Wedge-shaped microfluidic chip for circulating tumor cells isolation and its clinical significance in gastric cancer. *J Transl Med.* (2018) 16:139. doi: 10.1186/s12967-018-1521-8
25. Yang C, Zou K, Zheng L, Xiong B. Prognostic and clinicopathological significance of circulating tumor cells detected by RT-PCR in non-metastatic colorectal cancer: a meta-analysis and systematic review. *BMC Cancer.* (2017) 17:725. doi: 10.1186/s12885-017-3704-8
26. Yang C, Shi D, Wang S, Wei C, Zhang C, Xiong B. Prognostic value of pre- and post-operative circulating tumor cells detection in colorectal cancer patients treated with curative resection: a prospective cohort study based on ISET device. *Cancer Manag Res.* (2018) 10:4135–44. doi: 10.2147/CMAR.S176575
27. Yang C, Zou K, Yuan Z, Guo T, Xiong B. Prognostic value of circulating tumor cells detected with the CellSearch System in patients with gastric cancer: evidence from a meta-analysis. *Onco Targets Ther.* (2018) 11:1013–23. doi: 10.2147/OTT.S154114
28. Shahneh FZ. Sensitive antibody-based CTCs detection from peripheral blood. *Hum Antibodies.* (2013) 22:51–4. doi: 10.3233/HAB-130270
29. Pastuszak M, Groszewski K, Pastuszak M, Dyrla P, Wojtun S, Gil J. Cytokeratins in gastroenterology. Systematic review. *Prz Gastroenterol.* (2015) 10:61–70. doi: 10.5114/pg.2015.51182
30. Chaudry MA, Sales K, Ruf P, Lindhofer H, Winslet MC. EpCAM an immunotherapeutic target for gastrointestinal malignancy: current experience and future challenges. *Br J Cancer.* (2007) 96:1013–9. doi: 10.1038/sj.bjc.6603505
31. Kujawski R, Mik M, Przybyłowska-Sygut K, Majsterek I, Dziki A. Circulating tumor cells in colorectal cancer. *Pol Przegl Chir.* (2015) 87:277–81. doi: 10.1515/pjs-2015-0054
32. Galletti G, Sung MS, Vahdat LT, Shah MA, Santana SM, Altavilla G, et al. Isolation of breast cancer and gastric cancer circulating tumor cells by use of an anti HER2-based microfluidic device. *Lab Chip.* (2014) 14:147–56. doi: 10.1039/C3LC51039E
33. Gorges TM, Stein A, Quidde J, Hauch S, Rock K, Riethdorf S, et al. Improved detection of circulating tumor cells in metastatic colorectal cancer by the combination of the CellSearch(R) system and the adnatest(R). *PLoS ONE.* (2016) 11:e0155126. doi: 10.1371/journal.pone.0155126
34. Lin HC, Hsu HC, Hsieh CH, Wang HM, Huang CY, Wu MH, et al. A negative selection system PowerMag for effective leukocyte depletion and enhanced detection of EpCAM positive and negative circulating tumor cells. *Clin Chim Acta.* (2013) 419:77–84. doi: 10.1016/j.cca.2013.01.018
35. Wong LS, Bateman WJ, Morris AG, Fraser IA. Detection of circulating tumour cells with the magnetic activated cell sorter. *Br J Surg.* (1995) 82:1333–7. doi: 10.1002/bjs.1800821012
36. Nagrath S, Sequist LV, Maheswaran S, Bell DW, Irimia D, Ulkus L, et al. Isolation of rare circulating tumour cells in cancer patients by microchip technology. *Nature.* (2007) 450:1235–9. doi: 10.1038/nature06385
37. Xia J, Chen X, Zhou CZ, Li YG, Peng ZH. Development of a low-cost magnetic microfluidic chip for circulating tumour cell capture. *IET Nanobiotechnol.* (2011) 5:114–20. doi: 10.1049/iet-nbt.2011.0024
38. Andree KC, van Dalum G, Terstappen LW. Challenges in circulating tumor cell detection by the CellSearch system. *Mol Oncol.* (2016) 10:395–407. doi: 10.1016/j.molonc.2015.12.002
39. Murlidhar V, Rivera-Baez L, Nagrath S. Affinity versus label-free isolation of circulating tumor cells: who wins? *Small.* (2016) 12:4450–63. doi: 10.1002/smll.201601394
40. Jin C, McFaul SM, Duffy SP, Deng X, Tavassoli P, Black PC, et al. Technologies for label-free separation of circulating tumor cells: from historical foundations to recent developments. *Lab Chip.* (2014) 14:32–44. doi: 10.1039/C3LC50625H
41. Nordgard O, Tjensvoll K, Gilje B, Soreide K. Circulating tumour cells and DNA as liquid biopsies in gastrointestinal cancer. *Br J Surg.* (2018) 105:e110–20. doi: 10.1002/bjs.10782
42. Hao SJ, Wan Y, Xia YQ, Zou X, Zheng SY. Size-based separation methods of circulating tumor cells. *Adv Drug Deliv Rev.* (2018) 125:3–20. doi: 10.1016/j.addr.2018.01.002
43. Khamenehfar A, Li PC. Microfluidic devices for circulating tumor cells isolation and subsequent analysis. *Curr Pharm Biotechnol.* (2016) 17:810–21. doi: 10.2174/1389201017666160301103509
44. Shields CWt, Reyes CD, Lopez GP. Microfluidic cell sorting: a review of the advances in the separation of cells from debulking to rare cell isolation. *Lab Chip.* (2015) 15:1230–49. doi: 10.1039/C4LC01246A
45. Xu Y, Qin T, Li J, Wang X, Gao C, Xu C, et al. Detection of circulating tumor cells using negative enrichment immunofluorescence and an *in situ* hybridization system in pancreatic cancer. *Int J Mol Sci.* (2017) 18:E622. doi: 10.3390/ijms18040622
46. Chen JY, Tsai WS, Shao HJ, Wu JC, Lai JM, Lu SH, et al. Sensitive and specific biomimetic lipid coated microfluidics to isolate viable circulating tumor cells and microemboli for cancer detection. *PLoS ONE.* (2016) 11:e0149633. doi: 10.1371/journal.pone.0149633
47. Valladares-Ayerbes M, Diaz-Prado S, Reboredo M, Medina V, Iglesias-Diaz P, Lorenzo-Patino MJ, et al. Bioinformatics approach to mRNA markers discovery for detection of circulating tumor cells in patients with gastrointestinal cancer. *Cancer Detect Prev.* (2008) 32:236–50. doi: 10.1016/j.cdp.2008.08.002
48. Valladares-Ayerbes M, Diaz-Prado S, Reboredo M, Medina V, Lorenzo-Patino MJ, Iglesias-Diaz P, et al. Evaluation of plakophilin-3 mRNA as a biomarker for detection of circulating tumor cells in gastrointestinal cancer patients. *Cancer Epidemiol Biomarkers Prev.* (2010) 19:1432–40. doi: 10.1158/1055-9965.EPI-10-0123
49. Wang S, Zheng G, Cheng B, Chen F, Wang Z, Chen Y, et al. Circulating tumor cells (CTCs) detected by RT-PCR and its prognostic role in gastric cancer: a meta-analysis of published literature. *PLoS ONE.* (2014) 9:e99259. doi: 10.1371/journal.pone.0099259

50. Mansilla C, Soria E, Ramirez N. The identification and isolation of CTCs: a biological Rubik's cube. *Crit Rev Oncol Hematol.* (2018) 126:129–34. doi: 10.1016/j.critrevonc.2018.03.027
51. Rawal S, Yang YP, Cote R, Agarwal A. Identification and quantitation of circulating tumor cells. *Annu Rev Anal Chem.* (2017) 10:321–43. doi: 10.1146/annurev-anchem-061516-045405
52. Lampignano R, Schneck H, Neumann M, Fehm T, Neubauer H. Enrichment, isolation and molecular characterization of EpCAM-negative circulating tumor cells. *Adv Exp Med Biol.* (2017) 994:181–203. doi: 10.1007/978-3-319-55947-6_10
53. Song Y, Tian T, Shi Y, Liu W, Zou Y, Khajvand T, et al. Enrichment and single-cell analysis of circulating tumor cells. *Chem Sci.* (2017) 8:1736–51. doi: 10.1039/C6SC04671A
54. Zhu Z, Qiu S, Shao K, Hou Y. Progress and challenges of sequencing and analyzing circulating tumor cells. *Cell Biol Toxicol.* (2018) 34:405–15. doi: 10.1007/s10565-017-9418-5
55. Ramskold D, Luo S, Wang YC, Li R, Deng Q, Faridani OR, et al. Full-length mRNA-Seq from single-cell levels of RNA and individual circulating tumor cells. *Nat Biotechnol.* (2012) 30:777–82. doi: 10.1038/nbt.2282
56. Pantel K, Alix-Panabieres C. Liquid biopsy in 2016: circulating tumour cells and cell-free DNA in gastrointestinal cancer. *Nat Rev Gastroenterol Hepatol.* (2017) 14:73–4. doi: 10.1038/nrgastro.2016.198
57. Abdallah EA, Braun AC, Flores B, Senda L, Urvanegia AC, Calsavara V, et al. The potential clinical implications of circulating tumor cells and circulating tumor microemboli in gastric cancer. *Oncologist.* (2019) 24:e854–63. doi: 10.1634/theoncologist.2018-0741
58. Brungs D, Lynch D, Luk AW, Minaei E, Ranson M, Aghmesheh M, et al. Cryopreservation for delayed circulating tumor cell isolation is a valid strategy for prognostic association of circulating tumor cells in gastroesophageal cancer. *World J Gastroenterol.* (2018) 24:810–8. doi: 10.3748/wjg.v24.i7.810
59. Ito H, Sato J, Tsujino T, Yamaguchi N, Kimura S, Gohda K, et al. Long-term prognostic impact of circulating tumour cells in gastric cancer patients. *World J Gastroenterol.* (2016) 22:10232–41. doi: 10.3748/wjg.v22.i46.10232
60. Lee SJ, Lee J, Kim ST, Park SH, Park JO, Park YS, et al. Circulating tumor cells are predictive of poor response to chemotherapy in metastatic gastric cancer. *Int J Biol Markers.* (2015) 30:e382–6. doi: 10.5301/jbm.5000151
61. Li Y, Gong J, Zhang Q, Lu Z, Gao J, Li Y, et al. Dynamic monitoring of circulating tumour cells to evaluate therapeutic efficacy in advanced gastric cancer. *Br J Cancer.* (2016) 114:138–45. doi: 10.1038/bjc.2015.417
62. Li Y, Zhang X, Gong J, Zhang Q, Gao J, Cao Y, et al. Aneuploidy of chromosome 8 in circulating tumor cells correlates with prognosis in patients with advanced gastric cancer. *Chin J Cancer Res.* (2016) 28:579–88. doi: 10.21147/j.issn.1000-9604.2016.06.04
63. Liu Y, Ling Y, Qi Q, Lan F, Zhu M, Zhang Y, et al. Prognostic value of circulating tumor cells in advanced gastric cancer patients receiving chemotherapy. *Mol Clin Oncol.* (2017) 6:235–42. doi: 10.3892/mco.2017.1125
64. Meulendijks D, de Groot JW, Los M, Boers JE, Beerepoot LV, Polee MB, et al. Bevacizumab combined with docetaxel, oxaliplatin, and capecitabine, followed by maintenance with capecitabine and bevacizumab, as first-line treatment of patients with advanced HER2-negative gastric cancer: a multicenter phase 2 study. *Cancer.* (2016) 122:1434–43. doi: 10.1002/cncr.29864
65. Okabe H, Tsunoda S, Hosogi H, Hisamori S, Tanaka E, Tanaka S, et al. Circulating tumor cells as an independent predictor of survival in advanced gastric cancer. *Ann Surg Oncol.* (2015) 22:3954–61. doi: 10.1245/s10434-015-4483-6
66. Uenosono Y, Arigami T, Kozono T, Yanagita S, Hagihara T, Haraguchi N, et al. Clinical significance of circulating tumor cells in peripheral blood from patients with gastric cancer. *Cancer.* (2013) 119:3984–91. doi: 10.1002/cncr.28309
67. Zhang Q, Shan F, Li Z, Gao J, Li Y, Shen L, et al. A prospective study on the changes and clinical significance of pre-operative and post-operative circulating tumor cells in resectable gastric cancer. *J Transl Med.* (2018) 16:171. doi: 10.1186/s12967-018-1544-1
68. Zheng X, Fan L, Zhou P, Ma H, Huang S, Yu D, et al. Detection of circulating tumor cells and circulating tumor microemboli in gastric cancer. *Transl Oncol.* (2017) 10:431–41. doi: 10.1016/j.tranon.2017.02.007
69. Wang L, Zhou S, Zhang W, Wang J, Wang M, Hu X, et al. Circulating tumor cells as an independent prognostic factor in advanced colorectal cancer: a retrospective study in 121 patients. *Int J Colorectal Dis.* (2019) 34:589–97. doi: 10.1007/s00384-018-03223-9
70. Bahnassy AA, Salem SE, Mohanad M, Abulezz NZ, Abdellateif MS, Hussein M, et al. Prognostic significance of circulating tumor cells (CTCs) in Egyptian non-metastatic colorectal cancer patients: a comparative study for four different techniques of detection (Flowcytometry, CellSearch, Quantitative Real-time PCR and Cytomorphology). *Exp Mol Pathol.* (2019) 106:90–101. doi: 10.1016/j.yexmp.2018.12.006
71. Delgado-Urena M, Ortega FG, de Miguel-Perez D, Rodriguez-Martinez A, Garcia-Puche JL, Ilyine H, et al. Circulating tumor cells criteria (CyCAR) versus standard RECIST criteria for treatment response assessment in metastatic colorectal cancer patients. *J Transl Med.* (2018) 16:251. doi: 10.1186/s12967-018-1624-2
72. Messaritakis I, Sfakianaki M, Papadaki C, Koulouridi A, Vardakis N, Koinis F, et al. Prognostic significance of CEACAM5mRNA-positive circulating tumor cells in patients with metastatic colorectal cancer. *Cancer Chemother Pharmacol.* (2018) 82:767–75. doi: 10.1007/s00280-018-3666-9
73. Wang W, Wan L, Wu S, Yang J, Zhou Y, Liu F, et al. Mesenchymal marker and LGR5 expression levels in circulating tumor cells correlate with colorectal cancer prognosis. *Cell Oncol.* (2018) 41:495–504. doi: 10.1007/s13402-018-0386-4
74. Zhang Y, Zarrabi K, Hou W, Madajewicz S, Choi M, Zucker S, et al. Assessing clinical outcomes in colorectal cancer with assays for invasive circulating tumor cells. *Biomedicines.* (2018) 6:E69. doi: 10.3390/biomedicines6020069
75. Hashimoto M, Tanaka F, Yoneda K, Takuwa T, Kuroda A, Matsumoto S, et al. The clinical value of circulating tumour cells (CTCs) in patients undergoing pulmonary metastasectomy for metastatic colorectal cancer. *J Thorac Dis.* (2018) 10:1569–77. doi: 10.21037/jtd.2018.03.05
76. Chou WC, Wu MH, Chang PH, Hsu HC, Chang GJ, Huang WK, et al. A prognostic model based on circulating tumour cells is useful for identifying the poorest survival outcome in patients with metastatic colorectal cancer. *Int J Biol Sci.* (2018) 14:137–46. doi: 10.7150/ijbs.23182
77. Fang C, Fan C, Wang C, Huang Q, Meng W, Yu Y, et al. Prognostic value of CD133(+) CD54(+) CD44(+) circulating tumor cells in colorectal cancer with liver metastasis. *Cancer Med.* (2017) 6:2850–7. doi: 10.1002/cam4.1241
78. Zhang D, Zhao L, Zhou P, Ma H, Huang F, Jin M, et al. Circulating tumor microemboli (CTM) and vimentin+ circulating tumor cells (CTCs) detected by a size-based platform predict worse prognosis in advanced colorectal cancer patients during chemotherapy. *Cancer Cell Int.* (2017) 17:6. doi: 10.1186/s12935-016-0373-7
79. Hinz S, Hendricks A, Wittig A, Schafmayer C, Tepel J, Kalthoff H, et al. Detection of circulating tumor cells with CK20 RT-PCR is an independent negative prognostic marker in colon cancer patients - a prospective study. *BMC Cancer.* (2017) 17:53. doi: 10.1186/s12885-016-3035-1
80. Bork U, Rahbari NN, Scholch S, Reissfelder C, Kahlert C, Buchler MW, et al. Circulating tumour cells and outcome in non-metastatic colorectal cancer: a prospective study. *Br J Cancer.* (2015) 112:1306–13. doi: 10.1038/bjc.2015.88
81. Sotelo MJ, Sastre J, Maestro ML, Veganzones S, Vieitez JM, Alonso V, et al. Role of circulating tumor cells as prognostic marker in resected stage III colorectal cancer. *Ann Oncol.* (2015) 26:535–41. doi: 10.1093/annonc/mdu568
82. Seeberg LT, Waage A, Brunborg C, Hugenschmidt H, Renolen A, Stav I, et al. Circulating tumor cells in patients with colorectal liver metastasis predict impaired survival. *Ann Surg.* (2015) 261:164–71. doi: 10.1097/SLA.0000000000000580
83. Musella V, Pietrantonio F, Di Buduo E, Iacovelli R, Martinetti A, Sottotetti E, et al. Circulating tumor cells as a longitudinal biomarker in patients with advanced chemorefractory, RAS-BRAF wild-type colorectal cancer receiving cetuximab or panitumumab. *Int J Cancer.* (2015) 137:1467–74. doi: 10.1002/ijc.29493
84. van Dalum G, Stam GJ, Scholten LF, Mastboom WJ, Vermes I, Tibbe AG, et al. Importance of circulating tumor cells in newly diagnosed colorectal cancer. *Int J Oncol.* (2015) 46:1361–8. doi: 10.3892/ijo.2015.2824

85. Kuboki Y, Matsusaka S, Minowa S, Shibata H, Suenaga M, Shinozaki E, et al. Circulating tumor cell (CTC) count and epithelial growth factor receptor expression on CTCs as biomarkers for cetuximab efficacy in advanced colorectal cancer. *Anticancer Res.* (2013) 33:3905–10.
86. Gazzaniga P, Raimondi C, Gradilone A, Biondi Zoccai G, Nicolazzo C, Gandini O, et al. Circulating tumor cells in metastatic colorectal cancer: do we need an alternative cutoff? *J Cancer Res Clin Oncol.* (2013) 139:1411–6. doi: 10.1007/s00432-013-1450-0
87. Sastre J, Maestro ML, Gomez-Espana A, Rivera F, Valladares M, Massuti B, et al. Circulating tumor cell count is a prognostic factor in metastatic colorectal cancer patients receiving first-line chemotherapy plus bevacizumab: a Spanish Cooperative Group for the Treatment of Digestive Tumors study. *Oncologist.* (2012) 17:947–55. doi: 10.1634/theoncologist.2012-0048
88. Matsusaka S, Suenaga M, Mishima Y, Kuniyoshi R, Takagi K, Terui Y, et al. Circulating tumor cells as a surrogate marker for determining response to chemotherapy in Japanese patients with metastatic colorectal cancer. *Cancer Sci.* (2011) 102:1188–92. doi: 10.1111/j.1349-7006.2011.01926.x
89. Iinuma H, Watanabe T, Mimori K, Adachi M, Hayashi N, Tamura J, et al. Clinical significance of circulating tumor cells, including cancer stem-like cells, in peripheral blood for recurrence and prognosis in patients with Dukes' stage B and C colorectal cancer. *J Clin Oncol.* (2011) 29:1547–55. doi: 10.1200/JCO.2010.30.5151
90. Tol J, Koopman M, Miller MC, Tibbe A, Cats A, Creemers GJ, et al. Circulating tumour cells early predict progression-free and overall survival in advanced colorectal cancer patients treated with chemotherapy and targeted agents. *Ann Oncol.* (2010) 21:1006–12. doi: 10.1093/annonc/mdp463
91. Cohen SJ, Punt CJ, Iannotti N, Saidman BH, Sabbath KD, Gabrail NY, et al. Relationship of circulating tumor cells to tumor response, progression-free survival, and overall survival in patients with metastatic colorectal cancer. *J Clin Oncol.* (2008) 26:3213–21. doi: 10.1200/JCO.2007.15.8923
92. Yang C, Wei C, Wang S, Han S, Shi D, Zhang C, et al. Combined features based on preoperative controlling nutritional status score and circulating tumour cell status predict prognosis for colorectal cancer patients treated with curative resection. *Int J Biol Sci.* (2019) 15:1325–35. doi: 10.7150/ijbs.33671
93. Zou K, Yang S, Zheng L, Wang S, Xiong B. Prognostic role of the circulating tumor cells detected by cytological methods in gastric cancer: a meta-analysis. *Biomed Res Int.* (2016) 2016:2765464. doi: 10.1155/2016/2765464
94. Alix-Panabieres C, Pantel K. Challenges in circulating tumour cell research. *Nat Rev Cancer.* (2014) 14:623–31. doi: 10.1038/nrc3820
95. Hinz S, Roder C, Tepel J, Hendricks A, Schafmayer C, Becker T, et al. Cytokeratin 20 positive circulating tumor cells are a marker for response after neoadjuvant chemoradiation but not for prognosis in patients with rectal cancer. *BMC Cancer.* (2015) 15:953. doi: 10.1186/s12885-015-1989-z
96. Kubisch I, de Albuquerque A, Schuppan D, Kaul S, Schaich M, Stolzel U. Prognostic role of a multimarker analysis of circulating tumor cells in advanced gastric and gastroesophageal adenocarcinomas. *Oncology.* (2015) 89:294–303. doi: 10.1159/000437373
97. Magni E, Botteri E, Ravenda PS, Cassatella MC, Bertani E, Chiappa A, et al. Detection of circulating tumor cells in patients with locally advanced rectal cancer undergoing neoadjuvant therapy followed by curative surgery. *Int J Colorectal Dis.* (2014) 29:1053–9. doi: 10.1007/s00384-014-1958-z
98. Mishima Y, Matsusaka S, Chin K, Mikuniya M, Minowa S, Takayama T, et al. Detection of HER2 amplification in circulating tumor cells of HER2-negative gastric cancer patients. *Target Oncol.* (2017) 12:341–51. doi: 10.1007/s11523-017-0493-6
99. Tang L, Zhao S, Liu W, Parchim NF, Huang J, Tang Y, et al. Diagnostic accuracy of circulating tumor cells detection in gastric cancer: systematic review and meta-analysis. *BMC Cancer.* (2013) 13:314. doi: 10.1186/1471-2407-13-314
100. Lee AW, Lin FX, Wei PL, Jian-Wei G, Chen JK. Binary-blend fibber-based capture assay of circulating tumor cells for clinical diagnosis of colorectal cancer. *J Nanobiotechnol.* (2018) 16:4. doi: 10.1186/s12951-017-0330-1
101. Chen CJ, Sung WW, Chen HC, Chern YJ, Hsu HT, Lin YM, et al. Early assessment of colorectal cancer by quantifying circulating tumor cells in peripheral blood: ECT2 in diagnosis of colorectal cancer. *Int J Mol Sci.* (2017) 18:743. doi: 10.3390/ijms18040743

6

The Effectiveness of Gastrectomy with Chemoradiotherapy Among Stage IV Gastric Adenocarcinoma

Shuchun Li [1,2] ***and Lu Zang*** [1,2*]

[1] *Department of Surgery, Ruijin Hospital, Shanghai Jiaotong University School of Medicine, Shanghai, China,*

[2] *Shanghai Minimally Invasive Surgery Center, Shanghai, China*

Correspondence:
Lu Zang
zanglu@yeah.net

Objectives: The strategy for the treatment of stage IV gastric cancer remains controversial. The objective of this study was to assess whether tumor resection is beneficial to survival in gastric cancer patients with incurable stage IV disease.

Methods: This is a retrospective cohort study of gastric cancer patients in the Surveillance, Epidemiology, and End Results (SEER) database between 2010 and 2015. Due to the baseline bias, 1:1 propensity score matching (PSM) was used in this cohort. Patients were grouped by treatment, (1) gastrectomy with chemoradiotherapy (CRT), or (2) CRT only, and a Cox proportional hazards regression model was used to identify predictors of survival. Overall survival was compared between the two groups using the Kaplan-Meier method.

Result: After propensity score matching, 162 stage IV gastric cancer patients diagnosed from 2010 to 2015 were identified. Among these patients, half underwent gastrectomy with CRT, while the others received CRT only. The median overall survival rates were 22 months from the date of surgery for the gastrectomy with CRT group and 9.0 months for CRT only group. In the multivariable Cox regression analysis, surgery was associated with a significant improvement in overall survival [hazard ratio (HR) of death = 0.31, 95% confidence interval (CI) = 0.21–0.46, $P < 0.0001$].

Conclusion: In conclusion, stage IV gastric cancer is still a fatal disease. This population-based study found that compared with CRT alone, CRT with gastrectomy may be associated with a survival benefit in patients with metastatic GC. In selected patients' survival can be prolonged when the primary tumor is removed. Prospective, randomized trials are required to determine the best strategy for metastatic GC and to describe the characteristics of the selected patients.

Keywords: gastric cancer, metastasis, gastrectomy, chemoradiotherapy, survival

INTRODUCTION

Gastric cancer (GC) is an aggressive cancer and the third leading cause of cancer-related death worldwide (1). Since it is usually diagnosed when the tumor is locally advanced or metastatic, it has a poor prognosis. However, the standard treatment strategy for metastatic gastric cancer remains controversial. Many clinical trials have proven that combination chemotherapy improves the overall survival (OS) and quality of life of metastatic gastric cancer compared that in patients treated with supportive care (2, 3). For patients with a good general condition, current practice guidelines recommend palliative chemotherapy in the European Society for Medical Oncology (ESMO) guidelines (4) and chemoradiotion or systemic therapy in the National Comprehensive Cancer Network (NCCN) guidelines (5). Due to the poor prognosis, it is crucial to look for innovative methods or the appropriate combination of treatments.

The value of surgery in metastatic GC remains controversial. Recently, REGATTA, a randomized controlled trial, has denied the effectiveness of palliative gastrectomy for metastatic GC (6). However, some studies indicated that many patients with unresectable tumors survived for a long period when they underwent curative resection after chemotherapy. Curative surgery after chemotherapy is called as conversion surgery. It is defined as a surgical treatment aiming at R0 resection after systemic therapy in initially unresectable tumors (7). This approach has been shown to be a potential option for some metastatic GC patients.

The aim of this population-based cohort study was to determine the efficacy of chemoradiotherapy with gastrectomy and whether it could prolong survival in patients with stage IV gastric cancer.

MATERIALS AND METHODS

Data Source

A retrospective cohort study was carried out using the Surveillance, Epidemiology, and End Results (SEER) database[1], which is a population-based cancer registry covering ~34.6% of the U.S. population. The SEER database has collected cancer incidence, prevalence, and survival data from 18 registries of the U.S. since 1973 (www.seer.cancer.gov). The SEER database includes data on patient demographics, cancer site, histologic type, stage, dates of diagnosis and survival. SEER*Stat version 8.3.5 was used to extract the patient data. The chemotherapy and radiation therapy (RT) status was obtained after an additional authorization and informed the potential bias related to these data (8).

Patient Selection

Patients with gastric adenocarcinoma diagnosed in 2010–2015 were included in this study. Histologically diagnosed cases were identified by the specific codes of the International Classification of Diseases for Oncology, 3rd edition (ICD-O-3), including 8140/3, 8144/3, 8145/3, 8255/3, 8260/3, 8480/3, 8481/3, and 8490/3. The primary sites with ICD-O-3 topography codes from C16.0 to C16.9 were used in this study. The workflow for patient selection is shown in **Figure 1**. We identified 32,008 patients 18 years or older with gastric cancer. Among these, 6,215 patients were excluded because GC was not the initial diagnosis, and we subsequently also removed patients who were diagnosed at autopsy or from death certificate or who were missing baseline information. To prevent the limitation of missing treatment records, we only enrolled patients who had both chemotherapy and radiotherapy. Finally, 249 cases were enrolled for further analysis.

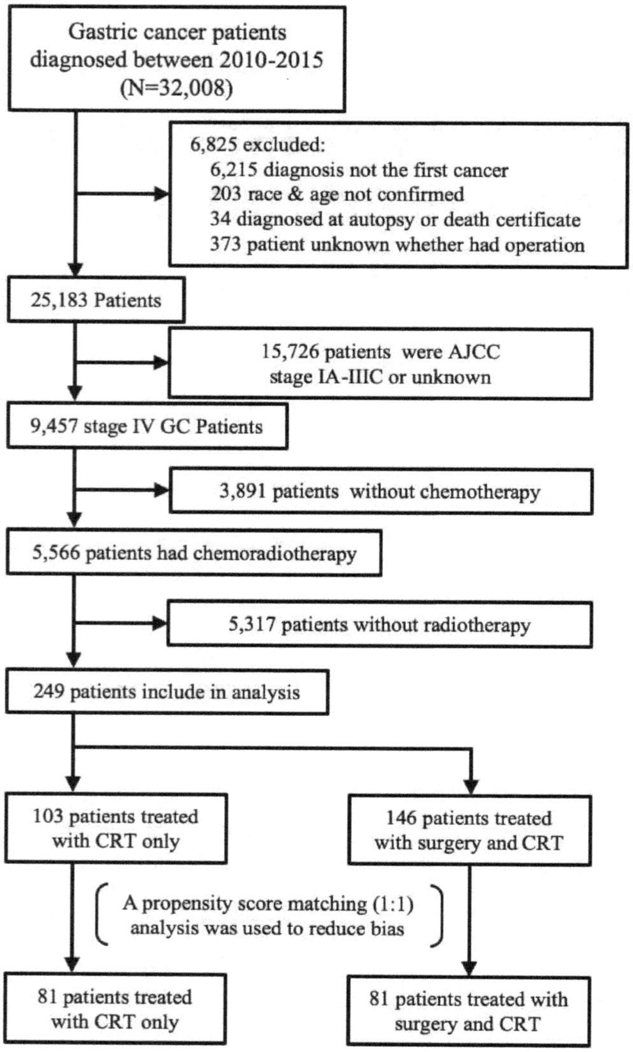

FIGURE 1 | Flowchart of data extraction from SEER database.

Statistical Analysis

Chi-square tests were used to compare categorical variables. In an observational study, a propensity score matching analysis can be used to balance the distribution of observed baseline covariates between treated and untreated subjects and reduce the bias of selection (9, 10). By applying propensity score matching to adjust for group differences in this cohort, we first used demographic parameters, including age, sex, race, tumor location, primary site invasion depth, regional lymph nodes

[1]Surveillance, Epidemiology, and End Results (SEER) Program (www.seer.cancer.gov) SEERStat Database: Incidence - SEER 9 Regs Research Data, Nov 2017 Sub (1973–2015) <Katrina/Rita Population Adjustment> - Linked To County Attributes - Total U.S., 1969–2016 Counties, National Cancer Institute, DCCPS, Surveillance Research Program, released April 2018, based on the November 2017 submission.

TABLE 1 | Clinical characteristics of patients who were diagnosed with stage IV gastric cancer involved in study.

	Patient characteristics in raw data			Patient characteristics after propensity score weighting		
	CRT only $n = 103$	Gastrectomy + CRT $n = 146$	p	CRT only $n = 81$	Gastrectomy + CRT $n = 81$	p
Age at diagnosis (years)			0.924			0.926
20–39	12 (11.65)	14 (9.58)		10 (12.35)	10 (12.35)	
40–59	43 (41.75)	64 (43.84)		34 (41.98)	30 (37.04)	
60–79	46 (44.66)	64 (43.84)		35 (43.21)	39 (48.15)	
>=80	2 (1.94)	4 (2.74)		2 (2.47)	2 (2.47)	
Sex			0.883			0.863
Male	73 (70.87)	101 (69.19)		58 (71.60)	57 (70.37)	
Female	30 (29.13)	45 (30.82)		23 (28.40)	24 (29.63)	
Race			0.224			0.240
White	77 (75.76)	102 (69.86)		62 (76.54)	61 (75.31)	
Black	7 (6.80)	20 (13.70)		3 (3.70)	8 (9.88)	
Others	19 (18.45)	24 (16.44)		16 (19.75)	12 (14.81)	
T stage			<0.001			<0.001
T1	15 (14.56)	6 (4.11)		15 (18.52)	2 (2.47)	
T2	3 (2.91)	12 (8.22)		3 (3.70)	5 (6.17)	
T3	28 (27.18)	60 (41.10)		27 (33.33)	38 (46.91)	
T4	17 (16.50)	63 (43.15)		14 (17.28)	31 (38.27)	
TX	40 (38.83)	5 (3.42)		22 (27.16)	5 (6.17)	
N Stage			<0.001			0.001
N0	29 (28.16)	21 (14.38)		16 (19.75)	18 (22.22)	
N1	49 (47.57)	40 (27.40)		40 (49.38)	28 (34.57)	
N2	11 (10.68)	38 (26.03)		11 (13.58)	20 (24.69)	
N3	4 (3.88)	45 (30.82)		4 (4.94)	14 (17.28)	
NX	10 (9.71)	2 (1.37)		10 (12.35)	1 (1.23)	
Location			<0.001			0.165
Cardia & Fund	74 (71.84)	58 (39.73)		54 (66.67)	44 (54.32)	
Body	10 (9.71)	11 (7.53)		9 (11.11)	8 (9.88)	
Antrum & Pylorus	6 (5.83)	33 (22.60)		6 (7.41)	15 (18.52)	
Others	13 (12.62)	44 (30.14)		12 (14.81)	14 (17.28)	
Year of diagnosis			0.108			0.245
2010–2011	27 (26.21)	57 (39.04)		24 (29.63)	32 (39.51)	
2012–2013	38 (36.89)	44 (30.14)		29 (35.80)	20 (24.69)	
2014–2015	38 (36.89)	45 (30.82)		28 (34.57)	29 (35.80)	
Lauren classification			0.154			0.170
Intestinal	78 (75.73)	94 (64.38)		64 (79.01)	58 (71.60)	
Diffuse	24 (23.30)	49 (33.56)		17 (20.99)	20 (24.69)	
Others	1 (0.97)	3 (2.05)		0 (0)	3 (3.70)	
Extend of gastrectomy			–			–
Total	–	67 (45.89)		–	39 (48.15)	
Partial/sub-total	–	79 (54.11)		–	42 (51.85)	
Regional node examined			–			–
<15	–	59 (40.41)		–	31 (38.27)	
15–25	–	45 (30.82)		–	27 (33.33)	
>25	–	27 (18.50)		–	14 (17.28)	
UK	–	15 (10.27)		–	9 (11.11)	

In the tables, the number in parentheses is the constituent ratio.

involved, Lauren classification and marital status, to create a logistic regression model. Then, every patient had a propensity score, which was utilized to match between the CRT with surgery group and the CRT only group (1:1 matching). The median overall survival duration was measured by the Kaplan-Meier method. The survival durations in the CRT group and the CRT with surgery group were compared by the log-rank test. Multivariable Cox proportional hazards regression models were assessed to determine the factors that were associated with survival. Statistical analyses were performed with SPSS, version 23 (IBM Corporation, Armonk, NY, USA), and R, version 3.5.1 (R Foundation for Statistical Computing, Vienna, Austria. https://www.R-project.org/). All statistical tests were two-sided, and $p < 0.05$ was considered statistically significant.

RESULTS

Demographics and Clinical Parameters of the Cohort

There were 32,008 gastric adenocarcinoma patients extracted from the SEER database from 2010 to 2015. Finally, we identified 249 patients who met the inclusion criteria (**Figure 1**). Among the unmatched cohort, 103 underwent CRT only, and 146 had CRT with gastrectomy. Chi-square tests revealed a significant difference between the two groups. Compared with the CRT group, the CRT with gastrectomy group had a higher proportion of patients with more lymph node metastasis, especially for N3 grade (30.82 vs. 3.88%; $p < 0.001$). The primary site of the lesion was more likely located in the lower third of the stomach in the CRT with gastrectomy group (22.6 vs. 5.83; $p < 0.001$) (**Table 1**). The mean number of regional lymph nodes examined in the CRT with gastrectomy group was 18.40 ± 13.08. Approximately 43% of the patients had more than 15 lymph nodes examined. For the data on the surgical methods, the extent of gastrectomy was classified as total or partial/subtotal gastrectomy. The information on distant metastasis is shown in **Table 2**. The reasons for diagnosing stage IV gastric cancer varied, including liver involvement (23.29%), distant lymph nodes (22.49%), brain involvement (11.24%), bone involvement (13.65%), and lung involvement (12.05%). A propensity score matched analysis was used to partially reduce the baseline imbalance between the groups. Finally, 81 pairs of patients were generated by PSM one-to-one matching. For the patients who underwent surgery, 39 (48.15%), and 42 (51.85%) underwent total and partial/subtotal gastrectomy, respectively. A detailed comparison of the demographics and clinical characteristics of unmatched and matched patients is shown in **Table 1**.

Survival Outcomes

In the unmatched cohort, the median overall survival was 10 months for patients in the CRT group vs. 17 months for patients in the CRT with gastrectomy group. The Kaplan-Meier curves for overall survival are shown in **Figure 2A**. The log-rank test showed that the CRT with gastrectomy group had better overall survival than the CRT only group ($p < 0.0001$). After matching, the results were similar between the two groups (**Figure 2B**). The CRT with gastrectomy group had a 13-month longer median overall survival than the CRT only group (22 vs. 9 months for OS, $p < 0.0001$ log-rank test).

Evaluation of Prognostic Factors

The multivariate analysis of all patients indicated that surgery (HR = 0.23, 95% CI 0.14–0.36, $p < 0.0001$) and primary site located in antrum & pylorus (HR = 1.82, 95% CI 1.00–3.30, $p = 0.05$) were related to reduced mortality (**Table 3**). In the 81 paired cases, the Cox proportional hazards model was used to evaluate the prognostic factors for overall survival. Surgery was the only independent prognostic factor for OS (HR = 0.31, 95% CI 0.21–0.46, $p < 0.001$). The influence of surgery on mortality remained robust with adjustment for age, sex, race, tumor invasion depth, lymph node metastasis and primary site location. The details are illustrated in **Figure 3**.

TABLE 2 | Type of distant metastasis in the cohort before matching.

Distant metastasis organ involved	Patient number[a] N = 25183	Patient number[b] N = 249
Liver	3909 (15.52)	58 (23.29)
Distant lymph nodes	2960 (11.75)	56 (22.49)
Lung	1369 (5.44)	30 (12.05)
Bone	1208 (4.80)	34 (13.65)
Brain	189 (0.75)	28 (11.24)

[a] The gastric cancer patients extracted from SEER database. [b] The patients enrolled in this study. In the tables, the number in parentheses is the constituent ratio.

DISCUSSION

Stage IV gastric cancer remains a lethal disease, and the median overall survival of metastatic or unresectable GC is ~4.6–13.1 months, as reported in previous studies (11–13). In this population-based analysis, the medial OS was 14 months, which is similar to that in a previous report. Interestingly, our investigation provides evidence of a strong association between surgery and decreased overall mortality in metastatic gastric cancer patients who received chemoradiotherapy in a large population-based study. The sensitivity analysis showed that surgery was a prognostic factor for overall survival in both the unmatched and matched cohorts. Gastric cancer disseminates principally through hematic flow or peritoneal spread. The most common metastatic distribution is to the liver and peritoneal surfaces. In previous reports, the overall rates of metastasis to the liver and peritoneum were 9.9–18.7% and 12.3%, respectively, (14, 15). In our study, the hepatic metastatic rate was 15.52%, which is similar to that in a previous study. However, there is little information on other metastatic sites in the SEER database, especially peritoneal metastasis.

The primary aim of treatment for stage IV GC is to delay disease progression and relieve symptoms such as tumor-related hemorrhage or obstruction. Systemic therapy is the primary treatment for metastatic gastric cancer. Surgery is only performed when bleeding or obstruction occurs (16). However, whether the addition of gastrectomy to chemotherapy improves survival for metastatic GC remains controversial. The Dutch Gastric Cancer Group reported that palliative resection may increase the survival rate (8.1 vs. 5.4 months, $p < 0.001$) in patients with incurable GC, especially in patients with only one metastatic site who are under 70 years old (17). A retrospective study including 288 patients also showed that the median overall survival rates were 12 months and 7.8 months for patients with and without primary

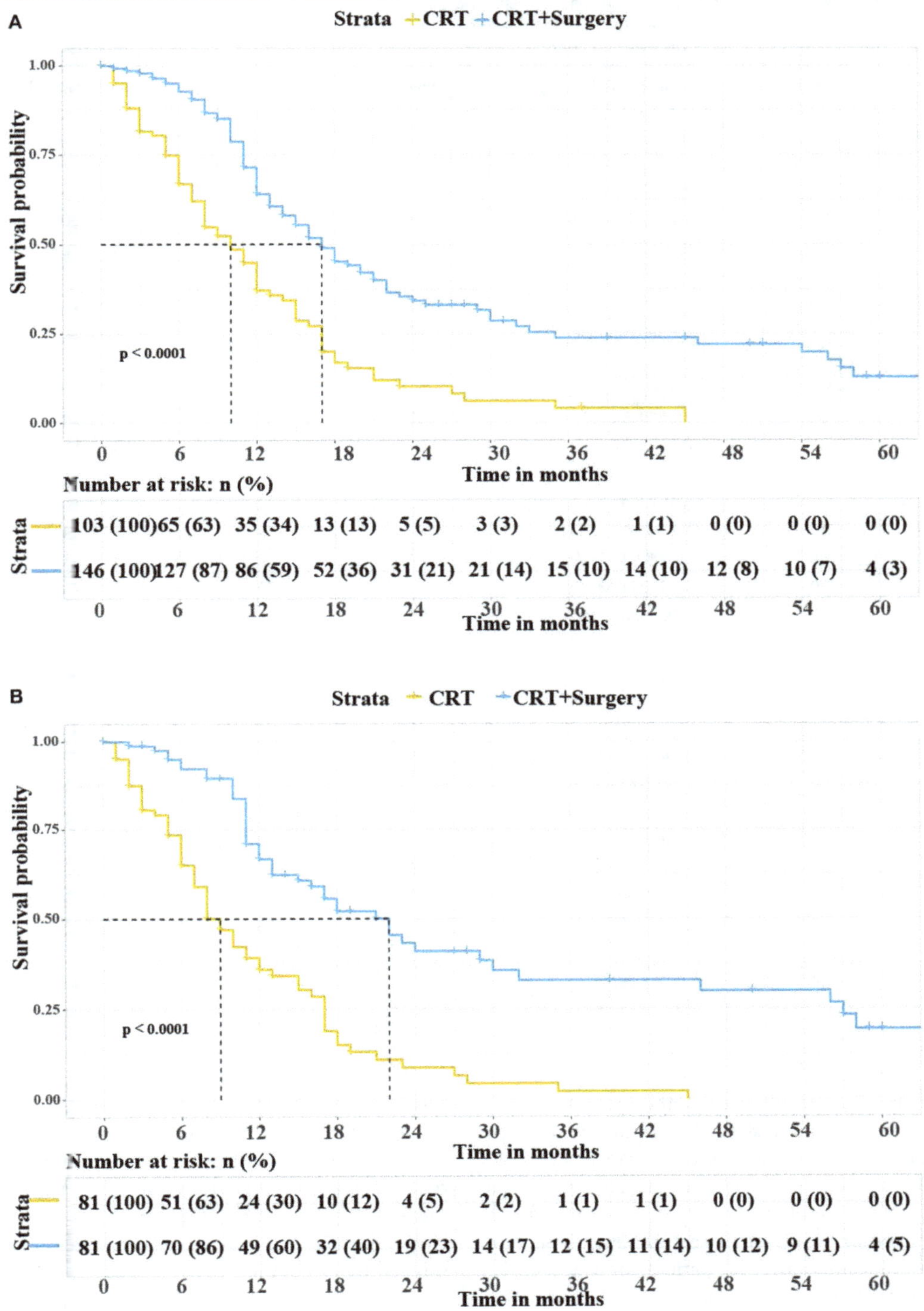

FIGURE 2 | (A) Overall survival rate according to the treatment modalities in all patients. **(B)** Overall survival rate according to the treatment modalities in matched patients. CRT, chemoradiotherapy.

tumor resection, respectively ($p < 0.001$) (18). Leonardo et al. used the GIRGC database and analyzed stage IV unresectable tumors. These tumors became resectable after chemotherapy. Further analysis showed that these patients could benefit from radical gastrectomy. More than one type of metastatic lesion was the main prognostic factor in these patients (HR 4.41, 95% CI 1.72–11.3, $p = 0.002$) (19).

These results indicate that tumor burden reduction was correlated with prolonged OS in patients with metastatic GCs. Moreover, circulating tumor cells (CTCs) are the tumor cells

TABLE 3 | Multivariable cox regression analysis predicting mortality risk for metastatic GC both in unmatched and matched cohorts.

	Unmatched cohort			Matched cohort		
Characteristics	***n***	**HR (95CI%)**	***p*-Value**	***n***	**HR (95CI%)**	***p*-Value**
Age at diagnosis (years)						
20–39	26	1[Reference]	NA	20	1[Reference]	NA
40–59	107	1.28 (0.73–2.24)	0.39	64	1.16 (0.64–2.12)	0.62
60–79	109	1.27 (0.71–2.28)	0.42	74	1.10 (0.60–2.02)	0.75
>=80	7	0.92 (0.29–2.95)	0.89	4	0.52 (0.12–2.30)	0.39
Sex						
Male	174	1[Reference]	NA	115	1[Reference]	NA
Female	75	0.85 (0.58–1.24)	0.39	47	0.85 (0.56–1.29)	0.45
Race						
White	179	1[Reference]	NA	123	1[Reference]	NA
Black	27	1.05 (0.59–1.86)	0.86	11	0.74 (0.34–1.59)	0.44
Others	43	0.85 (0.53–1.37)	0.51	28	0.89 (0.54–1.49)	0.67
T stage						
T1	21	1[Reference]	NA	17	1[Reference]	NA
T2	15	1.74 (0.72–4.25)	0.22	8	0.97 (0.34–2.75)	0.95
T3	88	1.07 (0.56–2.04)	0.84	65	0.59 (0.31–1.13)	0.11
T4	80	1.13 (0.56–2.33)	0.71	45	0.77 (0.40–1.49)	0.43
TX	45	0.90 (0.47–1.72)	0.76	27	1.17 (0.57–2.40)	0.67
N Stage						
N0	50	1[Reference]	NA	34	1[Reference]	NA
N1	89	1.22 (0.76–1.95)	0.41	68	1.21 (0.73–2.03)	0.46
N2	49	1.22 (0.69–2.17)	0.49	31	0.81 (0.43–1.54)	0.53
N3	49	1.74 (1.00–3.04)	0.05	18	1.55 (0.77–3.1)	0.22
NX	12	1.24 (0.61–2.55)	0.55	11	1.73 (0.81–3.68)	0.16
Location						
Cardia & Fund	132	1[Reference]	NA	98	1[Reference]	NA
Body	21	0.85 (0.44–1.65)	0.63	17	0.68 (0.36–1.26)	0.22
Antrum & Pylorus	39	1.82 (1.00–3.30)	0.05	21	0.87 (0.49–1.56)	0.64
Others	57	2.10 (1.20–3.68)	0.01	26	1.14 (0.68–1.91)	0.62
Surgery						
No	103	1[Reference]	NA	81	1[Reference]	NA
Yes	146	0.23 (0.14–0.36)	<0.0001	81	0.31 (0.21–0.46)	<0.0001

left from the primary site, and they enter the bloodstream. It has recently been a topic of interest in clinical cancer research (20). In other solid tumors, such as colorectal cancer (21) and ovarian cancer (22), a reduction in tumor burden was related to longer survival. Recent research on CTCs in gastric cancer provides some evidence for the positive effects of tumor resection because the OS is significantly lower for patients in whom CTCs are identified than for those without them (23).

The REGATTA trial, an open label, randomized, phase 3 trial, was designed to determine the value of gastrectomy in unresectable advanced GC, providing the highest level of evidence about this question (6). This study demonstrated that gastrectomy followed by chemotherapy did not show any survival benefit compared with chemotherapy alone. This conclusion was adopted in the new version of the Japanese gastric cancer treatment guidelines (16). Reduction surgery is not recommended for GC with a single non-cured factor. Although this study represents the highest level of evidence for gastrectomy for metastatic GC, there remain some limitations that deserve discussion. First, this study started in 2008. The chemotherapy regimen used in this study was S-1 plus cisplatin, which is the standard treatment for advanced GC in East Asia (24). However, with the development of chemotherapy, it has been showed that SOX (S-1 plus oxaliplatin) is a preferable regimen in terms of the safety profile (13). Second, the gastrectomy arm in this study had neither D2 lymphadenectomy nor adjacent organ resection, which suggested that it did not achieve R0 resection. D2 lymphadenectomy has been the standard procedure for resectable advanced GC for a long time (25). At the same time, previous studies demonstrated that R0 resection was a significant independent predictor of overall survival in patients who underwent conversion surgery (26, 27). D2 lymphadenectomy is related to higher post-operative mortality and morbidity, which may have negative effects on stage IV GC patients. Even so,

Characteristics	n	HR(95CI%)	p Value
Age at diagnosis(years)			
20–39	20	1[Reference]	
40–59	64	1.16(0.64–2.12)	0.620
60–79	74	1.10(0.60–2.02)	0.752
>=80	4	0.52(0.12–2.30)	0.389
Sex			
Male	115	1[Reference]	
Female	47	0.85(0.56–1.29)	0.446
Race			
White	123	1[Reference]	
Black	11	0.74(0.34–1.59)	0.438
Others	28	0.89(0.54–1.49)	0.666
T stage			
T1	17	1[Reference]	
T2	8	0.97(0.34–2.75)	0.948
T3	65	0.59(0.31–1.13)	0.110
T4	45	0.77(0.40–1.49)	0.432
TX	27	1.17(0.57–2.40)	0.666
N Stage			
N0	34	1[Reference]	
N1	68	1.21(0.73–2.03)	0.460
N2	31	0.81(0.43–1.54)	0.528
N3	18	1.55(0.77–3.1)	0.218
NX	11	1.73(0.81–3.68)	0.155
Location			
Cardia & Fund	98	1[Reference]	
Body	17	0.68(0.36–1.26)	0.218
Antrun & Pylorus	21	0.87(0.49–1.56)	0.644
Others	26	1.14(0.68–1.91)	0.617
Surgery			
No	81	1[Reference]	
Yes	81	0.31(0.21–0.46)	<0.0001

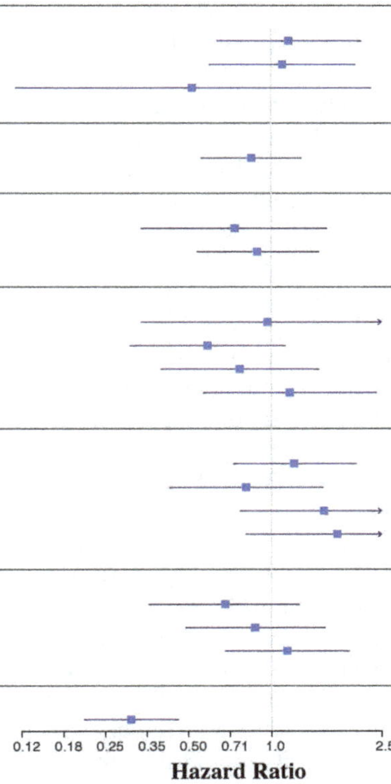

FIGURE 3 | Forest plot of overall survival stratified analysis in the matched cohort.

R0 resection is important for prolonging OS. Furthermore, in the subgroup analyses of overall survival, the median number of chemotherapy cycles was decreased in gastrectomy with chemotherapy group compared with the chemotherapy alone group in patients with upper-third tumor (3 vs. 6 cycles). All of the points mentioned above had side effects on achieving the positive results for the trial. Besides, in the chemotherapy alone group, 5 patients underwent curable gastrectomy and get a long-term survival since complete disappearance of incurable factors after chemotherapy. Therefore, the value of gastrectomy in patients with metastatic GC should not be denied absolutely.

Conversion surgery is defined as a surgical treatment aiming at R0 resection after systemic therapy for tumors that were initially incurable (28). In recent years, positive progress for conversion surgery has been made in clinical trials. AIO-FLOT3 is an II-phase clinical study which is designed to investigate the efficacy of chemotherapy and surgery in patients with advanced gastric cancer (29). The study consisted of 3 arms. A total of 51 patients with resectable gastric cancer were included in arm A, who underwent radical surgery after 4 cycles of FLOT neoadjuvant chemotherapy and were treated with 4 cycles of FLOT chemotherapy after surgery. A total of 60 patients with localized metastatic gastric cancer were included in arm B. The localized metastasis refers to single organ metastasis with or without retroperitoneal lymph node metastasis. The patients in arm B received at least 4 cycles of FLOT chemotherapy and proceeded to surgery if it was possible to achieve a R0 resection for the primary tumor and metastatic lesions after re-evaluation. Otherwise systemic chemotherapy will be continued (8 cycles in total). A total of 127 patients with extensive metastasis were included in arm C, who underwent at least 8 cycles of FLOT palliative chemotherapy. The study endpoint was overall survival (OS). Finally, with a median follow-up time of 28.6 months, more than half of the patients in arm A were still alive. 36 (60%) patients in arm B underwent surgery, and their overall survival was significantly longer than that of arm C (22.9 vs. 10.7 months, $p < 0.001$). Even within arm B, the overall survival of the patients underwent surgery was significantly longer than those who could not undergo surgery (31.3 vs. 15.9 months, $p < 0.001$). The results of the study indicated that long-term survival benefit could be obtained for patients with advanced gastric cancer through full-course comprehensive treatment and the tumor curative resection. In our cohort, the CRT with gastrectomy group had a significantly longer median overall survival than CRT only group (22 vs. 9 months).

In terms of the value of radiotherapy, it is usually used patients with stage IB to IIIB GC to downstage or downsize the primary site, increasing the possibility for radical resection (30). However, patients with stage IV GC has remote organ involvement, which is not appropriate for radiotherapy.

Therefore, the main purpose was to control bleeding and improve quality of life (QoL) (31). However, concurrent chemoradiotherapy shows superiority to chemotherapy or radiotherapy alone in prolonging the survival of patients with metastatic GC (32, 33).

We acknowledge that our study still has some limitations. First, as a retrospective cohort study, although PSM was used to minimize the effect of the differences between the groups, selection bias is still a potential limitation of this study. Patients who underwent surgery were likely to have a potentially resectable disease when it was diagnosed, which might be one source of selection bias as well. In addition, due to the limitations of the SEER database, some information was not available to access, such as: removal of the metastatic sites, surgical margin status, D1/D2 node dissection, the chemotherapy regimen and the dose/field/intent of radiotherapy. In this study, the CRT with gastrectomy group had total or partial gastrectomy, which means the primary site was removed. However, it is unknown whether the metastatic sites were removed, which is a prognostic factor in stage IV GC as well. In terms of lymph node dissection extent, among the 146 patients who underwent surgery, the mean number of regional lymph nodes examined was 18.40, which was more than 15 lymph nodes minimum, as recommended by NCCN gastric cancer guidelines, to avoid stage migration (5). Therefore, considering the importance of these factors, the prolonged survival in the CRT with gastrectomy group that was observed in the current results should be interpreted with caution.

CONCLUSIONS

In summary, stage IV gastric cancer remains a fatal disease. This study was a population-based study that revealed that, compared with CRT alone, CRT with gastrectomy may achieve a survival benefit in patients with metastatic GC. This indicated that selected metastatic gastric cancer patients may experience prolonged survival with primary tumor removal. Although its characteristics cannot be described currently, a further well-designed investigation is required to determine the best treatment strategy. Conversion therapy may provide a direction for the treatment of stage IV gastric cancer patients.

AUTHOR CONTRIBUTIONS

All authors listed had made a great contribution to the work. LZ: came up with the concept/hypothesis, designed the study, and revised the manuscript. SL: collected and analyzed the data, drafted the manuscript. Finally, all the authors took responsible to the final manuscript and approved it for publication.

ACKNOWLEDGMENTS

The authors acknowledge and sincerely appreciate the efforts of the Surveillance, Epidemiology, and End Results (SEER) Program tumor registries in the establishment of the SEER database.

REFERENCES

1. Global Burden of Disease Cancer C, Fitzmaurice C, Allen C, Barber RM, Barregard L, Bhutta ZA, et al. Global, regional, and national cancer incidence, mortality, years of life lost, years lived with disability, and disability-adjusted life-years for 32 cancer groups, 1990 to 2015: a systematic analysis for the global burden of disease study. *JAMA Oncol.* (2017) 3:524–48. doi: 10.1001/jamaoncol.2016.5688
2. Glimelius B, Ekstrom K, Hoffman K, Graf W, Sjoden PO, Haglund U, et al. Randomized comparison between chemotherapy plus best supportive care with best supportive care in advanced gastric cancer. *Ann Oncol.* (1997) 8:163–8. doi: 10.1023/A:1008243606668
3. Kang JH, Lee SI, Lim DH, Park KW, Oh SY, Kwon HC, et al. Salvage chemotherapy for pretreated gastric cancer: a randomized phase III trial comparing chemotherapy plus best supportive care with best supportive care alone. *J Clin Oncol.* (2012) 30:1513–8. doi: 10.1200/JCO.2011.39.4585
4. Smyth EC, Verheij M, Allum W, Cunningham D, Cervantes A, Arnold D, et al. Gastric cancer: ESMO clinical practice guidelines for diagnosis, treatment and follow-up. *Ann Oncol.* (2016) 27(Suppl. 5):v38–49. doi: 10.1093/annonc/mdw350
5. National Comprehensive Cancer Network. *NCCN Clinical Practice Guidelines in Oncology.* Gastric cancer (version 1. 2020): National Comprehensive Cancer Network (2020). Available online at: https://www.nccn.org/professionals/physician_gls/pdf/gastric.pdf
6. Fujitani K, Yang HK, Mizusawa J, Kim YW, Terashima M, Han SU, et al. Gastrectomy plus chemotherapy versus chemotherapy alone for advanced gastric cancer with a single non-curable factor (REGATTA): a phase 3, randomised controlled trial. *Lancet Oncol.* (2016) 17:309–18. doi: 10.1016/S1470-2045(15)00553-7
7. Yoshida K, Yamaguchi K, Okumura N, Tanahashi T, Kodera Y. Is conversion therapy possible in stage IV gastric cancer: the proposal of new biological categories of classification. *Gastric Cancer.* (2016) 19:329–38. doi: 10.1007/s10120-015-0575-z
8. Noone AM, Lund JL, Mariotto A, Cronin K, McNeel T, Deapen D, et al. Comparison of SEER treatment data with medicare claims. *Med Care.* (2016) 54:e55–64. doi: 10.1097/MLR.0000000000000073
9. Rubin DB. Estimating causal effects from large data sets using propensity scores. *Ann Intern Med.* (1997) 127(8 Pt 2):757–63. doi: 10.7326/0003-4819-127-8_Part_2-199710151-00064
10. Austin PC. An introduction to propensity score methods for reducing the effects of confounding in observational studies. *Multivariate Behav Res.* (2011) 46:399–424. doi: 10.1080/00273171.2011.568786
11. Chang YR, Han DS, Kong SH, Lee HJ, Kim SH, Kim WH, et al. The value of palliative gastrectomy in gastric cancer with distant metastasis. *Ann Surg Oncol.* (2012) 19:1231–9. doi: 10.1245/s10434-011-2056-x
12. Koizumi W, Kim YH, Fujii M, Kim HK, Imamura H, Lee KH, et al. Addition of docetaxel to S-1 without platinum prolongs survival of patients with advanced gastric cancer: a randomized study (START). *J Cancer Res Clin Oncol.* (2014) 140:319–28. doi: 10.1007/s00432-013-1563-5
13. Yamada Y, Higuchi K, Nishikawa K, Gotoh M, Fuse N, Sugimoto N, et al. Phase III study comparing oxaliplatin plus S-1 with cisplatin plus S-1 in chemotherapy-naive patients with advanced gastric cancer. *Ann Oncol.* (2015) 26:141–8. doi: 10.1093/annonc/mdu472
14. Cheon SH, Rha SY, Jeung HC, Im CK, Kim SH, Kim HR, et al. Survival benefit of combined curative resection of the stomach (D2 resection) and liver in gastric cancer patients with liver metastases. *Ann Oncol.* (2008) 19:1146–53. doi: 10.1093/annonc/mdn026
15. Riihimaki M, Hemminki A, Sundquist K, Sundquist J, Hemminki K. Metastatic spread in patients with gastric cancer. *Oncotarget.* (2016) 7:52307–16. doi: 10.18632/oncotarget.10740
16. Association JGC. Japanese gastric cancer treatment guidelines 2014 (ver. 4). *Gastric Cancer.* (2017) 20:1–19. doi: 10.1007/s10120-016-0622-4

17. Hartgrink HH, Putter H, Klein Kranenbarg E, Bonenkamp JJ, van de Velde CJ, Dutch Gastric Cancer G. Value of palliative resection in gastric cancer. *Br J Surg.* (2002) 89:1438–43. doi: 10.1046/j.1365-2168.2002.02220.x
18. Musri FY, Mutlu H, Karaagac M, Eryilmaz MK, Gunduz S, Artac M. Primary tumor resection and survival in patients with stage IV gastric cancer. *J Gastric Cancer.* (2016) 16:78–84. doi: 10.5230/jgc.2016.16.2.78
19. Solaini L, Ministrini S, Bencivenga M, D'Ignazio A, Marino E, Cipollari C, et al. Conversion gastrectomy for stage IV unresectable gastric cancer: a GIRCG retrospective cohort study. *Gastric Cancer.* (2019) 22:1285–93. doi: 10.1007/s10120-019-00968-2
20. Nordgard O, Tjensvoll K, Gilje B, Soreide K. Circulating tumour cells and DNA as liquid biopsies in gastrointestinal cancer. *Br J Surg.* (2018) 105:e110–20. doi: 10.1002/bjs.10782
21. Rosen SA, Buell JF, Yoshida A, Kazsuba S, Hurst R, Michelassi F, et al. Initial presentation with stage IV colorectal cancer: how aggressive should we be? *Arch Surg.* (2000) 135:530–4; discussion 4–5. doi: 10.1001/archsurg.135.5.530
22. Dauplat J, Le Bouedec G, Pomel C, Scherer C. Cytoreductive surgery for advanced stages of ovarian cancer. *Semin Surg Oncol.* (2000) 19:42–8. doi: 10.1002/1098-2388(200007/08)19:1<42::AID-SSU7>3.0.CO;2-M
23. Uenosono Y, Arigami T, Kozono T, Yanagita S, Hagihara T, Haraguchi N, et al. Clinical significance of circulating tumor cells in peripheral blood from patients with gastric cancer. *Cancer-Am Cancer Soc.* (2013) 119:3984–91. doi: 10.1002/cncr.28309
24. Koizumi W, Narahara H, Hara T, Takagane A, Akiya T, Takagi M, et al. S-1 plus cisplatin versus S-1 alone for first-line treatment of advanced gastric cancer (SPIRITS trial): a phase III trial. *Lancet Oncol.* (2008) 9:215–21. doi: 10.1016/S1470-2045(08)70035-4
25. Songun I, Putter H, Kranenbarg EM, Sasako M, van de Velde CJ. Surgical treatment of gastric cancer: 15-year follow-up results of the randomised nationwide Dutch D1D2 trial. *Lancet Oncol.* (2010) 11:439–49. doi: 10.1016/S1470-2045(10)70070-X
26. Fukuchi M, Ishiguro T, Ogata K, Suzuki O, Kumagai Y, Ishibashi K, et al. Prognostic role of conversion surgery for unresectable gastric cancer. *Ann Surg Oncol.* (2015) 22:3618–24. doi: 10.1245/s10434-015-4422-6
27. Yabusaki H, Nashimoto A, Matsuki A, Aizawa M. Significance of surgical treatment in multimodal therapy for stage IV highly advanced gastric cancer. *Hepatogastroenterology.* (2013) 60:377–81. doi: 10.5754/hge12653
28. Terashima M. Conversion therapy for gastric cancer: who can make conversion as successful as Goromaru? *Gastric Cancer.* (2016) 19:685–6. doi: 10.1007/s10120-016-0609-1
29. Al-Batran SE, Homann N, Pauligk C, Illerhaus G, Martens UM, Stoehlmacher J, et al. Effect of neoadjuvant chemotherapy followed by surgical resection on survival in patients with limited metastatic gastric or gastroesophageal junction cancer: the AIO-FLOT3 trial. *JAMA Oncol.* (2017) 3:1237–44. doi: 10.1001/jamaoncol.2017.0515
30. Min C, Bangalore S, Jhawar S, Guo Y, Nicholson J, Formenti SC, et al. Chemoradiation therapy versus chemotherapy alone for gastric cancer after R0 surgical resection: a meta-analysis of randomized trials. *Oncology.* (2014) 86:79–85. doi: 10.1159/000354641
31. Izuishi K, Mori H. Recent strategies for treating stage IV gastric cancer: roles of palliative gastrectomy, chemotherapy, and radiotherapy. *J Gastrointestin Liver Dis.* (2016) 25:87–94. doi: 10.15403/jgld.2014.1121.251.rv2
32. Group GTS. A comparison of combination chemotherapy and combined modality therapy for locally advanced gastric carcinoma. gastrointestinal tumor study group. *Cancer Am Cancer Soc.* (1982) 49:1771–7. doi: 10.1002/1097-0142(19820501)49:9<1771::AID-CNCR2820490907>3.0.CO;2-M
33. Smalley SR, Benedetti JK, Haller DG, Hundahl SA, Estes NC, Ajani JA, et al. Updated analysis of SWOG-directed intergroup study 0116: a phase III trial of adjuvant radiochemotherapy versus observation after curative gastric cancer resection. *J Clin Oncol.* (2012) 30:2327–33. doi: 10.1200/JCO.2011.36.7136

7

Recent Status of Laparoscopic Distal Gastrectomy in Korea: A Multicenter Retrospective Cohort Study (Pre-study Survey of KLASS-07 Trial)

Chang In Choi[1], *Chang Min Lee*[2], *Ji Ho Park*[3], *Ye Seob Jee*[4], *Han Hong Lee*[5], *Oh Jeong*[6] *and Sungsoo Park*[7]*

[1] *Department of Surgery, Biomedical Research Institute, Pusan National University College of Medicine, Busan, South Korea,* [2] *Department of Surgery, Korea University College of Medicine, Seoul, South Korea,* [3] *Department of Surgery, Gyeongsang National University School of Medicine, Jinju, South Korea,* [4] *Department of Surgery, Dankook University College of Medicine, Cheonan, South Korea,* [5] *Department of Surgery, College of Medicine, The Catholic University of Korea, Seoul, South Korea,* [6] *Department of Surgery, Chonnam National University Medical School, Gwangju, South Korea,* [7] *Department of Surgery, Korea University Medical Center Anam Hospital, Seoul, South Korea*

Correspondence:
Sungsoo Park
kugspss@korea.ac.kr

Purpose: To analyze the surgical trend and brief postoperative results of laparoscopic distal gastrectomy (LDG) in Korea on the basis of a multicenter cohort.

Materials and Methods: Data of 812 patients who underwent LDG between January and December 2016 were collected from 14 surgeons at 7 institutions. Patients were divided into laparoscopy-assisted distal gastrectomy (LADG) group and totally laparoscopic distal gastrectomy (TLDG) group. Perioperative and clinicopathologic outcomes were compared retrospectively.

Results: Among the patients [$n = 222$ (27.3%) LADG; $n = 590$ (72.7%) TLDG], there are no significant differences in patient's demographics (sex, age, body mass index, and American Society of Anesthesiologists score). Billroth-I anastomosis (84.7%) was most performed in the LADG group, but Billroth-II anastomosis (59.0%) in the TLDG group ($p < 0.001$). The mean operative time was longer in the TLDG group (197.3 ± 44.4 min vs. 222.0 ± 60.2 min, $p < 0.001$), and there was no statistical difference in the hospital stay between the two groups (9.6 ± 4.8 days vs. 8.9 ± 7.1 days, $p = 0.149$). There were no significant differences in morbidity and mortality between the two groups. The length of proximal margin was longer in the TLDG group (4.3 ± 3.1 cm vs. 6.0 ± 3.4 cm, $p < 0.001$), but the distal margin was longer in the LADG group (6.5 ± 3.7 cm vs. 5.5 ± 3.1 cm, $p < 0.001$). The distribution of operations among each institution was shown very heterogeneously.

Conclusion: There was no significant difference related to surgical outcome between LADG and TLDG in pre-study survey prior to KLASS-07 trial. Therefore, to obtain more reliable data, well designed prospective randomized controlled study is needed.

Keywords: gastric cancer, gastrectomy, laparoscopic surgery, baseline survey, multicenter study

INTRODUCTION

Since the first report of laparoscopic gastrectomy for gastric cancer by Kitano et al. minimally invasive surgery has been developed steadily in the recent two decades. Laparoscopic surgery has various advantages such as less postoperative pain, inflammatory response, rapid recovery, early discharge, and excellent cosmetic result compared with conventional open laparotomy (1–4). Several studies have demonstrated that the oncologic safety of laparoscopic gastrectomy is similar to conventional open gastrectomy for early gastric cancer (5, 6), and laparoscopic gastrectomy was already accepted as the standard treatment option for early gastric cancer as well as benign gastric tumor. In addition, laparoscopic gastrectomy widens its boundary with the development of surgical skill and instruments even to locally advanced gastric cancer on the basis of evidence from several retrospective studies (7–9). With this, large-scale prospective studies are ongoing, and the final results are being awaited (KLASS-02, JLSSG0901) (10, 11).

Laparoscopy-assisted gastrectomy required a mini-laparotomy on the epigastrium for gastric division and anastomosis after laparoscopic gastric mobilization (extracorporeal anastomosis). In cases that a patient is obese or has short duodenum, the anastomosis could not be easy under the narrow working space of the mini-incision, whereas in the totally laparoscopic gastrectomy, the whole procedure from the gastric division including lymphadenectomy to the anastomosis is performed intracorporeally. It has various advantages, such as the superiority of the cosmetic result due to umbilical incision and convenient anastomosis under good operative view even in obese patients. According to accumulated laparoscopic surgical experience, the recent surgical trend shifted from laparoscopy-assisted gastrectomy to totally laparoscopic gastrectomy (12).

However, a prospective randomized controlled study (RCT) comparing the postoperative outcome and patient's life of quality (QoL) is still rare, although there were several retrospective studies between these two procedures. Thus, authors are preparing for a multicenter prospective study comparing the QoL and postoperative outcome between laparoscopy-assisted distal gastrectomy (LADG) and totally laparoscopic distal gastrectomy (TLDG) and conducted a brief survey regarding the surgical trend among Korean gastric surgeons as reference for a subsequent study (KLASS-07 trial). Therefore, this study aimed to analyze the current status and surgical trend of laparoscopic distal gastrectomy in Korea.

METHODS

This study was designed as a multicenter retrospective cohort study. Medical data of 812 patients were collected retrospectively using the same case report form provided by 14 gastric surgeons of seven institutions, which are affiliated to the KLASS-07 trial organizing committee. Between January and December 2016, patients who were diagnosed with gastric adenocarcinoma or neuroendocrine carcinoma underwent laparoscopic distal gastrectomy. All patients were compared by dividing them into two groups: LADG and TLDG group. Pylorus-preserving gastrectomy (PPG) was excluded in this database as it is not a distal gastrectomy despite a partial gastrectomy.

Patients' demographics, postoperative outcome, and pathologic data were analyzed, and all continuous data are expressed as mean ± standard deviation. Categorial variables were assessed by Pearson's chi-square test and Fisher's exact test, and continuous variables were assessed by Student's *t*-test. American Society of Anesthesiologists (ASA) scores between the two groups were compared (1 vs. others). We described all anastomosis methods separately. However, in the statistical analysis, we included Billroth II with Braun anastomosis (B-IIb) to Billroth II anastomosis (B-II), and uncut Roux-en-Y anastomosis (REY) to Roux-en-Y anastomosis to reduce the errors. In a comparison of the resectability, complete resection case was compared with incomplete resection case (R1 and R2). Moreover, in the analysis of the World Health Organization classification, most common tubular adenocarcinoma was compared with signet ring cell carcinoma because the pathologic entities of other gastric cancers were very rare. Subgroup analysis was performed for the operation time according to the reconstruction method in each group. For this, one-way analysis of variance and Bonferroni *post-hoc* analysis were used. In the LADG group, uncut REY anastomosis was included in REY anastomosis for the statistical calculation.

To visualize patients' distribution according to each institution, jittered scatterplot was applied using the following formula: (measured value) + (R-0.5) X 0.3, where "R" is a random number from zero to one. For all analyses, $p < 0.05$ was considered significant statistically and SPSS version 22.0 for Windows (SPSS, Inc., Chicago, IL) was used for statistical analysis. This study was reviewed and approved by the Institutional Review Board of Pusan National University Hospital (H-1803-023-064). And informed written consent in terms of using their medical records was provided to all patients and their legal guardian before study enrollment.

RESULTS

Patient Demographics and Perioperative Data

A total of 222 (27.3%) patients underwent LADG and 590 (72.7%) patients underwent TLDG. Of the 812 patients, 511 (62.9%) were men, with a mean age of 61.9 ± 11.4 years and mean body mass index (BMI) of 24.6 ± 13.4 kg/m2. There were no significant differences in sex, age, BMI, and ASA scores between the two groups (**Table 1**).

Postoperative data are presented in **Table 2**. In all patients, B-II was most performed in 357 (44.0%) patients and Billroth I anastomosis (B-I) was performed in 213 (26.1%) patients. With regard to the anastomosis method, B-I was performed in 188 (84.7%) patients in the LADG group and 24 (4.1%) patients in the TLDG group. B-II was performed in 9 (4.1%) patients in the LADG group and 348 (59.0%) patients in the TLDG group. Moreover, REY was performed in 18 (8.1%) patients in the LADG group and in 114 (19.4%) patients in the TLDG group. There was

TABLE 1 | Patients' demographics.

Variables	LADG (n = 222)	TLDG (n = 590)	Overall (n = 812)	p-value
Sex				0.569
Male	136 (61.3)	375 (63.6)	511 (62.9)	
Female	86 (38.7)	215 (36.4)	301 (37.1)	
Age (years)	61.5 ± 10.3	62.0 ± 11.8	61.9 ± 11.4	0.558
BMI (kg/m^2)	23.9 ± 3.0	24.8 ± 15.6	24.6 ± 13.4	0.367
ASA score				0.637[a]
1	52 (23.5)	129 (22.0)	184 (22.4)	
2	165 (74.7)	406 (69.2)	571 (70.7)	
3	4 (1.8)	50 (8.5)	54 (6.7)	
4	0	2 (0.3)	2 (0.2)	

LADG, laparoscopy-assisted distal gastrectomy; TLDG, totally laparoscopic distal gastrectomy; ASA, American Society of Anesthesiologists.
[a]ASA score 1 vs. Others.

TABLE 2 | Postoperative data.

Variables	LADG (n = 222)	TLDG (n = 590)	Overall (n = 812)	p-value
Reconstruction method				<0.001[a]
Billoth-I	188 (84.7)	24 (4.1)	212 (26.1)	
Billoth-II	9 (4.1)	348 (59.0)	357 (44.0)	
Billoth-II + Braun	6 (2.7)	50 (8.5)	56 (6.9)	
Uncut Roux-en-Y	1 (0.5)	54 (9.2)	55 (6.8)	
Roux-en-Y	18 (8.1)	114 (19.3)	132 (16.3)	
Reconstruction manner				1.000
Stapling	222 (100.0)	589 (99.8)	811 (99.9)	
Manual	0	1 (0.2)	1 (0.1)	
LND extent				<0.001
D1	2 (0.9)	17 (2.9)	19 (2.3)	
D1+	40 (18.0)	466 (79.0)	506 (62.3)	
≥D2	180 (81.1)	107 (18.1)	287 (35.3)	
Co-resection				0.009
Yes	33 (14.9)	49 (8.3)	82 (10.1)	
No	189 (85.1)	541 (91.7)	730 (89.9)	
Curability				0.199[b]
R0	222 (100.0)	583 (98.8)	805 (99.1)	
R1	0	4 (0.7)	4 (0.5)	
R2	0	3 (0.5)	3 (0.4)	
Operative time (min)	197.3 ± 44.4	222.0 ± 60.2	215.2 ± 57.4	<0.001
Hospital stay (days)	9.6 ± 4.8	8.9 ± 7.1	9.1 ± 6.6	0.149
Morbidity[c]	18 (10.6)	63 (11.8)	81 (11.5)	0.783
Mortality	1 (0.5)	2 (0.3)	3 (0.4)	1.000

LADG, laparoscopic assisted distal gastrectomy; TLDG, totally laparoscopic distal gastrectomy; DG, distal gastrectomy; LND, lymph node dissection.
[a]B-I vs. B-II (+Braun) vs. Roux-en-Y (+Uncut).
[b]R0 vs. R1 and R2.
[c]There were 106 missing values of total 812 cases.

a significant difference in the anastomosis method between the two groups ($p < 0.001$). Both groups were mostly anastomosed with the stapling method.

D2 lymphadenectomy (180 patients, 81.1%) in the LADG group and D1+ lymphadenectomy in the TLDG groups (466 patients, 79.0%) were mostly performed ($p < 0.001$). Frequency of co-resection was higher in the LADG group than in the TLDG (14.9% vs. 8.3%, $p = 0.009$). The mean operative time was longer in the TLDG group than in the LADG group (197.3 ± 44.4 min vs. 222.0 ± 60.2 min, $p < 0.001$). Morbidity was slightly higher in the TLDG group; however, it was not significant statistically (18 patients, 10.6% vs. 63 patients, 11.8%, $p = 0.783$). One patient died (0.5%) in the LADG and two (0.3%) in the TLDG, and no difference was found between the two groups.

Pathological Data

Overall, the mean tumor size was 3.0 ± 2.1 cm, and tumor size was larger in the LADG group, but no difference was shown between the two groups (3.3 ± 2.1 cm vs. 2.9 ± 2.1 cm, $p = 0.058$). In the LADG group, the tumor located in mid-part of the stomach was 115 (51.8%) patients and in the lower part was 95 (42.8%) patients, whereas the middle tumor was 36.9% and the lower tumor was 62.5% in the TLDG group ($p < 0.001$). Moderately differentiated tubular adenocarcinoma (tub MD) was the most common in 239 (29.4%) of all patients, poorly differentiated tubular adenocarcinoma (tub PD) was confirmed in 218 (26.5%) patients, and cohesive carcinoma (SRC) was identified in 172 (21.2%) patients. In the LADG group, tub MD and SRC were diagnosed finally in each 70 (31.5%) patient and 66 (29.7%). In the TLDG group, tub MD and tub PD were confirmed in 169 (28.6%) and 163 (27.6%) patients, respectively. In Lauren's classification, the incidence of intestinal and diffuse type was comparable (45.4% vs. 46.3%) in the LADG group. In the TLDG group, the intestinal type was greater than the diffuse type (59.0% vs. 23.8%), and there was a significant difference in the final pathologic finding ($p<0.001$). The retrieved lymph node was significantly greater in the TLDG group (42.6 vs. 46.3, $p = 0.008$), and there were no differences in metastatic lymph nodes between the two groups. Resection margin showed significant differences in both groups. The length of the proximal margin (PRM) was longer in the TLDG group (4.3 ± 3.1 cm vs. 6.0 ± 3.4cm, $p < 0.001$) and distal margin (DRM) was longer in the LADG group (6.5 ± 3.7 cm vs. 5.5 ± 3.1 cm, $p < 0.001$). All pathologic data are presented in **Table 3**.

Distribution of Patients According to the Institution

Collected patients' data by each institution shows very heterogeneous distribution, and it was difficult to find any regularity. B-I was performed in 212 patients, of which 24 (4.1%) underwent intracorporeal B-I (delta anastomosis) in the TLDG group and 188 (84.7%) patients underwent extracorporeal B-I in the LADG group. B-II was performed in 357 patients, but it was performed in only 9 (4.1%) patients through LADG and most patients underwent intracorporeal B-II through TLDG. B-IIb, REY, and uncut REY were performed in 56, 132, and 55

TABLE 3 | Pathological data.

Variables	LADG (*n* = 222)	TLDG (*n* = 590)	Overall (*n* = 812)	*p*-value
Tumor size (cm)	3.3 ± 2.1	2.9 ± 2.1	3.1 ± 2.1	0.058
Tumor location				<0.001
Upper	12 (5.4)	3 (0.5)	15 (1.8)	
Middle	115 (51.8)	218 (36.9)	333 (41.0)	
Lower	95 (42.8)	369 (62.5)	464 (57.1)	
WHO classification				<0.001[a]
Papillary	3 (1.4)	2 (0.3)	5 (0.6)	
Tub WD	29 (13.1)	128 (21.7)	157 (19.3)	
Tub MD	70 (31.5)	169 (28.6)	239 (29.4)	
Tub PD	52 (23.4)	163 (27.6)	215 (26.5)	
Mucinous	0	9 (1.5)	9 (1.1)	
Cohesive (SRC)	66 (29.7)	106 (18.0)	172 (21.2)	
Others	1 (0.5)	10 (1.7)	11 (1.4)	
Unknown	1 (0.5)	3 (0.5)	4 (0.5)	
Lauren				<0.001
Intestinal	99 (45.4)	329 (59.0)	428 (55.2)	
Diffuse	101 (46.3)	133 (23.8)	234 (30.2)	
Mixed	181 (8.3)	96 (17.2)	114 (14.7)	
Retrived lymph nodes	42.6 ± 15.9	46.3 ± 17.9	45.3 ± 17.5	0.008
Metastatic lymph nodes	0.5 ± 2.1	0.9 ± 3.6	0.8 ± 3.3	0.149
T stage				0.002
T1a	115 (52.0)	273 (46.7)	388 (48.1)	
T1b	87 (39.4)	193 (33.0)	282 (35.0)	
T2	10 (4.5)	58 (9.9)	67 (8.3)	
T3	2 (0.9)	33 (5.6)	34 (4.2)	
T4a	7 (3.2)	28 (4.8)	35 (4.3)	
N stage				0.267
N0	193 (86.9)	492 (83.4)	685 (84.4)	
N1	16 (7.2)	54 (9.2)	70 (8.6)	
N2	9 (4.1)	19 (3.2)	28 (3.4)	
N3	4 (1.8)	25 (4.2)	29 (3.6)	
TNM stage[b]				0.031[c]
IA	182 (82.4)	430 (73.5)	612 (75.9)	
IB	18 (8.1)	65 (11.1)	83 (10.3)	
IIA	9 (4.1)	32 (5.5)	41 (5.1)	
IIB	8 (3.6)	23 (3.9)	31 (3.8)	
IIIA	1 (0.5)	10 (1.7)	11 (1.4)	
IIIB	2 (0.9)	10 (1.7)	12 (1.5)	
IIIC	1 (0.5)	15 (2.6)	16 (2.0)	
Proximal margin (cm)	4.3 ± 3.1	6.0 ± 3.4	5.5 ± 3.4	<0.001
Distal margin (cm)	6.5 ± 3.7	5.5 ± 3.1	5.8 ± 3.3	<0.001
ESD before surgery	18 (8.1)	29 (4.9)	47 (5.8)	0.092

LADG, laparoscopy-assisted distal gastrectomy; TLDG, totally laparoscopic distal gastrectomy; Tub, tubular adenocarcinoma; WD, well-differentiated; MD, moderate-differentiated; PD, poorly-differentiated; SRC, signet-ring cell; ESD, endoscopic submucosal dissection. Some missing values were excluded in a calculation.

[a] Tub vs. SRC.

[b] TNM stage was analyzed with AJCC 7th edition.

[c] Stage I vs. II vs. III.

patients, respectively. This may show various results according to the policy of the institutions. laparoscopy-assistedDetails of the patient distribution are visualized in **Figure 1**.

Comparison of the Operation Time According to the Reconstruction Methods in Each Group

In the LADG group, the overall operation time of B-I and B-II reconstruction is relatively shorter than others (191.4 and 187.1 min). B-I and B-II groups in LADG showed significant differences compared with REY group (including uncut REY, $p < 0.001$ and 0.001). In the TLDG group, there were no big numerical differences in the operation time among each reconstruction methods. The overall operation time was longest in B-I reconstruction (delta anastomosis) group (236.5 min). And there was a significant difference between B-II and REY group in Bonferroni *post-hoc* analysis (216.3 min vs. 236.2 min, $p = 0.022$). The statistical difference was presented as the lowercase a, b, and c in **Figure 2**.

DISCUSSIONS

Laparoscopy-assisted gastrectomy has been used for a long time with increasing popularity from an era of early laparoscopic surgery until the present. In this procedure, gastric mobilization and lymph node dissection are carried out laparoscopically, and the anastomosis is performed extracorporeally through the mini-laparotomy in the epigastrium. However, anastomosis of intestines in very obese patients or patients with thick abdominal wall could be difficult because excessive traction is needed and the operative visual field is poor in narrow and restricted space of the upper abdominal cavity. Totally laparoscopic gastrectomy, in which the whole operation is carried out intracorporeally, enables anastomosis of intestine more safely and conveniently, as the anastomosis site can be monitored directly under the laparoscopic view.

The term totally laparoscopic gastrectomy was first used in 1999 by Mayers in his report of intracorporeal B-I anastomosis (13). Thereafter, intracorporeal anastomoses using various methods have been reported, and the recent surgical trend has progressed to totally laparoscopic gastrectomy with high interest in minimally invasive surgery. Ikeda et al. compared LADG with TLDG for 80 gastric cancer patients, and they reported no significant difference in operation time, harvested lymph node, and morbidity; however, TLDG showed less blood loss and rapid recovery compared with LADG (12). Kim et al. compared the postoperative outcome related to BMI between LADG and TLDG. They reported that there was no difference in major complication in an obese patient with BMI more than 25 kg/m2 between two groups, but in the LADG group, the overall complication was higher, and recovery after surgery (such as dietary progression, first flatus, and hospital stay) was slower than that in the TLDG group (14). Kanaji also anticipated that TLDG with a short hospital stay, wide working space, and small wound size could replace LADG via a prospective randomized controlled study (15). Han et al. suggested that TLDG is superior to LADG in terms of operative time, blood loss, hospital stay, and cosmetic result (16). Lee et al. reported that the inflammatory response might be lower in TLDG by less tissue damage because it does not require excessive traction of the stomach through

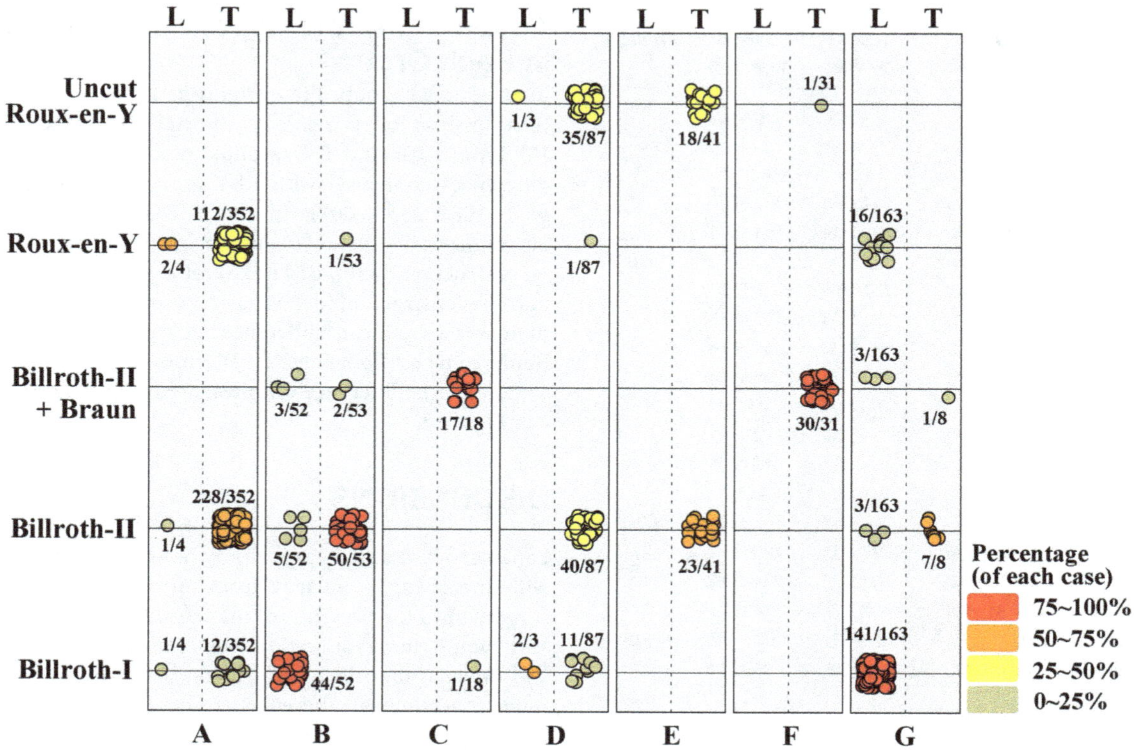

FIGURE 1 | Distribution of surgical procedures in each institution. The value was colored and visualized according to its percentage. L, laparoscopy-assisted distal gastrectomy; T, totally laparoscopic distal gastrectomy.

the mini-laparotomy for anastomosis (17). Recently, Lin et al. suggested that the number of harvested lymph node was higher in TLDG, but there were no differences in other factors related to postoperative outcome and recovery (18). Similarly, numerous studies compared TDLG with LADG. However, those were mostly single-sectional retrospective study with inconsistent and varied results.

In a recent meta-analysis by Zhang et al. there were no differences in the operative time, analgesic use, first flatus, and overall complication between LADG and TLDG, but TLDG was superior to LADG in terms blood loss, number of harvested lymph node, and hospital stay (19). However, high-level evidences are difficult to obtain through meta-analysis because of the rarity of prospective RCTs for TLDG. Through their prospective RCT for 110 gastric cancer patients in 2015, Woo et al. reported that early surgical outcome (including the complication) and QoL did not show differences between LADG and TLDG. This was only a single-institution trial, but a markedly valuable study. As mentioned above, there have been some papers comparing the TDLG and LADG. And many authors have emphasized the feasibility or superiority of the TLDG. However, the LADG is still performed in some institutions although recent surgical trend moves to the TLDG. To obtain more reliable data for the postoperative outcome (including quality of life), a well-designed multicenter prospective RCT is needed.

The KLASS-07 trial is a multicenter prospective RCT which compares the QoL of patients who underwent LADG and TLDG. At this time, recruiting researcher was closed with support of the Korean Laparoscopic Gastrointestinal Surgery Study Group and a review of the institutional review board for the study is in progress. This brief survey of the current status of domestic gastric cancer surgery was performed as reference for the study protocol. Of the total 891 patients, 591 (71.4%) underwent TLDG, and there were no significant differences in patients' demographics. This reflects that the recent trend of the laparoscopic gastrectomy shifted from LADG to TLDG. laparoscopy-assisted.

In LADG, B-I was the most common anastomosis (84.7%). In the TLDG group, B-I (delta anastomosis) was only 4.1%, B-II was 59.0%, and REY was 19.3%. Delta anastomosis was first introduced by Kanaya et al. in 2002, and many later studies concluded that it was a safe and feasible procedure clinically (20). However, our result implies that the delta anastomosis has still many difficulties to be accepted as the standard anastomosis technique for TLDG.

The co-resection was higher in the LADG group than in the TLDG group, but most cases were cholecystectomy and it may not have clinical significance. The operation time was longer in the TLDG because intracorporeal gastrojejunostomy, such as B-II or REY anastomosis, is a time-consuming procedure. The hospital stay in the TLDG group was shorter, but it was

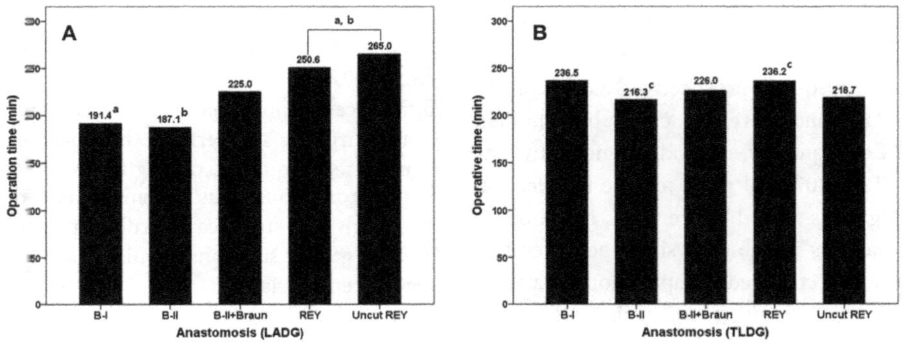

FIGURE 2 | Comparison of the operation time according to the reconstruction methods in each group. Bonferroni *post-hoc* analysis was used and statistical different values were marked lowercase a, b, and c.

not statistically significant, and there were no differences in the morbidity and mortality between the two groups. This result is consistent with other studies.

The number of harvested lymph node was significantly higher in the TLDG group. However, lymph node dissection during the LADG and TLDG is performed in the same manner. Because more than 40 lymph nodes were resected in both groups, it could be not a factor affecting the clinical course. In a comparison of TNM stage, T1, N0, and stage I were most frequent for all patients. This could mean that many surgeons are still selecting patients for laparoscopic approach for gastric cancer. This may be due to the lack of results regarding the safety and long-term outcome of laparoscopic gastrectomy for advanced gastric cancer (KLASS-02, JLSSG0901). Moreover, in this study, there were more early cancer cases in the LADG group, and we think that has affected the result from the institutional policy for the indication of laparoscopic gastrectomy.

In the TLDG group, PRM was longer and DRM was shorter than that in the LADG group. This may be associated to the tumor location of the TLDG group, which was lower than that in the LADG group, and lesion localization is known to be difficult in the intracorporeal anastomosis during TLDG because surgeons cannot manually palpate the lesion directly. Therefore, the surgeon's concern about obtaining clear margin leads to wider resection, and preference to gastrojejunostomy rather than gastroduodenostomy during TLDG could also influence the result (16, 21). However, Shinohara et al. suggested no significant differences in the length of PRM between the two groups, and Jeong et al. reported that PRM was rather shorter in the TLDG group (22, 23). In these studies, gastroduodenostomy (B-I, delta anastomosis) was mostly performed after TLDG. We speculated that the results could be affected by the difference in the anastomosis method.

The patient distribution according to participant institution is visualized in **Figure 1**, which indicates that five of the seven institutions preferred TLDG and one toward LADG. In addition, one institution which performed LADG mostly chose gastroduodenostomy as the standard anastomosis procedure, it may cause a deviation of the extracorporeal B-I anastomosis in the LADG group. REY is known to increase gradually in Korea; however, B-II is more commonly used than REY as an alternative method to intracorporeal gastroduodenostomy (delta anastomosis) after TLDG, and uncut REY or B-IIb is also performed in some cases. Although super high-volume centers, with around 1,000 gastrectomies performed, were excluded in this study, we think that the heterogeneity of the results in this study might reflect the current status of the gastric surgeon's society in Korea, because the anastomosis method after the TLDG was not standardized among institutions and surgeons. These points emphasize the necessity of a multicenter RCT for comparing TLDG with LADG. While many previous studies have focused on the postoperative outcomes, this study shows an aspect of the recent laparoscopic gastrectomy including the perioperative data between two groups. It can be one of the strengths of the multicenter cohort study.

There are some differences in the operation time according to the anastomosis methods in each group. Overall operation time was higher in the TLDG group than the LADG group. This may cause to take more time for tumor localization and anastomosis in TLDG. Although we couldn't evaluate pure anastomosis time in each group, LADG with B-I and B-II showed relatively short operation time. We think that it is a reasonable result because Braun anastomosis and Roux-en-Y need additional jejunojejunostomy. Whereas, TLDG with intracorporeal B-I (delta) anastomosis showed the longest operation time. Delta anastomosis uses more stapler compared with extracorporeal B-I anastomosis, however, it has been known as not time-consuming procedure. Finally, delta anastomosis might be the unfamiliar or not preferred method to participants in this study. This deviation between extra- and intracorporeal B-I anastomosis became the background to exclude the B-I anastomosis.

This preliminary study has several limitations. First, the number of 812 cases is relatively small to represent the surgical trend in Korea, even if it was not a small cohort. However, it could be significant data as they were from various institutions. Second, as mentioned, the anastomosis methods are very heterogeneous among institutions. However, it will be thoroughly controlled by the study protocol in a subsequent prospective RCT (KLASS-07), from which more reasonable results could be obtained for TLDG and LADG. Consequently, gastroduodenostomy was finally excluded from KLASS-07 trial protocol due to selection deviation between two groups. Third, there were 107 missing values among the 812 patients in the analysis of postoperative complications. Moreover, the collected complication data were not classified according to severity grade, such as Clavien-Dindo classification. However, the overall complication rate in this study was around 10%, and we believe that this could be an acceptable result comparing other studies. Because the surgical technique and postoperative management have been shared among surgeons within the surgical society, the morbidity rate of missed values would not show a big difference in the collected data.

CONCLUSION

This is a preliminary study conducted before starting the KLASS-07 trial and our data shows there were no significant differences in postoperative results between LADG and TLDG. Many surgeons still perform the laparoscopic gastrectomy using various techniques according to their own policy because there is no strong consensus statement related to LADG and TLDG. Although this study can hardly represent the surgical trend of Korean gastric surgeons, it might be a meaningful reference for a multicenter trial.

AUTHOR CONTRIBUTIONS

CC performed the statistical analysis, prepared the manuscript, and drafted this manuscript. SP supervised and organized the study. CL, JP, YJ, HL, and OJ contributed to manuscript modification. All authors contributed to data acquisition and read and approved the final manuscript.

REFERENCES

1. Adachi Y, Suematsu T, Shiraishi N, Katsuta T, Morimoto A, Kitano S, et al. Quality of life after laparoscopy-assisted Billroth I gastrectomy. *Ann Surg.* (1999) 229:49–54. doi: 10.1097/00000658-199901000-00006
2. Mochiki E, Nakabayashi T, Kamimura H, Haga N, Asao T, Kuwano H. Gastrointestinal recovery and outcome after laparoscopy-assisted versus conventional open distal gastrectomy for early gastric cancer. *World J Surg.* (2002) 26:1145–9. doi: 10.1007/s00268-002-6286-8
3. Lee JH, Han HS, Lee JH. A prospective randomized study comparing open vs laparoscopy-assisted distal gastrectomy in early gastric cancer: early results. *Surg Endosc.* (2005) 19:168–73. doi: 10.1007/s00464-004-8808-y
4. Kim YW, Baik YH, Yun YH, Nam BH, Kim DH, Choi IJ, et al. Improved quality of life outcomes after laparoscopy-assisted distal gastrectomy for early gastric cancer: results of a prospective randomized clinical trial. *Ann Surg.* (2008) 248:721–7. doi: 10.1097/SLA.0b013e318185e62e
5. Kim H-H, Han S-U, Kim M-C, Hyung WJ, Kim W, Lee H-J, et al. Prospective randomized controlled trial (phase III) to comparing laparoscopic distal gastrectomy with open distal gastrectomy for gastric adenocarcinoma (KLASS 01). *J Korean Surg Soc.* (2013) 84:123. doi: 10.4174/jkss.2013.84.2.123
6. Katai H, Mizusawa J, Katayama H, Takagi M, Yoshikawa T, Fukagawa T, et al. Short-term surgical outcomes from a phase III study of laparoscopy-assisted versus open distal gastrectomy with nodal dissection for clinical stage IA/IB gastric cancer: Japan Clinical Oncology Group Study JCOG0912. *Gastric Cancer.* (2017) 20:699–708. doi: 10.1007/s10120-016-0646-9
7. Hamabe A, Omori T, Tanaka K, Nishida T. Comparison of long-term results between laparoscopy-assisted gastrectomy and open gastrectomy with D2 lymph node dissection for advanced gastric cancer. *Surg Endosc.* (2012) 26:1702–9. doi: 10.1007/s00464-011-2096-0
8. Hu Y, Huang C, Sun Y, Su X, Cao H, Hu J, et al. Morbidity and mortality of laparoscopic versus open D2 distal gastrectomy for advanced gastric cancer: a randomized controlled trial. *J Clin Oncol.* (2016) 34:1350–7. doi: 10.1200/JCO.2015.63.7215
9. Park DJ, Han SU, Hyung WJ, Kim MC, Kim W, Ryu SY, et al. Long-term outcomes after laparoscopy-assisted gastrectomy for advanced gastric cancer: a large-scale multicenter retrospective study. *Surg Endosc.* (2012) 26:1548–53. doi: 10.1007/s00464-011-2065-7
10. Kim HH, Hyung WJ, Cho GS, Kim MC, Han SU, Kim W, et al. Morbidity and mortality of laparoscopic gastrectomy versus open gastrectomy for gastric cancer: an interim report–a phase III multicenter, prospective, randomized Trial (KLASS Trial). *Ann Surg.* (2010) 251:417–20. doi: 10.1097/SLA.0b013e3181cc8f6b
11. Lee S-W, Etoh T, Ohyama T, Inaki N, Sakuramoto S, Yoshida K, et al. Short-term outcomes from a multi-institutional, phase III study of laparoscopic versus open distal gastrectomy with D2 lymph node dissection for locally advanced gastric cancer (JLSSG0901). *J Clin Oncol.* (2017) 35(suppl. 15):4029. doi: 10.1200/JCO.2017.35.15_suppl.4029
12. Ikeda O, Sakaguchi Y, Aoki Y, Harimoto N, Taomoto J, Masuda T, et al. Advantages of totally laparoscopic distal gastrectomy over laparoscopically assisted distal gastrectomy for gastric cancer. *Surg Endosc.* (2009) 23:2374–9. doi: 10.1007/s00464-009-0360-3
13. Mayers TM, Orebaugh MG. Totally laparoscopic Billroth I gastrectomy. *J Am Coll Surg.* (1998) 186:100–3. doi: 10.1016/S1072-7515(97)00142-7
14. Kim MG, Kawada H, Kim BS, Kim TH, Kim KC, Yook JH, et al. A totally laparoscopic distal gastrectomy with gastroduodenostomy (TLDG) for improvement of the early surgical outcomes in high BMI patients. *Surg Endosc.* (2011) 25:1076–82. doi: 10.1007/s00464-010-1319-0
15. Kanaji S, Harada H, Nakayama S, Yasuda T, Oshikiri T, Kawasaki K, et al. Surgical outcomes in the newly introduced phase of intracorporeal anastomosis following laparoscopic distal gastrectomy is safe and feasible compared with established procedures of extracorporeal anastomosis. *Surg Endosc.* (2013) 28:1250–5. doi: 10.1007/s00464-013-3315-7
16. Han G, Park JY, Kim YJ. Comparison of short-term postoperative outcomes in totally laparoscopic distal gastrectomy versus laparoscopy-assisted distal gastrectomy. *J Gastric Cancer.* (2014) 14:105–10. doi: 10.5230/jgc.2014.14.2.105
17. Lee SH, Kim IH, Kim IH, Kwak SG, Chae HD. Comparison of short-term outcomes and acute inflammatory response between laparoscopy-assisted and totally laparoscopic distal gastrectomy for early gastric cancer. *Ann Surg Treat Res.* (2015) 89:176–82. doi: 10.4174/astr.2015.89.4.176
18. Lin M, Zheng CH, Huang CM, Li P, Xie JW, Wang JB, et al. Totally laparoscopic versus laparoscopy-assisted Billroth-I anastomosis for gastric cancer: a case-control and case-matched study. *Surg Endosc.* (2016) 30:5245–54. doi: 10.1007/s00464-016-4872-3
19. Zhang YX, Wu YJ, Lu GW, Xia MM. Systematic review and meta-analysis of totally laparoscopic versus laparoscopic assisted distal gastrectomy for gastric cancer. *World J Surg Oncol.* (2015) 13:116. doi: 10.1186/s12957-015-0532-7
20. Kanaya S, Gomi T, Momoi H, Tamaki N, Isobe H, Katayama T, et al. Delta-shaped anastomosis in totally laparoscopic Billroth I gastrectomy: new technique of intraabdominal gastroduodenostomy. *J Am Coll Surg.* (2002) 195:284–7. doi: 10.1016/S1072-7515(02)01239-5
21. Woo J, Lee JH, Shim KN, Jung HK, Lee HM, Lee HK. Does the difference of invasiveness between totally laparoscopic distal gastrectomy and laparoscopy-assisted distal gastrectomy lead to a difference in early surgical

outcomes? A prospective randomized trial. *Ann Surg Oncol.* (2015) 22:1836–43. doi: 10.1245/s10434-014-4229-x

22. Shinohara T, Kawano S, Tanaka Y, Fujisaki M, Watanabe A, Yamamoto K, et al. Comparison of the cost and outcomes following totally laparoscopic and laparoscopy-assisted distal gastrectomies for gastric cancer: a single-institution comparison. *Surg Endosc.* (2016) 30:3573–81. doi: 10.1007/s00464-015-4656-1
23. Jeong O, Jung MR, Park YK, Ryu SY. Safety and feasibility during the initial learning process of intracorporeal Billroth I (delta-shaped) anastomosis for laparoscopic distal gastrectomy. *Surg Endosc.* (2015) 29:1522–9. doi: 10.1007/s00464-014-3836-8

8

Surgery Strategies for Gastric Cancer with Liver Metastasis

*Zai Luo, Zeyin Rong and Chen Huang**

Department of General Surgery, Shanghai General Hospital, School of Medicine, Shanghai Jiao Tong University, Shanghai, China

***Correspondence:**
Chen Huang
richard-hc@hotmail.com

Gastric cancer with liver metastasis is defined as advanced gastric cancer and remains one of the deadliest diseases with poor prognosis. Approximately 4–14% of patients with gastric cancers presented with liver metastases at the initial diagnosis. Owing to its incurability, first-line treatment for gastric cancer with liver metastases is systematic chemotherapy, whereas surgery is usually performed to alleviate severe gastrointestinal symptoms. However, continuously emerging retrospective studies confirmed the role of surgery in gastric cancer with liver metastases and showed significantly improved survival rate in patients assigned to a group of surgery with or without chemotherapy. Therefore, more and more convincing data that resulted from prospective randomized clinical trials is in need to clarify the surgery strategies in patients with gastric cancer with liver metastasis.

Keywords: gastric cancer, liver metastasis, surgery, strategy, R0 resection

INTRODUCTION

Gastric cancer (GC), as the third most frequent cause of cancer-related death for human cancers in the world, continues to carry a noticeably higher fatality-to-case ratio, accounting for exceeding 782,000 confirmed cases died in 2018 worldwide (1). Especially in China, based on data from National Central Cancer Registry of China (NCCR) in 2015, gastric cancer was the most common cancer and the leading cause of cancer death except for lung cancer (2). Predominantly due to late-onset and non-specific symptoms and lack of active screening programs, ~34% of patients have distant metastases according to the Surveillance, Epidemiology, and End Results (SEER) Database (3), and nearly 4–14% of patients present with liver metastases at the initial presentation (4). In fact, the leading causes of death for gastric cancer include local recurrence, gross peritoneal dissemination, direct invasion to other organs, and extensive distant organ metastases. Anatomically speaking, the liver is the most common site of hematogenous metastases for advanced gastric cancer. Gastric cancer with liver metastases (GCLM) is generally classified into two types: one is synchronous metastases, which defined as metastases occurring before or during surgery or within 6 months after gastrectomy, and the other is metachronous metastases, which defined as metastases identified at least 6 months after gastrectomy (5). Synchronous GCLM is detected in nearly 5–10% of gastric cancer patients at diagnosis (6), whereas metachronous GCLM is in up to 37% after "curative" resection of primary gastric cancer (7).

According to practical clinical guidelines, such as the National Comprehensive Cancer Network (NCCN), GCLM was regarded as stage IVb disease and unresectable tumor, which not only showed aggressive oncological behavior but also accompanied by distant metastases. And it was traditionally recommended with systemic chemotherapy including CF (cisplatin and fluorouracil) or ECF (epirubicin, cisplatin, and fluorouracil) chemotherapeutic regimens

(8). Recently, accumulating clinical trials have achieved significant progress in chemotherapy. For example, for HER2-negative advanced gastric cancer, the findings of the SPIRITS trial revealed the superiority of S-1 plus cisplatin to S-1 alone in advanced gastric cancer (9). Furthermore, results of the G-SOX trial found that S-1 plus oxaliplatin was non-inferior to S-1 plus cisplatin in advanced gastric cancer, mainly in less toxic and more convenient clinically (10). For HER2-positive advanced gastric cancer, discoveries of the ToGA trial found that chemotherapy regimen consisting of capecitabine plus or fluorouracil plus cisplatin in combination with trastuzumab was a promising option for patients with HER2-positive advanced gastric cancer (11). In addition, results of the ATTRACTION-2 trial indicated the survival benefits of nivolumab in patients with advanced gastric or gastroesophageal junction cancer (12). Although major progress was made in chemotherapy and molecularly targeted biological therapy (13, 14), until now, the median survival time (MST) of patients with GCLM was between 7 and 14.1 months (9–12). Given the dismal prognosis of patients with GCLM, there was an urgent need to develop better treatment strategies for GCLM in the absence of institutional guidelines or protocols.

Inspired by substantial survival benefits and compelling evidence of surgery in patients with colorectal cancer liver metastases (15, 16), many clinical surgeons explored the role of surgery in GCLM, which was considered as a crucial intervention and the most essential step to cure disease and to prolong patient life (17). Increasing systemic and aggressive oncological behaviors were shown in GCLM (18), compared with colorectal cancer liver metastases; gastrectomy was reserved for the palliation of severe gastrointestinal symptoms such as refractory hemorrhage and obstruction in patients with GCLM based on NCCN (8). On the contrary, the Guidelines Committee of the Japan Gastric Cancer Association was in favor of surgical resection of potentially resectable M1 disease (19), and recent studies showed that the potential of surgical resection in selected GCLM, which can bring MST between 9 and 67.5 months and 5-year survival, varies from 0 to 42%, inspiringly (5, 20, 21). This review aims to summarize recent studies underpinning the surgical resection for GCLM and to explain the surgery strategies in different clinical classifications of GCLM.

CURRENT EVIDENCE

Controversies in the Surgical Resection of Gastric Cancer With Liver Metastasis

From the perspective of the routine clinical application, objective assessments of clinical data about surgical resection in GCLM are essential to investigate the surgery strategies in GCLM. Although surgery is recommended to alleviate severe gastrointestinal symptoms in consensus, the utility of surgery in GCLM still remains highly controversial. More recently, inconsistent and contradictory findings of surgical resection in GCLM have emerged in published literature (22, 23).

A public clinical trial (REGATTA) (22) failed to improve the overall survival (OS) rate in advanced gastric cancer patients assigned to gastrectomy plus post-operative chemotherapy than in those assigned to chemotherapy alone (14.3 vs. 16.6 months). However, evidence from a clinical trial (AIO-FLOT3) (23) showed different outcomes. Compared with patients who experienced chemotherapy alone, patients who experienced neoadjuvant chemotherapy followed by surgical resection had superior OS (22.9 vs. 10.7 months). Notably, the design of the REGATTA trial differed from the design of the AIO-FLOT3 trial in some respects, which possibly had influenced outcomes of the trial. First, most GCLM patients enrolled in the REGATTA trial were accompanied by peritoneal metastases, who were recognized as the worst kind in advanced GC patients in prognosis. Second, the surgical management in the REGATTA trial was restricted to D1 lymphadenectomy only, whereas in the AIO-FLOT3 trial, the surgical management adopted gastrectomy with D2 lymphadenectomy, which was recommended for total or subtotal distal gastrectomy (24). Third, compared with gastrectomy plus chemotherapy adopted in the REGATTA trial, the AIO-FLOT3 trial utilized neoadjuvant chemotherapy followed by surgical resection in the treatment plan. Collectively, the above evidence reveals the crucial factors including patient selection, surgical procedures, and treatment options in a multimodality approach to GCLM.

Potential Superiority of Surgery in Gastric Cancer With Liver Metastasis

Available evidence of surgery for patients with GCLM mostly relies on retrospective studies, systematic reviews, and prospective trials. Data published after 2000 mostly showed significant and prognostic benefits of surgical resection for GCLM (**Table 1**) (5, 6, 20, 21, 25, 73), and the benefits were in continuous increase owing to advancements in accurate diagnosis, patient selection, perioperative nutritional support, anesthetic techniques, surgery approaches, management of post-operative complications, and enhanced recovery after surgery.

Recently, principally from East Asia and Europe, large retrospective studies on the surgical resection of GCLM have shown continuously acceptable survival outcomes for selected patients. Nishi et al. (51) demonstrated that the overall 1- and 3-year survival rates after hepatic resection for GCLM were 88.9 and 17.8% in 10 selected patients, respectively, with an MST of 21.5 months and no post-operative mortality. Similarly, in a retrospective single-center study involving 34 patients with GCLM, Ryu et al. (59) investigated the significance of surgical procedures including hepatic resection for more massive metastases and surgical microwave ablation for patients who had a high operative risk and identified prognostic factors. The results showed acceptable morbidity and favorable long-term outcomes, as the 1-, 3-, and 5-year OS rates after surgery were 86.5, 51.4, and 42.1%, respectively, and the 1-, 3-, and 5-year recurrence-free survival (RFS) rates were 38.5, 28.0, and 28.0%, respectively, with no significant survival differences for varied surgical treatments ($P = 0.213$).

Meanwhile, a nationwide retrospective study from England also showed that gastrectomy combined with hepatectomy for synchronous GCLM might carry survival benefits in

TABLE 1 | Demographics and survival in GCLM patients underwent surgical resection.

References	Year	Country	Type	Study interval	No. of Patients	Median Age	Post-operative 30-day mortality (%)	Overall survival			
								1 year (%)	3 years (%)	5 years (%)	MST (months)
Adam et al. (25)	2006	France	Retro	1983–2004	64	NR	NR	NR	NR	27	15
Aizawa et al. (26)	2014	Japan	Retro	1997–2010	53	66	NR	NR	NR	18.6	27.4
Ambiru et al. (27)	2001	Japan	Retro	1975–1999	40	63	0	NR	NR	18	12
Baek et al. (28)	2013	Korea	Retro	2003–2010	12	61	0	65	NR	39	31
Chen et al. (29)	2013	China	Retro	2007–2012	20	57	0	NR	NR	15	22.3
Cheon et al. (30)	2008	Korea	Retro	1995–2005	41	60	1.72	75	32	21	17
Choi et al. (31)	2010	Korea	Retro	1986–2007	14	65	NR	67	38.3	NR	NR
Dittmar et al. (32)	2012	Germany	Retro	1995–2009	15	57	0	NR	NR	27	48
Fukami et al. (33)	2017	Japan	Retro	2001–2012	14	66	NR	71.4	42.9	42.9	27.9
Fuji et al. (34)	2001	Japan	Retro	1979–1999	10	58.5	10	60	20	10	NR
Garancini et al. (35)	2012	Italy	Retro	1998–2007	21	64	0	68	31	19	11
Guner et al. (36)	2016	Korea	Retro	1998–2013	68	61	NR	79.1	40.6	30	NR
Hirai et al. (37)	2006	Japan	Retro	1993–2004	14	NR	NR	NR	NR	41.6	NR
Hwang et al. (38)	2009	Korea	Retro	1995–2005	73	59	NR	NR	NR	NR	20
Imanura et al. (39)	2001	Japan	Retro	1990–1997	17	NA	NR	60	25	NR	NR
Kinoshita et al. (40)	2015	Japan	Retro	1990–2010	256	64	NR	77.3	41.9	31.1	31.1
Koga et al. (41)	2007	Japan	Retro	1985–2005	42	64	0	76	48	42	34
Kokkola et al. (42)	2012	Finland	Retro	2000–2009	23	61.4	NR	NR	NR	NR	14.3
Komeda et al. (43)	2014	Japan	Retro	2000–2012	24	69.5	0	78.3	40.1	40.1	22.3
Lee et al. (20)	2017	Korea	Retro	2000–2014	7	59.2	NR	NR	NR	68.6	67.5
Li et al. (6)	2015	China	Retro	2008–2011	25	61.4	NR	72	NR	NR	20.5
Li et al. (44)	2017	China	Retro	1996–2012	34	62	NR	73.5	36.9	24.5	26.2
Liu et al. (45)	2012	China	Retro	1995–2010	35	NR	NR	58.1	21.7	NR	15
Liu et al. (46)	2015	China	Retro	1990–2009	35	56	0	NR	NR	14.3	33
Makino et al. (47)	2010	Japan	Retro	1992–2007	16	NA	0	82.3	46.4	37.1	31.2
Markar et al. (48)	2016	UK	Retro	1997–2012	78	NR	7.2	64.1	NR	38.5	NR
Miki et al. (49)	2012	Japan	Retro	1995–2009	25	72	NR	73.9	42.8	36.7	33.4
Morise et al. (50)	2008	Japan	Retro	1989–2004	18	64	NR	56.3	27.3	27.3	13
Nishi et al. (51)	2018	Japan	Retro	1996–2008	39	64	0	56.4	17.9	10.3	14
Nomura et al. (52)	2009	Japan	Retro	1991–2005	17	65.8	NR	NR	NR	30.8	21
Ohkura et al. (53)	2015	Japan	Retro	1985–2014	9	66	NR	88.9	29.6	NR	NR
Okano et al. (54)	2002	Japan	Retro	1986–1999	19	69	NR	77	34	34	21
Oki et al. (55)	2016	Japan	Retro	2000–2010	94	70	NR	86.5	51.4	42.1	40.8
Qiu et al. (56)	2013	China	Retro	1998–2009	25	NR	0	96	70.4	29.4	38
Roh et al. (et al. (57)	2005	Korea	Retro	1988–1996	11	61	0	73	NR	27	19
Rudloff et al. (58)	2014	USA	Pro	2009–2012	9	45	NR	44.4	33.3	22.2	11.3
Ryu et al. (59)	2017	Japan	Retro	1997–2015	14	NR	NR	84.6	51.3	51.3	NR
Saiura et al. (60)	2002	Japan	Retro	1981–1998	10	60.5	30	50	30	20	25
Sakamoto et al. (61)	2007	Japan	Retro	1990–2005	37	64	0	NR	NR	11	31
Schildberg et al. (62)	2012	Germany	Retro	1972–2008	31	65	6	NR	NR	13	NR
Shinohara et al. (63)	2015	Japan	Retro	1995–2010	22	NR	0	86	26	26	22
Shirabe et al. (64)	2003	Japan	Retro	1979–2001	36	66	0	64	26	26	NR
Song et al. (65)	2017	China	Retro	2001–2012	96	63	0	87.5	47.6	21.7	34
Takemura et al. (66)	2012	Japan	Retro	1993–2011	64	65	0	84	50	37	34
Thelen et al. (5)	2008	Germany	Retro	1988–2002	24	64	4.2	38	16	10	9
Tiberio et al. (67)	2016	Italy	Retro	1990–2013	105	68	0.9	58.2	20.3	13.1	14.6
Tsujimoto et al. (68)	2010	Japan	Retro	1980–2007	17	66	NR	75	37.5	31.5	34
Turanli et al. (21)	2010	Turkey	Pro	2005–2008	18	NR	NR	NR	0	0	14.1
Ueda et al. (69)	2009	Japan	Retro	1991–2005	15	NR	0	80	NR	60	13.4
Viganò et al. (70)	2013	Italy	Retro	1997–2008	20	61.5	0	95	63.2	33.2	52.3
Wang et al. (71)	2012	China	Retro	2003–2008	30	60	0	43.3	16.7	16.7	11
Wang et al. (72)	2014	China	Retro	1996–2008	39	64	0	56	17.9	10.3	14
Zacherl et al. (73)	2002	Austria	Retro	1980–1999	15	62	0	36	14.3	0	8.8

Retro indicates retrospective study; NR, not reported; MST, median survival time.

selected patients (48). Kaplan–Meier curve analyses showed that patients who were selected to have gastrectomy with additional hepatectomy for liver metastases (GGH group) had survival similar to that of patients who had gastrectomy in the absence of liver metastases (GG group) ($P = 0.196$) and improved survival than did patients who had gastrectomy without liver resection for liver metastases (GGNH group) ($P < 0.001$) and patients with GCLM who had no surgery (GNS group) ($P < 0.001$). As for mortality, the GGH group and GGNH group had similar 30-day mortality ($P = 0.246$), whereas the former had significantly improved 90-day mortality ($P = 0.009$), 1-year mortality ($P < 0.001$), and 5-year mortality ($P < 0.001$); and the GNS group had the worst OS and highest mortality at 30, 90 days, 1, and 5 years ($P < 0.001$) in the four groups. The results of this study revealed that gastrectomy combined with additional surgical resection of liver metastases was better than palliative treatment or gastrectomy without resection of liver metastases for patients with GCLM in survival benefits.

To reassess this bias problem in full measure, many systematic reviews and pooled analyses were conducted. A systematic review launched by Liao et al. (74) included eight non-randomized studies, representing a total of 677 patients with GCLM. The median OS time in patients who underwent gastrectomy combined with hepatectomy was significantly prolonged, as compared with the median OS time of those who underwent palliative therapy (23.7 vs. 7.6 months), with survival rates of the two arms of 69, 40, 33%, and 27, 8, 4% at 1, 2, and 3 years, respectively. Compared with palliative therapy, hepatectomy was associated with significantly lower mortality at 1-year (OR 0.17, $P < 0.001$) and 2-year (OR 0.15, $P < 0.001$). Owing to the disparity in the stage of disease, differences of the regimen of chemotherapy, and preference of surgery of surgeons (75), patients who underwent hepatectomy in Western countries showed lower median rates of OS at 1 year (60 vs. 76%), 2 years (30 vs. 47%), and 3 years (23 vs. 39%) than did those in Asian countries.

As previously stated, most of the published papers on surgical resection in patients with GCLM came from retrospective data, whereas only four randomized controlled trials (RCTs) investigated the role of surgery for patients with GCLM so far. The REGATTA trial was the first RCT to compare gastrectomy followed by chemotherapy with chemotherapy alone concerning OS in patients with GCLM (22). Findings from this trial denied the survival efficacy of palliative gastrectomy followed by chemotherapy from an interim analysis, which had caused the interruption of this trial in 2016. However, to some extent, results from the AIO-FLOT3 trial countered those of the REGATTA trial by strict inclusion criteria, surgical approaches, and treatment regimens (23). The AIO-FLOT3 trial exhibited favorable survival in patients with GCLM who received neoadjuvant chemotherapy and later underwent surgical resection, which had provided a rationale for the ongoing AIO-FLOT5 trial (NCT02578368) (76). Compared with the REGATTA trial, the AIO-FLOT5 trial excludes the enrolment of patients with clinically visible tumors of the peritoneum and >P1 peritoneal tumors, adopts a complete resection of a primary tumor including standardized lymphadenectomy (R0 and at least D2), and adjusts the place of chemotherapy and surgery. Hopefully, if this trial was proved to be effective, it could potentially lead to a new standard of therapy. Another ongoing trial named SURGIGAST (NCT03042169), which has not recruited patients, aims to compare the OS of palliative surgical resection plus chemotherapy with that of chemotherapy alone for stage IV gastric cancer including GCLM (77).

Despite the significant survival benefits from gastrectomy combined with hepatectomy over non-resectional management in patients with GCLM, as well as favorable published outcomes from chemotherapy followed by surgery over chemotherapy alone, it must be stressed that most of data came from retrospective studies and systematic reviews. Thus, outcome data from the AIO-FLOT5 trial and the SURGIGAST trial are awaited to verify the survival benefit of surgical resection suggested by retrospective studies and systematic reviews.

Prognostic Factors and Patient Selection in Gastric Cancer With Liver Metastasis

A considerable amount of published literature about surgery in GCLM illustrates the ascendency of surgery. However, it is conspicuous that not every patient will benefit from surgery. Hence, prognostic evaluation is crucial to identify the suitable candidates for radical surgery, which are of gastric cancer, liver metastases (synchronous disease), and liver metastases alone (metachronous disease), from those who will not benefit from surgery.

Lately, in a multicenter retrospective study, Tiberio et al. (78) compared the application of radical surgery vs. palliative gastrectomy or palliative surgery without resection in GCLM, in which radical surgery had achieved better long-term results than others in the 5-year survival rate (9.3, 2.1, and 0%, respectively). In light of this, they further recognized the best candidates for radical surgery through systematically investigating the patient-related, gastric cancer-related, metastasis-related, and treatment-related prognostic factors. Results confirmed that the invasive depth of primary tumor ($P < 0.001$), curative surgical procedure (R0 resection; $P = 0.001$), timing of hepatic involvement ($P < 0.001$), and adjuvant chemotherapy ($P < 0.001$) were associated with long-term survival, independently. Especially in R0 resection, results implied that it can significantly reduce the possibility of recurrence in GC patients with liver oligometastasis, even in patients with multiply scattered metastases in both lobes of the liver.

Accordingly, in the metachronous disease, Tiberio et al. (79) also revealed that T4 gastric cancer ($P = 0.019$), the presence of lymph node metastases ($P = 0.05$), and grade 3 GC ($P = 0.018$) displayed negative prognostic factors. Moreover, a multivariate analysis demonstrated that a therapeutic strategy of liver metastases was highly associated with survival as well, in particular when R0 resection was performed ($P < 0.001$).

Likewise, based on real-world data, the AGAMENON registry involving 1,792 patients with advanced GC (80), distal esophagus, or gastroesophageal junction revealed higher 3-year survival rate after metastasectomy than non-metastasectomy (30.6 vs. 8.4%; $P < 0.001$) and median OS since metastasectomy of 16.7 months.

With the use of a state-arrival extended Markov proportional hazard (PH) model, a multivariate analysis indicated the presence of a HER2-positive tumor treated with trastuzumab ($P = 0.001$) and chemotherapy followed by surgical procedure ($P < 0.001$) as favorable predictors of survival. Moreover, they also found that the unreasonable interval time between the initiation of chemotherapy and surgery appeared to worsen outcomes. Their results also recommended that 5 months as interval time benefits most patients, which is consistent with the AIO-FLOT3 trial.

Also, Takemura et al. (66) reported the overall 5-year survival rate of 37% and the MST of 34 months in 64 patients achieved macroscopically complete (R0 or R1) resections. Among 64 patients, 50 patients had the largest hepatic metastasis of more than 5 cm in diameter, and 14 patients had <5 cm in diameter ($P = 0.07$). Results demonstrated that patients with a maximum diameter of hepatic metastasis >5 cm had poorer long-term survival ($P = 0.018$).

Above all, most of identified prognostic factors were similar with those in various literature through multivariate analyses, which could be roughly divided into five major categories that consisted of primary tumor-associated, liver metastasis-associated, extrahepatic metastasis-associated, and treatment-associated prognostic factors and others, as shown in **Table 2**. However, these factors were mainly identified from retrospective studies in single center or multicenter, which need to be validated in prospective clinical studies to further confirm their prognostic role.

SURGERY IN DIFFERENT CATEGORIES OF GASTRIC CANCER WITH LIVER METASTASIS

New Classified Evaluation for Gastric Cancer With Liver Metastasis

Although the Lauren classification and the WHO classification are popular in pathological grading of GCs, they are insufficient to guide personalized treatments, especially in GCLM. New classified evaluation for GCLM is thus required. Encouragingly, recent advancements in retrospective studies and prospective studies have greatly facilitated the identification of potential candidates.

Referring to the clinical study on GCLM and classification of stage IV GC (83), we divided GCLM patients into three categories, as shown in **Figure 1**. First, GCLM could be divided into the potentially resectable tumor (category I), marginally resectable tumor (category II), and unresectable tumor (category III) according to the analysis of clinical decision making in multidisciplinary treatment. For example, macroscopic peritoneal dissemination was considered an essential factor during the classification process, because patients with peritoneal dissemination or positive peritoneal cytology had significantly poor prognosis (84). Second, patients of category I were recommended to undergo surgery followed by post-operative chemotherapy or to receive neoadjuvant chemotherapy combined with surgery. Patients in category II were suggested to adopt conversion therapy aimed to an R0 resection after combined chemotherapy. Patients in category III, who also had obstruction and bleeding of the gastrointestinal tract in some cases, were advised to receive palliative chemotherapy.

Surgery Strategies in Different Categories of Gastric Cancer With Liver Metastasis

Surgery in Resectable Liver Metastases (Category I)

Potentially resectable liver metastases (category I) were characterized by <5 metastasis (better for solitary metastasis), with the diameter of the largest metastatic lesion measuring <5 cm and metastasis occurring in one liver lobe, which was regarded as a technically resectable metastasis.

For patients who conformed to the defining characteristics of category I, evidence from clinical trials and retrospective studies recommended them to undergo neoadjuvant chemotherapy followed by R0 resection of hepatic metastasis with or without primary GC and D2 lymphadenectomy and post-operative chemotherapy. Komeda et al. (43) indicated that the overall 5-year survival rate and MST of patients with GCLM who underwent gastrectomy followed by curative hepatectomy were 40.1% and 22.3 months, respectively. Especially in patients with a maximum size of liver metastasis ≤5 cm, they had higher overall 5-year survival than had patients with a maximum size of liver metastasis > 5 cm (51.7 vs. 14.3%). Furthermore, in a retrospective study that enrolled 24 patients with GC with two or three liver-limited metastases, Shirasu et al. (81) found no survival benefit for patients who experienced hepatectomy only compared with chemotherapy only ($P = 0.146$). However, recurrence and death occurred in none of the patients who received initial chemotherapy followed by surgery. Despite small sample size of patients, this study still should be regarded as a direction for further study.

Similarly, in a prospectively comparative study involving 49 patients with synchronous GCLM, Li et al. (6) compared patients assigned to R0 resection of primary tumor and liver metastasis as well as D2 lymphadenectomy followed by post-operative chemotherapy with patients assigned to chemotherapy only. Results revealed that the MST of surgery group was significantly longer than that of the control group (20.5 vs. 9.1 months). Moreover, the response to chemotherapy was indicated by the prognostic factors only through their multivariate analysis. Remarkably, the AIO-FLOT3 trial (23) enrolled 60 patients with liver metastases of <5 to receive eight cycles of the FOLT (fluorouracil, oxaliplatin, leucovorin, and docetaxel) chemotherapy in total, 36 of whom underwent surgery to achieve margin-free (R0) resection after the first four cycles of neoadjuvant chemotherapy. Compared with 24 patients assigned to chemotherapy only, 36 patients with surgery had more favorable MST (31.3 vs. 15.9 months) and progression-free survival (26.7 vs. 8.4 months).

In this case, initial gastrectomy and hepatectomy aimed to achieve R0 resection; otherwise, it should combined with neoadjuvant chemotherapy. Indeed, R0 resection was a microscopically margin-negative resection, in which no gross or microscopic tumor was kept in the primary tumor site,

TABLE 2 | Independent favorable prognostic factors for surgery in patients with GCLM.

Categories	Favorable prognostic factors	References
Primary tumor	No serosal invasion	(40, 66)
	Lower T stage	(33, 49, 65, 67, 78, 79)
	No lymphatic or venous invasion	(46, 55, 72, 79)
Liver metastases	Unilobar involvement	(26, 47, 61, 73, 78, 81)
	Number of metastatic lesions ≤ 3, especially for solitary metastasis	(30, 35, 40, 41, 46, 52–56, 61–63, 65, 69–72)
	Diameter of greatest lesion ≤ 5 cm	(36, 40, 43, 53, 66, 68)
	Metachronous metastases	(27, 51, 54, 62, 67)
Extrahepatic metastasis	Absence of peritoneal metastasis	(38, 39, 44, 69, 71)
Treatment	Negative margin (R0)	(5, 21, 30, 35, 62, 67, 69, 82)
	D2 Lymphadenectomy	(68)
	Neoadjuvant chemotherapy	(23)
	Post-operative chemotherapy	(42, 56, 67, 78)
	Response to chemotherapy	(6, 70)
Other	Lower CEA and CA 19-9 levels	(33, 59)
	HER2-positive tumor treated with trastuzumab	(23, 80)

GCLM, gastric cancer with liver metastases; CEA, carcinoembryonic antigen; CA 19-9, carbohydrate antigen 19-9.

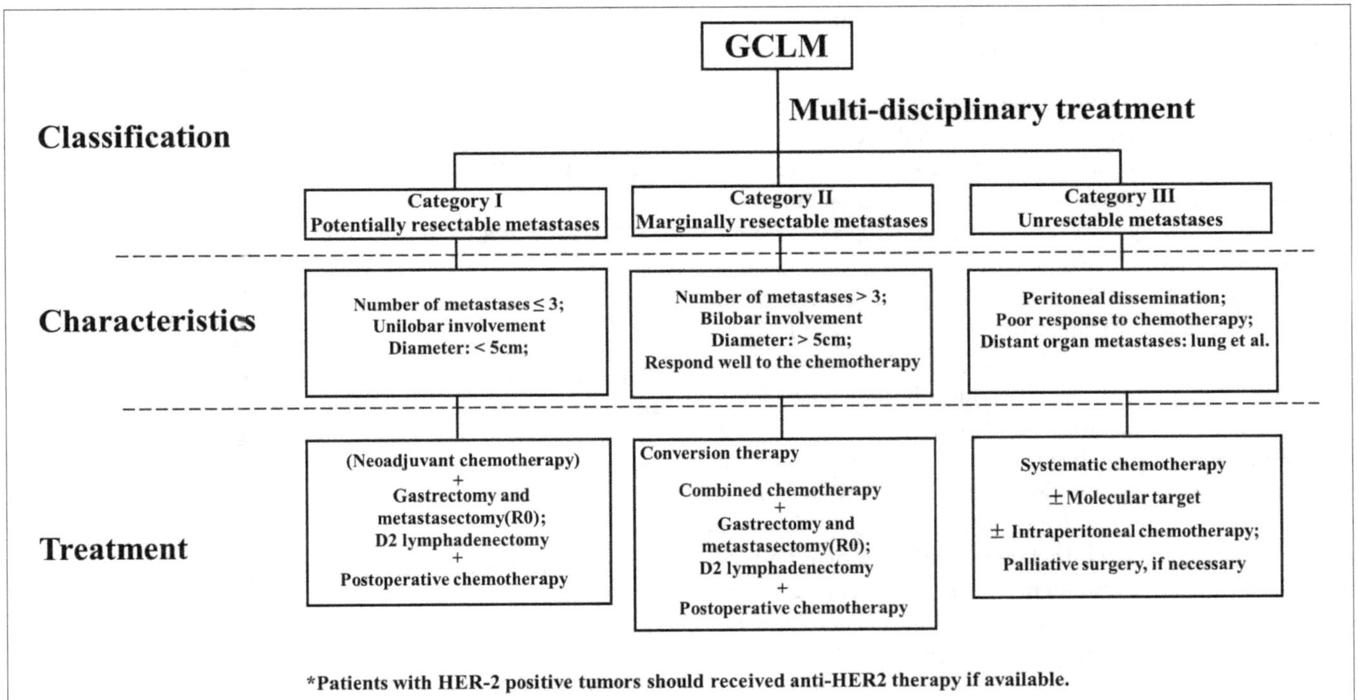

FIGURE 1 | Clinical classification, characteristics, and treatment of gastric cancer with liver metastases (GCLM).

which could remove the tumor and retain tissues to the hilt. Simultaneously, neoadjuvant chemotherapy was able to treat micrometastases at an early stage to downstage the primary tumor and obtained a higher R0 resection rate. Moreover, post-operative chemotherapy acted as a "supervisor" to maintain the state of R0 resection, for prevention of progression and recurrence of metastasis of gastric cancer. Thus, patients in this category were highly inclined to achieve R0 resection and obtain reduced recurrence rate.

Surgery in Marginally Resectable Liver Metastases (Category II)

Marginally resectable liver metastases (category II) was composed of patients with multiple liver metastases (>3), maximum tumor diameter that exceeds 5 cm, or bilobar invasion with the absence of peritoneal metastases. This category was regarded as oncologically and technically unresectable.

In clinical practice, surgery is controversial for these patients, as they are usually offered chemotherapy. However, existing evidence indicated that initially marginally resectable and unresectable gastric cancer could be converted into resectable gastric cancer by novel combined chemotherapy (83–85). Thus, recent studies begin to focus on surgery with an expectation of R0 resection performed in originally unresectable and marginally resectable GCLM that responded to chemotherapy. Fukuchi et al. (84) selected S-1 plus cisplatin or paclitaxel as initial combination chemotherapy for advanced gastric cancer including GCLM. Compared with patients who only received chemotherapy, patients treated with chemotherapy plus surgery had a prolonged survival at 5 years (43 vs. 1%).

Moreover, among patients who underwent conversion therapy, patients who underwent R0 resection had significantly more favorable survival as opposed to those who underwent R+ resections (49 vs. 15% in a 5-year survival rate). In a recent retrospective study involving patients with marginally resectable tumor, Yamaguchi et al. (82) reported that the MST of patients assigned to conversion therapy was 30.5 months, whereas that of patients assigned chemotherapy alone was 11.0 months ($P < 0.05$). In a group of conversion therapy, patients underwent R0 resection had prolonged survival time than had those who underwent R+ resection (56.2 vs. 16.3 months).

In spite of the encouraging outcomes mentioned, the limitations of the above studies should be noted. First, enrolled patients for most studies have experienced for a long period lack of consistencies in the decision making of diagnosis and in approaches of chemotherapeutic regimen and surgery. Second, inherent selection bias occurred in retrospective data including response to chemotherapy and performance status, which could affect outcomes. Third, in almost all retrospective studies, owing to the insufficiency in evidence of clinical characteristics including laboratory data and molecular classification, clinicopathological factors and response to chemotherapy were considered as major factors to predict the candidates for potential R0 surgical resection. Consequently, existing studies should accelerate the implementation of randomized clinical trials to determine the role of conversion therapy and to explore the effect of laboratory data and molecular classification on survival benefit to provide a guideline for patient stratification and personalized treatment in GCLM (86).

Surgery in Unresectable Liver Metastases (Category III)

Unresectable liver metastases (category III) contained patients with macroscopically peritoneal dissemination or extensive metastases in multiple organs, who carry a worse or less favorable prognosis.

According to recent studies, patients in category III could benefit from conversion therapy as well. However, only a small fraction of patients who responded well to chemotherapy were accessible to achieve R0 resection (87). Moreover, palliative chemotherapy remained as a mainstream treatment according to clinical guidelines. Consistent with palliative radiotherapy (88), palliative surgery also plays a vital role in coping with obstruction and bleeding of the gastrointestinal tract.

Above all, because most evidence came from retrospective studies, defining the role of surgery in different categories of GCLM was in need of more robust evidence from prospective randomized clinical trials. Furthermore, a combination of clinical classification and molecular classification of GCLM might accelerate the identification of novel therapeutic targets and formation of personalized treatment (89, 90).

PERSPECTIVES

In summary, despite the increasing evidence in favor of surgery in GCLM, the indication and extent of surgery, including the selection of patients and the potential to achieve R0 resection, should be carefully discussed and determined. Emerging research indicated that hepatic arterial infusion chemotherapy (HAIC), radiation therapy, and radiofrequency ablation (RFA) provided alternative treatment modalities for GCLM (36, 91, 92). Importantly, prospective randomized clinical trials are needed urgently to clarify the indication and the surgery strategies in GCLM.

AUTHOR CONTRIBUTIONS

ZL and CH were involved in the concept and design. ZL, ZR, and CH wrote, reviewed, and revised the manuscript. CH supervised the manuscript.

REFERENCES

1. Bray F, Ferlay J, Soerjomataram I, Siegel RL, Torre LA, Jemal A. Global cancer statistics 2018: GLOBOCAN estimates of incidence and mortality worldwide for 36 cancers in 185 countries. *Cancer J Clin.* (2018) 68:394–424. doi: 10.3322/caac.21492
2. Chen W, Zheng R, Baade PD, Zhang S, Zeng H, Bray F, et al. Cancer statistics in China, 2015. *Cancer J Clin.* (2016) 66:115–32. doi: 10.3322/caac.21338
3. Howlader N, Noone AM, Krapcho M, Garshell J, Neyman N, Altekruse SF, et al. *SEER Cancer Statistics Review, 1975–2010.* Bethesda, MD: National Cancer Institute (2013). Available online at: https://seer.cancer.gov/archive/csr/1975_2010/
4. Shin A, Kim J, Park S. Gastric cancer epidemiology in Korea. *J Gastr Cancer.* (2011) 11:135–40. doi: 10.5230/jgc.2011.11.3.135
5. Thelen A, Jonas S, Benckert C, Lopez-Hanninen E, Neumann U, Rudolph B, et al. Liver resection for metastatic gastric cancer. *Eur J Surg Oncol.* (2008) 34:1328–34. doi: 10.1016/j.ejso.2008.01.022

6. Li Z, Fan B, Shan F, Tang L, Bu Z, Wu A, et al. Gastrectomy in comprehensive treatment of advanced gastric cancer with synchronous liver metastasis: a prospectively comparative study. *World J Surg Oncol.* (2015) 13:212. doi: 10.1186/s12957-015-0627-1
7. D'Angelica M, Gonen M, Brennan MF, Turnbull AD, Bains M, Karpeh MS. Patterns of initial recurrence in completely resected gastric adenocarcinoma. *Ann Surg.* (2004) 240:808–16. doi: 10.1097/01.sla.0000143245.28656.15
8. National Comprehensive Cancer Network (NCCN). *Clinical Practice Guidelines in Oncology. Gastric Cancer, Version 5.* (2017). Available online at: https://www.nccn.org/professionals/physician_gls/f_guidelines.asp (accessed September 15, 2016).
9. Koizumi W, Narahara H, Hara T, Takagane A, Akiya T, Takagi M, et al. S-1 plus cisplatin versus S-1 alone for first-line treatment of advanced gastric cancer (SPIRITS trial): a phase III trial. *Lancet Oncol.* (2008) 9:215–21. doi: 10.1016/S1470-2045(08)70035-4
10. Yamada Y, Higuchi K, Nishikawa K, Gotoh M, Fuse N, Sugimoto N, et al. Phase III study comparing oxaliplatin plus S-1 with cisplatin plus S-1 in chemotherapy-naïve patients with advanced gastric cancer. *Ann Oncol.* (2015) 26:141–8. doi: 10.1093/annonc/mdu472
11. Bang YJ, Van Cutsem E, Feyereislova A, Chung HC, Shen L, Sawaki A, et al. Trastuzumab in combination with chemotherapy versus chemotherapy alone for treatment of HER2-positive advanced gastric or gastro-oesophageal junction cancer (ToGA): a phase 3, open-label, randomised controlled trial. *Lancet.* (2010) 376:687–97. doi: 10.1016/S0140-6736(10)61121-X
12. Kang YK, Boku N, Satoh T, Ryu MH, Chao Y, Kato K, et al. Nivolumab in patients with advanced gastric or gastro-oesophageal junction cancer refractory to, or intolerant of, at least two previous chemotherapy regimens (ONO-4538-12, ATTRACTION-2): a randomised, double-blind, placebo-controlled, phase 3 trial. *Lancet.* (2017) 390:2461–71. doi: 10.1016/S0140-6736(17)31827-5
13. de Hosson LD, van Veenendaal LM, Schuller Y, Zandee WT, de Herder WW, Tesselaar MET, et al. Clinical benefit of systemic treatment in patients with advanced pancreatic and gastrointestinal neuroendocrine tumours according to ESMO-MCBS and ASCO framework. *Ann Oncol.* (2017) 28:3022–27. doi: 10.1093/annonc/mdx547
14. Shah MA. Update on metastatic gastric and esophageal cancers. *J Clin Oncol.* (2015) 33:1760–9. doi: 10.1200/JCO.2014.60.1799
15. Quan D, Gallinger S, Nhan C, Auer RA, Biagi JJ, Fletcher GG, et al. The role of liver resection for colorectal cancer metastases in an era of multimodality treatment: a systematic review. *Surgery.* (2012) 151:860–70. doi: 10.1016/j.surg.2011.12.018
16. Hur H, Ko YT, Min BS, Kim KS, Choi JS, Sohn SK, et al. Comparative study of resection and radiofrequency ablation in the treatment of solitary colorectal liver metastases. *Am J Surg.* (2009) 197:728–36. doi: 10.1016/j.amjsurg.2008.04.013
17. Markar SR, Mikhail S, Malietzis G, Athanasiou T, Mariette C, Sasako M, et al. Influence of surgical resection of hepatic metastases from gastric adenocarcinoma on long-term survival: systematic review and pooled analysis. *Ann Surg.* (2016) 263:1092–101. doi: 10.1097/SLA.0000000000001542
18. Oguro S, Imamura H, Yoshimoto J, Ishizaki Y, Kawasaki S. Liver metastases from gastric cancer represent systemic disease in comparison with those from colorectal cancer. *J Hepato Biliary Pancr Sci.* (2016) 23:324–32. doi: 10.1002/jhbp.343
19. Kodera Y, Fujitani K, Fukushima N, Ito S, Muro K, Ohashi N, et al. Surgical resection of hepatic metastasis from gastric cancer: a review and new recommendation in the Japanese gastric cancer treatment guidelines. *Gastr Cancer.* (2014) 17:206–12. doi: 10.1007/s10120-013-0299-x
20. Lee JW, Choi MH, Lee YJ, Ali B, Yoo HM, Song KY, et al. Radiofrequency ablation for liver metastases in patients with gastric cancer as an alternative to hepatic resection. *BMC Cancer.* (2017) 17:185. doi: 10.1186/s12885-017-3156-1
21. Turanli S. The value of resection of primary tumor in gastric cancer patients with liver metastasis. *Ind J Surg.* (2010) 72:200–5. doi: 10.1007/s12262-010-0053-0
22. Fujitani K, Yang HK, Mizusawa J, Kim YW, Terashima M, Han SU, et al. Gastrectomy plus chemotherapy versus chemotherapy alone for advanced gastric cancer with a single non-curable factor (REGATTA): a phase 3, randomised controlled trial. *Lancet Oncol.* (2016) 17:309–18. doi: 10.1016/S1470-2045(15)00553-7
23. Al-Batran SE, Homann N, Pauligk C, Illerhaus G, Martens UM, Stoehlmacher J, et al. Effect of neoadjuvant chemotherapy followed by surgical resection on survival in patients with limited metastatic gastric or gastroesophageal junction cancer: the AIO-FLOT3 Trial. *JAMA Oncol.* (2017) 3:1237–44. doi: 10.1001/jamaoncol.2017.0515
24. Hu Y, Huang C, Sun Y, Su X, Cao H, Hu J, et al. Morbidity and mortality of laparoscopic versus open D2 distal gastrectomy for advanced gastric cancer: a randomized controlled trial. *J Clin Oncol.* (2016) 34:1350–7. doi: 10.1200/JCO.2015.63.7215
25. Adam R, Chiche L, Aloia T, Elias D, Salmon R, Rivoire M, et al. Hepatic resection fornoncolorectal nonendocrine liver metastases: analysis of 1,452 patients and development of a prognostic model. *Ann Surg.* (2006) 244:524–35. doi: 10.1097/01.sla.0000239036.46827.5f
26. Aizawa M, Nashimoto A, Yabusaki H, Nakagawa S, Matsuki A. Clinical benefit of surgical management for gastric cancer with synchronous liver metastasis. *Hepatogastroenterology.* (2014) 61:1439–45. doi: 10.5754/hge14149
27. Ambiru S, Miyazaki M, Ito H, Nakagawa K, Shimizu H, Yoshidome H, et al. Benefits and limits of hepatic resection for gastric metastases. *Am J Surg.* (2001) 181:279–83. doi: 10.1016/S0002-9610(01)00567-0
28. Baek HU, Kim SB, Cho EH, Jin SH, Yu HJ, Lee JI, et al. Hepatic resection for hepatic metastases from gastric adenocarcinoma. *J Gastr Cancer.* (2013) 13:86–92. doi: 10.5230/jgc.2013.13.2.86
29. Chen L, Song MQ, Lin HZ, Hao LH, Jiang XJ, Li ZY, et al. Chemotherapy and resection for gastric cancer with synchronous liver metastases. *World J Gastroenterol.* (2013) 19:2097–103. doi: 10.3748/wjg.v19.i13.2097
30. Cheon SH, Rha SY, Jeung HC, Im CK, Kim SH, Kim HR, et al. Survival benefit of combined curative resection of the stomach (D2 resection) and liver in gastric cancer patients with liver metastases. *Ann Oncol.* (2008) 19:1146–53. doi: 10.1093/annonc/mdn026
31. Choi SB, Song J, Kang CM, Hyung WJ, Kim KS, Choi JS, et al. Surgical outcome of metachronous hepatic metastases secondary to gastric cancer. *Hepatogastroenterology.* (2010) 57:29–34.
32. Dittmar Y, Altendorf-Hofmann A, Rauchfuss F, Götz M, Scheuerlein H, Jandt K, et al. Resection of liver metastases is beneficial in patients with gastric cancer: report on 15 cases and review of literature. *Gastr Cancer.* (2012) 15:131–6. doi: 10.1007/s10120-011-0080-y
33. Fukami Y, Kaneoka Y, Maeda A, Takayama Y, Takahashi T, Uji M, et al. Adjuvant hepatic artery infusion chemotherapy after hemihepatectomy for gastric cancer liver metastases. *Int J Surg.* (2017) 46:79–84. doi: 10.1016/j.ijsu.2017.08.578
34. Fujii K, Fujioka S, Kato K, Machiki Y, Kutsuna Y, Ishikawa A, et al. Resection of liver metastasis from gastric adenocarcinoma. *Hepatogastroenterology.* (2001) 48:368–71.
35. Garancini M, Uggeri F, Degrate L, Nespoli L, Gianotti L, Nespoli A, et al. Surgical treatment of liver metastases of gastric cancer: is local treatment in a systemic disease worthwhile? *HPB.* (2012) 14:209–15. doi: 10.1111/j.1477-2574.2011.00428.x
36. Guner A, Son T, Cho I, Kwon IG, An JY, Kim HI, et al. Liver-directed treatments for liver metastasis from gastric adenocarcinoma: comparison between liver resection and radiofrequency ablation. *Gastr Cancer.* (2016) 19:951–60. doi: 10.1007/s10120-015-0522-z
37. Hirai I, Kimura W, Fuse A, Isobe H, Hachiya O, Moriya T, et al. Surgical management for metastatic liver tumors. *Hepatogastroenterology.* (2006) 53:757–63.
38. Hwang SE, Yang DH, Kim CY. Prognostic factors for survival in patients with hepatic recurrence after curative resection of gastric cancer. *World J Surg.* (2009) 33:1468–72. doi: 10.1007/s00268-009-0034-2
39. Imamura H, Matsuyama Y, Shimada R, Kubota M, Nakayama A, Kobayashi A, et al. A study of factors influencing prognosis after resection of hepatic metastases from colorectal and gastric carcinoma. *Am J Gastroenterol.* (2001) 96:3178–84. doi: 10.1111/j.1572-0241.2001.05278.x
40. Kinoshita T, Kinoshita T, Saiura A, Esaki M, Sakamoto H, Yamanaka T. Multicentre analysis of long-term outcome after surgical resection for gastric cancer liver metastases. *Br J Surg.* (2015) 102:102–7. doi: 10.1002/bjs.9684

41. Koga R, Yamamoto J, Ohyama S, Saiura A, Seki M, Seto Y, et al. Liver resection for metastatic gastric cancer: experience with 42 patients including eight long-term survivors. *Jap J Clin Oncol.* (2007) 37:836–42. doi: 10.1093/jjco/hym113
42. Kokkola A, Louhimo J, Puolakkainen P. Does non-curative gastrectomy improve survival in patients with metastatic gastric cancer? *J Surg Oncol.* (2012) 106:193–6. doi: 10.1002/jso.23066
43. Komeda K, Hayashi M, Kubo S, Nagano H, Nakai T, Kaibori M, et al. High survival in patients operated for small isolated liver metastases from gastric cancer: a multi-institutional study. *World J Surg.* (2014) 38:2692–7. doi: 10.1007/s00268-014-2608-x
44. Li SC, Lee CH, Hung CL, Wu JC, Chen JH. Surgical resection of metachronous hepatic metastases from gastric cancer improves long-term survival: a population-based study. *PLoS ONE.* (2017) 12:e0182255. doi: 10.1371/journal.pone.0182255
45. Liu J, Li JH, Zhai RJ, Wei B, Shao MZ, Chen L. Predictive factors improving survival after gastric and hepatic surgical treatment in gastric cancer patients with synchronous liver metastases. *Chin Med J.* (2012) 125:165–71. doi: 10.3760/cma.j.issn.0366-6999.2012.02.001
46. Liu Q, Bi JJ, Tian YT, Feng Q, Zheng ZX, Wang Z. Outcome after simultaneous resection of gastric primary tumour and synchronous liver metastases: survival analysis of a single-center experience in China. *Asian Pac J Cancer Prev.* (2015) 16:1665–9. doi: 10.7314/APJCP.2015.16.4.1665
47. Makino H, Kunisaki C, Izumisawa Y, Tokuhisa M, Oshima T, Nagano Y, et al. Indication for hepatic resection in the treatment of liver metastasis from gastric cancer. *Anticancer Res.* (2010) 30:2367–76. Available online at: http://ar.iiarjournals.org/content/30/6/2367.long
48. Markar SR, Mackenzie H, Mikhail S, Mughal M, Preston SR, Maynard ND, et al. Surgical resection of hepatic metastases from gastric cancer: outcomes from national series in England. *Gastr Cancer.* (2017) 20:379–86. doi: 10.1007/s10120-016-0604-6
49. Miki Y, Fujitani K, Hirao M, Kurokawa Y, Mano M, Tsujie M, et al. Significance of surgical treatment of liver metastases from gastric cancer. *Anticancer Res.* (2012) 32:665–70. Available online at: http://ar.iiarjournals.org/content/32/2/665.long
50. Morise Z, Sugioka A, Hoshimoto S, Kato T, Ikeda M, Uyama I, et al. The role of hepatectomy for patients with liver metastases of gastric cancer. *Hepatogastroenterology.* (2008) 55:1238–41.
51. Nishi M, Shimada M, Yoshikawa K, Higashijima J, Tokunaga T, Kashihara H, et al. Results of hepatic resection for liver metastasis of gastric cancer. *J Med Invest.* (2018) 65:27–31. doi: 10.2152/jmi.65.27
52. Nomura T, Kamio Y, Takasu N, Moriya T, Takeshita A, Mizutani M, et al. Intrahepatic micrometastases around liver metastases from gastric cancer. *J Hepato Biliary Pancr Surg.* (2009) 16:493–501. doi: 10.1007/s00534-009-0081-y
53. Ohkura Y, Shinohara H, Haruta S, Ueno M, Hashimoto M, Sakai Y, et al. Hepatectomy offers superior survival compared with non-surgical treatment for </= 3 metastatic tumors with diameters < 3 cm from gastric cancer: a retrospective study. *World J Surg.* (2015) 39:2757–63. doi: 10.1007/s00268-015-3151-0
54. Okano K, Maeba T, Ishimura K, Karasawa Y, Goda F, Wakabayashi H, et al. Hepatic resection for metastatic tumors from gastric cancer. *Ann Surg.* (2002) 235:86–91. doi: 10.1097/00000658-200201000-00011
55. Oki E, Tokunaga S, Emi Y, Kusumoto T, Yamamoto M, Fukuzawa K, et al. Surgical treatment of liver metastasis of gastric cancer: a retrospective multicenter cohort study (KSCC1302). *Gastr Cancer.* (2016) 19:968–76. doi: 10.1007/s10120-015-0530-z
56. Qiu JL, Deng MG, Li W, Zou RH, Li BK, Zheng Y, et al. Hepatic resection for synchronous hepatic metastasis from gastric cancer. *Eur J Surg Oncol.* (2013) 39:694–700. doi: 10.1016/j.ejso.2013.03.006
57. Roh HR, Suh KS, Lee HJ, Yang HK, Choe KJ, Lee KU. Outcome of hepatic resection for metastatic gastric cancer. *Am Surg.* (2005) 71:95–9. Available online at: https://chinesesites.library.ingentaconnect.com/contentone/sesc/tas/2005/00000071/00000002/art00001
58. Rudloff U, Langan RC, Mullinax JE, Beane JD, Steinberg SM, Beresnev T, et al. Impact of maximal cytoreductive surgery plus regional heated intraperitoneal chemotherapy (HIPEC) on outcome of patients with peritoneal carcinomatosis of gastric origin: results of the GYMSSA trial. *J Surg Oncol.* (2014) 110:275–84. doi: 10.1002/jso.23633
59. Ryu T, Takami Y, Wada Y, Tateishi M, Matsushima H, Yoshitomi M, et al. Oncological outcomes after hepatic resection and/or surgical microwave ablation for liver metastasis from gastric cancer. *Asian J Surg.* (2019) 42:100–5. doi: 10.1016/j.asjsur.2017.09.005
60. Saiura A, Umekita N, Inoue S, Maeshiro T, Miyamoto S, Matsui Y, et al. Clinicopathological features and outcome of hepatic resection for liver metastasis from gastric cancer. *Hepatogastroenterology.* (2002) 49:1062–65.
61. Sakamoto Y, Sano T, Shimada K, Esaki M, Saka M, Fukagawa T, et al. Favorable indications for hepatectomy in patients with liver metastasis from gastric cancer. *J Surg Oncol.* (2007) 95:534–9. doi: 10.1002/jso.20739
62. Schildberg CW, Croner R, Merkel S, Schellerer V, Müller V, Yedibela S, et al. Outcome of operative therapy of hepatic metastatic stomach carcinoma: a retrospective analysis. *World J Surg.* (2012) 36:872–8. doi: 10.1007/s00268-012-1492-5
63. Shinohara T, Maeda Y, Hamada T, Futakawa N. Survival benefit of surgical treatment for liver metastases from gastric cancer. *J Gastrointest Surg.* (2015) 19:1043–51. doi: 10.1007/s11605-015-2775-6
64. Shirabe K, Shimada M, Matsumata T, Higashi H, Yakeishi Y, Wakiyama S, et al. Analysis of the prognostic factors for liver metastasis of gastric cancer after hepatic resection: a multi-institutional study of the indications for resection. *Hepatogastroenterology.* (2003) 50:1560–3.
65. Song A, Zhang X, Yu F, Li D, Shao W, Zhou Y. Surgical resection for hepatic metastasis from gastric cancer: a multi- institution study. *Oncotarget.* (2017) 8:71147–53. doi: 10.18632/oncotarget.16705
66. Takemura N, Saiura A, Koga R, Arita J, Yoshioka R, Ono Y, et al. Long-term outcomes after surgical resection for gastric cancer liver metastasis: an analysis of 64 macroscopically complete resections. *Langenbeck's Arch Surg.* (2012) 397:951–7. doi: 10.1007/s00423-012-0959-z
67. Tiberio GA, Ministrini S, Gardini A, Marrelli D, Marchet A, Cipollari C, et al. Factors influencing survival after hepatectomy for metastases from gastric cancer. *Eur J Surg Oncol.* (2016) 42:1229–35. doi: 10.1016/j.ejso.2016.03.030
68. Tsujimoto H, Ichikura T, Ono S, Sugasawa H, Hiraki S, Sakamoto N, et al. Outcomes for patients following hepatic resection of metastatic tumors from gastric cancer. *Hepatol Int.* (2010) 4:406–13. doi: 10.1007/s12072-009-9161-y
69. Ueda K, Iwahashi M, Nakamori M, Nakamura M, Naka T, Ishida K, et al. Analysis of the prognostic factors and evaluation of surgical treatment for synchronous liver metastases from gastric cancer. *Langenbeck's Arch Surg.* (2009) 394:647–53. doi: 10.1007/s00423-008-0311-9
70. Viganò L, Vellone M, Ferrero A, Giuliante F, Nuzzo G, Capussotti L. Liver resection for gastric cancer metastases. *Hepatogastroenterology.* (2013) 60:557–62. doi: 10.5754/hge11187
71. Wang YN, Shen KT, Ling JQ, Gao XD, Hou YY, Wang XF, et al. Prognostic analysis of combined curative resection of the stomach and liver lesions in 30 gastric cancer patients with synchronous liver metastases. *BMC Surg.* (2012) 12:20. doi: 10.1186/1471-2482-12-20
72. Wang W, Liang H, Zhang H, Wang X, Xue Q, Zhang R. Prognostic significance of radical surgical treatment for gastric cancer patients with synchronous liver metastases. *Med Oncol.* (2014) 31:258. doi: 10.1007/s12032-014-0258-3
73. Zacherl J, Zacherl M, Scheuba C, Steininger R, Wenzl E, Mühlbacher F, et al. Analysis of hepatic resection of metastasis originating from gastric adenocarcinoma. *J Gastrointest Surg.* (2002) 6:682–9. doi: 10.1016/S1091-255X(01)00075-0
74. Liao YY, Peng NF, Long D, Yu PC, Zhang S, Zhong JH, et al. Hepatectomy for liver metastases from gastric cancer: a systematic review. *BMC Surg.* (2017) 17:14. doi: 10.1186/s12893-017-0215-0
75. Kataoka K, Kinoshita T, Moehler M, Mauer M, Shitara K, Wagner AD, et al. Current management of liver metastases from gastric cancer: what is common practice? New challenge of EORTC and JCOG. *Gastr Cancer.* (2017) 20:904–12. doi: 10.1007/s10120-017-0696-7
76. Al-Batran SE, Goetze TO, Mueller DW, Vogel A, Winkler M, Lorenzen S, et al. The RENAISSANCE (AIO-FLOT5) trial: effect of chemotherapy alone vs. chemotherapy followed by surgical resection on survival and quality of life in patients with limited-metastatic adenocarcinoma of the stomach or esophagogastric junction - a phase III trial of the German AIO/CAO-V/CAOGI. *BMC Cancer.* (2017) 17:893. doi: 10.1186/s12885-017-3918-9
77. Zaanan A, Bouché O, Benhaim L, Buecher B, Chapelle N, Dubreuil O, et al. Gastric cancer: French intergroup clinical practice guidelines

for diagnosis, treatments and follow-up (SNFGE, FFCD, GERCOR, UNICANCER, SFCD, SFED, SFRO). *Digest Liver Dis.* (2018) 50:768–79. doi: 10.1016/j.dld.2018.04.025

78. Tiberio GA, Baiocchi GL, Morgagni P, Marrelli D, Marchet A, Cipollari C, et al. Gastric cancer 494 and synchronous hepatic metastases: is it possible to recognize candidates to R0 resection? *Ann Surg Oncol.* (2015) 22:589–96. doi: 10.1245/s10434-014-4018-6
79. Tiberio GA, Coniglio A, Marchet A, Marrelli D, Giacopuzzi S, Baiocchi L, et al. Metachronous hepatic metastases from gastric carcinoma: a multicentric survey. *Eur J Surg Oncol.* (2009) 35:486–91. doi: 10.1016/j.ejso.2008.12.017
80. Carmona-Bayonas A, Jiménez-Fonseca P, Echavarria I, Sánchez Cánovas M, Aguado G, Gallego J, et al. Surgery for metastases for esophageal-gastric cancer in the real world: data from the AGAMENON national registry. *Eur J Surg Oncol.* (2018) 44:1191–8. doi: 10.1016/j.ejso.2018.03.019
81. Shirasu H, Tsushima T, Kawahira M, Kawai S, Kawakami T, Kito Y, et al. Role of hepatectomy in gastric cancer with multiple liver-limited metastases. *Gastr Cancer.* (2018) 21:338–44. doi: 10.1007/s10120-017-0730-9
82. Yamaguchi K, Yoshida K, Tanahashi T, Takahashi T, Matsuhashi N, Tanaka Y, et al. The long-term survival of stage IV gastric cancer patients with conversion therapy. *Gastr Cancer.* (2018) 21:315–23. doi: 10.1007/s10120-017-0738-1
83. Yoshida K, Yamaguchi K, Okumura N, Tanahashi T, Kodera Y. Is conversion therapy possible in stage IV gastric cancer: the proposal of new biological categories of classification. *Gastr Cancer.* (2016) 19:329–38. doi: 10.1007/s10120-015-0575-z
84. Fukuchi M, Ishiguro T, Ogata K, Suzuki O, Kumagai Y, Ishibashi K, et al. Prognostic role of conversion surgery for unresectable gastric cancer. *Ann Surg Oncol.* (2015) 22:3618–24. doi: 10.1245/s10434-015-4422-6
85. Ikeguchi M, Miyake T, Matsunaga T, Yamamoto M, Fukumoto Y, Yamada Y, et al. Recent results of therapy for scirrhous gastric cancer. *Surg Today.* (2009) 39:290–4. doi: 10.1007/s00595-008-3860-1
86. Cancer Genome Atlas Research Network. Comprehensive molecular characterization of gastric adenocarcinoma. *Nature.* (2014) 513:202–9. doi: 10.1038/nature13480
87. Kitayama J, Ishigami H, Yamaguchi H, Yamashita H, Emoto S, Kaisaki S, et al. Salvage gastrectomy after intravenous and intraperitoneal paclitaxel (PTX) administration with oral S-1 for peritoneal dissemination of advanced gastric cancer with malignant ascites. *Ann Surg Oncol.* (2014) 21:539–46. doi: 10.1245/s10434-013-3208-y
88. Tey J, Zheng H, Soon YY, Leong CN, Koh WY, Lim K, et al. Palliative radiotherapy in symptomatic locally advanced gastric cancer: a phase II trial. *Cancer Med.* (2019) 8:1447–58. doi: 10.1002/cam4.2021
89. Bijlsma MF, Sadanandam A, Tan P, Vermeulen L. Molecular subtypes in cancers of the gastrointestinal tract. *Nat Rev Gastroenterol Hepatol.* (2017) 14:333–42. doi: 10.1038/nrgastro.2017.33
90. Van Cutsem E, Sagaert X, Topal B, Haustermans K, Prenen H. Gastric cancer. *Lancet.* (2016) 388:2654–64. doi: 10.1016/S0140-6736(16) 30354-3
91. Koukourakis GV. Evidence based radiation therapy for locally advanced resectable and unresectable gastric cancer. *World J Gastrointest Oncol.* (2011) 3:131–6. doi: 10.4251/wjgo.v3.i9.131
92. Seki H, Ohi H, Ozaki T, Yabusaki H. Hepatic arterial infusion chemotherapy using fluorouracil, epirubicin, and mitomycin C for patients with liver metastases from gastric cancer after treatment failure of systemic S-1 plus cisplatin. *Acta Radiol.* (2016) 57:781–8. doi: 10.1177/028418511 5603247

9

Effect of Biologic Material Reinforcement on Surgical Anastomosis After Gastrectomy

Won Jun Kim [1†], Chang Min Lee [2†], Liang An [1], Jong-Han Kim [3] and Sungsoo Park [4]*

[1] Korea University Medical Center, College of Medicine, Seoul, South Korea, [2] Department of Surgery, Korea University Medical Center, Ansan Hospital, Ansan, South Korea, [3] Department of Surgery, Korea University Medical Center, Guro Hospital, Seoul, South Korea, [4] Department of Surgery, Korea University Medical Center, Anam Hospital, Seoul, South Korea

***Correspondence:**
Sungsoo Park
kugspss@korea.ac.kr

† These authors have contributed equally to this work

Background: Acellular dermal matrix is a biologic material derived from the skin of human cadaveric donors. It has been used successfully in the past to reduce complications in breast surgery and hernia repair. This investigation was aimed at assessing the feasibility of using acellular dermal matrix to support the anastomosis after gastrectomy with the aim of reducing anastomotic site leakage complications.

Methods: Patients were randomly assigned to standard anastomotic reconstruction (control arm) or anastomotic reconstruction with acellular dermal matrix reinforcement (intervention arm). Surgical outcomes related to anastomotic complications were collected. Because actual anastomotic leaks found on imaging studies are infrequent and thus require a very high number of patient recruitment to detect statistically significant difference between the two groups, in this pilot investigation other clinical and laboratory measures that have been shown to correlate to or predict anastomotic leaks were also collected. Each surgical outcome was compared.

Results: A total of 94 patients (intervention arm: 50, control arm: 44), were included in the analysis. Two patients in the control arm (4.55%) and one patient in the intervention arm (2.00%) experienced anastomotic leakage ($p = 0.598$), a difference without statistical significance. However, average postoperative C-reactive protein (CRP) levels and NUn scores, both of which have been shown to reflect likelihood of progressing to anastomotic leakage, were significantly lower for the intervention arm. The control arm showed an average CRP level of 128.77 mg/dL (SD: 97.08) while the intervention arm showed 77.38 mg/dL (SD: 49.08, $p = 0.049$).

Conclusions: Leakage rate reduction with acellular dermal matrix reinforcement of anastomotic site was not detected in this investigation. However, postoperative inflammation levels and numerical predictors of anastomotic leakage development were significantly lower with acellular dermal matrix reinforcement of surgical anastomosis. This finding is worthy of further investigation, as reduction of inflammation with anastomotic site reinforcement is a novel finding, and more in-depth research may lead to discoveries on the physiologic role of the surgical anastomosis in post-gastrectomy patients. In addition, lower CRP and NUn scores for the intervention arm suggest potential for larger studies to detect reduction in clinical leak rates after acellular dermal matrix reinforcement.

Keywords: anastomotic leak, surgical anastomosis, gastrectomy, postoperative complications, gastric cancer, acellular dermal matrix

INTRODUCTION

Surgery of the gastrointestinal tract is most often concluded with anastomotic reconstruction of resection planes to restore gut continuity. Surgeons pay careful attention to these anastomotic sites as they are critical to procedure-related complications. The most dangerous and important anastomotic site complication is leakage, which is associated with increased morbidity and longer hospital stay as well as higher mortality (1). As the management of the anastomotic site during the reconstruction process is crucial in reducing these potentially fatal complications, the rates of such postoperative complications are often used as a surrogate marker for the quality of surgery (1–3). Although the surgical outcome for gastrointestinal surgeries has improved over time with experience and advancements in technique, the rate of postoperative complications remains high worldwide (4, 5). Various implements have been introduced in the surgical procedure, with the aim of reducing these complications: examples include the surgical stapler and bioabsorbable synthetic material scaffolds that support the anastomotic site (6–11). These new additions to the surgeon's arsenal have succeeded in reducing postoperative anastomotic complications to a certain degree (11, 12); but there is still much room for improvement, and various new approaches are being investigated by surgeons to further decrease anastomotic complication rates.

In contrast to the aforementioned bioabsorbable "synthetic" material, the acellular dermal matrix was developed as a "biologic" material scaffold for tissue reinforcement. The most prominent synthetic material reinforcement in use is the polyglycolic acid:trimethylene carbonate copolymer (Gore Seamguard®), which features an interconnected pore structure that allows the cells of the host to grow within it; it is then absorbed into host tissue around the staple line within six to seven months. It has been used to reduce postoperative complications in patients who have undergone gastrointestinal surgery. Biologic material like the acellular dermal matrix used in this investigation stands apart from the synthetic counterparts owing to its biologic origin. It is a connective tissue matrix of dermis harvested from the skin of human cadaveric donors, with the cellular components removed, based on the hypothesis that this may confer an advantage over synthetic material reinforcements as it can be revascularized with autologous tissue, resulting in reduced rates of infection and better maintenance of tissue strength, which have been shown to be true in animal studies (13, 14). Acellular dermal matrix is already being used in a number of applications, such as the repair of difficult hiatal hernias and the treatment of intestinal fistulization in patients with open peritoneal cavities (15, 16). The specific material used in this investigation (MegaDerm® - L&C Bio, SKN Techno Park, Sagimakgol-ro, Jungwon-gu, Seongnam-si, Gyeonggi-do, Korea) has also been used in plastic and reconstructive surgical applications (17–20). In this study, we aimed to assess the feasibility of using acellular dermal matrix reinforcement to reduce complications in patients who underwent gastrectomy, with a focus on anastomotic site leakage.

MATERIALS AND METHODS

Study Design

This pilot investigation is a randomized, double-arm, open-label, superiority study conducted in a single institute. Patients who had undergone total or subtotal gastrectomy for gastric adenocarcinoma were enrolled in this study. Enrollment took place from July of 2015 to April of 2016. Patients who provided their informed consent were randomized to either the control arm or the intervention arm: randomization sequence was created using Excel 2010 (Microsoft, Redmond, WA, USA) with a 1:1 allocation using simple randomization without stratification. Patients who underwent total or subtotal gastrectomy followed by standard anastomotic reconstruction without acellular dermal matrix reinforcement comprised the control arm, while those who underwent gastrectomy with the acellular dermal matrix reinforcement comprised the intervention arm. Data collected from the patients were analyzed by an independent investigator who was unaware of the allocation of each patient. The study protocol was approved by the institutional review board of Korea University Medical Center, Anam Hospital (Institutional Review Board number: MD15006). All procedures were conducted in accordance with the ethical standards of the institution's Committee on Human Experimentation and the Helsinki Declaration of 1975.

Patient Enrollment

The following inclusion and exclusion criteria were used for patient enrollment:
Inclusion criteria:

i) Patients between the ages of 20 and 90 years;
ii) Patients who were diagnosed with primary gastric adenocarcinoma by endoscopic biopsy;
iii) Patients who were fit for total or subtotal gastrectomy;
    A. ECOG (Eastern Cooperative Oncology Group) performance status 0 or 1
    B. ASA (American Society of Anesthesiologists) score between 1 and 3
    C. Patients who were not contraindicated for surgery based on the preoperative work-up

iv) Patients who provided informed consent by signing the IRB-approved consent form.

Exclusion criteria:

i) Patients who developed complications of gastric cancer (i.e., obstruction, perforation);
ii) Patients who received neoadjuvant chemotherapy or radiation therapy for the target gastric cancer of the surgery;
iii) Patients who received surgical or medical treatment for any other cancers in the last 5 years;
iv) Vulnerable patients (patients who are unable to make their own decisions, pregnant patients, patients planning on getting pregnant);
v) Patients who are currently or were enrolled in any time in the last 6 months in another clinical trial.

Operative Procedures and Postoperative Management

Patients were treated according to the standard guidelines for treatment of gastric cancer in Korea (21), which outlines the principles and standards of surgery for gastric cancer. All cases were laparoscopic with no conversion to open laparotomy. In all patients, lymphadenectomy was facilitated by an ultrasonic energy device (SOUND REACH®; Reach Surgical Inc., TEDA, Tianjin). Reconstruction procedures used were Billroth I, Billroth II, and Roux-en-Y esophagojejunostomy. Anastomotic reconstruction was conducted using the surgical stapler (ENDO REACH®; Reach Surgical Inc., TEDA, Tianjin); for patients in the intervention arm, acellular dermal matrix (MegaDerm® - L&C Bio, SKN Techno Park, Sagimakgol-ro, Jungwon-gu, Seongnam-si, Gyeonggi-do, Korea) was installed onto the surgical stapler with a hygroscopic suture fiber before use, after being moisturized to increase adhesiveness (**Figure 1**). Postoperative care was provided according to the institution's protocols.

Clavien-Dindo Classification Assessment

The main surgical outcome assessed in this investigation is the rate of anastomotic leakage. We primarily compared the severity of these postoperative anastomotic site complications in each group as measured by the modified Clavien-Dindo system, which is a widely adopted, objective classification system that grades the severity of surgical complications based on the level of intervention needed to resolve them (22). When the outlines proposed by the Clavien-Dindo classification were vague, the Japanese Clinical Oncology Group postoperative complications criteria (JCOG PC) criteria (23), which expands on the Clavien-Dindo system and more specifically delineates grades of each postoperative complication, were applied. As the potential for interpersonal variation remained, the classification process was conducted by two independent researchers who were unaware of each patient's treatment arm allocation. When discrepancies arose, the principal investigator (S.P.) was consulted to determine the final Clavien-Dindo classification for the patient.

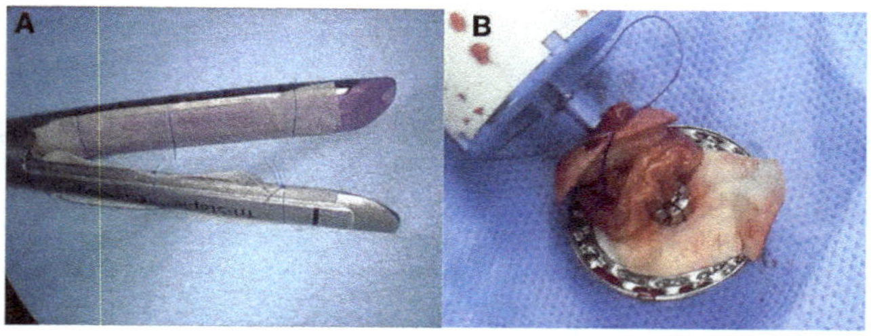

FIGURE 1 | Acellular dermal matrix loaded for use **(A)** linear stapler **(B)** circular stapler.

Anatomic Leakage Assessment

Computed tomography (CT), considered the best modality for the detection of gastrointestinal leakage (24), was the modality of choice when imaging was deemed clinically necessary. The clinical suspicion of leakage warranting imaging work-up was made by the patient's physician or the attending surgeon, with the basic consensus that episodes of fever peaking around 38.0°C constitute the most important clinical sign, as it has been designated a critical criterion for the suspicion of anastomotic leakage in previous studies (24–26). In addition, because post-gastrectomy leak rates are low and therefore difficult to statistically detect differences in leak rates between the two groups, other laboratory measurements that have been shown to predict anastomotic leak were also obtained. Inflammatory marker (e.g., white blood cell count, C-reactive protein) levels were obtained for patients when risk of leakage was even slightly suspected as there has been evidence that elevation of the C-reactive protein (CRP) level can be predictive of anastomotic leak complications (27–29). When multiple measurements were taken for a same patient, the highest value was used. In addition, Noble et al. showed that a combination of multiple laboratory values [the NUn score = 11.3894 + (0.005 × CRP) + (WCC × 0.186) - (0.174 × albumin); WCC refers to white blood cell count] can serve as a strong predictor of anastomotic leaks and other complications in esophageal resection (30); the NUn score was also obtained.

Statistical Analyses

Data were analyzed using IBM SPSS Statistics 24.0 (SPSS, Inc., Chicago, IL, USA). Continuous data were represented by their mean and standard deviation and the categorical data as frequencies and percentages. Student's t-test was used to compare continuous variables, and the χ^2 test and two-tailed Fisher's exact test were used to compare categorical variables. The average CRP values of postoperative days one, four, and seven were calculated for each treatment arm and plotted in a line graph.

RESULTS

A total of 94 patients were analyzed in the study. Of these patients, 50 were included in the intervention arm and 44 in the control arm. The scheme of enrollment is shown in **Figure 2**.

Patient demographics including age, sex, body mass index (BMI), comorbidities, American Society of Anesthesiologists (ASA) score, Eastern Cooperative Oncology Group (ECOG)

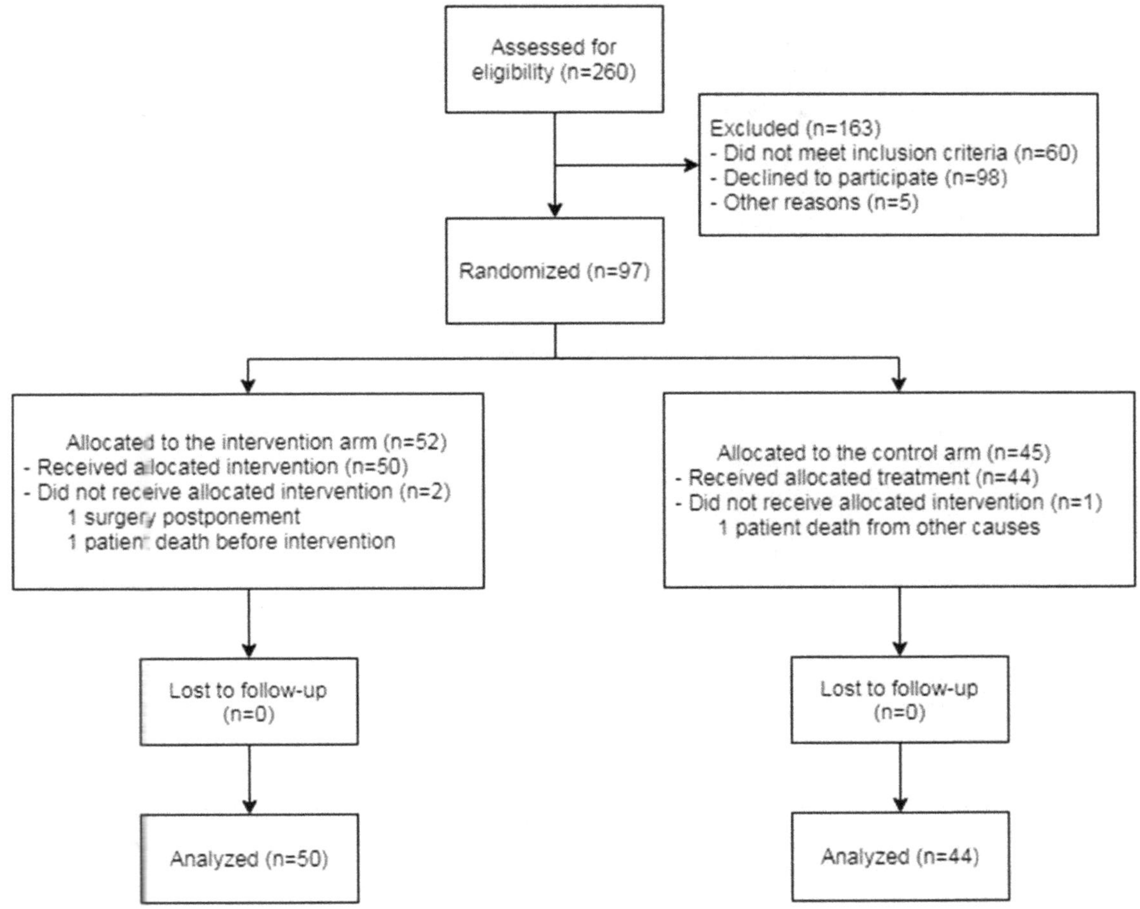

FIGURE 2 | Flow diagram of patient enrolment.

performance status, type of reconstruction received, and the extent of lymphadenopathy are described in **Table 1**. There were no significant differences in these baseline characteristics between the two groups.

Comparison of Clinicopathologic Outcomes

Postoperatively, data related to clinical outcomes including operation time, length of hospital stay, proximal resection margin, and complication rates were compared between the two groups (**Table 2**). There were no significant differences in the proximal resection margin, length of hospital stay, and operating time. The Clavien-Dindo (C-D) classification system was used for the comparison of complication rates. Of 44 patients in the control arm and 50 patients in the intervention arm, 19 (43.18%) and 20 (40.00%), respectively, experienced complications. No patients experienced complications of C-D class IIIb or higher. Although the control arm showed a tendency toward more severe (grade II or IIIa) complications, the difference was not statistically significant ($p = 0.1157$).

Comparison of Anastomotic Site Leakage Complications

The results of the comparison of anastomotic leak rates are shown in **Table 3**. Two of 44 patients in the control group developed leakage during the 6-month follow-up period, whereas one of the 50 suffered leakage in the intervention arm during the same period. The patients in the control arm developed 13 and 6 days after surgery; the patient in the intervention arm developed leakage 18 days after surgery. This difference did not have a statistically significant value ($p = 0.598$). There were also no significant differences in the number of episodes of fever, the clinical sign most commonly used to suspect leakage after gastrointestinal surgery. Postoperative CRP levels, on the other hand, were found to be significantly lower in patients who received acellular dermal matrix reinforcement. Comparison of average CRP levels of each patient showed that the control arm had an average CRP level of 128.77 mg/dL, compared to the average of 77.38 mg/dL in the intervention arm. The NUn score, developed by Noble et al. (30) to predict anastomotic leak in esophageal resection patients using postoperative CRP levels, white blood cell counts, and albumin levels, also showed

TABLE 1 | Baseline characteristics of patients.

Characteristics	Control (*n* = 44)	Biomaterial reinforcement (*n* = 50)	*P*
Age (years)(SD)	61.7 (10.6)	59.9 (10.4)	0.402
Sex ratio (M:F)			0.87
Male	28 (63.6%)	31 (62.0%)	
Female	16 (36.4%)	19 (38.0%)	
Body mass index (kg/m^2)	23.53 (2.93)	23.65 (2.92)	0.85
Comorbidities			0.225
None or 1	30	28	
>2	14	22	
Types of reconstruction			0.254
Billroth I	27	37	
Billroth II	6	7	
Esophagojejunostomy	11	6	
Extent of lymphadenopathy			0.694
D1+a	2	1	
D1+b	14	14	
D2	28	35	
T stage			0.365
T1a	12	18	
T1b	11	12	
T2	8	9	
T3	6	9	
T4a	7	2	
N stage			0.55
N0	22	32	
N1	11	8	
N2	5	6	
N3a	3	3	
N3b	3	1	
ECOG			0.544
0	41	48	
1	3	2	
ASA			0.231
1	2	5	
2	42	43	
3	0	2	

TABLE 2 | Comparison of clinicopathologic outcomes.

	Control no. (%)	Biomaterial reinforcement no. (%)	*P*
Proximal resection margin (cm)	4.45	4.47	0.974
Length of stay (days)	15.48	13.38	0.142
Postoperative fever			0.385
≥1 Fever episode	16 (36.4%)	14 (28.0%)	
No fever	28 (63.6%)	36 (72.0%)	
Operation time (minutes)	185.91	164.90	0.060
C-D class			
0	25 (56.8%)	30 (60.0%)	
I	6 (13.6%)	12 (24.0%)	
II	9 (20.5%)	5 (10.0%)	
IIIa	4 (9.1%)	3 (6.0%)	
IIIb	0	0	
IVa	0	0	
IVb	0	0	
V	0	0	
Total	44	50	
0 + I	31 (70.5%)	42 (84.0%)	0.1157
II + III	13 (29.5%)	8 (16.0%)	

TABLE 3 | Comparison of results related to anastomotic leakage.

Variables	Control	Biomaterial reinforcement	*P*
Leak found on imaging	2 (4.55%)	1 (2.00%)	(Fisher's) 0.598
Average CRP	128.77 (*n* = 17) (SD 97.08)	77.38 (*n* = 19) (SD 49.08)	0.049
NUn score	13.28 (*n* = 12) (SD 0.67)	12.71 (*n* = 13) (SD 0.67)	0.042

a statistically significant higher likelihood of progression to leakage for the control arm, with average scores of 13.29 (SD 0.667) and 12.71 (SD 0.667) for the control and intervention arms, respectively.

DISCUSSION

The primary endpoint of this study was clinically discovered episodes of anastomotic leakage. However, because we expected the number of these episodes to be low and our aim in this pilot investigation was to see the potential effect of acellular dermal matrix on postgastrectomy patients, clinical and laboratory measures that have been shown to predict anastomotic leaks were collected as secondary endpoints. These include cases of postoperative fever, inflammatory marker levels (i.e., CRP), and a scoring system developed to predict leaks in esophageal resection patients (i.e., NUn score). The severity of postoperative complications, as graded by the Clavien-Dindo classification system, was also collected as a secondary endpoint.

Acellular dermal matrix reinforcement of the anastomotic line after gastrectomy did not result in statistically significant improvements in either the occurrence of anastomotic site leakage. In addition, in terms of overall complication rates as represented by the Clavien-Dindo postoperative complication severity scale, there were no significant differences between the two treatment arms. However, the laboratory markers that reflect the likelihood of leakage, i.e., postoperative CRP levels and the NUn score, were significantly lower in the intervention arm.

The major limitation of our study is the small sample size. Because of the low rate of leakage complications, a large sample size—more than 1,500 patients in each arm based on the findings of this pilot investigation—is required for enough statistical power to demonstrate leak rate differences between the two arms. While an expected weakness, this pilot study is obviously underpowered to detect differences in clinical leak rates, and we have had to rely on extrapolation from secondary endpoints to draw conclusions about the effect of acellular dermal matrix reinforcement of the anastomotic site. However, the potential significance of our findings is discussed below, detailing findings that can serve as a reference for future studies of treatment for anastomotic leakage.

The most notable outcome of this investigation was the discrepancy in postoperative inflammation levels reflected by the CRP levels and NUn scores. Lower levels of these indicators have been shown to reflect lower likelihood of progressing to anastomotic leak (27–30). Studies have also shown that there is a correlation between overall postoperative complication rates and postoperative CRP levels as well (17, 31–33). Therefore, the reduced inflammatory levels in the acellular dermal matrix reinforcement group of this study may suggest that the anastomotic site reinforcement makes the operation more tolerable for the patient and has the potential to decrease likelihood of anastomotic leak development. In addition, the NUn score was specifically included in the analysis because while CRP is a nonspecific marker of inflammation and even CT images for leakage can be uncertain, the NUn score is a marker that is specifically designed to assess risk of leakage in the foregut. As such, it shows much less variance in either group compared to that of the nonspecific CRP. The lower NUn score in the intervention arm substantiates CRP findings. However because it is unknown how postoperative inflammation relates to each specific complication such as leakage, it must be noted that it is premature to firmly conclude on the clinical ramifications of lessened inflammation from these results alone.

Synthetic material reinforcements (as opposed to the biologic material acellular dermal matrix employed in this investigation) to anastomotic sites have been investigated in previous studies with positive results in reducing anastomotic complications. This material is already adopted for gastrectomy procedures. Similar to our investigation, Gayrel et al. have noted lower CRP levels in patients who received synthetic material reinforcement after sleeve gastrectomy than in those who did not, but this difference was without statistical significance (9). To the best of our knowledge, our investigation is the first to clinically show that a reinforcement material is able to statistically significantly reduce postoperative inflammation in upper gastrointestinal surgery. This may be related to the fundamental physiologic differences between biologic and synthetic materials. Acellular dermal matrix such as one used in this investigation is derived from human skin and treated with AlloClean® technology to leave only the extracellular matrix three-dimensional structure of the dermis. Synthetic buttress material, such as Gore Seamguard®, is made of polyglycolic acid:trimethylene carbonate (PGA:TMC) to form an interconnected pore structure to allow for cell infiltration and growth. Descriptions of both materials suggest they consist of comparable structures designed to perform similar functions. Synthetic buttress material is more integrated into the practice of current surgeons, but there were previous studies that have suggested superior performance of acellular dermal matrix over synthetic mesh reinforcement for hernia repairs and chest wall constructions (13, 14). A laboratory investigation found less inflammatory response in the integration of biologic materials compared to synthetic materials into tissue (34). We also speculate that the physiologic characteristic of biologic material has reduced postoperative inflammation as it leads to faster recovery of the anastomotic site, conferring a higher degree of protection against the development of anastomotic site weakness. However, we cannot yet draw conclusions on the difference between acellular dermal matrix reinforcement and synthetic reinforcements in the setting of gastrointestinal surgery, as no formal comparison between the two materials have been published to date.

In conclusion, this study was unable to detect any differences in leak rates or complication severity levels as measured by the Clavien-Dindo classification after application of acellular dermal matrix to reinforce the anastomotic site in patients who have undergone total or subtotal gastrectomy. The only notable difference between the intervention arm and the control arm was in the levels of postoperative inflammation. Findings from previous studies suggest that this decreased level of postoperative inflammation leads to more positive surgical outcomes in patients who received the biomaterial reinforcement, as these postoperative inflammatory marker levels are predictors of anastomotic leaks among other postoperative complications. Follow-up studies with larger sample sizes and longer follow-up periods may yield clinically significant differences in actual leak rates as well. In addition, further investigations into the mechanism behind postoperative inflammation after gastrointestinal surgery and the reason behind the decrease in inflammation with reinforcement of the anastomotic site with buttress materials may also uncover previously undiscovered surgical physiology.

ETHICS STATEMENT

The studies involving human participants were reviewed and approved by Korea University Institutional Review Board. The patients/participants provided their written informed consent to participate in this study.

AUTHOR CONTRIBUTIONS

SP first conceived, set up the parameters of the study, and was responsible for the oversight of the investigation as well as the manuscript production. He was also the surgeon responsible for operations detailed in the investigation. WK and CL further defined the patient enrollment criteria and data collection methods of the study, conducted the data analysis, and produced the final manuscript. LA and J-HK assisted in patient enrollment and led data collection. All authors contributed substantially to the study design and data analysis, revised the manuscript, and approved the current version of the paper. All authors contributed crucial intellectual information that made the production of this manuscript possible.

REFERENCES

1. Bruce J, Krukowski ZH, Al-Khairy G, Russell EM, Park KGM. Systematic review of the definition and measurement of anastomotic leak after gastrointestinal surgery. *Br J Surg.* (2001) 88:1157–68. doi: 10.1046/j.0007-1323.2001.01829.x
2. Lee JH, Park DJ, Kim HH, Lee HJ, Yang HK. Comparison of complications after laparoscopy-assisted distal gastrectomy and open distal gastrectomy for gastric cancer using the Clavien-Dindo classification. *Surg Endosc.* (2012) 26:1287–95. doi: 10.1007/s00464-011-2027-0
3. Jung MR, Park YK, Seon JW, Kim KY, Cheong O, Ryu SY. Definition and classification of complications of gastrectomy for gastric cancer based on the accordion severity grading system. *World J Surg.* (2012) 36:2400–11. doi: 10.1007/s00268-012-1693-y
4. Mickevicius A, Ignatavicius P, Markelis R, Parseliunas A, Butkute D, Kiudelis M, Endzinas Z, Maleckas A, and Dambrauskas Z. Trends and results in treatment of gastric cancer over last two decades at single East European centre: a cohort study. *BMC Surg.* (2014) 14:98. doi: 10.1186/1471-2482-14-98
5. Oh SJ, Choi WB, Song J, Hyung WJ, Choi SH, Noh SH, et al. Complications requiring reoperation after gastrectomy for gastric cancer: 17 years experience in a single institute. *J Gastrointest Surg.* (2009) 13:239–45. doi: 10.1007/s11605-008-0716-3
6. Loffler T, Rossion I, Goossen K, Saure D, Weitz J, Ulrich A, et al. Hand suture versus stapler for closure of loop ileostomy–a systematic review and meta-analysis of randomized controlled trials. *Langenbecks Arch Surg.* (2015) 400:193–205. doi: 10.1007/s00423-014-1265-8
7. Kimura M, Terashita Y. Use of bioabsorbable staple reinforcement material in side-to-side anastomoses: suture line reinforcement of the weak point of the anastomosis. *Ann Med Surg.* (2016) 6:50–5. doi: 10.1016/j.amsu.2016.01.034
8. Salgado W Jr, Rosa GV, Nonino-Borges CB, Ceneviva R. Prospective and randomized comparison of two techniques of staple line reinforcement during open Roux-en-Y gastric bypass: oversewing and bioabsorbable Seamguard(R). *J Laparoendosc Adv Surg Tech A.* (2011) 21:579–82. doi: 10.1089/lap.2010.0469
9. Gayrel X, Loureiro M, Skalli EM, Dutot C, Mercier G, Nocca D. Clinical and economic evaluation of absorbable staple line buttressing in sleeve gastrectomy in high-risk patients. *Obes Surg.* (2016) 26:1710–6. doi: 10.1007/s11695-015-1991-1
10. Alley JB, Fenton SJ, Harnisch MC, Angeletti MN, Peterson RM. Integrated bioabsorbable tissue reinforcement in laparoscopic sleeve gastrectomy. *Obes Surg.* (2011) 21:1311–5. doi: 10.1007/s11695-010-0313-x
11. Scott JD, Cobb WS, Carbonell AM, Traxler B, Bour ES. Reduction in anastomotic strictures using bioabsorbable circular staple line reinforcement in laparoscopic gastric bypass. *Surg Obes Relat Dis.* (2011) 7:637–42. doi: 10.1016/j.soard.2011.01.002
12. Placer C, Enriquez-Navascues JM, Elorza G, Timoteo A, Mugica JA, Borda N, et al. Preventing complications in colorectal anastomosis: results of a randomized controlled trial using bioabsorbable staple line reinforcement for circular stapler. *Dis Colon Rectum.* (2014) 57:1195–201. doi: 10.1097/DCR.0000000000000207
13. Holton LH III, Chung T, Silverman RP, Haerian H, Goldberg NH, Burrows WM, et al. Comparison of acellular dermal matrix and synthetic mesh for lateral chest wall reconstruction in a rabbit model. *Plast Reconstr Surg.* (2007) 119:1238–46. doi: 10.1097/01.prs.0000254347.36092.9c
14. Milburn ML, Holton LH, Chung TL, Li EN, Bochicchio GV, Goldberg NH, et al. Acellular dermal matrix compared with synthetic implant material for repair of ventral hernia in the setting of peri-operative *Staphylococcus aureus* implant contamination: a rabbit model. *Surg Infect.* (2008) 9:433–42. doi: 10.1089/sur.2007.044
15. Lee E, Frisella MM, Matthews BD, Brunt LM. Evaluation of acellular human dermis reinforcement of the crural closure in patients with difficult hiatal hernias. *Surg Endosc.* (2007) 21:641–5. doi: 10.1007/s00464-006-9117-4
16. Girard S, Sideman, M., Spain, D. A. A novel approach to the problem of intestinal fistulization arising in patients managed with open peritoneal cavities. *Am J Surg.* (2002) 184:166–7. doi: 10.1016/S0002-9610(02)00916-9
17. Suh MK, Lee KH, Harijan A, Kim HG, Jeong EC. Augmentation rhinoplasty with silicone implant covered with acellular dermal matrix. *J Craniofac Surg.* (2017) 28:445–8. doi: 10.1097/SCS.0000000000003225
18. Kim DY, Kang SW, Kim DS, Shin JU, Chung WY, Park CS, et al. Preventive effect of human acellular dermal matrix on post-thyroidectomy scars and adhesions: a randomized, double-blinded, controlled trial. *Dermatol Surg.* (2015) 41:812–20. doi: 10.1097/DSS.0000000000000410
19. Park GY, Yoon ES, Cho HE, Lee BI, Park SH. Acellular dermal matrix as a core strut for projection in nipple reconstruction: approaches for three different methods of breast reconstruction. *Arch Plast Surg.* (2016) 43:424–9. doi: 10.5999/aps.2016.43.5.424
20. Lee MC, Jang YJ, Yun IS, Lew DH, Lee WJ. Comparative skin evaluation after split-thickness skin grafts using 2 different acellular dermal matrices to cover composite forearm defects. *J Hand Surg Am.* (2017) 42:297 e1–10. doi: 10.1016/j.jhsa.2017.01.026
21. Lee JH, Kim JG, Jung HK, Kim JH, Jeong WK, Jeon TJ, et al. Clinical practice guidelines for gastric cancer in Korea: an evidence-based approach. *J Gastric Cancer.* (2014) 14:87–104. doi: 10.5230/jgc.2014.14.2.87
22. Dindo D, Demartines N, Clavien P-A. Classification of surgical complications. *Ann Surg.* (2004) 240:205–13. doi: 10.1097/01.sla.0000133083.54934.ae
23. Katayama H, Kurokawa Y, Nakamura K, Ito H, Kanemitsu Y, Masuda N, et al. Extended Clavien-Dindo classification of surgical complications: Japan Clinical Oncology Group postoperative complications criteria. *Surg Today.* (2016) 46:668–85. doi: 10.1007/s00595-015-1236-x
24. Abou Rached A, Basile M, El Masri H. Gastric leaks post sleeve gastrectomy: review of its prevention and management. *World J Gastroenterol.* (2014) 20:13904–10. doi: 10.3748/wjg.v20.i38.13904
25. Sakran N, Goitein D, Raziel A, Keidar A, Beglaibter N, Grinbaum R, et al. Gastric leaks after sleeve gastrectomy: a multicenter experience with 2,834 patients. *Surg Endosc.* (2013) 27:240–5. doi: 10.1007/s00464-012-2426-x
26. Li C, Zhao Y, Han Z, Zhou Y. Anastomotic leaks following gastrointestinal surgery: updates on diagnosis and interventions. *Int J Clin Exp Med.* (2016) 9:7031–40.
27. Dutta S, Fullarton GM, Forshaw MJ, Horgan PG, McMillan DC. Persistent elevation of C-reactive protein following esophagogastric cancer resection as a predictor of postoperative surgical site infectious complications. *World J Surg.* (2011) 35:1017–25. doi: 10.1007/s00268-011-1002-1
28. Ji L, Wang T, Tian L, Gao M. The early diagnostic value of C-reactive protein for anastomotic leakage post radical gastrectomy for esophagogastric junction carcinoma: a retrospective study of 97 patients. *Int J Surg.* (2016) 27:182–6. doi: 10.1016/j.ijsu.2016.02.021
29. Scepanovic MS, Kovacevic B, Cijan V, Antic A, Petrovic Z, Asceric R, et al. C-reactive protein as an early predictor for anastomotic leakage in elective abdominal surgery. *Tech Coloproctol.* (2013) 17:541–7. doi: 10.1007/s10151-013-1013-z
30. Noble F, Curtis N, Harris S, Kelly JJ, Bailey IS, Byrne JP, et al. Risk assessment using a novel score to predict anastomotic leak and major complications after oesophageal resection. *J Gastrointest Surg.* (2012) 16:1083–95. doi: 10.1007/s11605-012-1867-9
31. Spath C, Srinivasa S, Walsh M, Singh P, Rodgers M, Koea J. Role of post-operative serum C-reactive protein levels as a predictor of complications in upper gastrointestinal surgery. *ANZ J Surg.* (2019) 89:74–8. doi: 10.1111/ans.14789
32. Villard MA, Helm MC, Kindel TL, Goldblatt MI, Gould JC, Higgins RM. C-Reactive protein as a predictor of post-operative complications in bariatric surgery patients. *Surg Endosc.* (2018) 33:2479–84. doi: 10.1007/s00464-018-6534-0

33. Zhang K, Xi H, Wu X, Cui J, Bian S, Ma L, et al. Ability of serum C-reactive protein concentrations to predict complications after laparoscopy-assisted gastrectomy: a prospective cohort study. *Medicine.* (2016) 95:e3798. doi: 10.1097/MD.0000000000003798

34. Bryan N, Ashwin H, Smart N, Weyhe D, Wohlert S, Bayon Y, et al. Systemic inflammatory cytokine analysis to monitor biomaterial augmented tissue healing. *Int J Artif Organs.* (2015) 38:651–8. doi: 10.5301/ijao.5000450

10

COMplot, a Graphical Presentation of Complication Profiles and Adverse Effects for the Curative Treatment of Gastric Cancer

Tom van den Ende[1†], Frank A. Abe Nijenhuis[1†], Héctor G. van den Boorn[1], Emil ter Veer[1], Maarten C. C. M. Hulshof[2], Suzanne S. Gisbertz[3], Martijn G. H. van Oijen[1‡] and Hanneke W. M. van Laarhoven[1‡]*

[1] Department of Medical Oncology, Cancer Center Amsterdam, Amsterdam University Medical Centers (UMC), University of Amsterdam, Amsterdam, Netherlands,
[2] Department of Radiotherapy, Cancer Center Amsterdam, Amsterdam University Medical Centers (UMC), University of Amsterdam, Amsterdam, Netherlands,
[3] Department of Surgery, Cancer Center Amsterdam, Amsterdam University Medical Centers (UMC), University of Amsterdam, Amsterdam, Netherlands

Correspondence:
Hanneke W. M. van Laarhoven
h.vanlaarhoven@amsterdamumc.nl

† These authors have contributed equally to this work and share first authorship

‡ These authors share senior authorship

Background: For the curative treatment of gastric cancer, several neoadjuvant, and adjuvant treatment-regimens are available which have shown to improve overall survival. No overview is available regarding toxicity and surgery related outcomes. Our aim was to construct a novel graphical method concerning adverse events (AEs) associated with multimodality treatment and perform a meta-analysis to compare different clinically relevant cytotoxic regimens with each other.

Methods: The PubMed, EMBASE, CENTRAL, and ASCO/ESMO databases were searched up to May 2019 for randomized controlled trials investigating curative treatment regimens for gastric cancer. To construct single and bidirectional bar-charts (COMplots), grade 1–2 and grade 3–5 AEs were extracted per cytotoxic regimen. For surgery-related outcomes a pre-specified set of complications was used. Thereafter, treatment-arms comparing the same regimens were combined in a single-arm random-effects meta-analysis and pooled-proportions were calculated with 95% confidence-intervals. Comparative meta-analyses were performed based on clinical relevance and compound similarity.

Results: In total 16 RCTs (*n* = 4,526 patients) were included investigating pre-operative-therapy and 39 RCTs investigating adjuvant-therapy (*n* = 13,732 patients). Pre-operative COMplots were created for among others; 5-fluorouracil/leucovorin-oxaliplatin-docetaxel (FLOT), epirubicin-cisplatin-fluoropyrimidine (ECF), cisplatin-fluoropyrimidine (CF), and oxaliplatin-fluoropyrimidine (FOx). Pre-operative FLOT showed a minor increase in grade 1–2 and grade 3–4 AEs compared to pre-operative ECF, CF, and FOx. A pooled analysis of patients who had received pre-operative therapy compared to patients who underwent direct surgery did not reveal any significant difference in surgery related morbidity/mortality. When we compared three commonly used adjuvant regimens; S-1 had the lowest amount of grade 3–4 AEs compared to capecitabine with oxaliplatin (CAPOX) and 5-FU with radiotherapy (5-FU+RT).

Conclusion: COMplot provides a novel tool to visualize and compare treatment related AEs for gastric cancer. Based on our comparisons, pre-operative FLOT had a manageable toxicity profile compared to other pre-operative doublet or triplet regimens. We found no evidence indicating surgical outcomes might be hampered by pre-operative therapy. Adjuvant S-1 had a more favorable toxicity profile compared to CAPOX and 5-FU+RT.

Keywords: gastric cancer, chemotherapy, curative, toxicity, meta-analysis

INTRODUCTION

Gastric cancer treated with curative intent has a poor prognosis with a 5-year survival varying between 30 and 40% (1–3). There are several different treatment strategies for gastric cancer which have showed overall survival benefit in the perioperative, neoadjuvant or adjuvant setting, for example, the perioperative FLOT regimen (5-fluorouracil, leucovorin, oxaliplatin, and docetaxel) and the MAGIC regimen (epirubicin, 5-fluorouracil, and cisplatin) (2, 3), adjuvant chemotherapy, i.e., S-1 alone or capecitabine with oxaliplatin (4, 5) and adjuvant chemoradiotherapy, i.e., 5-fluorouracil with radiotherapy (6). Clinical practice varies between geographical regions due to local preferences and possibly differences in tumor biology. Perioperative chemotherapy is the preferred strategy in Europe, adjuvant chemotherapy is preferred in Asia and in the United States adjuvant chemo(radio)therapy is given with or without neoadjuvant chemotherapy (7–9).

Treatment related adverse events (AEs) during multimodality treatment may encompass toxicity due to conventional cytotoxic therapy but also surgery related mortality/morbidity. Toxicity is usually scored according to the Common Terminology Criteria for Adverse Events (CTCAE), in which AEs are graded from mild (grade 1 or 2) to severe (grade 3 or 4) and fatal (grade 5) (10). Furthermore, the occurrence of AEs may not only affect the period during systemic treatment with chemo(radio)therapy, but may also influence post-operative complications. As physicians may offer several curative treatment options to patients with gastric cancer, systemic treatment related AEs will play an important role in shared decision making between patients and physicians.

Well-informed decisions concerning treatment can improve adherence and quality of life (11). Currently, no graphical overview is available of systemic treatment related AEs pooled from multiple studies in the curative setting for gastric cancer. Our aim was to construct a comprehensive graphical overview of multimodality related AEs for the curative treatment of gastric cancer in the neo(adjuvant) setting and compare different clinically relevant regimens with each other (COMplots). Therefore, we conducted a systematic review with meta-analysis.

METHODS

Literature Search

PubMed, EMBASE, the Cochrane Central Register of Controlled Trials (CENTRAL), and the meeting abstracts from the American Society of Clinical Oncology (ASCO) and European Society for Medical Oncology (ESMO) were searched from 1977 up to May 2019. The search strategy consisted of medical subject headings (MeSH) and text words for gastric cancer and esophageal cancer (**Supplementary Methods**). Articles with esophageal adenocarcinoma patients where included if at least 20% of the total amount of patients had tumors located in the stomach. Two authors (TvdE, FaN) screened the titles, abstracts, and full articles independently. Article citations were cross-referenced to identify potentially missing articles. Discrepancies were discussed with a third arbiter (EtV or HvL) until consensus was reached.

Study Selection and Quality Assessment

Prospective phase II or III randomized controlled trials (RCTs) on the curative treatment of gastric cancer were included. Studies were eligible if patients were treated with one of the following intravenous or oral cytotoxic agents: a fluoropyrimidine (5-fluorouracil, capecitabine, UFT, tegafur, or S-1), a platinum compound (either cisplatin or oxaliplatin), a taxane (either docetaxel or paclitaxel), an anthracycline (either epirubicin or doxorubicin), irinotecan, mitomycin C, or methotrexate. Treatment could be administered in the neoadjuvant, perioperative, or adjuvant setting. Studies which investigated chemoradiotherapy were also included. Only studies that reported data on grade 1–2 or grade 3–5 AEs and/or on surgical morbidity/mortality were included. Trials which included patients with metastatic disease at baseline were excluded. The quality of the studies was assessed using the Cochrane Risk of Bias tool (version 5.1.0). Items were scored as low, high, or unknown risk of bias.

Data Extraction and Statistical Analysis

The incidence and severity of treatment related AEs, including the total number of patients who started treatment, were extracted from the study reports for each individual treatment arm. Moreover, surgery related complications were extracted.

A pre-specified set of AEs was constructed based on the available data to enable cross study comparisons based on individual regimens.

All statistical analyses were performed with the metafor 2.0-0 package in R version 3.5.1. For each treatment arm, the incidence of AEs or surgical complications was analyzed through meta-analysis with a random-effects model after application of the logit transformation. This resulted in pooled proportions with 95% confidence intervals (95% CI). A graphical representation of the data for each treatment arm was visualized in a bar chart with the 95% CI (COMplot). For each treatment arm, individual bar charts were constructed using the number of patients, number of events and the number of trials. Clinically relevant regimens were selected based on international guidelines and individual RCTs showing significant overall survival benefit compared to surgery alone (3–9, 12–14). AEs of RCTs investigating pre-operative regimens (as part of a neoadjuvant or perioperative scheme) were pooled together if they investigated the same regimen. The AEs of post-operative therapy as part of a perioperative scheme were pooled separately from purely adjuvant RCTs due to the inclusion of different patients groups (e.g., amount of patients with R0 resection, prior exposure to cytotoxic therapy). Relevant pre-operative regimens were cisplatin or oxaliplatin with a fluoropyrimidine (CF or FOx), 5-FU, leucovorin, oxaliplatin, and docetaxel (FLOT), taxane, cisplatin, and a fluoropyrimidine (TCF) or epirubicin, cisplatin, and a fluoropyrimidine (ECF). Clinically relevant post-operative regimens as part of a perioperative scheme were CF, FOx, FLOT, TCF, ECF, and CF with radiotherapy (CF+RT). Relevant adjuvant regimens were a fluoropyrimidine singlet (F), a fluoroprimidine doublet with either cisplatin (CF), oxaliplatin (FOx), or a taxane (TF). Relevant chemoradiotherapy regimens were 5-FU (5-FU+RT) and cisplatin with 5-FU (CF+RT). Less relevant regimens were included in the (**Supplementary Figures**).

Surgery related morbidity was grouped according to the following categories: total morbidity, any medical complication, any reintervention, abscess, anastomotic leakage, bleeding, infection, intestinal occlusion, pulmonary complications, sepsis, and wound healing disorders. Surgery related mortality was defined as death up to 90 days after surgery, depending on data presented.

Differences in adverse events proportions between several clinically relevant regimens were tested with a Wald test. Additional two-sided *post-hoc* testing, with Holm correction for multiple comparison, was performed if the Wald test was significant ($p < 0.05$). Comparisons between regimens were represented with bidirectional COMplot charts.

RESULTS

In total 4,139 unique references were retrieved from the PubMed, Embase, and CENTRAL databases. Sixty-eight references were selected for full text assessment after title and abstract screening. From the ASCO and ESMO conference meeting abstracts no additional data was identified as the publications of large RCTs were available in full text (e.g., FLOT-4, CRITICS). Finally, 55 original RCTs could be included. Sixteen studies (2, 3, 12, 15–27) investigated perioperative or neoadjuvant therapy and 39 only adjuvant therapy (**Figure 1**) (4–6, 28–63). An overview of all included studies including dosage of study medication is presented in (**Supplementary Table 1**).

Risk of Bias

The Cochrane Risk of bias tool was used to assess study quality (**Supplementary Figure 1**).

In 27 (49%) studies there was no risk of bias on any domain. Twelve (22%) studies were rated as unclear risk of bias on one domain and 10 (18%) studies on two domains. In six (11%) studies risk of bias was deemed unclear on three or more domains. There were no studies rated as having a high risk of bias.

COMplot for Pre-operative and Post-operative Therapy

For five clinically relevant pre-operative regimens, we constructed barcharts with confidence intervals and bidirectional charts with confidence intervals for adverse events (**Figures 2A,B**). The adverse events associated with systemic treatment, were subdivided for perioperative chemotherapy into different figures for pre-operative and post-operative therapy, if it was possible to identify this from individual RCTs. The AEs of trials investigating neoadjuvant therapy were pooled with the pre-operative arms of perioperative RCTs, if they investigated the same regimen. Comparisons were made between pre-operative FLOT, TCF, ECF, and two pre-operative fluoropyrmidine doublets; FOx and CF to identify any significant differences between grade 1–5 AEs (**Figures 3A,B**). In terms of grade 3–4 AEs, FLOT showed a minor increase in grade 3–4 AEs compared to ECF, CF, and FOx (mainly hematological toxicity: neutropenia and leukopenia). FLOT showed higher incidences of grade 1–2 AEs compared to CF and FOx (mainly gastrointestinal toxicity, stomatitis, and fatigue). FLOT also showed a higher amount of grade 1–2 AEs compared to ECF (diarrhea and neuropathy). Pre-operative TCF was associated with a higher incidence of grade 3–4 AEs compared to FLOT (anemia, febrile neutropenia, anorexia). Grade 1–2 AEs were higher with the FLOT regimen (mainly gastrointestinal toxicity). A full overview of significant differences in toxicity between the aforementioned regimens can be found in (**Supplementary Tables 2, 3**).

Post-operative ECF was not associated with an increase in grade 3–4 adverse events compared to CF+RT. However, post-operative CF+RT showed less grade 1–2 toxicity (neutropenia, mucositis, hand foot syndrome) compared to post-operative ECF. There was no toxicity data available on post-operative treatment with FLOT, TCF, FOx or CF.

Overall, a pooled analysis of patients randomized to a pre-operative therapy arm did not reveal any significant increase in surgery related morbidity/mortality compared to patients who underwent immediate surgery (**Figure 4**). An exploratory analysis was performed between several different pre-operative regimens; patients who received pre-operative CF experienced significantly less total surgery related morbidity compared to pre-operative FLOT and pre-operative ECF.

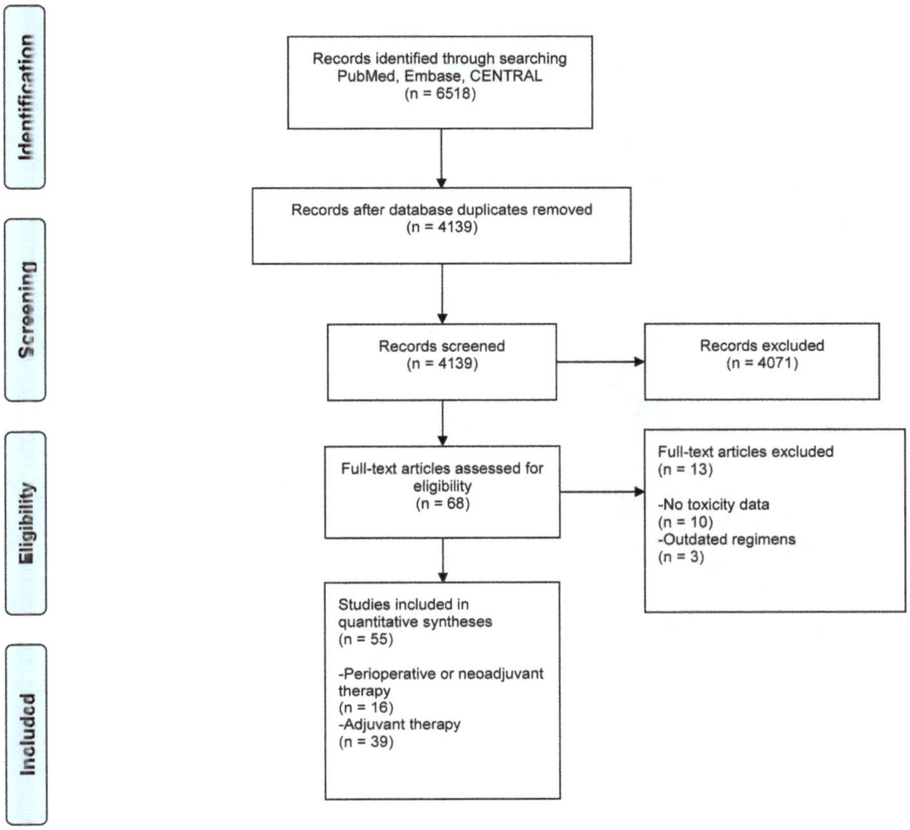

FIGURE 1 | PRISMA flowchart of included studies. CENTRAL, Cochrane Central Register of Controlled Trials; PRISMA, Preferred Reporting Items for Systematic Reviews and Meta-Analyses.

TOXplot for Adjuvant Therapy

For 19 adjuvant regimens, we constructed bar charts with confidence intervals for AEs. Comparisons were made between FOx and CF, F, F+RT, or TF. Compared to FOx, the regimens CF and F+RT showed higher incidences of grade 3–4 AEs (stomatitis, anorexia, fatigue, neutropenia). Compared to F monotherapy and the doublet TF, the doublet FOx showed higher incidences of grade 3–4 adverse events (hematological toxicity and neuropathy). TF was also associated with a reduction in grade 1–2 AEs compared to FOx (**Supplementary Table 4**).

To investigate regimens based on individual compounds; S-1 monotherapy, 5-FU+RT, and CAPOX were separately compared (**Figure 5**). In terms of grade 3–4 adverse events, 5-FU+RT was significantly more toxic than CAPOX and S-1 monotherapy (hematological toxicity, anorexia fatigue, mucositis). Treatment with S-1 monotherapy was associated with more grade 1–2 adverse events compared to CAPOX and 5-FU+RT (**Supplementary Table 5**).

Heterogeneity

For several pooled proportions with more than one RCT significant ($p < 0.05$) heterogeneity was observed using the *Q*-test. The I^2 values of these pooled AEs in the individual or bidirectional comparative COMplots ranged from 53 to 99%.

DISCUSSION

In this article, we have presented a novel overview of toxicity and surgical complications for the curative treatment of gastric cancer. The method in this paper is based on an article we published earlier on the toxicity profiles of first line chemotherapy in advanced gastroesophageal cancer (64). We conducted multiple random effect meta-analyses, based on individual treatment arms from RCTs. Using COMplot, we constructed a graphical presentation with pooled proportions and confidence intervals. Based on the performed analyses, we conclude that pre-operative therapy is not associated with an increase in surgery related morbidity or mortality compared to surgery alone. Pre-operative treatment with FLOT chemotherapy is not associated with a large increase in grade 3–4 AEs compared to pre-operative ECF, CF, or FOx. For adjuvant regimens, S-1 is associated with fewer grade 3–4 adverse events compared to CAPOX and 5-FU+RT.

A systematic review on shared decision making, across multiple types of cancer, found that in 19 out of 22 studies patients preferred a more active role regarding treatment decisions (65). The review highlighted that innovative interventions regarding improvement of shared decision making are lacking (65). For clinicians and patients, shared

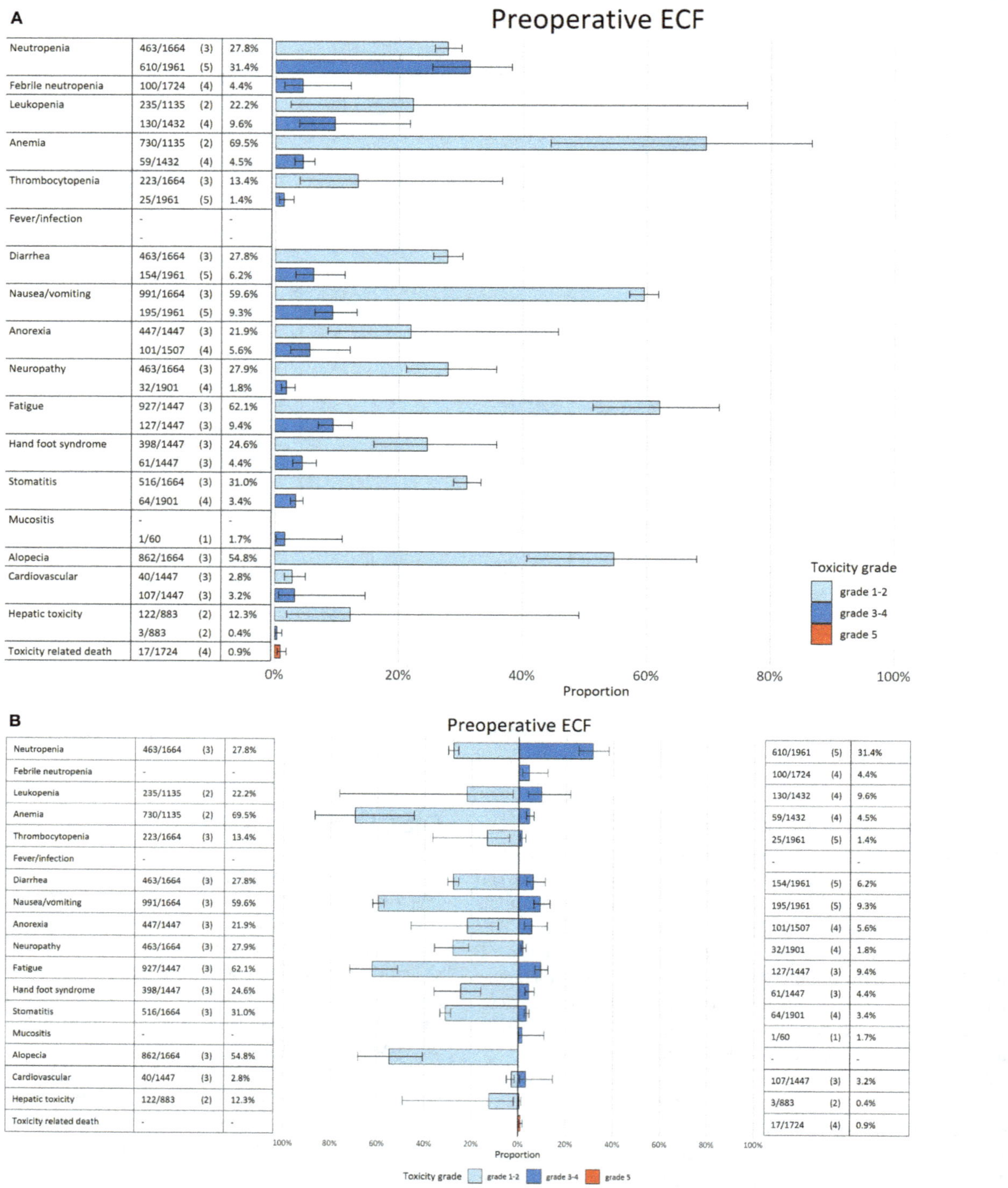

FIGURE 2 | (A) Bar chart for pre-operative epirubicin, cisplatin, and a fluoropyrimidine (ECF). In the first column the adverse events are mentioned per row. In the second column the amount of patients with the AE per grade are mentioned compared to the total amount of patients who were treated with the regimen. In brackets the amount of studies are mentioned. The pooled estimated incidence for each AE is mentioned in the third column. The bars in the figure give the pooled estimate with 95% CI (line in black in the bar). Every bar has a specific color which corresponds with the grade of the AE (light blue grade 1–2, dark blue grade 3–4, and red grade 5). **(B)** Bidirectional bar chart for pre-operative epirubicin, cisplatin and a fluoropyrimidine (ECF). In the first column the adverse events are mentioned per row. In the second column the amount of patients with the AE per grade are mentioned compared to the total amount of patients who were treated with the regimen. In brackets the amount of studies are mentioned. The pooled estimated incidence for each AE is mentioned in the third column. The bars in the figure give the pooled estimate with 95% CI (line in black in the bar). Every bar has a specific color which corresponds with the grade of the AE (light blue grade 1–2, dark blue grade 3–4 and red grade 5).

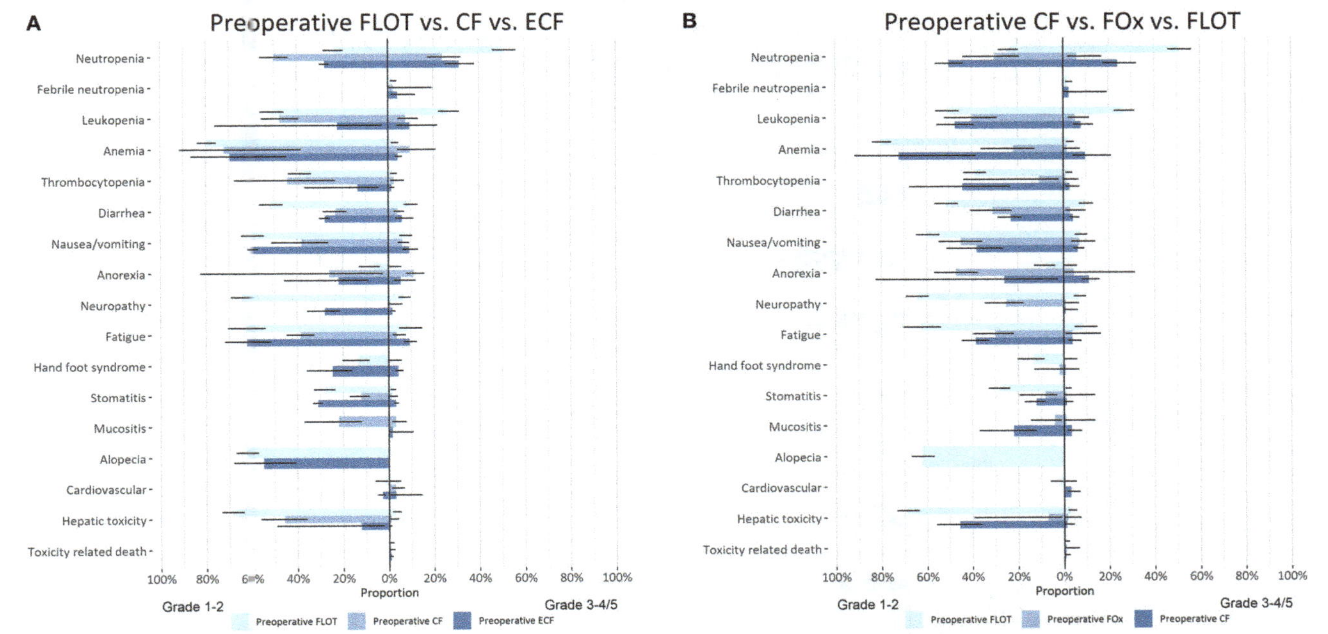

FIGURE 3 | (A) Bidirectional comparative meta-analysis of pre-operative 5-fluorouracil/leucovorin-oxaliplatin-docetaxel (FLOT), epirubicin-cisplatin-fluoropyrimidine (ECF), and cisplatin-fluoropyrimidine (CF). In the column on the left of the figure the adverse events are mentioned per group of bar charts. The bars in the figure give the pooled estimate with 95% CI (line in black in the bar). Grade 1–2 AEs are depicted on the left of the figure and grade 3–4/5 on the right of the figure. The color of the bar chart indicates which regimen is depicted. **(B)** Bidirectional comparative meta-analysis of pre-operative 5-fluorouracil/leucovorin-oxaliplatin-docetaxel (FLOT), cisplatin-fluoropyrimidine (CF), and oxaliplatin-fluoropyrimidine (FOx). In the column on the left of the figure the adverse events are mentioned per group of bar charts. The bars in the figure give the pooled estimate with 95% CI (line in black in the bar). Grade 1–2 AEs are depicted on the left of the figure and grade 3–4/5 on the right of the figure. The color of the bar chart indicates which regimen is depicted.

decision making can result in improved satisfaction with oncology care and communication with the physician (11). Unexpected and unrealistic views of patients on adverse effects of systemic treatment and surgical complications can result in decreased confidence in medical care, negative coping, and a deterioration in quality of life. It is well-known from phase I trials, that patients underestimate the potential toxicities that could result from oncological therapy (66). To improve awareness, recent efforts have focused on incorporating online information tools in oncology care. For example, an interactive online decision tool developed for breast cancer patients improved knowledge and preparation regarding treatment decisions (67). COMplots provide the physician with a graphical tool that could potentially facilitate the exchange of information on treatment effects between physician and patient. The data from COMplots and the method of analysis could be used in future online decision tools (68).

Graphical presentation of adverse effects of multimodality treatment is not yet available for use during consultation. COMplots provide pooled proportions with confidence intervals to give realistic estimates of the chance of occurrence of a certain adverse event. For clinicians, it can help in giving realistic estimates of the expected AEs (morbidity and mortality) regarding treatment with chemotherapy and surgery. Higher grade adverse events are deemed more acceptable to achieve curation. Therefore, clinicians might underestimate the value of informed decision making in the curative setting. However, even elderly curatively treated patients prefer an active or shared role above a passive role in oncological treatment decisions (69). Moreover, patients with a low health related quality of life reported more interest in shared decision making regarding cancer treatment (70). Clinicians can potentially use COMplots to actively engage patients in multimodality treatment decisions. Especially, for patients with co-morbidity or elderly patients COMplot can provide the means to weigh benefit of treatment, between regimens, or estimate the risks of undergoing major surgery. However, for this specific patient group, it should be realized that the estimates of adverse events from this pooled analysis are overall estimates and are not corrected for age or co-morbidity, these factors generally lead to an increase in toxicity.

In our COMplots we have performed several meta-analyses based on data from RCTs regarding the curative treatment of gastric cancer. Pre-operative therapy was not associated with an increase in surgery related morbidity or mortality compared to surgery alone. In several types of cancer, including esophageal and pancreatic cancer, neoadjuvant therapy was not associated with an increase in surgery related morbidity or mortality (71–73). Although, there is also evidence indicating the location and extent of the planning target volume of pre-operative radiotherapy

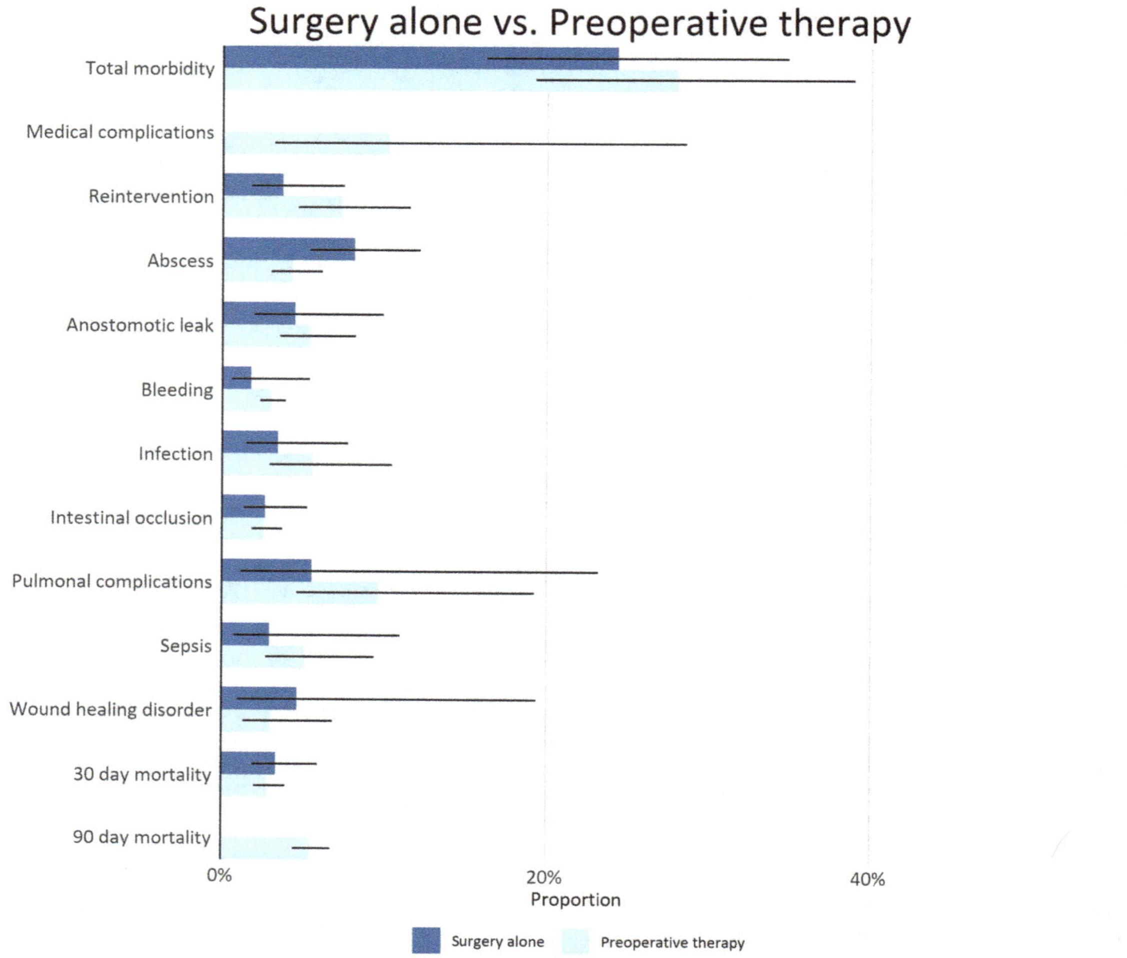

FIGURE 4 | Surgical morbidity and mortality in patients treated with pre-operative therapy or with surgery alone. In the column on the left of the figure surgical outcomes are mentioned per group of bar charts. The bars in the figure give the pooled estimate with 95% CI (line in black in the bar). The color of the bar chart indicates if patients received pre-operative therapy before surgery. There was not enough information to make a distinction in severity of the surgical complications. For surgery alone there was no information available on the amount of medical complications and 90 day mortality.

might increase post-operative morbidity in esophageal cancer (74, 75). Ongoing pre-operative trials for gastric cancer like the CRITICS-2 trial (NCT02931890) should take this into account when pre-operative chemoradiotherapy is given. Our meta-analysis primarily included pre-operative chemotherapy studies and only one pre-operative chemoradiotherapy study and could thus not effectively rule out an effect of chemoradiotherapy on post-operative morbidity. Moreover, due to the high degree of heterogeneity in studies: Asian vs. Western, surgical techniques, extent of lymph node dissection, no definite conclusions can be drawn on the impact of individual regimens on surgical outcomes. Therefore, our finding that pre-operative CF was associated with less surgery related morbidity compared to FLOT and ECF should be regarded as exploratory and should be further investigated.

Treatment with pre-operative FLOT chemotherapy was associated with a small increase in AEs compared to pre-operative ECF, FOx, and CF in the COMplot meta-analysis. In the FLOT-4 trial perioperative FLOT substantially improved overall survival compared to perioperative ECF for gastric cancer (13). Therefore, patients treated with curative intent in good condition should receive perioperative FLOT over ECF, FOx, and CF, as only a minor increase in AEs was found. Pre-operative doublet chemotherapy should be reserved for patients with treatment limiting co-morbidity.

Patients who receive an immediate resection and are eligible for adjuvant treatment experience less grade 3–4 AEs with S-1 monotherapy compared to CAPOX and 5-FU with radiotherapy. Therefore, S-1 monotherapy might be more attractive for patients with co-morbidity. However, it must be noted adjuvant S-1 has only been investigated in curatively resected Asian patients.

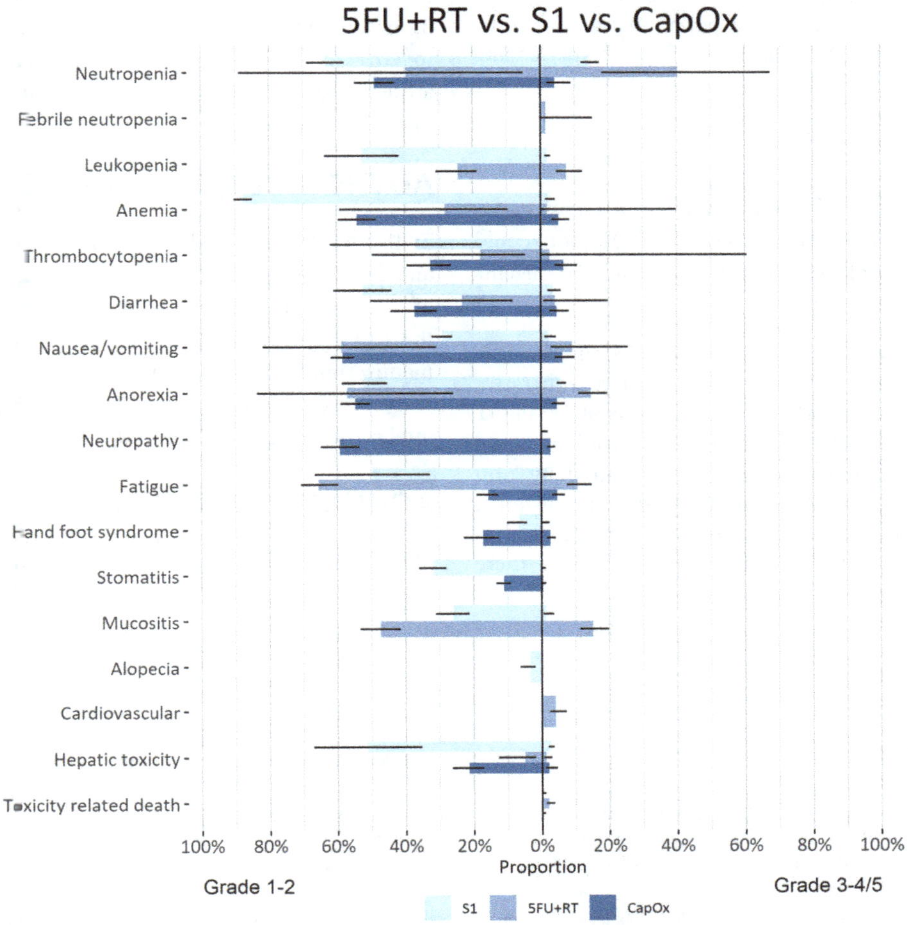

FIGURE 5 | Bidirectional comparative meta-analysis of adjuvant S-1, CAPOX or 5-FU+RT in patients who did not receive pre-operative therapy. In the column on the left of the figure the adverse events are mentioned per group of bar charts. The bars in the figure give the pooled estimate with 95% CI (line in black in the bar). Grade 1–2 AEs are depicted on the left of the figure and grade 3–4/5 on the right of the figure. The color of the bar chart indicates which regimen is depicted.

Effectivity in Western patients or patients with co-morbidity has not yet been investigated.

STRENGTHS AND LIMITATIONS

The main strength of COMplot is the graphical presentation of toxicity and surgery related outcomes through pooled proportion meta-analysis with confidence intervals. Moreover, data can easily be interpreted as the number of studies and patients is given for each pooled treatment arm. Data on which the individual COMplots are based, have been obtained from RCTs were adverse events have been systematically scored, using the CTCAE classification.

However, COMplots also have several limitations. First, the adverse events are scored according to their maximum grade in the RCTs (76). There is no information available on the duration of an adverse event and the impact on quality of life. A recent paper incorporated longitudinal data in graphic tables and histograms of two RCTs (77). For COMplots this was not possible as the included RCTs do not provide longitudinal data on toxicity over time. In the future, RCTs should include toxicity over time analyses and provide data on quality of life, also during curative treatment.

Second, trials only report adverse events which occur over a certain threshold (for example in 5% of all patients) and surgery related morbidity was, for most trials, only reported within 30 days after surgery. For a small amount of toxicity events, the COMplots underestimate occurrence. Moreover, the long-term morbidity or deterioration of quality of life is not incorporated in the COMplots. Large prospective cohorts can provide more accurate incidences of adverse events and provide data on long term morbidity after surgery (78).

Third, cross-study comparisons between perioperative and adjuvant trials was not possible due to heterogeneity in baseline characteristics. For example, patients in adjuvant trials were mostly included after a R0 resection.

Patients receiving post-operative chemotherapy in a perioperative trial were already pre-exposed to chemotherapy which could increase the likelihood of experiencing an AE.

CONCLUSION

COMplots were constructed for clinically relevant regimens for the curative treatment of gastric cancer. The COMplots could potentially be used to inform patients about adverse events related to multimodality treatment.

Based on our meta-analysis, pre-operative FLOT only showed a minor increase in AEs compared to pre-operative doublet or triplet regimens. Therefore, pre-operative FLOT should be the preferred regimen in the perioperative setting for fit patients. Surgical outcomes are not impaired by pre-operative chemotherapy and can thus be safely administered. Ongoing trials will shed more light on the impact of pre-operative chemoradiotherapy on surgical outcomes as there is not enough data on this yet. In the adjuvant setting, S-1 monotherapy had a more favorable toxicity profile compared to CAPOX and 5-FU with RT and could thus be an more attractive option for patients with co-morbidity limiting more intensive treatment.

AUTHOR CONTRIBUTIONS

TvdE and FA performed the search for the review, extracted data, and analyzed the results. HvdB and EtV devised the method of analysis. HvdB created the R software package to create the COMplots and perform a meta-analysis. TvdE wrote the manuscript. EtV, MvO, and HvL provided intellectual guidance and corrected several draft versions. SG and MH provided intellectual input and corrected the final draft.

ACKNOWLEDGMENTS

Mélanie Machiels for helping with creating the search strategy.

REFERENCES

1. Bray F, Ferlay J, Soerjomataram I, Siegel RL, Torre LA, Jemal A, et al. Global cancer statistics 2018: GLOBOCAN estimates of incidence and mortality worldwide for 36 cancers in 185 countries. *CA Cancer J Clin.* (2018) 68:394–424. doi: 10.3322/caac.21492
2. Al-Batran SE, Homann N, Pauligk C, Goetze TO, Meiler J, Kasper S, et al. Perioperative chemotherapy with fluorouracil plus leucovorin, oxaliplatin, and docetaxel versus fluorouracil or capecitabine plus cisplatin and epirubicin for locally advanced, resectable gastric or gastro-oesophageal junction adenocarcinoma (FLOT4): a randomised, phase 2/3 trial. *Lancet.* (2019) 393:1948–57. doi: 10.1016/S0140-6736(18)32557-1
3. Cunningham D, Allum WH, Stenning SP, Thompson JN, Van de Velde CJ, Nicolson M, et al. Perioperative chemotherapy versus surgery alone for resectable gastroesophageal cancer. *N Engl J Med.* (2006) 355:11–20. doi: 10.1056/NEJMoa055531
4. Sasako M, Sakuramoto S, Katai H, Kinoshita T, Furukawa H, Yamaguchi T, et al. Five-year outcomes of a randomized phase III trial comparing adjuvant chemotherapy with S-1 versus surgery alone in stage II or III gastric cancer. *J Clin Oncol.* (2011) 29:4387–93. doi: 10.1200/JCO.2011.36.5908
5. Noh SH, Park SR, Yang HK, Chung HC, Chung IJ, Kim SW, et al. Adjuvant capecitabine plus oxaliplatin for gastric cancer after D2 gastrectomy (CLASSIC): 5-year follow-up of an open-label, randomised phase 3 trial. *Lancet Oncol.* (2014) 15:1389–96. doi: 10.1016/S1470-2045(14)70473-5
6. Smalley SR, Benedetti JK, Haller DG, Hundahl SA, Estes NC, Ajani JA, et al. Updated analysis of SWOG-directed intergroup study 0116: a phase III trial of adjuvant radiochemotherapy versus observation after curative gastric cancer resection. *J Clin Oncol.* (2012) 30:2327–33. doi: 10.1200/JCO.2011.36.7136
7. Smyth EC, Verheij M, Allum W, Cunningham D, Cervantes A, Arnold D, et al. Gastric cancer: ESMO Clinical Practice Guidelines for diagnosis, treatment and follow-up. *Ann Oncol.* (2016) 27:v38–v49. doi: 10.1093/annonc/mdw350
8. National Comprehensive Cancer Network. *Gastric Cancer (Version 2.2018)* (2018). Retrieved from: https://www.nccn.org/professionals/physician_gls/pdf/gastric.pdf
9. Japanese Gastric Cancer. Japanese gastric cancer treatment guidelines 2014 (ver. 4). *Gastr Cancer.* (2017) 20:1–19. doi: 10.1007/s10120-016-0622-4
10. Colevas AD, Setser A. The NCI common terminology criteria for adverse events (CTCAE) v 3.0 is the new standard for oncology clinical trials. *J Clin Oncol.* (2004) 22:6098–8. doi: 10.1200/jco.2004.22.90140.6098
11. Kehl KL, Landrum MB, Arora NK, Ganz PA, van Ryn M, Mack JW, et al. Association of actual and preferred decision roles with patient-reported quality of care: shared decision making in cancer care. *JAMA Oncol.* (2015) 1:50–8. doi: 10.1001/jamaoncol.2014.112
12. Ychou M, Boige V, Pignon JP, Conroy T, Bouche O, Lebreton G, et al. Perioperative chemotherapy compared with surgery alone for resectable gastroesophageal adenocarcinoma: an FNCLCC and FFCD multicenter phase III trial. *J Clin Oncol.* (2011) 29:1715–21. doi: 10.1200/JCO.2010.33.0597
13. Al-Batran S-E, Homann N, Schmalenberg H, Kopp H-G, Haag GM, Luley KB, et al. Perioperative chemotherapy with docetaxel, oxaliplatin, and fluorouracil/leucovorin (FLOT) versus epirubicin, cisplatin, and fluorouracil or capecitabine (ECF/ECX) for resectable gastric or gastroesophageal junction (GEJ) adenocarcinoma (FLOT4-AIO): a multicenter, randomized phase 3 trial. *J Clin Oncol.* (2017) 35:4004. doi: 10.1200/JCO.2017.35.15_suppl.4004
14. NCC Network. *Gastric Cancer (Version 2.2018).* Available online at: https://www.nccn.org/professionals/physician_gls/pdf/gastric.pdf (accessed December 20, 2018).
15. Aoyama T, Nishikawa K, Fujitani K, Tanabe K, Ito S, Matsui T, et al. Early results of a randomized two-by-two factorial phase II trial comparing neoadjuvant chemotherapy with two and four courses of cisplatin/S-1 and docetaxel/cisplatin/S-1 as neoadjuvant chemotherapy for locally advanced gastric cancer. *Ann Oncol.* (2017) 28:1876–81. doi: 10.1093/annonc/mdx236
16. Cats A, Jansen EPM, van Grieken NCT, Sikorska K, Lind P, Nordsmark M, et al. Chemotherapy versus chemoradiotherapy after surgery and preoperative chemotherapy for resectable gastric cancer (CRITICS): an international,

open-label, randomised phase 3 trial. *Lancet Oncol.* (2018) 19:616–28. doi: 10.1016/S1470-2045(18)30132-3

17. Cunningham D, Stenning SP, Smyth EC, Okines AF, Allum WH, Rowley S, et al. Peri-operative chemotherapy with or without bevacizumab in operable oesophagogastric adenocarcinoma (UK Medical Research Council ST03): primary analysis results of a multicentre, open-label, randomised phase 2-3 trial. *Lancet Oncol.* (2017) 18:357–70. doi: 10.1016/S1470-2045(17)30043-8
18. Fazio N, Biffi R, Maibach R, Hayoz S, Thierstein S, Brauchli P, et al. Preoperative versus postoperative docetaxel-cisplatin- fluorouracil (TCF) chemotherapy in locally advanced resectable gastric carcinoma: 10-year follow-up of the SAKK 43/99 phase III trial. *Ann Oncol.* (2016) 27:668–73. doi: 10.1093/annonc/mdv620
19. Leong T, Smithers BM, Haustermans K, Michael M, Gebski V, Miller D, et al. TOPGEAR: a randomized, phase III trial of perioperative ECF chemotherapy with or without preoperative chemoradiation for resectable gastric cancer: interim results from an international, intergroup trial of the AGITG, TROG, EORTC and CCTG. *Ann Surg Oncol.* (2017) 24:2252–8. doi: 10.1245/s10434-017-5830-6
20. Schuhmacher C, Gretschel S, Lordick F, Reichardt P, Hohenberger W, Eisenberger CF, et al. Neoadjuvant chemotherapy compared with surgery alone for locally advanced cancer of the stomach and cardia: European Organisation for Research and Treatment of Cancer randomized trial 40954. *J Clin Oncol.* (2010) 28:5210–8. doi: 10.1200/JCO.2009.26.6114
21. Xue K, Ying X, Bu Z, Wu A, Li Z, Tang L, et al. Oxaliplatin plus S-1 or capecitabine as neoadjuvant or adjuvant chemotherapy for locally advanced gastric cancer with D2 lymphadenectomy: 5-year follow-up results of a phase II-III randomized trial. *Chin J Cancer Res.* (2018) 30:516–25. doi: 10.21147/j.issn.1000-9604.2018.05.05
22. Yoshikawa T, Morita S, Tanabe K, Nishikawa K, Ito Y, Matsui T, et al. Survival results of a randomised two-by-two factorial phase II trial comparing neoadjuvant chemotherapy with two and four courses of S-1 plus cisplatin (SC) and paclitaxel plus cisplatin (PC) followed by D2 gastrectomy for resectable advanced gastric cancer. *Eur J Cancer.* (2016) 62:103–11. doi: 10.1016/j.ejca.2016.04.012
23. Zhao Q, Li Y, Huang J, Fan L, Tan B, Tian Y, et al. Short-Term curative effect of S-1 plus oxaliplatin as perioperative chemotherapy for locally advanced gastric cancer: a prospective comparison study. *Pharmazie.* (2017) 72:236–40.
24. Hartgrink HH, van de Velde CJ, Putter H, Songun I, Tesselaar ME, Kranenbarg EK, et al. Neo-adjuvant chemotherapy for operable gastric cancer: long term results of the Dutch randomised FAMTX trial. *Eur J Surg Oncol.* (2004) 30:643–9. doi: 10.1016/j.ejso.2004.04.013
25. Imano M, Itoh T, Satou T, Sogo Y, Hirai H, Kato H, A, et al. Prospective randomized trial of short-term neoadjuvant chemotherapy for advanced gastric cancer. *Eur J Surg Oncol.* (2010) 36:963–8. doi: 10.1016/j.ejso.2010.06.012
26. Terashima M, Iwasaki Y, Mizusawa J, Katayama H, Nakamura K, Katai H, et al. Randomized phase III trial of gastrectomy with or without neoadjuvant S-1 plus cisplatin for type 4 or large type 3 gastric cancer, the short-term safety and surgical results: Japan Clinical Oncology Group Study (JCOG0501). *Gastric Cancer.* (2019). doi: 10.1007/s10120-019-00941-z
27. Zhao WH, Wang SF, Ding W, Sheng JM, Ma ZM, Teng LS, et al. Apoptosis induced by preoperative oral 5'-DFUR administration in gastric adenocarcinoma and its mechanism of action. *World J Gastroenterol.* (2006) 12:1356–61. doi: 10.3748/wjg.v12.i9.1356
28. Bajetta E, Buzzoni R, Mariani L, Beretta E, Bozzetti F, Bordogna G, et al. Adjuvant chemotherapy in gastric cancer: 5-year results of a randomised study by the Italian Trials in Medical Oncology (ITMO) Group. *Ann Oncol.* (2002) 13:299–307. doi: 10.1093/annonc/mdf040
29. Bajetta E, Floriani I, Di Bartolomeo M, Labianca R, Falcone A, Di Costanzo F, et al. Randomized trial on adjuvant treatment with FOLFIRI followed by docetaxel and cisplatin versus 5-fluorouracil and folinic acid for radically resected gastric cancer. *Ann Oncol.* (2014) 25:1373–8. doi: 10.1093/annonc/mdu146
30. Bamias A, Karina M, Papakostas P, Kostopoulos I, Bobos M, Vourli G, et al. A randomized phase III study of adjuvant platinum/docetaxel chemotherapy with or without radiation therapy in patients with gastric cancer. *Cancer Chemother Pharmacol.* (2010) 65:1009–21. doi: 10.1007/s00280-010-1256-6
31. Di Bartolomeo M, Buzzoni R, Mariani L, Ferrario E, Katia D, Gevorgyan A, et al. Feasibility of sequential therapy with FOLFIRI followed by docetaxel/cisplatin in patients with radically resected gastric adenocarcinoma. A randomized phase III trial.[Erratum appears in Oncology. 2007;73(5-6):406 Note: Ardizzoni, Antonio [corrected to Ardizzoia, Antonio]]. *Oncology.* (2006) 71:341–6. doi: 10.1159/000108575
32. Bouche O, Ychou M, Burtin P, Bedenne L, Ducreux M, Lebreton G, et al. Adjuvant chemotherapy with 5-fluorouracil and cisplatin compared with surgery alone for gastric cancer: 7-year results of the FFCD randomized phase III trial (8801). *Ann Oncol.* (2005) 16:1488–97. doi: 10.1093/annonc/mdi270
33. Cascinu S, Labianca R, Barone C, Santoro A, Carnaghi C, Cassano A, et al. Adjuvant treatment of high-risk, radically resected gastric cancer patients with 5-fluorouracil, leucovorin, cisplatin, and epidoxorubicin in a randomized controlled trial. *J Natl Cancer Inst.* (2007) 99:601–7. doi: 10.1093/jnci/djk131
34. Chang HM, Jung KH, Kim TY, Kim WS, Yang HK, Lee KU, et al. A phase III randomized trial of 5-fluorouracil, doxorubicin, and mitomycin C versus 5-fluorouracil and mitomycin C versus 5-fluorouracil alone in curatively resected gastric cancer. *Ann Oncol.* (2002) 13:1779–85. doi: 10.1093/annonc/mdf302
35. Chipponi J, Huguier M, Pezet D, Basso N, Hay JM, Quandalle P, et al. Randomized trial of adjuvant chemotherapy after curative resection for gastric cancer. *Am J Surg.* (2004) 187:440–5. doi: 10.1016/j.amjsurg.2003.12.014
36. Cirera L, Balil A, Batiste-Alentorn E, Tusquets I, Cardona T, Arcusa A, et al. Randomized clinical trial of adjuvant mitomycin plus tegafur in patients with resected stage III gastric cancer. *J Clin Oncol.* (1999) 17:3810–5. doi: 10.1200/JCO.1999.17.12.3810
37. Coombes RC, Schein PS, Chilvers CE, Wils J, Beretta G, Bliss JM, et al. A randomized trial comparing adjuvant fluorouracil, doxorubicin, and mitomycin with no treatment in operable gastric cancer. International Collaborative Cancer Group. *J Clin Oncol.* (1990) 8:1362–9. doi: 10.1200/JCO.1990.8.8.1362
38. De Vita F, Giuliani F, Orditura M, Maiello E, Galizia G, Di Martino N, et al. Adjuvant chemotherapy with epirubicin, leucovorin, 5-fluorouracil and etoposide regimen in resected gastric cancer patients: a randomized phase III trial by the Gruppo Oncologico Italia Meridionale (GOIM 9602 Study). *Ann Oncol.* (2007) 18:1354–8. doi: 10.1093/annonc/mdm128
39. Di Costanzo F, Gasperoni S, Manzione L, Bisagni G, Labianca R, Bravi S, et al. Adjuvant chemotherapy in completely resected gastric cancer: a randomized phase III trial conducted by GOIRC. *J Natl Cancer Inst.* (2008) 100:388–98. doi: 10.1093/jnci/djn054
40. Feng WM, Tang CW, Guo HH, Bao Y, Fei MY. Prolonged adjuvant capecitabine chemotherapy improved survival of stage IIIA gastric cancer after D2 gastrectomy. *Biomed Pharmacother.* (2015) 72:140–3. doi: 10.1016/j.biopha.2015.03.003
41. Fuchs CS, Niedzwiecki D, Mamon HJ, Tepper JE, Ye X, Swanson RS, et al. Adjuvant chemoradiotherapy with epirubicin, cisplatin, and fluorouracil compared with adjuvant chemoradiotherapy with fluorouracil and leucovorin after curative resection of gastric cancer: results from CALGB 80101 (Alliance). *J Clin Oncol.* (2017) 35:3671–7. doi: 10.1200/JCO.2017.74.2130
42. Kang YK, Chang HM, Yook JH, Ryu MH, Park I, Min YJ, et al. Adjuvant chemotherapy for gastric cancer: a randomised phase 3 trial of mitomycin-C plus either short-term doxifluridine or long-term doxifluridine plus cisplatin after curative D2 gastrectomy (AMC0201). *Br J Cancer.* (2013) 108:1245–51. doi: 10.1038/bjc.2013.86
43. Kim TH, Park SR, Ryu KW, Kim YW, Bae JM, Lee JH, et al. Phase 3 trial of postoperative chemotherapy alone versus chemoradiation therapy in stage III-IV gastric cancer treated with R0 gastrectomy and D2 lymph node dissection. *Int J Radiat Oncol Biol Phys.* (2012) 84:e585–92. doi: 10.1016/j.ijrobp.2012.07.2378
44. Krook JE, O'Connell MJ, Wieand HS, Beart RW Jr, Leigh JE, Kugler JW, et al. A prospective, randomized evaluation of intensive-course 5-fluorouracil plus doxorubicin as surgical adjuvant chemotherapy for resected gastric cancer. *Cancer.* (1991) 67:2454–8. doi: 10.1002/1097-0142(19910515)67:10<2454::AID-CNCR2820671010>3.0.CO;2-2

45. Kulig J, Kolodziejczyk P, Sierzega M, Bobrzynski L, Jedrys J, Popiela T, et al. Adjuvant chemotherapy with etoposide, adriamycin and cisplatin compared with surgery alone in the treatment of gastric cancer: a phase III randomized, multicenter, clinical trial. *Oncology*. (2010) 78:54–61. doi: 10.1159/000292360
46. Kwon HC, Kim MC, Kim KH, Jang JS, Oh SY, Kim SH, et al. Adjuvant chemoradiation versus chemotherapy in completely resected advanced gastric cancer with D2 nodal dissection. *Asia Pac J Clin Oncol.* (2010) 6:278–85. doi: 10.1111/j.1743-7563.2010.01331.x
47. Lee JJ, Kim SY, Shin I, Cho KS, Joo HZ, Yoon C. Randomized phase III trial of cisplatin, epirubicin, leucovorin, 5-Fluorouracil (PELF) combination versus 5-fluorouracil alone as adjuvant chemotherapy in curative resected Stage III gastric cancer. *Cancer Res Treat.* (2004) 36:140–5. doi: 10.4143/crt.2004.36.2.140
48. Lee CK, Jung M, Kim HS, Jung I, Shin DB, Kang SY, et al. S-1 Based doublet as an adjuvant chemotherapy for curatively resected stage III gastric cancer: results from the randomized phase III post trial. *Cancer Res.* (2019) 51:1–11. doi: 10.4143/crt.2018.028
49. Lise M, Nitti D, Marchet A, Sahmoud T, Buyse M, Duez N, et al. Final results of a phase III clinical trial of adjuvant chemotherapy with the modified fluorouracil, doxorubicin, and mitomycin regimen in resectable gastric cancer. *J Clin Oncol.* (1995) 13:2757–63. doi: 10.1200/JCO.1995.13.11.2757
50. Nakajima T, Nashimoto A, Kitamura M, Kito T, Iwanaga T, Okabayashi K, et al. Adjuvant mitomycin and fluorouracil followed by oral uracil plus tegafur in serosa-negative gastric cancer: a randomised trial. Gastric Cancer Surgical Study Group. *Lancet.* (1999) 354:273–7. doi: 10.1016/S0140-6736(99)01048-X
51. Nakajima T, Kinoshita T, Nashimoto A, Sairenji M, Yamaguchi T, Sakamoto J, et al. Randomized controlled trial of adjuvant uracil-tegafur versus surgery alone for serosa-negative, locally advanced gastric cancer. *Br J Surg.* (2007) 94:1468–76. doi: 10.1002/bjs.5996
52. Neri B, Cini G, Andreoli F, Boffi B, Francesconi D, Mazzanti R, et al. Randomized trial of adjuvant chemotherapy versus control after curative resection for gastric cancer: 5-year follow-up. *Br J Cancer.* (2001) 84:878–80. doi: 10.1054/bjoc.2000.1472
53. Nitti D, Wils J, Dos Santos JG, Fountzilas G, Conte PF, Sava C, et al. Randomized phase III trials of adjuvant FAMTX or FEMTX compared with surgery alone in resected gastric cancer. A combined analysis of the EORTC GI Group and the ICCG. *Ann Oncol.* (2006) 17:262–9. doi: 10.1093/annonc/mdj077
54. Park SH, Sohn TS, Lee J, Lim DH, Hong ME, Kim KM, et al. Phase III trial to compare adjuvant chemotherapy with capecitabine and cisplatin versus concurrent chemoradiotherapy in gastric cancer: final report of the adjuvant chemoradiotherapy in stomach tumors trial, including survival and subset analyses. *J Clin Oncol.* (2015) 33:3130–6. doi: 10.1200/JCO.2014.58.3930
55. Schwartz GK, Winter K, Minsky BD, Crane C, Thomson PJ, Anne P, et al. Randomized phase II trial evaluating two paclitaxel and cisplatin-containing chemoradiation regimens as adjuvant therapy in resected gastric cancer (RTOG-0114). *J Clin Oncol.* (2009) 27:1956–62. doi: 10.1200/JCO.2008.20.3745
56. Tentes AA, Markakidis SK, Karanikiotis C, Fiska A, Tentes IK, Manolopoulos VG, et al. Intraarterial chemotherapy as an adjuvant treatment in locally advanced gastric cancer. *Langenbecks Arch Surg.* (2006) 391:124–9. doi: 10.1007/s00423-006-0022-z
57. Tsavaris N, Tentas K, Kosmidis P, Mylonakis N, Sakelaropoulos N, Kosmas C, et al. A randomized trial comparing adjuvant fluorouracil, epirubicin, and mitomycin with no treatment in operable gastric cancer. *Chemotherapy.* (1996) 42:220–6. doi: 10.1159/000239446
58. Tsuburaya A, Yoshida K, Kobayashi M, Yoshino S, Takahashi M, Takiguchi N, et al. Sequential paclitaxel followed by tegafur and uracil (UFT) or S-1 versus UFT or S-1 monotherapy as adjuvant chemotherapy for T4a/b gastric cancer (SAMIT): a phase 3 factorial randomised controlled trial. *Lancet Oncol.* (2014) 15:886–93. doi: 10.1016/S1470-2045(14)70025-7
59. Tsujinaka T, Shiozaki H, Inoue M, Furukawa H, Hiratsuka M, Kikkawa N, et al. Evaluation of effectiveness of chemotherapy in patients with gastric cancer after curative resection. *Int J Clin Oncol.* (2000) 5:372–9. doi: 10.1007/PL00012066
60. Yoshikawa T, Terashima M, Mizusawa J, Nunobe S, Nishida Y, Yamada T, et al. Four courses versus eight courses of adjuvant S-1 for patients with stage II gastric cancer (JCOG1104): an open-label, phase 3, non-inferiority, randomised trial. *Lancet Gastroenterol Hepatol.* (2019) 4:208–16. doi: 10.1016/S2468-1253(18)30383-2
61. Yu C, Yu R, Zhu W, Song Y, Li T. Intensity-modulated radiotherapy combined with chemotherapy for the treatment of gastric cancer patients after standard D1/D2 surgery. *J Cancer Res Clin Oncol.* (2012) 138:255–9. doi: 10.1007/s00432-011-1085-y
62. Zhang XL, Shi HJ, Cui SZ, Tang YQ, Ba MC. Prospective, randomized trial comparing 5-FU/LV with or without oxaliplatin as adjuvant treatment following curative resection of gastric adenocarcinoma. *Eur J Surg Oncol.* (2011) 37:466–72. doi: 10.1016/j.ejso.2011.01.027
63. Zhu WG, Xua DF, Pu J, Zong CD, Li T, Tao GZ, et al. A randomized, controlled, multicenter study comparing intensity-modulated radiotherapy plus concurrent chemotherapy with chemotherapy alone in gastric cancer patients with D2 resection. *Radiother Oncol.* (2012) 104:361–6. doi: 10.1016/j.radonc.2012.08.024
64. Ngai LL, Ter Veer E, van den Boorn HG, van Herk EH, van Kleef JJ, van Oijen MGH, et al. TOXview: a novel graphical presentation of cancer treatment toxicity profiles. *Acta Oncol.* (2019) 1–11. doi: 10.1080/0284186X.2019.1601256
65. Tariman JD, Berry DL, Cochrane B, Doorenbos A, Schepp K. Preferred and actual participation roles during health care decision making in persons with cancer: a systematic review. *Ann Oncol.* (2010) 21:1145–51. doi: 10.1093/annonc/mdp534
66. Reeder-Hayes KE, Roberts MC, Henderson GE, Dees EC. Informed consent and decision making among participants in novel-design phase I oncology trials. *J Oncol Pract.* (2017) 13:e863–73. doi: 10.1200/JOP.2017.021303
67. Hawley ST, An LC, Li Y, Resnicow K, Morrow M, Jagsi R, et al. Primary outcomes analysis of a multicenter randomized controlled trial of an interactive decision tool for patients with breast cancer. *J Clin Oncol.* (2017) 35:6500. doi: 10.1200/JCO.2017.35.15_suppl.6500
68. Boorn Hvd, Abu-Hanna A, Veer Et, Kleef JJv, Lordick F, Stahl M, et al. Two novel registry-based prediction models for overall survival in patients with metastatic esophageal or gastric cancer. *J Clin Oncol.* (2018) 36:4021. doi: 10.1200/JCO.2018.36.15_suppl.4021
69. Hamelinck VC, Bastiaannet E, Pieterse AH, van de Velde CJH, Liefers GJ, Stiggelbout AM. Preferred and perceived participation of younger and older patients in decision making about treatment for early breast cancer: a prospective study. *Clin Breast Cancer.* (2018) 18:e245–53. doi: 10.1016/j.clbc.2017.11.013
70. Schaede U, Mahlich J, Nakayama M, Kobayashi H, Takahashi Y, Saito K H, et al. Shared decision-making in patients with prostate cancer in Japan: patient preferences versus physician perceptions. *J Glob Oncol.* (2018) 1-9. doi: 10.1200/JGO.2016.008045
71. Rajabi Mashhadi M, Bagheri R, Abdollahi A, Ghamari MJ, Shahidsales S, Salehi M, et al. The effect of neoadjuvant therapy on early complications of esophageal cancer surgery. *Iran J Otorhinolaryngol.* (2015) 27:279–84.
72. Czosnyka NM, Borgert AJ, Smith TJ. Pancreatic adenocarcinoma: effects of neoadjuvant therapy on post-pancreatectomy outcomes — an American College of Surgeons National Surgical Quality Improvement Program targeted variable review. *HPB.* (2017) 19:927–32. doi: 10.1016/j.hpb.2017.07.001
73. Mungo B, Molena D, Stem M, Yang SC, Battafarano RJ, Brock MV, et al. Does neoadjuvant therapy for esophageal cancer increase postoperative morbidity or mortality? *Dis Esophagus.* (2015) 28:644–51. doi: 10.1111/dote.12251
74. Juloori A, Tucker SL, Komaki R, Liao Z, Correa AM, Swisher SG, et al. Influence of preoperative radiation field on postoperative leak rates in esophageal cancer patients after trimodality therapy. *J Thorac Oncol.* (2014) 9:534–40. doi: 10.1097/JTO.0000000000000100

75. Koeter M, Kathiravetpillai N, Gooszen JA, van Berge Henegouwen MI, Gisbertz SS, van der Sangen MJ, et al. Influence of the extent and dose of radiation on complications after neoadjuvant chemoradiation and subsequent esophagectomy with gastric tube reconstruction with a cervical anastomosis. *Int J Radiat Oncol Biol Phys.* (2017) 97:813–21. doi: 10.1016/j.ijrobp.2016.11.054
76. Sivendran S, Latif A, McBride RB, Stensland KD, Wisnivesky J, Haines L, et al. Adverse event reporting in cancer clinical trial publications. *J Clin Oncol.* (2014) 32:83–9. doi: 10.1200/JCO.2013.52.2219
77. Thanarajasingam G, Atherton PJ, Novotny PJ, Loprinzi CL, Sloan JA, Grothey A. Longitudinal adverse event assessment in oncology clinical trials: the Toxicity over Time (ToxT) analysis of alliance trials NCCTG N9741 and 979254. *Lancet Oncol.* (2016) 17:663–70. doi: 10.1016/S1470-2045(16)00038-3
78. Coebergh van den Braak RRJ, van Rijssen LB, van Kleef JJ, Vink GR, Berbee M, van Berge Henegouwen MI, et al. Nationwide comprehensive gastro-intestinal cancer cohorts: the 3P initiative. *Acta Oncol.* (2018) 57:195–202. doi: 10.1080/0284186X.2017.1346381

11

GALC Triggers Tumorigenicity of Colorectal Cancer via Senescent Fibroblasts

Mengdi Yang[1†], Zhiyuan Jiang[1†], Guangyu Yao[1], Zhiyu Wang[1], Jing Sun[1], Huanlong Qin[2] and Hui Zhao[1*]*

[1] Department of Internal Oncology, Shanghai Jiao Tong University Affiliated Sixth People's Hospital, Shanghai, China,
[2] Department of Gastrointestinal Surgery, Shanghai Tenth People's Hospital Affiliated With Tongji University, Shanghai, China

***Correspondence:**
Huanlong Qin
qin_huanlong@126.com
Hui Zhao
zhao-hui@sjtu.edu.cn

† These authors have contributed equally to this work*

Colorectal cancer (CRC)-associated senescent fibroblasts may play a crucial role in tumor progression, but the mechanism remains unclear. In order to solve this complicated problem, we randomly collected 16 patients with CRC, who had been treated with oxaliplatin and capecitabine (XELOX). Hematoxylin-eosin (HE) staining revealed that the tumor-stroma ratio (TSR) of CRC was affected by XELOX treatment. Immunohistochemistry (IHC) and senescence-associated β-galactosidase (SAβG) staining were used to verify a stable model of senescent fibroblasts. IHC analysis showed that high expression levels of galactosylceramidase (GALC) and significant senescence-associated β-galactosidase (SAβG) staining were associated with CRC patient survival. We observed that fibroblasts overexpressing GALC underwent cell cycle arrest. Changes in cell morphology and cell cycle characteristics were accompanied by the upregulation of the *p16*, *p21*, and *p53* gene, and the downregulation of *hTERT* expression. In a co-culture system, fibroblasts overexpressing GALC significantly increased the proliferation of CRC cells. Transmission electron microscopy (TEM) analysis confirmed that GALC overexpression fibroblasts co-cultured with CRC caused changes in CRC cell morphology. The aging fibroblast co-culture group (70%) had a higher migration ability. *In vivo* experiments and transcriptomics analysis were performed to verify the effect of senescent fibroblasts on tumor formation and to identify the potential mechanisms for the above results. We found that a high expression of ATF3 was related to good survival rates. However, a high expression of KIAA0907 was bad for survival rates ($p < 0.05$). The knockdown of ATF3 can promote cell proliferation, migration, and clonogenic assays, while downregulation of KIAA0907 inhibits cell proliferation, migration, and clonogenic assays. The results demonstrate that senescent fibroblasts with a high level of GALC regulated several aspects of the tumor growth process, including migration and invasion.

Keywords: senescent fibroblasts, tumorigenicity, colorectal cancer, galactosylceramidase, tumor microenvironment

INTRODUCTION

Colorectal cancer (CRC) remains one of the leading causes of mortality worldwide, and it is a severe threat to public health (1, 2). Treatment of CRC is a critical challenge, since many patients do not respond to therapy and those that do respond can develop drug resistance after most advanced treatment strategies that are provided in the clinics (3, 4). Previous studies have demonstrated that senescent fibroblasts are abundant and heterogeneous in the tumor microenvironment (TME), and they are closely associated with cancer progression and resistance to therapy (5, 6). As fibroblasts are the most abundant cell type in the tumor stroma, the deregulation of secreted paracrine factors from fibroblasts has been shown to influence the growth, invasion, and metastasis of cancer cells (7). While several mechanisms have been reported for the regulation of cancers by senescent fibroblasts (8–10), it is clear that additional mechanisms also contribute to the stromal regulation of cancers, and thus, additional studies are warranted.

Senescent fibroblasts are thought to be precursors to cancer-associated fibroblasts (CAFs) (11, 12). They share the ability to stimulate proliferation and invasive behavior (13, 14). Senescence was originally used as a model to study the aging of fibroblasts both *in vitro* and *in vivo* (15). However, senescent cells induced by traditional methods are difficult to obtain in large quantities. In cell culture experiments and in aging humans, senescent fibroblasts have been associated with increased β-galactosidase (SAβG) activity (16). Galactosylceramidase (GALC) is a lysosomal protein that hydrolyzes the galactose ester bonds of galactosylceramide, galactosylsphingosine, lactosylceramide, and monogalactosyldiglyceride (17). High levels of GALC expression can increase the expression of β-galactosidase. Thus, the cell senescence status can be assessed by detecting GALC expression. Metastatic CRC remains one of the most malignant human gastrointestinal carcinomas, with one of the worst 5-year prognoses (18, 19). While there is known to be an interaction between fibroblasts and CRC cells (20), the mechanisms are yet to be fully elucidated. Hence, this study aims to examine the effect of senescent fibroblasts on various CRC cell phenotypes.

MATERIALS AND METHODS

Human Tissue Samples

The present study was reviewed and approved by the Ethics Committee of Shanghai Jiao Tong University Affiliated Sixth People's Hospital (2017-037). Written informed consent was obtained from all patients. The enrolling criteria included the following: (1) Colonoscopy diagnosed as CRC. (2) The preoperative imaging data were clearly T3-4N1-2M0, and the preoperative staging must have reached stage IIIB–IIIC (according to the American Cancer Society TNM staging standard) without distant metastasis. (3) Patients must be older than 18 years old and younger than 80 years old, and have a Kamofsky score of 70 or higher, with no history of tumor-related bleeding. (4) White blood cell count $>4 \times 10^9$/L, platelets $>100 \times 10^9$/L. The clearance rate of creatinine should be >60 ml/min, and there is sufficient liver function reserve: serum bilirubin <2.5 times the upper limit of normal, AS/ALT < 2.5 times the upper limit of normal. (5) The patient had no previous bowel surgery and no history of radiotherapy and chemotherapy. The patient does not have any other malignant diseases. All patients received at least three cycles of the XELOX regimen with a 3-week course (oxaliplatin 130 mg/m^2, day 1; capecitabine 1,250 mg/m^2 twice daily, days 1–14). (6) Puncture samples from patients enrolled should be usable to perform clinical IHC and TSR analysis. (7) Patients should be available for follow-ups. Sixteen patients undergoing surgery after neoadjuvant chemotherapy at Shanghai Sixth People's Hospital and Shanghai Tenth People's Hospital between January 2010 and December 2012 were selected for this study. Biopsy specimens were collected from each patient before and after chemotherapy. The colonoscopy results before chemotherapy confirmed the diagnosis of CRC, and the computed tomography (CT) and magnetic resonance imaging (MRI) data of all patients were available. The characteristics of the patients included in this study are listed in **Table 1**.

TABLE 1 | Basic information of clinical patients.

Characteristics			Number	Percent (%)
Gender	Man		9	56.25
	Woman		7	43.75
Tumor site				
	Colon			
		Ascending colon	4	25
		Sigmoid colon	3	18.75
	Rectum			
		High position (>10 cm)	3	18.75
		Median (7–10 cm)	2	12.5
		High position(<7 cm)	4	25
Surgical approach				
		Laparoscopic radical resection	10	62.5
		Dixon	3	18.75
		Miles	3	18.75
Pathology				
		Medium differentiated adenocarcinoma	5	31.25
		Low-grade adenocarcinoma	7	43.75
		Mucinous adenocarcinoma	4	25

Cell Culture

Fibroblasts HFL1 (ATCC® CCL-153), HFF-1 (ATCC® SCRC-1041), CRC cell lines LoVo (ATCC® CCL-229), RKO (ATCC® CRL-2577), HCT116 (ATCC® CCL-247), HT-29 (ATCC® HTB-38), and virus-packaging 293T (ATCC® CRL-11268) cells were all purchased from the Institute of Biochemistry and Cell Biology, Chinese Academy of Science (Shanghai, China). The details of these cell lines can be obtained from the American Type Culture Collection (https://www.atcc.org/products). HFL1, HFF-1, LoVo, RKO, HCT116, HT-29, and virus-packaging 293T cells were cultured in Dulbecco's Modified Eagle Medium (DMEM; Invitrogen, Carlsbad, CA, USA), supplemented with 10% fetal bovine serum (FBS) and 1% penicillin/streptomycin, at 37°C under 5% CO_2.

Lentivirus Packaging

The transfection mixture was prepared according to the following ratio: 600 μl OPTI-MEM plus, 72 μl PEI, and 24 μg plasmid [PLVX-GFP-GALC, PLVX-GFP, shCK, shATF3 (shATF3-1: TGCTGTTGACAGTGAGCGCAAAGAGGCGAC GAGAAAGAAATAGTGAAGCCACAGATGTATTTCTTTCTC GTCGCCTCTTTTTGCCTACTGCCTCGGA; shATF3-2:TGC TGTTGACAGTGAGCGCAAAGAGGCGACGAGAAAGAA ATAGTGAAGCCACAGATGTATTTCTTTCTCGTCGCCTCT TTTTGCCTACTGCCTCGGA), shKIAA0907(shKIAA0907-1:TGCTGTTGACAGTGAGCGACTGGTGGTAGCTGAAGT AGAATAGTGAAGCCACAGATGTATTCTACTTCAGCTACC ACCAGGTGCCTACTGCCTCGGA, shKIAA0907-2:TGCTGT TGACAGTGAGCGATAGATTTGTGAATCAGATTAATAGTG AAGCCACAGATGTATTAATCTGATTCACAAATCTAGTGC CTACTGCCTCGGA)], which included 12-μg target plasmid, 10.68-μg dR8.9, and 1.32-μg VSV-G. Then the mixture was allowed to stand for 10 min. Transfection occurred for 4–6 h, and the medium was then changed. The medium was collected at 48 and 72 h, respectively.

SAβG Staining

A Senescence β-Galactosidase Staining Kit (Beyotime, Shanghai, China; C0602) was used for SAβG staining. The SAβG staining efficiency was calculated as the number of positively stained cells divided by the total number of cells in a single field of view. Fibroblasts with a staining rate greater than 10% were used for subsequent experiments.

Cell Co-culture

CRC (LoVo, RKO, HCT116, HT29) cells were thawed and plated on 10-mm glass coverslips (Menzel Glaser; Braunschweig, Germany) in 24-well plates for co-culture experiments or directly onto Transwell chambers (24 wells, each with a 4 μm pore size polycarbonate membrane; Corning Incorporated, USA) for cell migration experiments. LoVo and RKO cells were separately added to a 24-well plate at 5×10^5 cells per well. LV-GALC and LV-NC HFL1 cells were then seeded in the lower chamber of the transwell chamber at 2×10^5 cells per well, with three replicate wells per group. Co-culture experiments were performed in duplicate and repeated on three independent occasions. Data from the three independent experiments were pooled.

Animal Experiments

Experimental animals were ordered through the Animal Ethics Committee of Shanghai Jiao Tong University Affiliated Sixth People's Hospital, and all animal experiments were performed under a protocol approved by the Committee (2016-0137). Two million viable LV-GALC, LV-NC, and LoVo cells were injected subcutaneously into the following two groups of 6-week-old nude male mice: (A) LoVo and LV-GALC ($n = 12$); and (B) LoVo and LV-NC ($n = 11$). Mice were sacrificed when the tumor volume in control mice reached 1,200 mm^3. Tumor volume (mm^3) was calculated based on the formula for approximating the volume of a spheroid. The tumor volume is calculated as V = (Length × width^2)/2.

Tumor-Stroma Ratio

The tumor-stroma ratio (TSR) was first used for the early evaluation of colon cancer in 2007 (21). The percentage of each field of view occupied by tumor cells was then evaluated under a microscope at 200× magnification, and the remaining area was considered as the percentage of stroma. At least two fields of view were selected for evaluation, and the highest percentage of stroma was used as the final value. TSR calculations were performed by at least two certified pathologists who were blind to the patients' information.

Immunofluorescence

The immunofluorescence assay was performed using the primary antibodies against Ki67 (Abcam, #ab15580, 1:100). The samples were then incubated with 1:200 for 1 h, and then incubated with 4′,6-diamidino-2-phenylindole (DAPI) (Santa Cruz TM) for 15 min. The images were captured and analyzed using Leica TCS SP8.

Immunohistochemical Studies

Paraffin-embedded sections were incubated with a primary antibody against ki-67 (Abcam, #ab15580, 1:100), GALC (Proteintech #21544-1-AP), p53 (CST #2527, 1:200), p21 (CST #2947, 1:100), and p16 (Abcam, #ab51243, 1:500), followed by incubation with a secondary biotinylated antibody (Kirkegaard & Perry Laboratories). The method used for immunohistochemistry has been described previously (22, 23).

Cell Cycle Analysis

Cell cycle analysis of LV-NC-HFL1/HFF-1, LV-GALC-HFL1/HFF-1, and/or HFL1/HFF-1 co-cultured with CRC cell lines was performed using propidium iodide (PI) staining (Beyotime, Shanghai, China; C1062). The experiment was performed according to the instructions of the reagent. The cells (5×10^5) were analyzed using a BD LSR Fortessa (BD Biosciences, USA), and the data were analyzed using the FlowJo software (TreeStar, USA).

Quantitative Reverse-Transcriptase PCR Analysis

Triplicate samples of total RNA were transcribed into complementary DNA (cDNA) using AMV Reverse Transcriptase (Promega, Madison, Wisconsin, USA). qPCR was performed on the cDNA samples using gene-specific primers, the Maxima TM SYBR Green/ROX qPCR Master Mix (Fermentas, Glen Burnie, Maryland), and a 7300HT real-time PCR instrument (Applied Biosystems, Foster City, CA, USA). PCR results were evaluated by melting curve analysis and by confirming the expected PCR products on 2% (w/v) agarose gels. The following equation was used for the analysis: $\Delta C_T = C_{T targetgene} - C_{T\ Internalreferencegene}$; the comparison between samples:

TABLE 2 | RT-PCR primers in this study.

Genes	Sequences
galc Forward	TATTTCCGAGGATACGAGTGGT
galc Reverse	CCAGTCGAAACCTTTTCCCAG
p16 Forward	GATCCAGGTGGGTAGAAGGTC
p16 Reverse	CCCCTGCAAACTTCGTCCT
p21 Forward	GGGGACCTAGAGCAACTTACT
p21 Reverse	CAGCGCAGTCCTTCCAAAT
tert Forward	GGCACGGCTTTTGTTCAGAT
tert Reverse	TCCGGGCATAGCTGGAGTAG
p53 Forward	AGCTTGATCGCCTCTATAAGGA
p53 Reverse	CCCTCAGCTCATTAACACGCT

$\Delta\Delta C_T = \Delta C_{T\ Experimentalgroup} - \Delta C_{T\ Controlgroup}$; foldchange = $2^{-\Delta\Delta CT}$. The sequences of all PCR primers are listed in **Table 2**.

Western Blotting Analysis

Total cell lysates were prepared using a RIPA buffer. Equal amounts of protein were separated by electrophoresis, transferred onto polyvinylidene fluoride membranes, and incubated with primary antibodies against anti-p53 (CST #2527, 1:1,000), anti-p21 (CST #2947, 1:1,000), anti-p16 (Abcam, #ab51243, 1:1,000), and anti-GADPH (Abcam #8245, 1:2,000), and a Horseradish peroxidase-conjugated secondary antibody (Jackson ImmunoResearch, West Grove, PA, USA, 1:5,000) was used; blots were developed with the ECL Plus reagent (Millipore, Burlington, MA, USA).

Transmission Electron Microscope Analysis

Samples were placed into 5-ml centrifuge tubes, fixed in glutaraldehyde for 1 h at room temperature, and then stored at 4°C for 4 h. After fixation, the samples were washed three times with 0.2 M phosphate buffer (pH 7.4) for 10 min each wash. The samples were then serially dehydrated in ethanol at concentrations of 30, 50, 75, 90, 95, and 100% for 10 min at each concentration. After desiccation in a drying oven for 12 h, the samples were fixed on the copper plates of the microscope for analysis by transmission electron microscopy (TEM).

RNA-Seq

After 24 h of co-culture, as described above, the Transwell chamber was discarded and RNA was extracted from co-cultured LoVo cells in a 6-well plate for RNA-seq analysis. The samples were sent to Genechem (Shanghai, China) for RNA-seq library preparation. The library quality was assessed on the Agilent Bioanalyzer 2100 system. Three biological replicates were used for RNA-seq experiments. Sequencing libraries were generated using a NEBNext Ultra^{TM} RNA Library Prep Kit for Illumina (NEB, USA). The clustering of the index-coded samples was performed on a cBot Cluster Generation System using a TruSeq PE Cluster Kit v4-cBot-HS (Illumia), following the manufacturer's instructions.

Transwell Assays

In total, 1×10^5 cells were seeded into the upper Transwell chambers (Corning, NY, USA), and media with 10% FBS were added to the lower chamber. After incubation for 24 h, the chamber was fixed in methanol and then stained using crystal violet (Beyotime). Using a light microscope, at least five randomly selected fields were photographed, after which the counts were averaged. All experiments were performed in triplicate.

Cell Count Kit-8

The cells were cultured in a 96-well plate for 0, 24, 48, 72, and 96 h. Thereafter, a Cell Count Kit-8 (CCK-8, Dojindo, Japan) with a medium volume of 10% was added into the wells and incubated for 2–4 h at 37°C. The absorbance (OD) of the solution was then measured using a microplate reader (Biorad, USA) at 450 nm. The experiments were carried out in sextuplicate.

Colony Formation Assay

Cells were plated in a six-well plate and incubated at 37 °C for 2 weeks. Colonies were fixed with 4% phosphate-buffered formalin (pH 7.4) and stained with Giemsa for 15 min. Each experiment was performed in triplicate.

Statistical Analysis

Data were analyzed by ANOVA, the chi-square test, or the two-tailed Student's t-test, the Fisher-exact test, and the Mann–Whitney U-test, as appropriate, using SPSS version 20.0 (SPSS Inc., Chicago, IL, USA). All data are presented as the mean ± SD, and $^*p < 0.05$, $^{**}p < 0.01$, $^{***}p < 0.001$ was considered to be statistically significant. All experiments were performed on three independent occasions.

RESULTS

Analysis of Interstitial Cell Senescence and Related Pathological Parameters in Patients Undergoing Neoadjuvant Chemotherapy for Advanced CRC

To understand the changes that occur in the tumor stroma in patients undergoing neoadjuvant chemotherapy for CRC, 16 patients with locally advanced CRC, who had been treated with oxaliplatin and capecitabine (XELOX), were randomly selected. HE staining was performed on tumor samples to determine TSR before and after (**Figure 1A**) neoadjuvant chemotherapy. The characteristics of the patients included in the study are listed in **Table 1**. We found that 37.50% of patients ($n = 6$) had increased TSR after chemotherapy; however, changes in total TSR had no significant effect on the prognosis of patients ($p = 0.3$) (**Table 3**). We also stained tumor tissue samples for GALC, Ki67, p53, and E-cadherin (**Figures 1B–E**) to explore the relationship between these markers and prognosis. The results showed that high levels of GALC expression were associated with a poor prognosis ($p < 0.01$; **Table 4**).

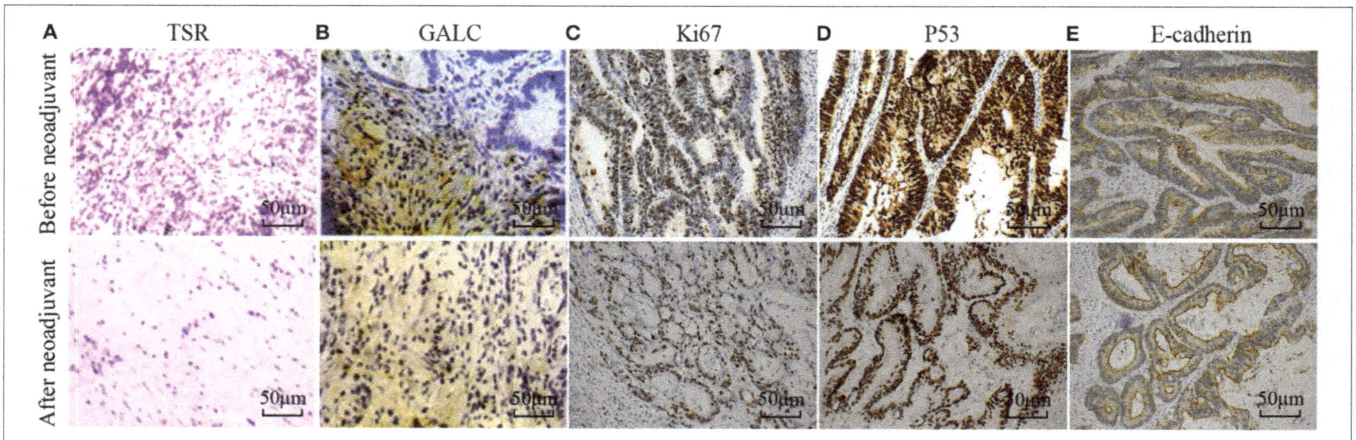

FIGURE 1 | Disease-related indicators before and after neoadjuvant chemotherapy for colorectal cancer. **(A)** Hematoxylin-eosin (HE) staining showing the tumor-stroma ratio before and after neoadjuvant chemotherapy. Immunohistochemical staining of GALC **(B)**, Ki67 **(C)**, p53 **(D)**, and E-cadherin **(E)** was performed to explore the relationship between these markers and prognosis. $p < 0.05$ was considered statistically significant.

TABLE 3 | The relationship between the clinical pathological factors and prognosis.

TSR	State		p
	Survival ($n = 11$)	Died ($n = 5$)	
Up	3	3	0.3
Down or not change	8	2	

TABLE 4 | The relationship between the immunohistochemical markers and prognosis.

Proteins	Expression	State		P
		Survival ($n = 11$)	Died ($n = 5$)	
GALC	H	1	5	<0.01**
	L	10	0	
Ki67	H	7	4	0.6
	L	4	1	
p53	H	5	2	1
	L	6	3	
E-cadherin	H	4	2	1
	L	7	3	

Generation of Senescent Fibroblasts Through GALC Overexpression

To explore the mechanism for the association between high GALC expression fibroblasts and poor prognosis in CRC patients, we transfected fibroblast cells with PLVX-GFP (LV-NC) or PLVX-GFP-GALC (LV-GALC) vectors (**Figure 2A**). We then determined the expression of GALC in LV-NC, LV-GALC, and un-transfected HFF1/HFL1 cells (NC) using qRT-PCR ($p < 0.05$, **Figure 2B**). These results demonstrated the successful overexpression of GALC in LV-GALC HFL1/HFF-1 fibroblasts. We also observed senescent features (24), including increased SAβG staining (**Figure 2C**) and morphological changes to larger, more flattened, and more irregularly shaped cells in LV-GALC HFF1/HFL1 cells, not observed in LV-NC HFF-1/HFL1 cells.

GALC-Overexpressing Senescence Fibroblast Cells

Relative to LV-NC and NC fibroblast cells, there was a significant increase in the number of LV-GALC HFF1/HFL1 fibroblasts in the G0/G1 phase and a significant decrease in the number of cells in the G2/M phase (**Figure 2D**). We further examined the cell cycle profile and the expression of additional protein markers associated with senescence, including *p16*, *p21*, and *p53*. LV-GALC HFF1/ HFL1 fibroblast cells had elevated *p16*, *p21*, and *p53* mRNA levels (**Figures 2E,F**, $p < 0.05$), while LV-GALC cells had lower ($p < 0.05$) levels of *hTERT* mRNA. The protein expression of P16, P21, and P53 was found to be higher in LV-GALC HFF1/HFL1 fibroblast cells than in LV-NC and NC fibroblast cells (**Figures 2G,H**). Overall, our results demonstrated that GALC overexpression led to the senescence of HFF1/HFL1 fibroblast cells.

Impact of Senescent Fibroblasts on CRC Cells

We sought to determine the effects of LV-GALC fibroblast cells on several aspects of tumor regulation in co-culture models with CRC cells. Through cell cycle profile analysis, we observed a decreased percentage of RKO and HCT116 cells in the G0/G1 phase, but an increased percentage in the G2/M phase, when they were co-cultured with LV-GALC fibroblast cells. The most significant effect was seen in RKO cells at 48 h ($p < 0.05$). A similar phenomenon was observed in LoVo cells after 24 and 48 h of co-culture ($p < 0.05$); however, there was no enrichment of HT29 cells in the G2/M phase (**Figure 3A**). In the Transwell migration assays, RKO and LoVo cells co-cultured with LV-GALC HFL1 fibroblast cells had significantly enhanced cell mobility ($p < 0.05$). The mobility of HT29 cells co-cultured with LV-GALC HFL1 fibroblast cells was not different from

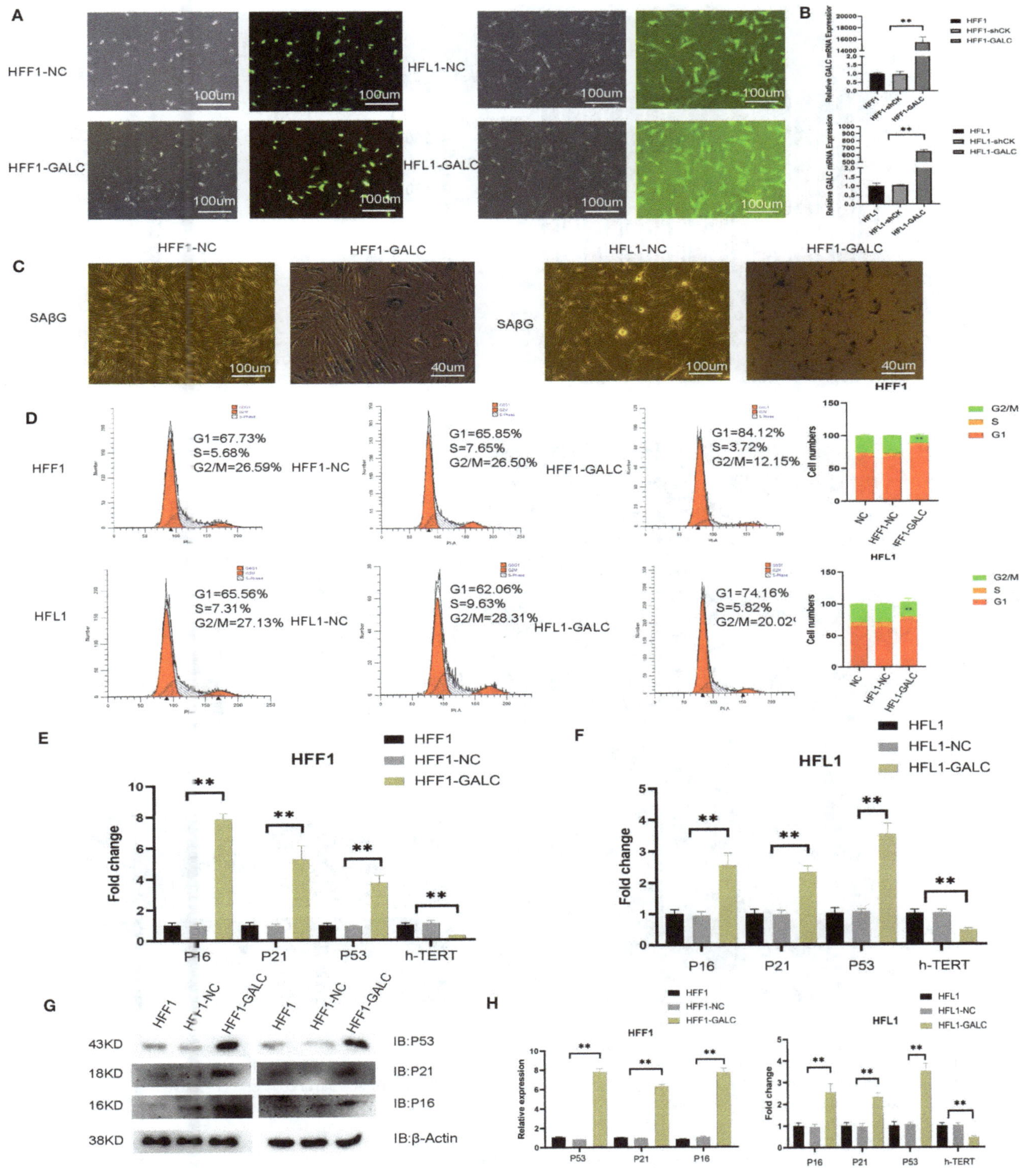

FIGURE 2 | Generation of senescent fibroblasts, and the cell cycle and senescence-associated markers in LV-GALC HFF1/HFL1 fibroblasts cells. **(A)** Construction of the LV-GALC HFF1/HFL1 fibroblasts cells. **(B)** The expression of GALC in normal HFF1/HFL1 cells (NC), LV-NC HFF1/HFL1 fibroblasts, and LV-GALC HFF1/HFL1 fibroblast cells. **(C)** β-galactosidase staining of LV-NC HFF1/HFL1 fibroblasts and LV-GALC HFF1/HFL1 fibroblast cells. **(D)** Cell cycle analysis of NC, LV-NC HFF1/HFL1 fibroblasts, and LV-GALC HFF1/HFL1 fibroblast cells. **(E,F)** qRT-PCR analysis of *hTERT*, *p16*, *p21*, and *p53* expression in NC, LV-NC HFF1/HFL1 fibroblasts, and LV-GALC HFF1/HFL1 fibroblast cells. **(G)** The expression of p53, p21, and p16 proteins in NC, LV-NC, and LV-GALC HFF1/HFL1 cells. **(H)** Quantitative analysis of the expression of p16, p53, and p21 proteins in NC, LV-NC, and LV-GALC HFF1/HFL1 cells.

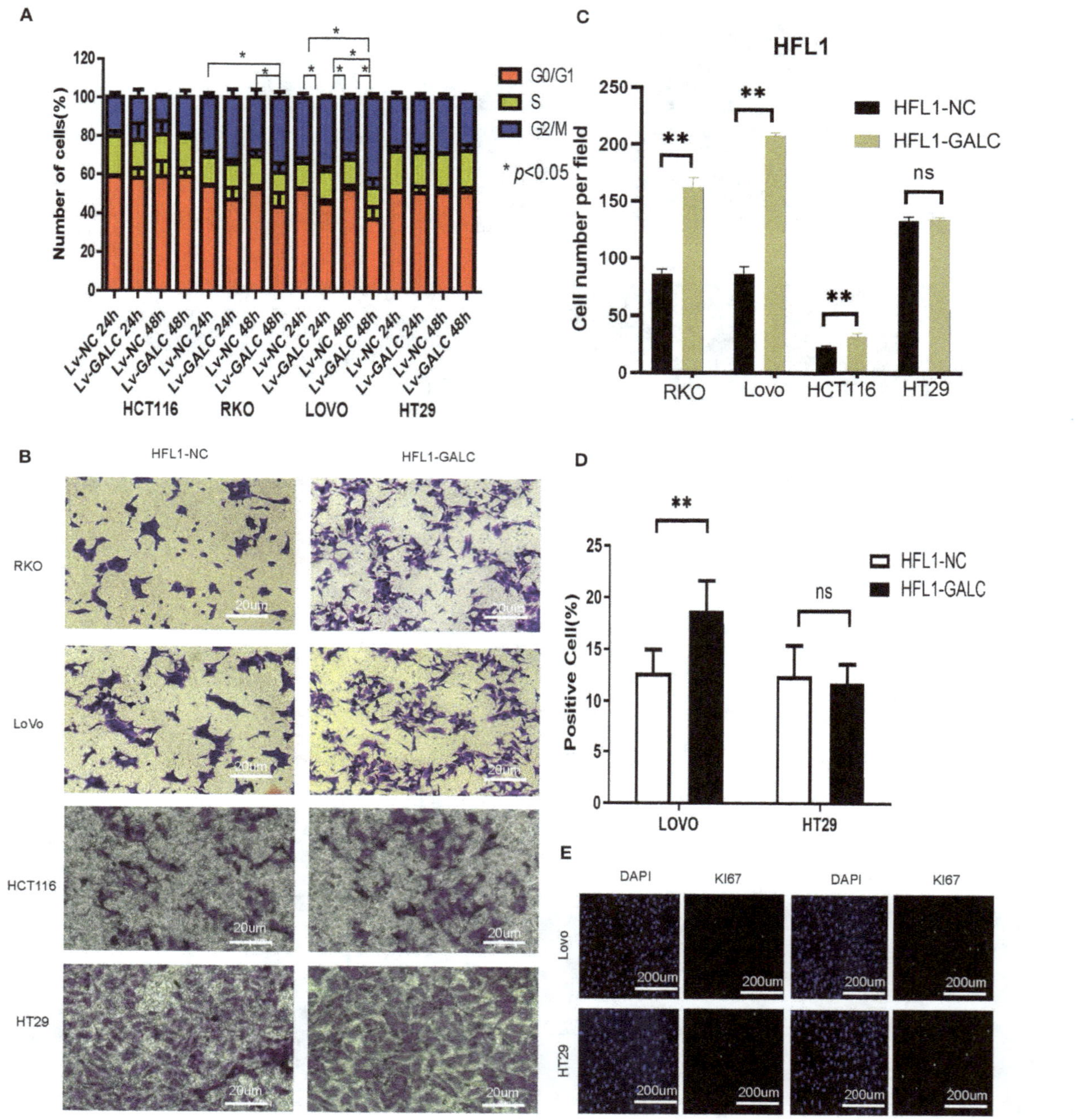

FIGURE 3 | *In vitro* impact of senescent fibroblasts on CRC cells. **(A)** After co-culture with LV-GALC fibroblasts cells, the proportion of G0/G1 phase LoVo cells shown at 24 and 48 h ($p < 0.05$) and the proportion of G0/G1 phase RKO cells shown at 48 h ($p < 0.05$). **(B,C)** Migration ability in a Transwell migration assay for RKO, LoVo, HCT116, and HT29 cells co-cultured with LV-GALC fibroblast cells and control cells ($p < 0.05$). **(D,E)** Ki-67 staining of LoVo cells co-cultured with LV-GALC fibroblast cells ($p < 0.05$). $p < 0.05$ was considered statistically significant.

their mobility when co-cultured with LV-NC HFL1 fibroblast cells (**Figures 3B,C**). We also examined the proliferation indices represented by Ki67 expression in LoVo and HT29 cells. The proliferation indices for LoVo cells when co-cultured with LV-NC and LV-GALC fibroblast cells were 12.72 ± 2.26% and 18.71 ± 2.88%, respectively ($p < 0.05$). However, no apparent changes were seen in the proliferation of HT29 cells (**Figures 3D,E**).

Changes in the Structure of CRC Cells Co-cultured With Senescent Fibroblasts

We utilized TEM to examine the structure of CRC cells co-cultured with senescent LV-GALC HFL1 fibroblasts (**Figures 4A–C**) or LV-NC HFL1 fibroblasts (**Figures 4D–F**). We observed 10 cells in each group and found that seven of the aging fibroblast co-culture group (70%) contained cell

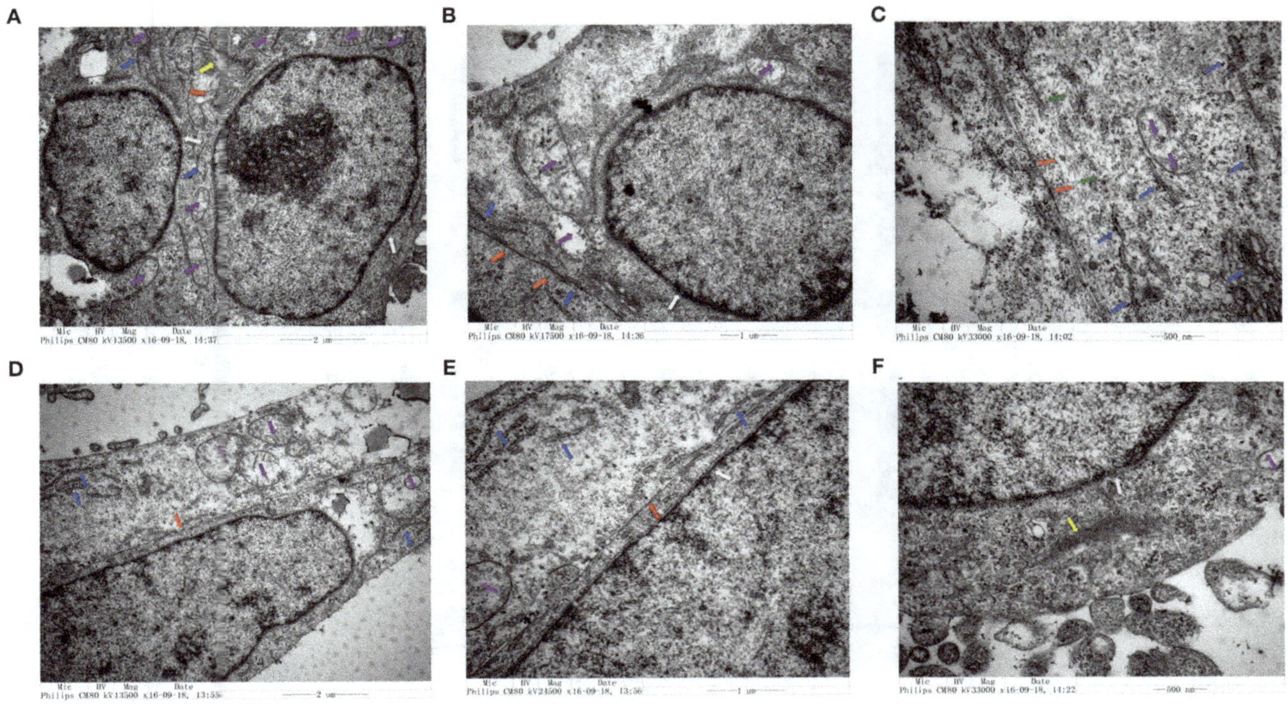

FIGURE 4 | Transmission electron microscopy analysis of colorectal cell lines in the presence and absence of senescent fibroblasts. **(A–C)** Structural characteristics of the LoVo cells that co-cultured with LV-GALC fibroblasts and **(D–F)** LoVo cells that co-cultured with LV-NC fibroblasts. Nuclear membrane (white arrow), mitochondria (purple arrow), visible increase in rough endoplasmic reticulum ribosomes (blue arrow), tight connection between cells (red arrow), microfilament (yellow), and microtube (green).

morphological changes, compared with only two in the control group (20%). The aging fibroblast co-culture group (70%) had a higher migration ability: large nuclear heteromorphism, nuclear chromatin accumulation, increased mitochondria (Purple arrow), visible increase in rough endoplasmic reticulum ribosomes (Blue arrow), fewer tight connection between cells (Red Arrow), microfilament (Yellow), microtube (Green), changes in cell polarity, with more elongated protrusions and foot processes, and an increase in the number of extracellular microvilli, which are not easily observed in attached and centrifuged cells. We observed that senescent fibroblasts induced notable morphological changes in the cancer cell cytoskeletal structure, with an increased number of microfilament structures. These changes may contribute to the mobility of the cancer cells and potentially enhance their metastatic capacity.

In vivo Impacts of Senescent Fibroblasts on CRC

To further investigate the *in vivo* effects of senescent fibroblasts on CRC, we also implanted xenografts of LV-GALC HFL1 fibroblasts co-cultured LoVo cells into nude mice. Seven days after the subcutaneous injection of cancer cells, 12 group A mice (LV-GALC HFL1 fibroblasts and LoVo cells) and 11 group B mice (LV-NC HFL1 fibroblasts and LoVo cells) demonstrated tumor formation (**Figure 5A**) Group A mice showed a statistically significant increase in tumor volume compared to group B mice. In the first 2 weeks, there was no significant difference in the tumor volume between the tumors of group A mice and those of group B. After the third week, in concordance with tumor growth, mice in group A demonstrated significantly greater weight loss compared to mice in group B (**Figure 5B**). When senescent fibroblast and tumor cells were first inoculated in mice, senile fibroblasts promoted tumor growth. However, the phenotype of senile fibroblasts was lost as the cells were inoculated for a longer period. Finally, we investigated the expression of p16, p21, and p53 (**Figure 5C**) in groups A and B mice. We found that P16, P21, and P53 were more highly expressed in group A mice (LV-GALC fibroblasts and LoVo cells) than group B mice (LV-NC fibroblasts and LoVo cells). Overall, our results suggested that exogenous senescent fibroblasts likely contribute to the grafting and growth of tumor cells.

Transcriptomics and Biochemical Analysis Revealed the Putative Mechanism Underlying the Impact of Senescent Fibroblasts on CRC

To elucidate the mechanism by which senescent fibroblasts promote the tumor properties of CRC cells, we performed transcriptomics and biochemical analysis of CRC co-cultured with LV-GALC and LV-NC fibroblast cells. First, we constructed

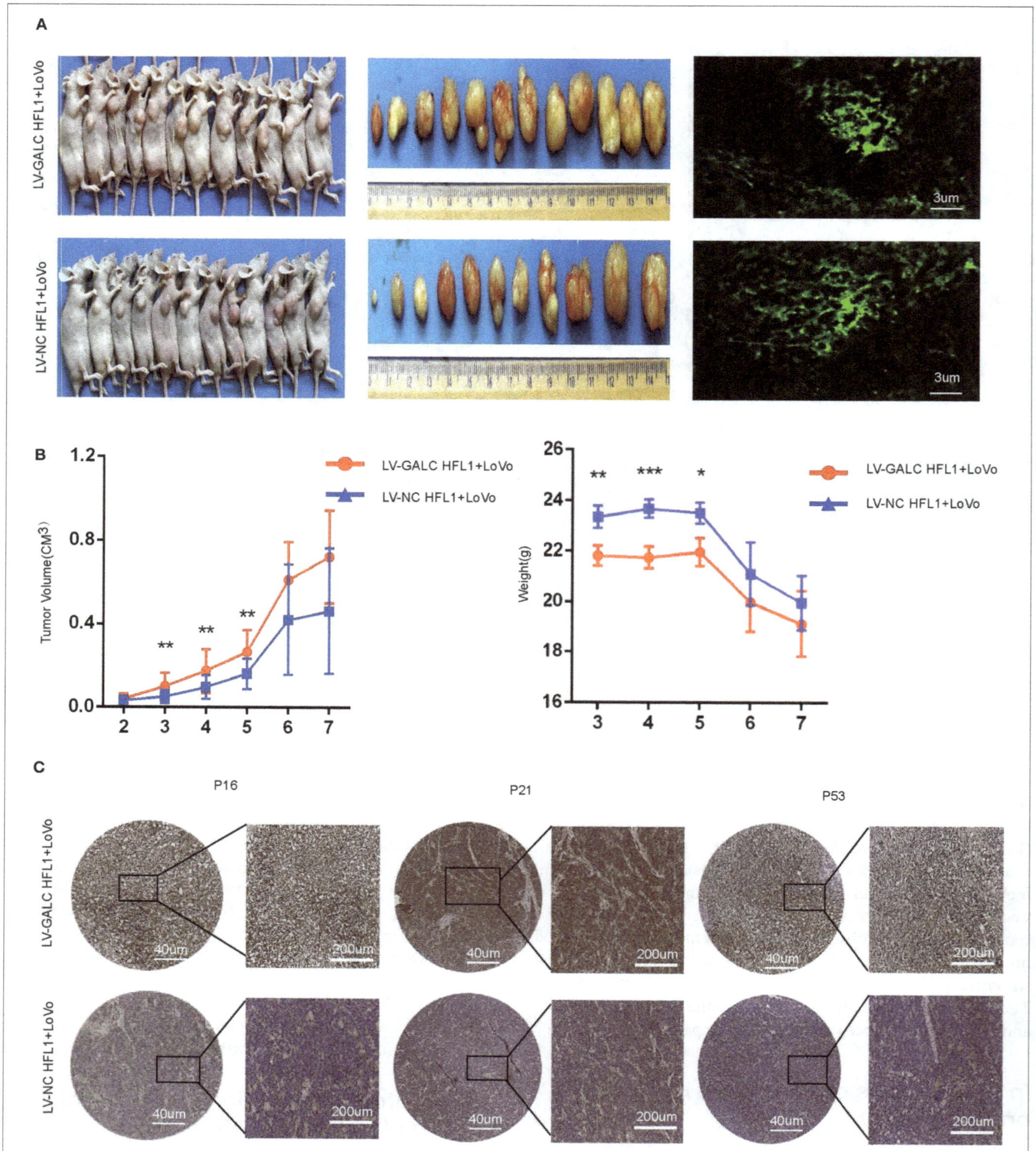

FIGURE 5 | *In vivo* impact of senescent fibroblasts on cancer cells. **(A)** Group A (LoVo and LV-GALC fibroblast cells) and Group B (LoVo and LV-NC fibroblast cells) mice, tumors sizes, and green fluorescence staining were shown. Tumor volume **(B)** and weight data for the two groups of mice. $p < 0.05$ was considered statistically significant. **(C)** Group A (LoVo and LV-GALC fibroblast cells) and group B (LoVo and LV-NC fibroblast cells) mice tumors were stained with P16, P21, and P53 using IHC.

Volcano maps (**Figure 6A**) and Heat maps (**Figure 6B**) to identify the genes differentially expressed between these two groups. Next, we examined the expression of several genes using the TCGA database and found that low levels of ATF3 expression and high levels of KIAA0907, LOC388152, and ZNF529 expression contributed to tumorigenicity. Furthermore, based on TCGA follow-up and statistical analyses, we found that low levels of ATF3 expression and high levels of KIAA0907, LOC388152, and ZNF529 expression were significantly associated with reduced survival ($p < 0.05$, **Figure 6C**). Gene ontology (GO) pathway enrichment analysis [biological process (BP), molecular function (MF), and cellular component (CC)] suggested that co-culturing with senescent fibroblasts led to the activation of several pathways associated with tumor cell survival and metastasis (**Figure 6D**). We also analyzed the expression of ATF3 and KIAA0907 in CRC using The Human Protein Atlas (www.proteinatlas.org). Compared with normal tissues, ATF3 is weakly expressed in CRC, while KIAA0907 is highly expressed in CRC (**Figure 6E**).

ATF3 and KIAA0907 Are Closely Related to Tumorigenesis and Metastasis

In order to verify the transcriptome results, we knocked down KIAA0907 (**Figure 7A**), which was highly expressed, and ATF3 (**Figure 7B**), which was weakly expressed. We then conducted the CCK8 (**Figures 7C,D**) and colony formation (**Figures 7E,F**) assay to explore the influence of ATF3 and KIAA0907 on CRC. We found that the knockdown of ATF3 promoted cell proliferation and the knockdown of KIAA0907 inhibited cell proliferation. The Transwell assay found that the knockdown of KIAA0907 (**Figure 7G**) inhibited cell migration, and the deregulation of ATF3 (**Figure 7H**) promoted it. These results revealed that LV-GALC fibroblast cells co-cultured with CRC upregulates oncogenes and downregulates tumor suppressor genes, thereby affecting tumor progression.

DISCUSSION

CRC is the fourth most common cancer diagnosed in adults and the second leading cause of death from cancer in the United States (25). Neoadjuvant systemic chemotherapy is advocated by current treatment guidelines (26). However, not all neoadjuvant chemotherapies are effective for all patients. A better understanding of the biology of CRC is imperative for the development of more effective therapeutic approaches (27).

Cellular senescence is a stable state of proliferative arrest that provides a barrier to malignant transformation and contributes to the antitumor activity of certain chemotherapies (28, 29). Senescent fibroblasts are already highly resistant to chemotherapy (30). Specifically, senescent stromal cells have been shown to play a role in carcinogenesis (31). Senescent fibroblasts can stimulate cancer cell proliferation and invasion (32). The results from this study demonstrated that tumors treated with chemotherapy were enriched in these stromal cells and this, in turn, worsened patient outcomes. These findings led us to subsequently examine the effect of senescent fibroblasts on the regulation of several phenotypes that are key to CRC tumorigenesis by GALC.

First, we established a stable model of senescent fibroblasts and we then used co-culture experiments to examine the effects of LV-GALC fibroblast effects on several tumor phenotypes relevant to CRC biology. The overexpression of GALC in HFL1/HFF-1 fibroblasts cells resulted in positive SAβG staining and the morphological changes to larger, more flattened, and more irregularly shaped cells that closely resembled senescent cells compared to LV-NC HFF1/HFL1 fibroblasts. We found that the percentage of LV-GALC cells in the G0/G1 phase was significantly higher than the percentage of control cells in the G0/G1 phase, whereas the percentage of LV-GALC cells in the G2/M phase was significantly lower, suggesting that cells have undergone cell cycle arrest. Notably, p53/P21/P16 is a vital signal axis that can induce cell senescence (33). We further identified LV-GALC senescent fibroblasts with higher G0/G1 cell cycle characteristics, which were accompanied by the upregulation of p16, p21, and p53 not only at the gene level but also in proteins. In co-culture experiments, LV-GALC fibroblast cells significantly increased the proliferation of LoVo cells and, expectedly, reduced the number of LoVo cells in the G0/G1 phase, while increasing those in the G2/M phase. *In vivo* experiments assessing subcutaneous tumor formation in mice showed that both tumor volume and tumor weight were greater in group A than in group B. In the early period when LV-GALC fibroblasts possess senescent properties ($p < 0.05$), P16, P21, and P53 were more highly expressed in group A mice (LV-GALC fibroblasts and LoVo cells) than group B mice (LV-NC fibroblasts and LoVo cells). This indicates that senescent interstitial fibroblasts can increase the tumorigenic ability of human CRC cells *in vivo*.

Understanding the transcriptome is essential for understanding development and disease processes (34, 35). In the present study, we performed RNA-seq experiments to further analyze the effects of co-culture on cell function and tumorigenesis. Furthermore, transcriptomics and biochemical analysis of CRC cells showed that there are many genes that are differentially expressed between co-cultures of LV-GALC senescent fibroblasts and LV-NC fibroblast cells. GO pathway enrichment analysis suggested that co-culturing CRC cells with senescent fibroblasts led to the activation of several pathways associated with tumor cell survival and metastasis. Cellular Component Ontology (CC) revealed that the co-culture group had more desmosome components. This is consistent with our TEM results, which further illustrated that CRC cell co-cultured with LV-GALC senescent fibroblasts had an increased number of microfilament structures, which may contribute to the mobility of cancer cells and potentially enhance metastatic capacity. ATF3 and KIAA0907 potentially contribute to tumorigenicity, and these factors were significantly associated with survival in the TCGA. We further explored the roles of ATF3 and KIAA0907 in CRC cells. We found that the knockdown of ATF3 promoted cell proliferation, migration, and clonogenic formation, while the deregulation of KIAA0907 inhibited it, which may explain the above results that senescent fibroblasts and CAFs share the ability to stimulate proliferation and invasive

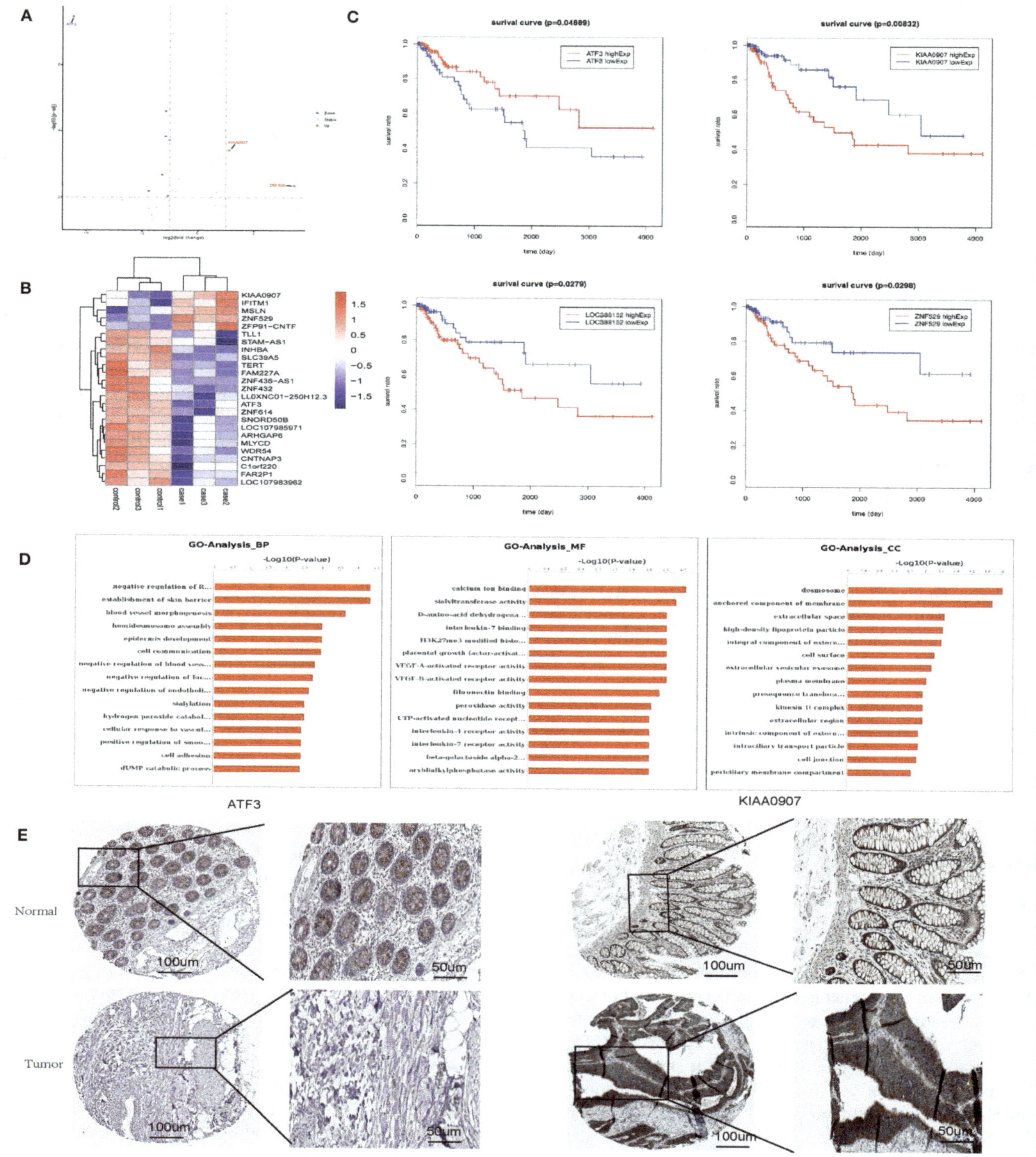

FIGURE 6 | Transcriptomics and biochemical analysis revealed the putative mechanism for the impact of senescent fibroblasts on CRC. **(A)** Volcano map and **(B)** heat map analyses were performed to identify genes that were differentially expressed between LV-GALC and LV-NC fibroblast cells co-cultured with LoVo cells. **(C)** Survival analysis of ATF3, KIAA0907, LOC388152, and ZNF529 using datasets from the TCGA database. **(D)** Gene ontology pathway enrichment analysis suggested that co-culture LV-GALC fibroblasts with LoVo led to the activation of several pathways. **(E)** The expression of ATF3 and KIAA0907 in CRC and normal colon tissue by IHC [data from The Human Protein Atlas (www.proteinatlas.org)]. $p < 0.05$ was considered statistically significant.

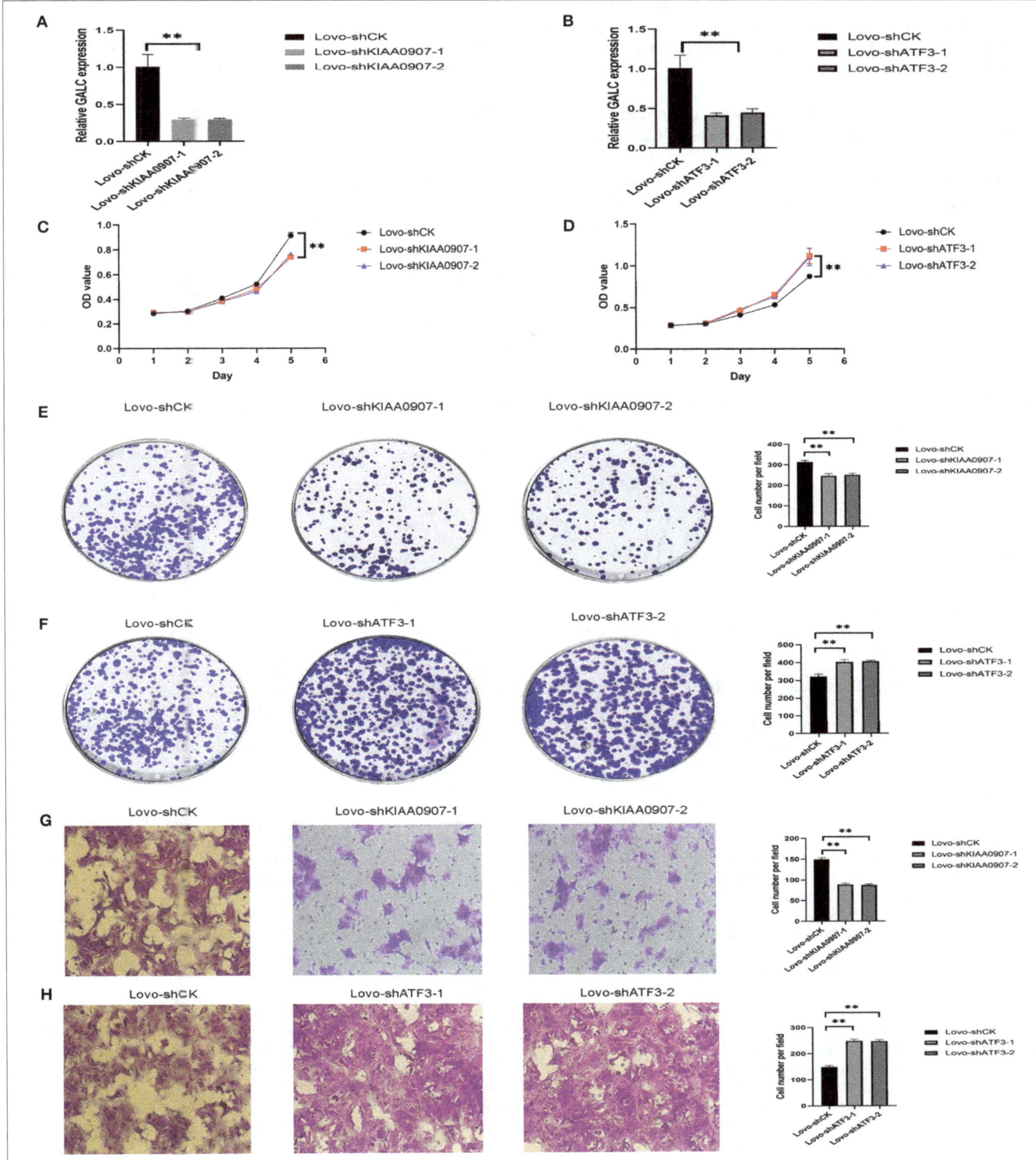

FIGURE 7 | ATF3 and KIAA0907 are closely related to tumorigenesis and metastasis. Knockdown efficiency of KIAA0907 **(A)** and ATF3 **(B)**. CCK8 assays showed the cell proliferation after Knockdown KIAA0907 **(C)** and ATF3 **(D).** Colony formation assays showed the proliferation after Knockdown KIAA0907 **(E)** and ATF3 **(F).** Transwell assay revealed the cell migration after Knockdown KIAA0907 **(G)** and ATF3 **(H)**.

behavior and also indicate the potential mechanisms. Taken together, these results showed that senescent fibroblasts regulate the tumorigenicity of CRC cells and play important roles in tumor biology.

Herein, we demonstrated that senescent fibroblasts regulated several aspects of the survival and metastasis of CRC. Targeting these processes may improve the efficacy of clinical treatment. New therapeutic strategies should be developed based on our understanding of the regulatory roles of the TME in CRC.

ETHICS STATEMENT

The studies involving human participants were reviewed and approved by The present study was reviewed and approved by the Ethics Committee of Shanghai Jiao Tong University Affiliated Sixth People's Hospital (2017-037). The patients/participants provided their written informed consent to participate in this study. The animal study was reviewed and approved by the Animal Ethics Committee of Shanghai Jiao Tong University Affiliated Sixth People's Hospital and all animal experiments were performed under a protocol approved by the Committee (2016-0137).

AUTHOR CONTRIBUTIONS

MY: data curation, project administration, management, coordination responsibility for the research activity planning and execution and writing. ZJ: methodology, application of statistical, mathematical, and computational. GY: collected clinical samples and investigation. ZW: validation experiments and other research outputs. JS: provision of study materials, patients, laboratory samples, and instrumentation tools. HQ and HZ: formulation of overarching research goals and aims, supervision.

ACKNOWLEDGMENTS

We thank all individuals who participated in this work.

REFERENCES

1. Bray F, Ferlay J, Soerjomataram I, Siegel RL, Torre LA, Jemal A. Global cancer statistics 2018: GLOBOCAN estimates of incidence and mortality worldwide for 36 cancers in 185 countries. *CA Cancer J Clin.* (2018) 68:394–424. doi: 10.3322/caac.21492
2. Siegel RL, Miller KD, Jemal A. Cancer statistics, 2018. *CA Cancer J Clin.* (2018) 68:7–30. doi: 10.3322/caac.21442
3. Siravegna G, Mussolin B, Buscarino M, Corti G, Cassingena A, Crisafulli G, et al. Clonal evolution and resistance to EGFR blockade in the blood of colorectal cancer patients. *Nat Med.* (2015) 21:795–801. doi: 10.1038/nm.3870
4. Punt CJ, Koopman M, Vermeulen L. From tumour heterogeneity to advances in precision treatment of colorectal cancer. *Nat Rev Clin Oncol.* (2017) 14:235. doi: 10.1038/nrclinonc.2016.171
5. Alspach E, Flanagan KC, Luo X, Ruhland MK, Huang H, Pazolli E, et al. p38MAPK plays a crucial role in stromal-mediated tumorigenesis. *Cancer Discov.* (2014) 4:716–29. doi: 10.1158/2159-8290.CD-13-0743
6. Schubeler D. Function and information content of DNA methylation. *Nature.* (2015) 517:321–6. doi: 10.1038/nature14192
7. Bhowmick NA, Neilson EG, Moses HL. Stromal fibroblasts in cancer initiation and progression. *Nature.* (2004) 432:332–337. doi: 10.1038/nature03096
8. Kim E, Rebecca V, Fedorenko IV, Messina JL, Mathew R, Maria-Engler SS, et al. Senescent fibroblasts in melanoma initiation and progression: an integrated theoretical, experimental, and clinical approach. *Cancer Res.* (2013) 73:6874–85. doi: 10.1158/0008-5472.CAN-13-1720
9. Coppe JP, Desprez PY, Krtolica A, Campisi J. The senescence-associated secretory phenotype: the dark side of tumor suppression. *Annu Rev Pathol.* (2010) 5:99–118. doi: 10.1146/annurev-pathol-121808-102144
10. Wang H, Tian L, Goldstein A, Liu J, Lo HC, Sheng K, et al. Bone-in-culture array as a platform to model early-stage bone metastases and discover anti-metastasis therapies. *Nat Commun.* (2017) 8:15045. doi: 10.1038/ncomms15045
11. Ohtani N, Hara E. Roles and mechanisms of cellular senescence in regulation of tissue homeostasis. *Cancer Sci.* (2013) 104:525–30. doi: 10.1111/cas.12118
12. Jayatilaka H, Tyle P, Chen JJ, Kwak M, Ju J, Kim HJ, et al. Synergistic IL-6 and IL-8 paracrine signalling pathway infers a strategy to inhibit tumour cell migration. *Nat Commun.* (2017) 8:15584. doi: 10.1038/ncomms15584
13. Gorgoulis V, Adams PD, Alimonti A, Bennett DC, Bischof O, Bishop C, et al. Cellular senescence: defining a path forward. *Cell.* (2019) 179:813–27. doi: 10.1016/j.cell.2019.10.005
14. Taddei ML, Cavallini L, Comito G, Giannoni E, Folini M, Marini A, et al. Senescent stroma promotes prostate cancer progression: the role of miR-210. *Mol Oncol.* (2014) 8:1729–46. doi: 10.1016/j.molonc.2014.07.009
15. Campisi J, Robert L. Cell senescence: role in aging and age-related diseases. *Interdiscip Top Gerontol.* (2014) 39:45–61. doi: 10.1159/000358899
16. Dimri GP, Lee X, Basile G, Acosta M, Scott G, Roskelley C, et al. A biomarker that identifies senescent human cells in culture and in aging skin *in vivo*. *Proc Natl Acad Sci USA.* (1995) 92:9363–7. doi: 10.1073/pnas.92.20.9363
17. Visigalli I, Ungari S, Martino S, Park H, Cesani M, Gentner B, et al. The galactocerebrosidase enzyme contributes to the maintenance of a functional hematopoietic stem cell niche. *Blood.* (2010) 116:1857–66. doi: 10.1182/blood-2009-12-256461
18. Loupakis F, Cremolini C, Masi G, Lonardi S, Zagonel V, Salvatore L, et al. Initial therapy with FOLFOXIRI and bevacizumab for metastatic colorectal cancer. *N Engl J Med.* (2014) 371:1609–18. doi: 10.1056/NEJMoa1403108
19. Grothey A, Van Cutsem E, Sobrero A, Siena S, Falcone A, Ychou M, et al. Regorafenib monotherapy for previously treated metastatic colorectal cancer (CORRECT): an international, multicentre, randomised, placebo-controlled, phase 3 trial. *Lancet.* (2013) 381:303–12. doi: 10.1016/S0140-6736(12)61900-X
20. Calon A, Lonardo E, Berenguer-Llergo A, Espinet E, Hernando-Momblona X, Iglesias M, et al. Stromal gene expression defines poor-prognosis subtypes in colorectal cancer. *Nat Genet.* (2015) 47:320–9. doi: 10.1038/ng.3225
21. Mesker WE, Junggeburt JM, Szuhai K, de Heer P, Morreau H, Tanke HJ, et al. The carcinoma-stromal ratio of colon carcinoma is an independent factor for survival compared to lymph node status and tumor stage. *Cell Oncol.* (2007) 29:387–98. doi: 10.1155/2007/175276
22. Yang M, Sun Y, Sun J, Wang Z, Zhou Y, Yao G, et al. Differentially expressed and survival-related proteins of lung adenocarcinoma with bone metastasis. *Cancer Med.* (2018) 7:1081–92. doi: 10.1002/cam4.1363
23. Fromowitz FB, Viola MV, Chao S, Oravez S, Mishriki Y, Finkel G, et al. ras p21 expression in the progression of breast cancer. *Hum Pathol.* (1987) 18:1268–75. doi: 10.1016/S0046-8177(87)80412-4
24. Gu K, Xu Y, Li H, Guo Z, Zhu S, Zhu S, et al. Real-time tracking and *in vivo* visualization of beta-galactosidase activity in colorectal tumor with a ratiometric near-infrared fluorescent probe. *J Am Chem Soc.* (2016) 138:5334–40. doi: 10.1021/jacs.6b01705

25. Wolf AMD, Fontham ETH, Church TR, Flowers CR, Guerra CE, LaMonte SJ, et al. Colorectal cancer screening for average-risk adults: 2018 guideline update from the American Cancer Society. *CA Cancer J Clin.* (2018) 68:250–81. doi: 10.3322/caac.21457
26. Siriwardena AK, Mason JM, Mullamitha S, Hancock HC, Jegatheeswaran S. Management of colorectal cancer presenting with synchronous liver metastases. *Nat Rev. Clin Oncol.* (2014) 11:446–59. doi: 10.1038/nrclinonc.2014.90
27. Lu J, Ye X, Fan F, Xia L, Bhattacharya R, Bellister S, et al. Endothelial cells promote the colorectal cancer stem cell phenotype through a soluble form of Jagged-1. *Cancer Cell.* (2013) 23:171–85. doi: 10.1016/j.ccr.2012.12.021
28. Narita M, Narita M, Krizhanovsky V, Nunez S, Chicas A, Hearn SA, et al. A novel role for high-mobility group a proteins in cellular senescence and heterochromatin formation. *Cell.* (2006) 126:503–14. doi: 10.1016/j.cell.2006.05.052
29. De Castro J, Garcia R, Garrido P, Isla D, Massuti B, Blanca B, et al. Therapeutic potential of denosumab in patients with lung cancer: beyond prevention of skeletal complications. *Clin Lung Cancer.* (2015) 16:431–46. doi: 10.1016/j.cllc.2015.06.004
30. Fane M, Weeraratna AT. How the ageing microenvironment influences tumour progression. *Nat Rev Cancer.* (2020) 20:89–106. doi: 10.1038/s41568-019-0222-9
31. Agrawal K, Das V, Taborska N, Gursky J, Dzubak P, Hajduch M. Differential regulation of methylation-regulating enzymes by senescent stromal cells drives colorectal cancer cell response to DNA-demethylating Epi-drugs. *Stem Cells Int.* (2018) 2018:6013728. doi: 10.1155/2018/6013728
32. Krtolica A, Parrinello S, Lockett S, Desprez PY, Campisi J. Senescent fibroblasts promote epithelial cell growth and tumorigenesis: a link between cancer and aging. *Proc Natl Acad Sci USA.* (2001) 98:12072–7. doi: 10.1073/pnas.211053698
33. Yang F, Yi M, Liu Y, Wang Q, Hu Y, Deng H. Glutaredoxin-1 silencing induces cell senescence via p53/p21/p16 signaling axis. *J Proteome Res.* (2018) 17:1091–100. doi: 10.1021/acs.jproteome.7b00761
34. Wang Z, Gerstein M, Snyder M. RNA-Seq: a revolutionary tool for transcriptomics. *Nat Rev Genet.* (2009) 10:57–63. doi: 10.1038/nrg2484
35. Dijkstra KK, Voabil P, Schumacher TN, Voest EE. Genomics- and transcriptomics-based patient selection for cancer treatment with immune checkpoint inhibitors: a review. *JAMA Oncol.* (2016) 2:1490–5. doi: 10.1001/jamaoncol.2016.2214

12

Long-Term Outcomes Comparison of Endoscopic Resection with Gastrectomy for Treatment of Early Gastric Cancer

Liangliang An [1†], *Sharen Gaowa* [2†], *Haidong Cheng* [1*] *and Mingxing Hou* [1*]

[1] *Department of General Surgery, Affiliated Hospital of Inner Mongolia Medical University, Hohhot, China,*
[2] *Department of Pathology, College of Basic Medicine, Inner Mongolia Medical University, Hohhot, China*

***Correspondence:**
Haidong Cheng
chenghaidongbj@163.com
Mingxing Hou
houmingxingnmghhht@163.com

† *These authors have contributed equally to this work*

Background: Endoscopic resection (ER) and gastrectomy have been both accepted as curative treatments for early gastric cancer. We intended to compare ER with gastrectomy treatments on safety of patients, disease-free survival and overall survival for early gastric cancer through this systematic review.

Methods: A literature search was performed in Pubmed, Embase, and Cochrane Library databases. Studies that have compared ER with gastrectomy for early gastric cancer were included in this meta-analysis. We searched for clinical studies published before March 2019. Stata 12.0 software was used for systematic analysis.

Results: Nine studies were included in this systematic review, ER treatment was associated with a shorter length of stay (WMD = −8.53, 95% CI −11.56 to −5.49), fewer postoperative complications (OR = 0.47, 95% CI 0.34–0.65). ER can be performed safely with shorter hospital stay and fewer postoperative complications than gastrectomy. Recurrence rate was higher for ER than for gastrectomy treatment (HR = 3.56, 95% CI 1.86–6.84), mainly because metachronous gastric cancers developed only in the ER treatment. However, most of the metachronous gastric cancers could be curatively treated with ER again, and it didn't affect overall survival of patients with early gastric cancer. There was no difference in overall survival rate between ER and gastrectomy (HR = 0.84, 95% CI 0.63–1.13).

Conclusions: ER and gastrectomy are both acceptable for curative treatment of early gastric cancer. However, due to the comparable overall survival and lower postoperative complications and shorter length of stay, ER is better than gastrectomy for early gastric cancer, who met the indication for ER treatment.

Keywords: endoscopic resection, gastrectomy, recurrence, overall survival, systematic review

INTRODUCTION

Gastric cancer is one of the most gastrointestinal tract tumors worldwide (1, 2). Even if the incidence of gastric cancer has been declining in the world, it remains one of the most causes of cancer-related mortality in China (3–5). For minimal invasive surgery, the Japanese Gastric Cancer Association's gastric cancer treatment guide lines recommended endoscopic resection (ER) for early gastric cancer (6). ER includes endoscopic mucosal resection (EMR) and endoscopic submucosal dissection (ESD). And, ER is an effective treatment for gastric cancer, but the clinical outcomes of ER in treatment of gastric cancer were controversial (7).

As we know, there were no multi-center studies, which compared the survival benefit between ER and gastrectomy treatments. Only several single-center studies have compared ER with gastrectomy in early gastric cancer (6, 8–15). However, the results of studies were inconsistent. Systematic review and meta-analysis was a powerful and effective method, which could overcome the limitation of small sample sizes of study through combining results from several individual studies, then conduct and achieve a systematic assessment (16). Although, studies comparing ER and gastrectomy in early gastric cancer were most retrospective studies, there is evidence that pooling of high-quality non-randomized comparative studies (NRCTs) is as comparable as pooling randomized comparative studies (RCTs) when assessing clinical surgical outcomes (17). Therefore, we systematically analyzed high-quality clinical researches that have compared ER with gastrectomy in this study and conducted systematic review of combined NRCTs.

The aim of the study was to compare long-term outcomes of ER and gastrectomy treatments for early gastric cancer, and explore whether ER is superior to gastrectomy in early gastric cancer, and we systematically compared length of stay, postoperative complications, disease-free survival and overall survival between ER with gastrectomy treatments in early gastric cancer.

METHODS

Search Strategy

We conducted and reported this systematic review and meta-analysis following the PRISMA statement (18). The retrieval words are "early gastric cancer," "early stomach cancer," "early stomach neoplasm," "ESD," "EMR," "endoscopic resection," and "gastrectomy." A search was performed in Pubmed, Embase, and Cochrane Library databases. The studies that have compared ER with gastrectomy for early gastric cancer were included in this meta-analysis. We searched for clinical studies published before March 2019. Meanwhile, we tried to find relevant literature through references of clinical studies. Then we read the full text and determine the eligible studies. Finally, a total of nine studies were included in the analysis.

Include and Exclude Standards

Studies were acceptable in systematic review if they met these standards: Research compared the outcomes of ER and gastrectomy; Research reported at least one of the following clinical outcomes, including length of stay, postoperative

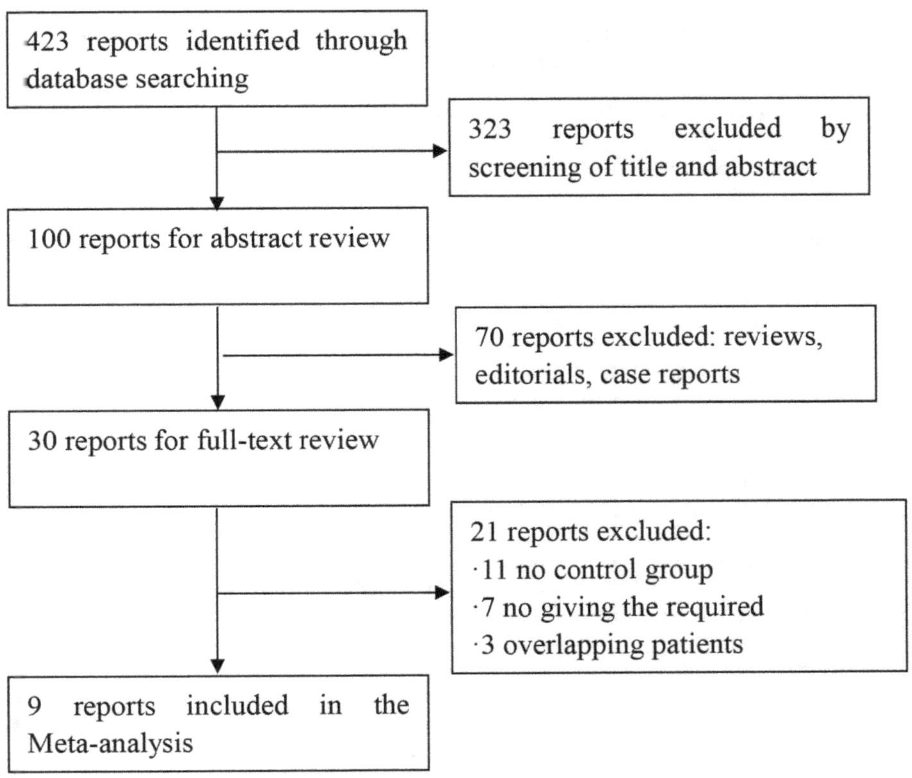

FIGURE 1 | Flow chart for article screening.

complications, disease-free survival and overall survival; Research was published as a full text in the English language. Research that failed to extract effective data or provide the full text was excluded.

The inclusion criteria of patients: who were newly diagnosed as early gastric cancer, histologically confirmed adenocarcinoma limited to the mucosa or submucosa (TNM stage 0-IIIB), and received gastrectomy or ER for treatment. The exclusion criteria of patients: who had undergone previous gastrectomy. Postoperative pathological evaluation was performed in all included studies. A clear surgical margin was confirmed through pathological evaluation. If a clear surgical margin was not achieved in patients, these patients needed additional ER or gastrectomy. And, patients needed additional gastrectomy were excluded from the study.

Data Extraction

Two reviewers (Liangliang An, Haidong Cheng) extracted the data of included studies independently and reached consensus on all data. The following data was extracted: authors' name, year of publication, study location, number of patients, length of stay, postoperative complications, disease-free survival and overall survival. HR and 95% CI were used to calculate the disease-free survival and overall survival. Some of the studies included in this meta-analysis provided HR and 95% CI explicitly. If HR and 95% CI were not directly reported in the included studies, we evaluated the HR and 95% CI in the original studies by the methods which illustrated by Parmar et al. (19). Moreover, if the original studies included the median, range and the number of patients, we estimated the mean and variance by the methods illustrated by Hozo et al. (20).

Assessment of Quality of Included Studies

Quality assessment was peer-reviewed by two reviewers (Liangliang An, Haidong Cheng) independently. Quality scores of the included clinical studies were assessed by the Methodological Index for Nonrandomized Studies (MINORS) (21). We assessed the quality of a study by evaluating 12 items. Studies with $\geq$18 scores were considered high quality, and were included in the systematic review.

Statistical Analysis

Systematic review was performed by using statistical Stata 12.0 software (StatCorp, College Station, TX, USA) (22, 23). The test for heterogeneity used the Q-test statistic and I^2 statistics. Based on the combined test for heterogeneity, we chose the appropriate method. If there is no heterogeneity among studies ($P \geq 0.1$), we used the fixed effects model for data consolidation. While there is the heterogeneity ($P < 0.1$) between the results of the study, the random effects model for data

TABLE 1 | Characteristics of studies included in the meta-analysis.

Study	Year	Type of study	Study period	ER indication	ER	Group	Number	Age	Gender
Tsuyoshi Etoh	2005	Retrospective study	1085–1999	Absolute indication	EMR(49)	ER Gastrectomy	49 44	84.2 82.2	27/17 31/18
Kwi-Sook Choi	2011	Retrospective analysis with propensity-score matching	1997–2002	Intramucosal gastric cancer	EMR(172)	ER Gastrectomy	172 379	59.3 (9.1) 58.4 (10.3)	127/45 286/93
Philip Chiu	2012	Retrospective cohort study	1993–2010	Mucosal or submucosal involvement	ESD(74)	ER Gastrectomy	74 40	66 (14–88) 67 (33–84)	49/25 23/17
Dae Yong Kim	2014	Retrospective study	2004–2007	Absolute criteria(35) Expanded criteria(107)	ESD(142)	ER Gastrectomy	142 71	62.0 (10.3) 56.7 (12.0)	94/48 58/13
Takeshi Yamashina	2014	Retrospective study	1998–2012	Mucosal or submucosal involvement	EMR(27) ESD(15)	ER Gastrectomy	42 13	71.5 (54–89) 69 (39–76)	40/2 12/1
Ju Choi	2014	Retrospective cohort study	2002–2007	Absolute indication	EMR(86) ESD(175)	ER Gastrectomy	261 114	62 (54–68) 62 (54–66)	195/66 88/26
Chan Park	2014	Retrospectively analyzed the clinical data	2007–2012	Expanded indication	ESD(307)	ER Gastrectomy	307 200	74.5 (3.8) 74.1 (3.5)	211/96 133/67
Young Kim	2014	Prospectively collected clinical data	2001–2009	Expanded indication	EMR(18) ESD(147)	ER Gastrectomy	165 292	62 (54–70) 60 (52–68)	122/43 217/75
Sara Najmeh	2016	Prospectively collected database	2007–2014	Expanded indication	ESD(30)	ER Gastrectomy	30 37	74 (40–86) 75 (34–86)	23/7 24/13

analysis would be used. We also explored reasons for inter-study heterogeneity using subgroup analysis by the indication for ER treatment and the endoscopic procedure EMR or ESD. Sensitivity analysis was also conducted by omission of each single study to evaluate stability of the results. Publication bias was evaluated with the Begg's test. A *P*-value of < 0.05 was regarded as significant.

RESULTS

Study Selection and Quality Assessment

Four hundred twenty-three potential articles were generated through our search strategy. After screening the title and abstract, 323 reports were excluded. After reading the research, 70 reports were excluded because they were a review, editorial, or case report. After reading the full text, 11 reports were excluded because there was no control group. Seven were excluded for no giving the required outcomes. Three reports were excluded owing to overlapping patients in multiple studies. The process of our study selection was shown in **Figure 1**. Nine articles, which were considered to be of high quality, were enrolled in the study. The main characteristics and quality scores of studies are presented in **Tables 1, 2**.

TABLE 2 | Quality scores of the included clinical studies were assessed by the Methodological Index for Nonrandomized Studies (MINORS).

Study	A	B	C	D	E	F	G	H	I	J	K	L	Quality scores
Tsuyoshi Etoh	2	2	1	2	2	2	2	0	2	2	2	1	20
Kwi-Sook Choi	2	2	0	2	1	2	1	0	2	2	2	2	18
Philip Chiu	2	2	1	2	2	2	2	0	2	2	2	2	21
Dae Yong Kim	2	2	1	2	1	2	2	0	2	2	2	1	19
Takeshi Yamashina	2	2	0	2	1	2	2	0	2	2	2	2	19
Ju Choi	2	2	1	2	1	1	2	0	2	2	2	1	18
Chan Park	2	2	2	2	2	2	2	0	2	2	2	2	22
Young Kim	2	2	2	2	1	2	2	1	2	2	2	2	22
Sara Najmeh	2	2	0	2	1	2	2	0	2	2	2	1	18

A, Clearly stated aim; B, Inclusion of consecutive patients; C, Prospective collection of data; D, Endpoints appropriate to the aim of the study; E, Unbiased assessment of the study endpoint; F, Follow-up period appropriate to the aim of the study; G, Loss to follow up <5%; H, Prospective calculation of the study size; I, An adequate control group; J, Contemporary groups; K, Baseline equivalence of groups; L, Adequate statistical analyses. The items are scored 0 (not reported), 1 (reported but inadequate), or 2 (reported and adequate).

Length of Stay

As show in **Figure 2**, five studies reported data on the length of stay. Because of significant heterogeneity ($I^2 = 91.2\%$, $P = 0.000$), a random-effect model was used. There was significant difference in length of stay between the ER and gastrectomy treatment for early gastric cancer. ER treatment was associated with shorter length of stay than gastrectomy treatment (WMD = −8.53, 95% CI −11.56 to −5.49). In the subgroup of expanded indication, the difference of length of stay between ER and gastrectomy was also statistically significant (WMD = −6.2, 95% CI −9.45 to −2.94; **Figure 3**). In the subgroup of ESD, there was also a significant difference in length of stay (WMD = −5.63, 95% CI −7.05 to −4.21; **Figure 4**).

Postoperative Complications

As show in **Figure 5**, all nine researches included postoperative complications. There was no significant heterogeneity ($I^2 = 46.9\%$, $P = 0.058$), and a fixed-effect model was used. The incidence of postoperative complications of gastrectomy treatment were higher than that of ER treatment (OR = 0.47, 95% CI 0.34–0.65). In the subgroup of expanded indication and ESD, there was also a significant difference in complications (**Figures 3, 4**).

Disease-Free Survival

In this meta-analysis, five studies included the disease-free survival. Because of no significant heterogeneity ($I^2 = 45.1\%$, $P = 0.122$), a fixed-effect model was used. Patients who underwent ER treatment had higher recurrence rate than that of gastrectomy treatment (HR = 3.56, 95% CI 1.86–6.84; **Figure 6**). The results demonstrated that the recurrence rate of ER treatment was significantly higher than that of gastrectomy treatment. This was most likely because of residual gastric mucosa, which may contain areas at high risk of the development of metachronous gastric cancer. Additional

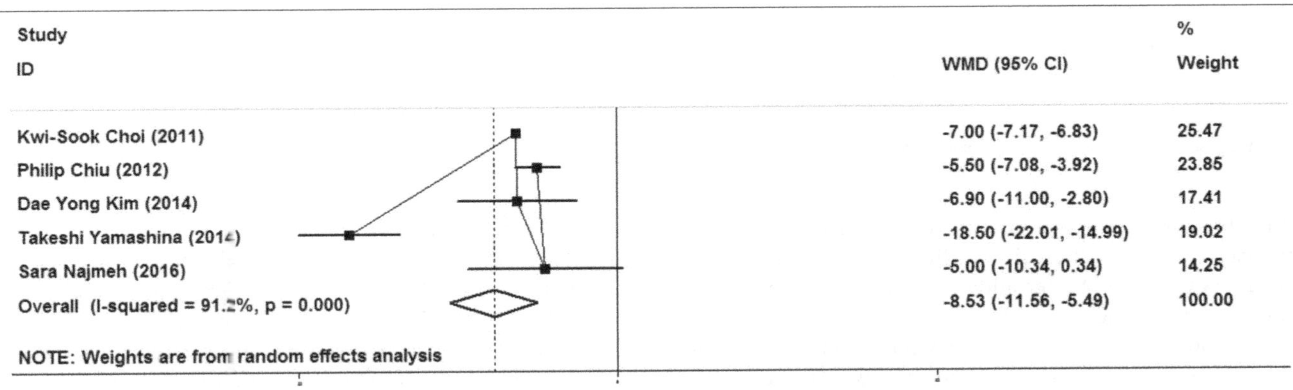

FIGURE 2 | Meta-analysis on length of stay, there was significant difference in length of stay between the ER and gastrectomy treatments.

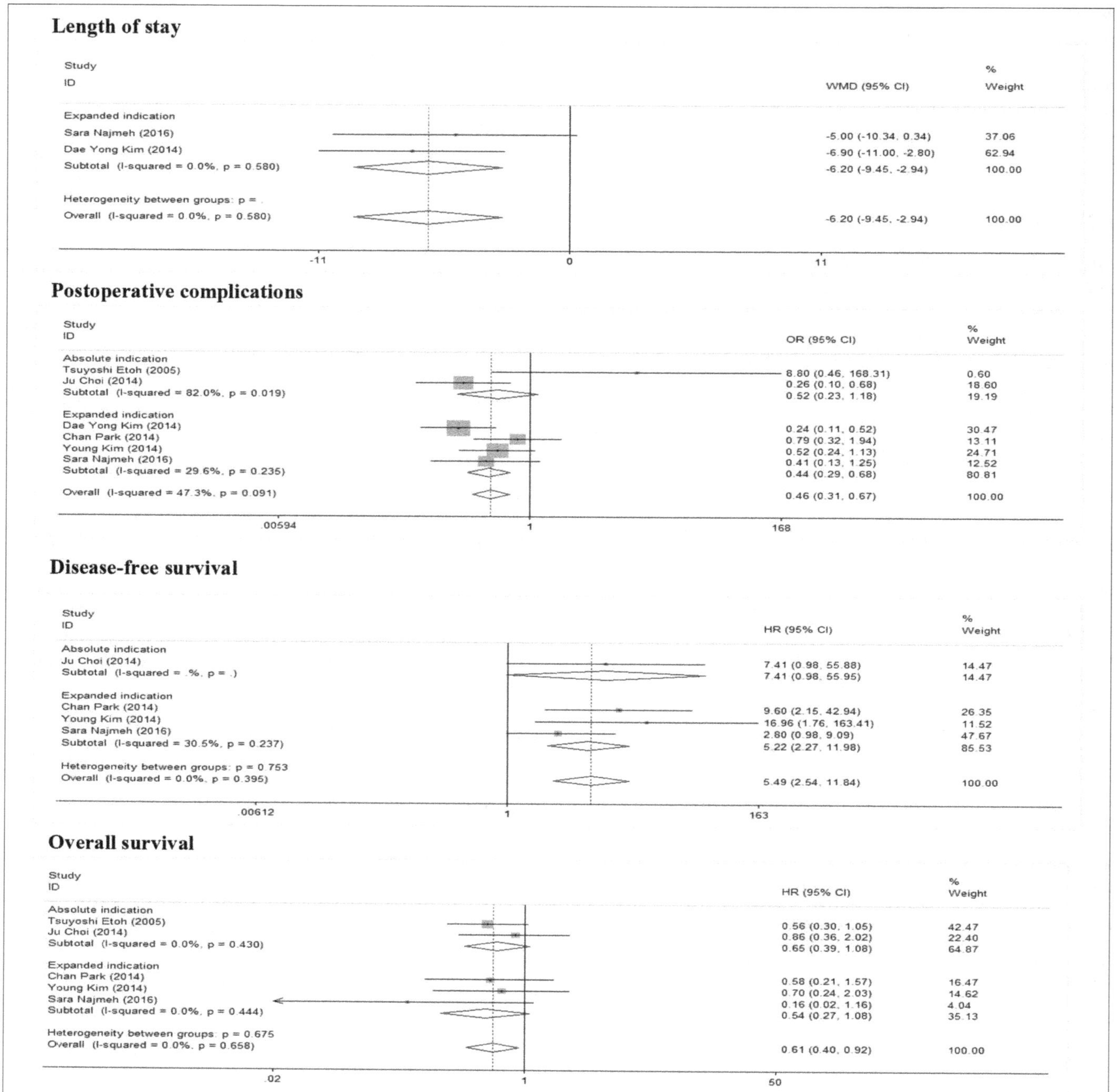

FIGURE 3 | Subgroup meta-analysis of indication for ER treatment.

treatments for recurrence lesions should be considered in early gastric cancer patients after ER, but the current studies did not show any adverse event after additional endoscopic treatments for metachronous lesions, and the overall survival of early gastric cancer was no significant difference between ER and gastrectomy. In the subgroup of expanded indication and ESD, there was also a significant difference in disease-free survival between ER and gastrectomy (**Figures 3, 4**).

Overall Survival

As show in **Figure 7**, the data of overall survival was reported in eight studies. Because of no significant heterogeneity ($I^2 = 26.5\%$, $P = 0.217$), a fixed-effect model was used. Overall survival did not differ between ER and gastrectomy treatment (HR = 0.84, 95% CI 0.63–1.13). In the subgroup analysis, there was also no significant difference in overall survival (**Figures 3, 4**).

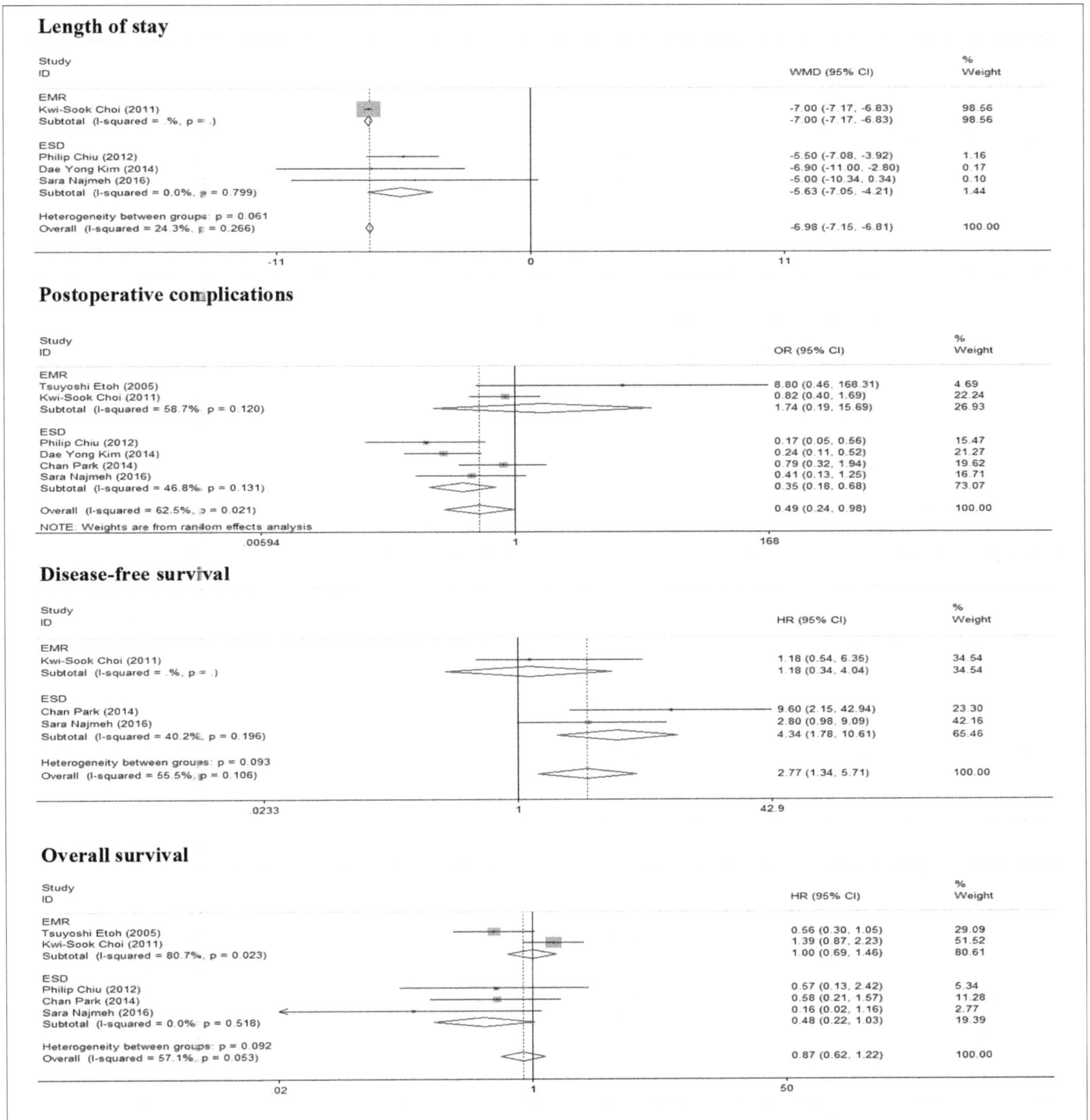

FIGURE 4 | Subgroup meta-analysis of ER procedure.

Publication Bias

Publication bias was evaluated based on postoperative complications by using Begg's test. There was no publication bias in nine studies of this meta-analysis ($P = 0.835$). Funnel plot analysis of the studies is shown in **Figure 8**. Sensitivity analysis also indicated that omitting any single study did not affect the pooled overall survival HR significantly (**Figure 9**).

DISCUSSION

In recent years, with the development of digestive endoscopic techniques, more and more early gastric cancer in the absence of any symptoms was found (24, 25). Gastrectomy treatment has been conducted as the conventional treatment for early gastric cancer (26). However, in selected early gastric cancer, ER is

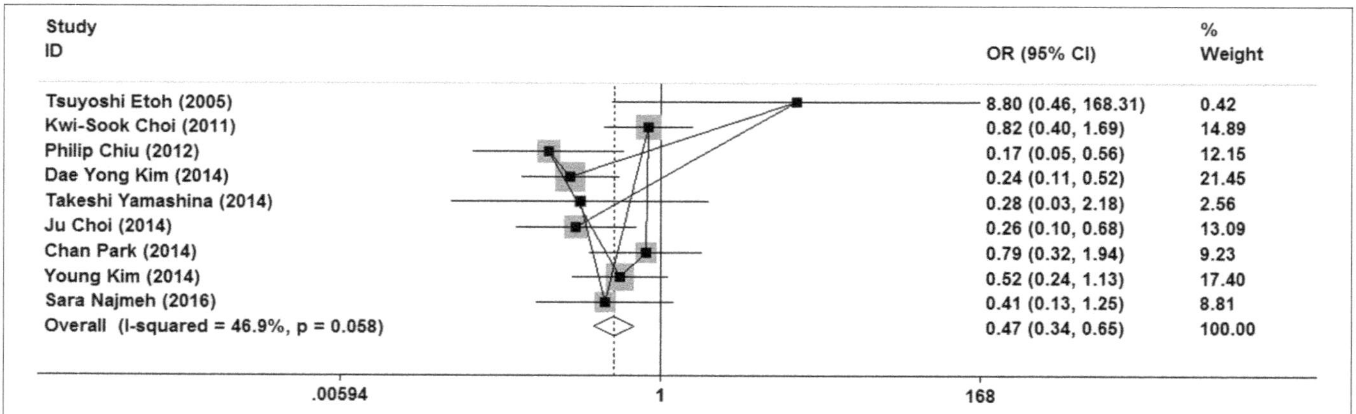

FIGURE 5 | Meta-analysis on postoperative complication, postoperative complications of gastrectomy treatment were higher than that of ER treatment.

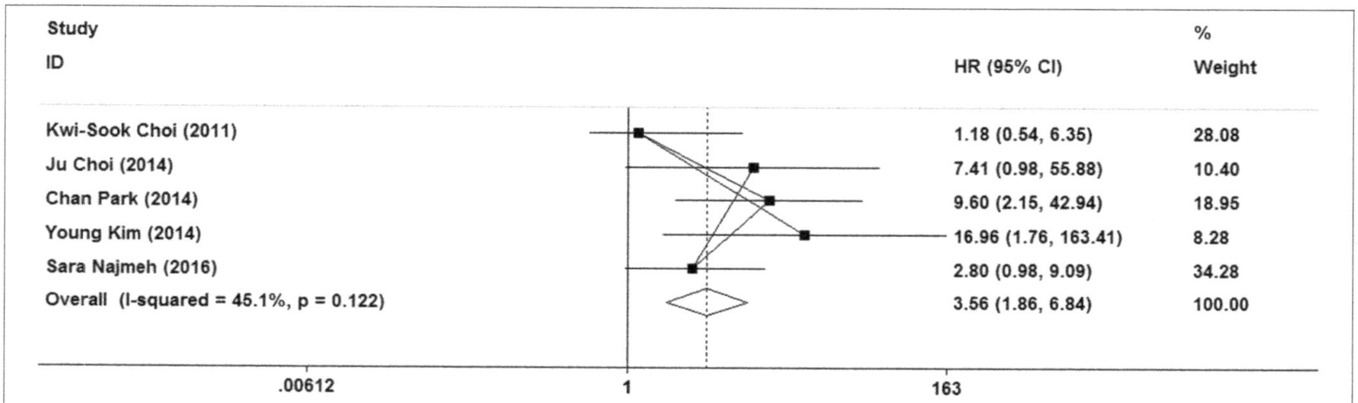

FIGURE 6 | Meta-analysis on disease-free survival, patients who underwent ER treatment had higher recurrence rate than that of gastrectomy treatment.

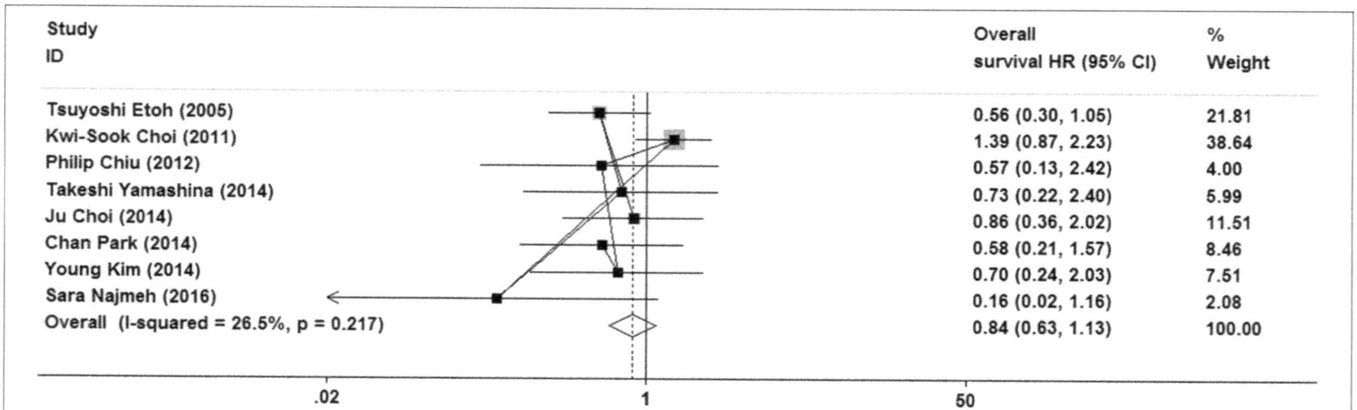

FIGURE 7 | Meta-analysis on overall survival, overall survival did not differ between ER and gastrectomy treatments.

accepted due to its minimal invasiveness and better quality of life after the procedure (27). In recent years, ER has become the minimal treatment for early gastric cancer (28–30).

According to the Japanese gastric cancer treatment guidelines, ER includes EMR and ESD (31). And ER is indicated as a standard treatment for the following tumor: a differentiated-type adenocarcinoma without ulcerative findings UL(−), of which the depth of invasion is clinically diagnosed as T1a and the diameter is ≤2 cm. The expanded indication is that Tumors clinically diagnosed as T1a and: (a) of differentiated-type, UL(−), but >2 cm in diameter. (b) of differentiated-type, UL(+), and ≤3 cm in

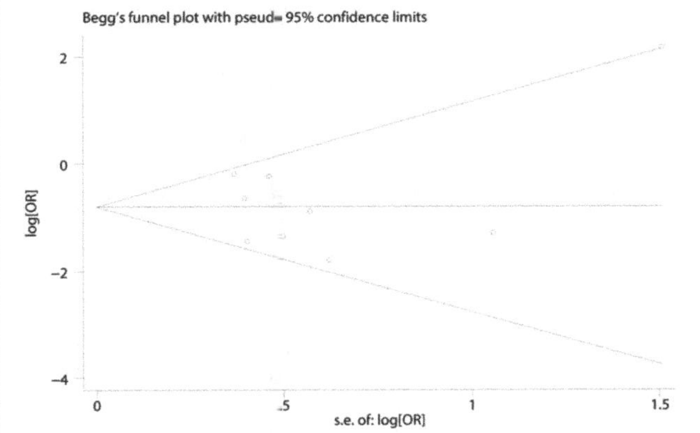

FIGURE 8 | Funnel plot depicting standard error by log relative risk.

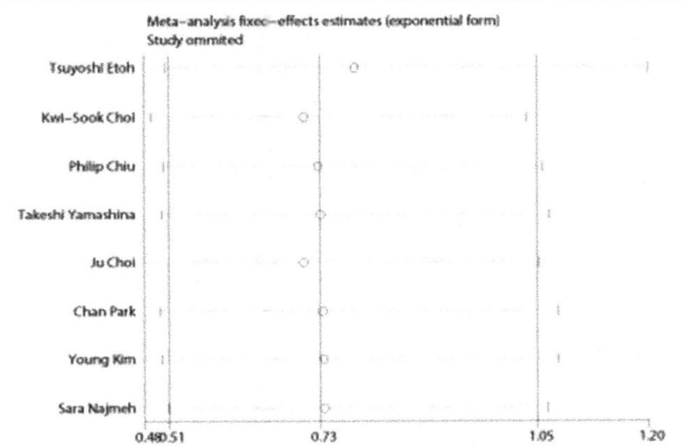

FIGURE 9 | Sensitivity analysis of overall survival.

diameter. (c) of undifferentiated-type, UL(−), and ≤2 cm in diameter.

ER was minimally invasive treatment for early gastric cancer, which met guideline or expanded criteria (32). However, clinical outcomes of ER remain controversial, several recent reports suggest that lymph node metastasis may occur after ER treatment in early gastric cancer (33–35). Therefore, treatment outcomes of ER are still controversial for early gastric cancer (36, 37). This meta-analysis combined results from several individual studies to evaluate the outcomes of ER.

In this meta-analysis, a total of nine studies analyzing the ER and gastrectomy treatment were included. This meta-analysis showed that ER treatment showed some advantages, it had a significantly shorter length of stay, and a lower postoperative complication rates. And there were no significant difference between ER and gastrectomy treatments in the overall survival of early gastric cancer. These results of length of stay, postoperative complications, and overall survival were consistent with those of other meta-analyses (38, 39).

There was much evidence to show that the recurrence rate of ER treatment was significantly higher than that of gastrectomy treatment, and the recurrence rates of ER was 4.7–11.1%, and the recurrence rates of gastrectomy was 0.0–1.1%. In this results, the risk of tumor recurrence was significantly higher in the ER group than in the surgery group. This was most likely because of residual gastric mucosa, which may contain areas at high risk of the development of metachronous gastric cancer, such as mucosa with atrophic gastritis and intestinal metaplasia (40). Additional treatments for recurrence lesions should be considered in early gastric cancer patients after ER, but the current studies did not show any adverse event after additional endoscopic treatments for metachronous lesions, and the overall survival of early gastric cancer was no significant difference between ER and gastrectomy treatment. And, metachronous gastric cancer did not affect overall survival (6, 11, 15).

There are some limitations of this meta-analysis. The approach of extrapolating the HR of overall survival was a potential factor might lead to heterogeneity of outcomes. Moreover, this meta-analysis only included fully published studies. Unpublished researches were not included in meta-analysis. In addition, this study was searched with language restriction, so this analysis only included studies in English.

In conclusion, ER and gastrectomy are both acceptable for curative treatments of early gastric cancer. However, ER is better than gastrectomy for early gastric cancer, who met the indication for ER treatment, due to the comparable overall survival and lower postoperative complications and shorter hospital stay.

AUTHOR CONTRIBUTIONS

LA and SG: development of methodology. SG and HC: acquisition of data (acquired and managed patients, provided facilities, etc.). LA, SG, and HC: analysis and interpretation of data (e.g., statistical analysis, computational analysis). HC and MH: writing, review, and/or revision of the manuscript. MH: study supervision.

REFERENCES

1. Kamangar F, Dores GM, Anderson WF. Patterns of cancer incidence, mortality, and prevalence across five continents: defining priorities to reduce cancer disparities in different geographic regions of the world. *J Clin Oncol.* (2006) 24:2137–50. doi: 10.1200/JCO.2005.05.2308
2. Ferlay J, Steliarova-Foucher E, Lortet-Tieulent J, Rosso S, Coebergh JW, Comber H, et al. Cancer incidence and mortality patterns in Europe: estimates for 40 countries in 2012. *Eur J Cancer.* (2013) 49:1374–403. doi: 10.1016/j.ejca.2012.12.027
3. Kelley JR, Duggan JM. Gastric cancer epidemiology and risk factors. *J Clin Epidemiol.* (2003) 56:1–9. doi: 10.1016/S0895-4356(02)00534-6

4. Parkin DM. International variation. *Oncogene.* (2004) 23:6329–40. doi: 10.1038/sj.onc.1207726
5. Ferlay J, Shin HR, Bray F, Forman D, Mathers C, Parkin DM. Estimates of worldwide burden of cancer in 2008: GLOBOCAN 2008. *Int J Cancer.* (2010) 127:2893–917. doi: 10.1002/ijc.25516
6. Choi KS, Jung HY, Choi KD, Lee GH, Song HJ, Kim DH, et al. EMR versus gastrectomy for intramucosal gastric cancer: comparison of long-term outcomes. *Gastrointest Endosc.* (2011) 73:942–8. doi: 10.1016/j.gie.2010.12.032
7. Japanese Gastric Cancer Association. Japanese gastric cancer treatment guidelines 2014 (ver. 4). *Gastric Cancer.* (2017) 20:1–19. doi: 10.1007/s10120-016-0622-4
8. Kim YI, Kim YW, Choi IJ, Kim CG, Lee JY, Cho SJ, et al. Long-term survival after endoscopic resection versus surgery in early gastric cancers. *Endoscopy.* (2015) 47:293–301. doi: 10.1055/s-0034-1391284
9. Choi IJ, Lee JH, Kim YI, Kim CG, Cho SJ, Lee JY, et al. Long-term outcome comparison of endoscopic resection and surgery in early gastric cancer meeting the absolute indication for endoscopic resection. *Gastrointest Endosc.* (2015) 81:333–41.e331. doi: 10.1016/j.gie.2014.07.047
10. Chiu PW, Teoh AY, To KF, Wong SK, Liu SY, Lam CC, et al. Endoscopic submucosal dissection (ESD) compared with gastrectomy for treatment of early gastric neoplasia: a retrospective cohort study. *Surg Endosc.* (2012) 26:3584–91. doi: 10.1007/s00464-012-2371-8
11. Park CH, Lee H, Kim DW, Chung H, Park JC, Shin SK, et al. Clinical safety of endoscopic submucosal dissection compared with surgery in elderly patients with early gastric cancer: a propensity-matched analysis. *Gastrointest Endosc.* (2014) 80:599–609. doi: 10.1016/j.gie.2014.04.042
12. Kim DY, Hong SJ, Cho GS, Jeong GA, Kim HK, Han JP, et al. Long-term efficacy of endoscopic submucosal dissection compared with surgery for early gastric cancer: a retrospective cohort study. *Gut Liver.* (2014) 8:519–25. doi: 10.5009/gnl13061
13. Yamashina T, Uedo N, Dainaka K, Aoi K, Matsuura N, Ito T, et al. Long-term survival after endoscopic resection for early gastric cancer in the remnant stomach: comparison with radical surgery. *Ann Gastroenterol.* (2015) 28:66–71.
14. Etoh T, Katai H, Fukagawa T, Sano T, Oda I, Gotoda T, et al. Treatment of early gastric cancer in the elderly patient: results of EMR and gastrectomy at a national referral center in Japan. *Gastrointest Endosc.* (2005) 62:868–71. doi: 10.1016/j.gie.2005.09.012
15. Najmeh S, Cools-Lartigue J, Mueller C, Ferri LE. Comparing laparoscopic to endoscopic resections for early gastric cancer in a high volume North American Center. *J Gastrointest Surg.* (2016) 20:1547–53. doi: 10.1007/s11605-016-3176-1
16. Rundhaug JE. Matrix metalloproteinases and angiogenesis. *J Cell Mol Med.* (2005) 9:267–85. doi: 10.1111/j.1582-4934.2005.tb00355.x
17. Abraham NS, Byrne CJ, Young JM, Solomon MJ. Meta-analysis of well-designed nonrandomized comparative studies of surgical procedures is as good as randomized controlled trials. *J Clin Epidemiol.* (2010) 63:238–45. doi: 10.1016/j.jclinepi.2009.04.005
18. Moher D, Liberati A, Tetzlaff J, Altman DG, PRISMA Group. Preferred reporting items for systematic reviews and meta-analyses: the PRISMA statement. *PLoS Med.* (2009) 6:e1000097. doi: 10.1371/journal.pmed.1000097
19. Parmar MK, Torri V, Stewart L. Extracting summary statistics to perform meta-analyses of the published literature for survival endpoints. *Stat Med.* (1998) 17:2815–34. doi: 10.1002/(SICI)1097-0258(19981230)17:24<2815::AID-SIM110>3.0.CO;2-8
20. Hozo SP, Djulbegovic B, Hozo I. Estimating the mean and variance from the median, range, and the size of a sample. *BMC Med Res Methodol.* (2005) 5:13. doi: 10.1186/1471-2288-5-13
21. Slim K, Nini E, Forestier D, Kwiatkowski F, Panis Y, Chipponi J. Methodological index for non-randomized studies (minors): development and validation of a new instrument. *ANZ J Surg.* (2003) 73:712–6. doi: 10.1046/j.1445-2197.2003.02748.x
22. Shen W, Xi H, Zhang K, Cui J, Li J, Wang N, et al. Prognostic role of EphA2 in various human carcinomas: a meta-analysis of 23 related studies. *Growth Factors.* (2014) 32:247–53. doi: 10.3109/08977194.2014.984806
23. Shen WS, Xi HQ, Wei B, Chen L. Effect of gastrectomy with bursectomy on prognosis of gastric cancer: a meta-analysis. *World J Gastroenterol.* (2014) 20:14986–91. doi: 10.3748/wjg.v20.i40.14986
24. Carter KJ, Schaffer HA, Ritchie WP. Early gastric cancer. *Ann Surg.* (1984) 199:604–9. doi: 10.1097/00000658-198405000-00016
25. Waisberg J, Bromberg SH, Franco MI, Stephani SM, Zanotto A, de Godoy AC, et al. The role of surgery in the treatment of primary gastric lymphoma. *Int Surg.* (2000) 85:219–25.
26. Pak KH, Hyung WJ, Son T, Obama K, Woo Y, Kim HI, et al. Long-term oncologic outcomes of 714 consecutive laparoscopic gastrectomies for gastric cancer: results from the 7-year experience of a single institute. *Surg Endosc.* (2012) 26:130–6. doi: 10.1007/s00464-011-1838-3
27. Lian J, Chen S, Zhang Y, Qiu F. A meta-analysis of endoscopic submucosal dissection and EMR for early gastric cancer. *Gastrointest Endosc.* (2012) 76:763–70. doi: 10.1016/j.gie.2012.06.014
28. Lee H, Yun WK, Min BH, Lee JH, Rhee PL, Kim KM, et al. A feasibility study on the expanded indication for endoscopic submucosal dissection of early gastric cancer. *Surg Endosc.* (2011) 25:1985–93. doi: 10.1007/s00464-010-1499-7
29. Park YM, Cho E, Kang HY, Kim JM. The effectiveness and safety of endoscopic submucosal dissection compared with endoscopic mucosal resection for early gastric cancer: a systematic review and metaanalysis. *Surg Endosc.* (2011) 25:2666–77. doi: 10.1007/s00464-011-1627-z
30. Park CH, Min JH, Yoo YC, Kim H, Joh DH, Jo JH, et al. Sedation methods can determine performance of endoscopic submucosal dissection in patients with gastric neoplasia. *Surg Endosc.* (2013) 27:2760–7. doi: 10.1007/s00464-013-2804-z
31. Japanese Gastric Cancer Association. Japanese gastric cancer treatment guidelines 2010 (ver. 3). *Gastric Cancer.* (2011) 14:113–23. doi: 10.1007/s10120-011-0042-4
32. Soetikno R, Kaltenbach T, Yeh R, Gotoda T. Endoscopic mucosal resection for early cancers of the upper gastrointestinal tract. *J Clin Oncol.* (2005) 23:4490–8. doi: 10.1200/JCO.2005.19.935
33. Kang HJ, Kim DH, Jeon TY, Lee SH, Shin N, Chae SH, et al. Lymph node metastasis from intestinal-type early gastric cancer: experience in a single institution and reassessment of the extended criteria for endoscopic submucosal dissection. *Gastrointest Endosc.* (2010) 72:508–15. doi: 10.1016/j.gie.2010.03.1077
34. Chung JW, Jung HY, Choi KD, Song HJ, Lee GH, Jang SJ, et al. Extended indication of endoscopic resection for mucosal early gastric cancer: analysis of a single center experience. *J Gastroenterol Hepatol.* (2011) 26:884–7. doi: 10.1111/j.1440-1746.2010.06611.x
35. Oya H, Gotoda T, Kinjo T, Suzuki H, Yoshinaga S, Taniguchi H, et al. A case of lymph node metastasis following a curative endoscopic submucosal dissection of an early gastric cancer. *Gastric Cancer.* (2012) 15:221–5. doi: 10.1007/s10120-011-0111-8
36. Nakamoto S, Sakai Y, Kasanuki J, Kondo F, Ooka Y, Kato K, et al. Indications for the use of endoscopic mucosal resection for early gastric cancer in Japan: a comparative study with endoscopic submucosal dissection. *Endoscopy.* (2009) 41:746–50. doi: 10.1055/s-0029-1215010
37. Min BH, Lee JH, Kim JJ, Shim SG, Chang DK, Kim YH, et al. Clinical outcomes of endoscopic submucosal dissection (ESD) for treating early gastric cancer: comparison with endoscopic mucosal resection after circumferential precutting (EMR-P). *Dig Liver Dis.* (2009) 41:201–9. doi: 10.1016/j.dld.2008.05.006

38. Meng FS, Zhang ZH, Wang YM, Lu L, Zhu JZ, Ji F. Comparison of endoscopic resection and gastrectomy for the treatment of early gastric cancer: a meta-analysis. *Surg Endosc.* (2016) 30:3673–83. doi: 10.1007/s00464-015-4681-0
39. Sun W, Han X, Wu S, Yang C. Endoscopic resection versus surgical resection for early gastric cancer: a systematic review and meta-analysis. *Medicine.* (2015) 94:e1649. doi: 10.1097/MD.0000000000001649
40. Correa P. Human gastric carcinogenesis: a multistep and multifactorial process–First American Cancer Society Award Lecture on Cancer Epidemiology and Prevention. *Cancer Res.* (1992) 52:6735–40.

13

Conversion Surgery for Stage IV Gastric Cancer

*Fei Zhang[†], Xuanzhang Huang[†], Yongxi Song, Peng Gao, Cen Zhou, Zhexu Guo, Jinxin Shi, Zhonghua Wu and Zhenning Wang**

Key Laboratory of Precision Diagnosis and Treatment of Gastrointestinal Tumors, Ministry of Education, Department of Surgical Oncology and General Surgery, The First Affiliated Hospital of China Medical University, Shenyang, China

Correspondence:
Zhenning Wang
josieon826@sina.cn

[†] These authors have contributed equally to this work

The prognosis of stage IV gastric cancer (GC) is poor, with palliative chemotherapy remaining the main therapeutic option. Studies increasingly indicate that patients with unresectable stage IV GC, who undergo gastrectomy with radical intention after responding to several regimens of combined chemotherapy, can achieve good survival outcomes. Thus, surgery aiming at radical resection for unresectable stage IV GC after combined chemotherapy has received increasing attention in recent years. This novel therapeutic strategy was defined as conversion surgery in patients with unresectable stage IV GC and it can associate with significant improved survival when R0 resection can be achieved. Despite the recent advances in conversion surgery for patients with unresectable stage IV GC, selection criteria for combination chemotherapy regimens, indications for conversion surgery, optimal timing to surgery, and postoperative chemotherapy all remain controversial. This article reviews the current state of conversion surgery for unresectable stage IV GC.

Keywords: conversion surgery, conversion therapy, metastatic gastric cancer, unresectable gastric cancer, combined chemotherapy, stage IV gastric cancer

INTRODUCTION

Despite early screening and improved intensive therapy, gastric cancer (GC) remains to be the fifth most common cancer and third most common cause of cancer-related deaths worldwide, leading to increased health care burden (1, 2). The prognosis for patients with stage IV gastric cancer is poor, and palliative chemotherapy remains the main therapeutic approach for this cohort (3, 4). Despite recent developments in chemotherapy, the median overall survival (OS) of stage IV GC patients remains to be 9–11 months (5, 6). For unresectable stage IV GC patients, only surgeries to relieve symptoms, such as a palliative resection or bypass operations, are commonly considered (7–9). The possibility of additional survival benefits achieved by chemotherapy following palliative surgery has been controversial. Recently, the REGATTA trial randomized 175 stage IV GC patients with a single incurable factor (liver metastases, peritoneal metastases, or para-aortic lymph node metastases) to chemotherapy alone or to initial gastrectomy followed by chemotherapy, but the surgery-first approach failed to show improvements in survival (10). Even with the greater advances achieved by adding a targeted monoclonal antibody to conventional chemotherapy (11–13), the prognosis for unresectable stage IV GC is still unsatisfactory. Thus, novel therapeutic strategies are required for treating unresectable stage IV GC patients.

Several combined S-1 based chemotherapy regimens may allow for conversion of initially unresectable GC to resectable cancer in clinical trials, and additional surgery following this chemotherapy was associated with long-term survival in selected patients (14–16). These advances raise new clinical issues in the treatment of unresectable stage IV GC patients. In some patients, incurable factors apparently disappear or are well-controlled during chemotherapy. For such patients, surgery with curable intent may be possible. Previous reviews investigating the effects of surgery for unresectable stage IV GC patients after chemotherapy also indicate that surgery with curable intention after chemotherapy is associated with prolonged survival in selected patients with a single incurable factor (17, 18), such as liver metastases, peritoneal metastases, or para-aortic lymph node metastases (19, 20). Thus, "conversion surgery" is defined as a surgical treatment aiming at a curable intention after tumors initially deemed technically or oncologically unresectable or only marginally resectable respond to chemotherapy (21, 22). Notably, conversion surgery refers to a radical cure and is different from palliative surgery or other terms concerning surgical resection for advanced incurable tumors such as "salvage," "adjuvant," or "secondary" surgery (23–27). Furthermore, there is no consensus on a clear border between curative surgery scheduled after neoadjuvant chemotherapy and conversion surgery (28, 29). Neoadjuvant chemotherapy can be used for initially resectable advanced GC to reduce tumor size and eradicate micrometastases to improve survival (30, 31), whereas chemotherapy for conversion surgery is used for unresectable advanced GC patients (18, 21).

Developments in conversion surgery have improved life expectancy in patients with incurable advanced GC, attracting increasing attention to conversion surgery for unresectable advanced GC in recent years (18, 32–34). However, selection criteria for combination chemotherapy regimens, indications for conversion surgery, optimal time to surgery, and postoperative chemotherapy all remain controversial. Therefore, we summarize the current state of the field regarding conversion surgery for stage IV GC in this review.

SEARCH STRATEGY AND SELECTION CRITERIA

We searched PubMed for articles published in English from 1997 to 2019 using the search terms "gastric cancer", "conversion therapy," "conversion surgery," "stage IV gastric cancer," "incurable advanced GC," and "unresectable advanced GC." No other parameters were applied. Case reports were excluded. Ultimately, 20 articles were included (shown in **Table 1**).

Abbreviations: CRS, cytoreductive surgery; CR, complete response; EIPL, extensive intraoperative peritoneal lavage; GC, gastric cancer; HIPEC, hyperthermic intraperitoneal chemotherapy; IP, intraperitoneal; LM, liver metastases; MST, median survival time; NAC, neoadjuvant chemotherapy; NLHIPEC, neoadjuvant laparoscopic hyperthermic intraperitoneal chemoperfusion; NIPS, neoadjuvant intraperitoneal and systemic chemotherapy; OS, overall survival; PAN, para-aortic lymph node; PM, Peritoneal metastases; PR, partial response; RR, response rate.

CONVERSION SURGERY OF PERITONEAL DISSEMINATION

Peritoneal metastases (PM), or peritoneal carcinomatosis, is the most common type of metastasis in stage IV GC with poor prognosis (38, 50, 51). Although GC patients with PM undergo combined intensive chemotherapy, the prognosis for this cohort was still unsatisfactory due to their relative resistance to systemic chemotherapy and low drug delivery into the abdominal cavity (35, 36). Developments in S-1 based chemotherapeutic regimens (S-1 plus cisplatin, SP; docetaxel plus cisplatin and S-1, DCS) for advanced GC patients (52–55) resulted in improved overall survival (OS) rate for advanced GC patients with PM. Thus, these advances in chemotherapy are expected to improve survival in unresectable stage IV GC patients with PM. A phase II trial of preoperative S-1 plus cisplatin (SP, oral S-1 plus intravenous cisplatin) chemotherapy, followed by gastrectomy with curable intention in unresectable stage IV GC patients with PM, showed a high response rate to SP with a longer OS over chemotherapy alone. Although most of the eligible patients in this trial had PM, R0 resection was still achieved in 51% of patients after preoperative SP chemotherapy, suggesting that controlling peritoneal dissemination is extremely important in conversion surgery for this cohort (15). Similarly, a trial of SP induction chemotherapy, followed by curative resection in unresectable stage IV GC patients with PM, showed a good response to SP chemotherapy followed by R0 resection with a high median survival time (MST) relative to chemotherapy alone (39). Despite advances in intravenous chemotherapy for unresectable stage IV GC patients with PM (22, 38–40, 55), drug delivery into the abdominal cavity remained low and sustained intraperitineal concentrations were still relatively poor with limited controlled efficacy (56).

Since intraperitoneal (IP) delivery of chemotherapy can attain higher drug exposure in the peritoneal cavity with reduced systemic toxicity (57), intraperitoneal administration of paclitaxel can provide sustained high local concentrations to increase its antitumor effects in GC patients with PM (58). Although promising results have been achieved for combination chemotherapy of IP paclitaxel with S-1 for patients with unresectable GC and PM, yielding a MST of 17.6 months and a 1-year OS of 77.1%(59), salvage gastrectomy on advanced GC patients with PM after disappearance or apparent shrinkage of PM yielded a MST of 26.4 months and a 1-year OS of 82%(60), indicating that conversion surgery may be considered in the cohort with a favorable response after IP paclitaxel plus systemic chemotherapy (50). A single-arm phase II study of conversion surgery following eight cycles of IP paclitaxel with systemic oxaliplatin and capecitabine (XELOX) in unresectable GC patients with PM and/or positive peritoneal washing cytology showed that six patients who underwent conversion gastrectomy, after a favorable response rate to combined XELOX and IP paclitaxel experienced a MST of 21.6 months, compared to patients receiving systemic chemotherapy alone in other trials who had MST of 3.1–10.6 months (50). Additionally, a recent meta-analysis indicated that there are survival benefits associated with hyperthermic intraperitoneal chemotherapy

TABLE 1 | Unresectable characteristics and conversion surgical treatments.

Year	References	Unresectable criteria					Chemotherapy	Surgery type	≥D2	Conversion surgery (%)*	R0 *n* (%)**
		T4	P1	H1	PAN/N3	Other					
1997	Nakajima et al. (35)	8 (27%)	9 (30%)	11 (37%)	23 (77%)	3 (10%)	FLEP	NS	NS	19/30 (63.33%)	9 (47%)
2002	Yano et al. (36)	12 (35%)	26 (76%)	4 (12%)	10 (3.4%)	1 (3.4%)	FEMTXP or THP-FLPM	NS	NS	14/34 (41.17%)	8 (57%)
2012	Satoh et al. (15)	–	24 (49%)	3 (6%)	7 (14%)	17 (33%)	S1+Cisplatin	TG (58.0%) DG (21.5%)	82%	44/51(86.27%)	26 (59%)
2012	Kanda et al. (16)	9 (32%)	7 (25%)	4 (14.3%)	15 (54%)	–	S1 + Cisplatin or Paclitaxel or Irinotecan	TG (42.89%) DG (57.1%)	96.30%	28/31 (90.32%)	26 (93%)
2013	Han et al. (37)	–	7 (14%)	5 (10%)	15 (29.4%)	7 (14%)	5-FU ± Platinum or Taxane ± 5-FU ± Platinum	NS	NS	34/34 (100%)	26 (76%)
2014	Kim et al. (38)	–	43 (100%)	–	–	–	5-FU + Cisplatin or S1 + Cisplatin	TG (72.2%) DG (27.7%)	100%	18/43 (41.86%)	10 (55%)
2014	Saito et al. (39)	9 (10.22%)	26 (29.54%)	7 (7.95%)	21 (23.86%)	7 (7.95%)	S-1 + cisplatin	TG (38.4%) DG (61.6%)	100%	59/88 (67.04%)	13 (22%)
2015	Fukuchi et al. (22)	6 (15%)	11 (28%)	5 (13%)	–	29 (73%)	S1 + Cisplatin or S1 + Paclitaxel	TG (72.5%) DG (27.5%)	NS	40/151 (26.49%)	32 (80%)
2015	Kinoshita et al. (40)	–	15 (26%)	18 (32%)	23 (40%)	2 (3.5%)	DCS	TG (64.7%) DG (26.5%)	50%	34/57 (59.64%)	27 (79%)
2017	Sato et al. (41)	14 (14%)	33 (33%)	29 (29%)	61 (61%)	11 (11%)	DCS Iline, CPT-11 II line	TG (84.8%) DG (12.1%)	100%	33/100 (33%)	28 (85%)
2017	Mieno et al. (42)	8 (25.8%)	8 (25.8%)	5 (16%)	18 (58%)	–	DCS + DS	TG (74.2%) DG (22.6%)	77%	31	23 (74%)
2017	Uemura (43)	6 (13.9%)	16 (37.2%)	14 (32.6%)	22 (51.2%)	4 (9.3%)	Modified DCS	NS	100%	43/49 (87.75%)	15 (35%)
2017	Einama et al. (44)	1 (10%)	3 (30%)	1 (10%)	4 (40%)	1 (10%)	S1 + CDDP or DOC	TG (40%) DG (30%)	100%	10	10 (100%)
2017	Maeda et al. (45)	–	–	3 (37.5%)	8 (100%)	–	Modified DCX	NS	100%	3/8 (37.5%)	3 (100%)
2017	Yamaguchi et al. (46)	–	35 (41%)	–	37 (44%)	34 (40%)	DCS or S1 or S1 + Cisplatin or S1 + Taxane	TG (82.1%) DG (17.9%)	NS	84/259 (32.43%)	43 (51%)
2017	AIO-FLOT3 (29)	13 (21.8%)	4 (6.7%)	11 (18.3%)	36 (60.1%)	2 (3.3%)	FLOT	NS	NS	36/60 (60%)	29 (80%)
2018	Morgagni et al. (47)	8 (36.36%)	2 (9.09%)	2 (9.09%)	11 (50%)	–	Epirubicin + Cisplatinum + 5-FU or Oxaliplatin + 5-FU or Docetaxel + Oxaliplatin + 5-FU or Other	TG (72.7%) DG (22.7%)	91.9%	33/57 (57.89%)	22 (67%)
2018	Beom et al. (32)	2 (2.0%)	33 (32.7%)	11 (10.9%)	35 (34.7%)	20 (19.8%)	Platinum + 5-FU or Taxane + 5-FU or Platinum + Taxane + 5-FU or Taxane + Platinum or Others	TG (56.4%) DG (43.6%)	75.2%	101	57 (56%)

(Continued)

TABLE 1 | Continued

Year	References	Unresectable criteria					Chemotherapy	Surgery type	≥D2	Conversion surgery (%)*	R0 n (%)**
		T4	P1	H1	PAN/N3	Other					
2019	Solaini et al. (48)	–	38 (84.4%)	4 (8.8%)	3 (6.6%)	–	Cisplantin + 5-FU or Epirubicin + Cisplatinum + 5-FU or Docetaxel + Oxaliplatin + 5-FU or Other	TG (73.3%) DG (26.7%)	91.1%	45	30 (67%)
2019	Li et al. (49)	–	8 (9.8%)	10 (12.2%)	60 (74.1%)	3 (3.7%)	Oxaliplatin + 5-FU (Capecitabne or S-1) or Oxaliplatin + 5-FU + Docetaxel/Anthracyclines	NS	NS	81/414 (19.5%)	66 (81.4%)

*P1, Peritoneal carcinomatosis; H1, Hepatic metastases; PAN, Para-aortic node metastases; TG, Total gastrectomy; DG, Distal gastrectomy; DCS/DS: Docetaxel-Cisplatin-S1/Docetaxel-Cisplatin; FEMTXP: Fluorouracil, epirubicin, methotrexate, cisplatin; THP-FLPM: Pirarubicin, 5-FU, Leucovorin, Cisplatin, mitomycin C; FLEP: 5-FU + Leucovorin + Etoposide; CDDP: Cisplatin; DOC: Docetaxel; FLOT: fluorouracil, leucovorin, oxaliplatin, and docetaxel; *Conversion surgery rate: (conversion surgery number)/population ×100%; ** R0 resection rate: (R0 resection number)/(conversion surgery number) ×100%; NS: Not specified.*

(HIPEC), delivering a high drug concentration for advanced GC patients with PM involvement compared with systemic chemotherapy alone (61). A cohort study of conversion surgery after HIPEC, plus chemotherapy in a small cohort of stage IV GC patients with PM, showed good long-term outcomes, suggesting that combination HIPEC may represent a useful and feasible technique to improve survival in GC patients with PM undergoing conversion surgery (47). In a GIRCG retrospective cohort study, 23 unresectable stage IV GC patients with PM received conversion gastrectomy after HIPEC plus chemotherapy, with a conversion rate of 60.5%(48).

A phase III trial was conducted (PHOENIX-GC), with the IP arm showing a better response in the amount of ascites and a high negative conversion rate of 78% for peritoneal cytology, further supporting the clinical benefit of the IP regimen for advanced GC with PM. However, OS was not significantly affected, indicating that further studies might be necessary to explore favorable candidate selection and new therapeutic strategies for intraperitoneal therapy (62). On the other hand, cytoreductive surgery plus hyperthermic intraperitoneal chemotherapy (CRS+HIPEC) has been applied in GC with PM (63, 64). Although a large retrospective study showed that long-term survival could only be achieved in GC patients with limited PM, it is still expected to explore in unresectable GC patients with advanced PM (63). Therefore, additional trials involving various combinations of therapeutic options for GC patients with PM including cytoreductive surgery plus hyperthermic intraperitoneal chemotherapy (CRS+HIPEC), neoadjuvant intraperitoneal and systemic chemotherapy (NIPS), and neoadjuvant laparoscopic hyperthermic intraperitoneal chemoperfusion (NLHIPEC) are still needed to explore their feasibility and efficacy for conversion.

CONVERSION SURGERY OF LIVER METASTASES

Stage IV GC patients present with various metastatic sites, and the liver is one of the most common sites of synchronous and metachronous GC metastases through the hematogenous pathway (65, 66). For unresectable advanced GC patients with liver metastases (LM), conversion surgery options encompass surgical therapies including liver resection, radiofrequency ablation (RFA), or microwave coagulation therapy (MCT) combined with systemic chemotherapy. Han et al. retrospectively reviewed clinicopathological data for surgery aiming at curative resection in GC patients with LM who responded well to induction chemotherapy. Of these, five GC patients with LM underwent radical gastric resection plus liver metastectomy after Docetaxel-Cisplatin-5-FU (DCF) chemotherapy, with a R0 resection rate of 100% (37). A retrospective trial conducted by Kinoshita et al. included 18 stage IV GC patients with LM receiving DCS chemotherapy. Among them, 11 underwent conversion gastrectomy (including 5 liver metastectomy) after DCS chemotherapy, with a MST of 18.9 months and a 3-year OS rate of 40.4%, whereas the MST was 15.6 months and 3-year OS rate was 27.5% for the 7 patients who did not achieve conversion surgery (40). Following this, a multi-institutional retrospective study conducted by Sato et al. included 29 GC patients with LM, among whom six underwent conversion surgery after DCS chemotherapy. Importantly, among the six patients with liver metastases, two underwent partial hepatectomies with a complete pathological response and two were treated with RFA, and after chemotherapy the metastatic lesions completely disappeared in two cases. Interestingly, DCS treatment led to conversion therapy in these patients with synchronous unresectable LM, and this cohort had good prognosis with a MTS of 22 months compared with chemotherapy alone (41). Additionally, Yamaguchi et al. reported that 20 stage IV GC patients with LM underwent conversion surgery plus liver metastasectomy after chemotherapy with a conversion rate of 21.5% (20/93), and suggested that metastasectomy along with primary tumor resection might be feasible for this population, provided that the metastases respond well to chemotherapy (46). Similarly, Beom et al. reported that three stage IV GC patients with LM who received radical gastrectomy plus hepatectomy after a better response (CR/PR, complete response/partial response) to chemotherapy had a good MST of 49.2 months compared with other types of distant metastasis with a MST of 13.6 months (32). Furthermore, Li et al. reported that stage IV GC patients with LM saw remarkable survival benefit from simultaneous liver resection or RFA after a good response to chemotherapy relative to chemotherapy alone, which may relate to their nearly tumor-free status after simultaneous surgery or RFA of LMs (49).

Although there is good prognosis for multiple conversion options in stage IV GC patients with LM, a multi-institutional retrospective study of conversion surgery after DCS chemotherapy in GC patients with LM showed a recurrence rate was 50% (41). Furthermore, previous studies of incurable GC patients with LM undergoing liver resection or RFA without preoperative therapy found recurrence rates up to 63.6–91.0% (65–67). Therefore, postoperative chemotherapy should be accompanied by cautious follow up (37). Despite promising indications for conversion surgery in unresectable GC patients with LM, the potential benefits of surgical resection and best treatment regimens in this cohort remain to be determined by further prospective studies and randomized controlled trials.

CONVERSION SURGERY OF LYMPH NODE METASTASES

GC patients with extensive lymph node metastases, including para-aortic lymph node (PAN) metastases or bulky nodes around the hepatic, splenic, or celiac arteries, are often considered to be unresectable and have poor prognosis (68). However, an adequate lymphadenectomy during surgical treatment is crucial for GC treatment, especially for unresectable GC patients with PAN metastases who undergo combined chemotherapy. A study conducted by Park et al. followed outcomes of GC patients with isolated PAN metastases following palliative chemotherapy, finding a 3-year OS of only 13.1% (69). Even when GC patients with PAN metastases can undergo gastrectomy, these patients still had poor survival outcomes, with a 3-year OS of 5% (68). Therefore, a preoperative chemotherapy approach has been recommended as a treatment strategy for GC patients with PAN metastases. Alternatively, a randomized controlled trial of JCOG9501 indicated that D2 lymphadenectomy plus preventative PAN dissection (PAND) does not improve survival rate in patients with curable GC compared with D2 lymphadenectomy alone (70), however cases with macroscopic PAN metastases at surgery were excluded from analysis, leading to a low incidence of metastatic PAN in patients with PAND. Therefore, the prognostic efficacy of PAND after chemotherapy for GC patients with PAN metastases is still unclear (71). Thus, further studies are necessary to clarify the importance of PAND after induction chemotherapy.

Two phase II trials (JCOG0001and JCOG0405) were conducted to evaluate the safety and efficacy of gastrectomy with D2 lymphadenectomy plus PAND for GC patients with PAD metastases after preoperative combined chemotherapy. In JCOG001 and JCOG0405, GC patients with PAD metastases who received two or three cycles of irinotecan and cisplatinor cisplatin and S-1 chemotherapy, followed by gastrectomy with D2 lymphadenectomy plus PAND yielded a 3-year survival of 27.0 and 58.5%, respectively (72, 73). Therefore, combined chemotherapy followed by gastrectomy with D2 lymphadenectomy plus PAND are considered as safe and effective treatments for GC patients with PAD metastases. Since S-1 based chemotherapy was indicated to improve outcomes for advanced unresectable GC patients with PAD metastases (53, 54, 74), recent trials have seen encouraging outcomes for conversion gastrectomy with D2 lymphadenectomy plus PAND after chemotherapy in stage IV GC patients with PAN metastases. Saito et al. reported that unresectable stage IV GC patients with PAN metastases, who underwent radical gastrectomy with D2 lymphadenectomy plus PAND after induction CS chemotherapy, yielded a conversion surgery rate of 25.0% (4/16) (39). Additionally, a multi-institutional retrospective study of unresectable advanced GC patients with PAN metastases who underwent radical gastrectomy with D2 lymphadenectomy plus PAND after DCS chemotherapy showed a good conversion surgery rate of 33.3% (9/27) and a good median OS of 47.8 months, over the median OS of 15.7 months for chemotherapy alone (41). Furthermore, a retrospective study of stage IV GC patients with PAN metastases undergoing conversion surgery with D2 lymphadenectomy plus PAND after DCS chemotherapy showed a high conversion surgery rate of 73.9% (17/23) and a good 3-year OS over chemotherapy alone (72.9 vs. 15.2%) (40).

Although, unresectable stage IV GC patients with PAN metastases, receiving induction chemotherapy followed by conversion surgery with D2 lymphadenectomy plus PAND, have achieved better conversion resection rates and survival outcomes compare to chemotherapy alone, the prognosis for this cohort is still unsatisfactory. Based on the promising outcomes of radiotherapy combined with chemotherapy for locally advanced GC patients with lymph node metastases (75–77), preoperative radiotherapy may improve the long-survival of unresectable stage IV GC patients with PAN metastases. Therefore, further research must identify optimal preoperative multimodal treatments of radiotherapy combined with chemotherapy for this cohort and further explore its feasibility and efficacy in the near future.

FUTURE WORK AND PERSPECTIVES

Selecting Stage IV GC Patients That Can Benefit From Conversion Surgery

It is extremely important to identify stage IV GC patients that can benefit from conversion surgery. Although palliative gastrectomy followed by chemotherapy showed no survival benefit for these patients, compared with chemotherapy alone in the REGATTA trial (10), this trial helped oncological surgeons to select eligibility criteria for surgery in unresectable advanced GC. Further studies also indicated that unresectable stage IV GC patients with a single incurable factor (liver metastases, peritoneal metastases, or para-aortic lymph node metastases) receiving combined chemotherapy followed by conversion surgery have achieved high R0 resection rates and good prognosis (32, 41–43, 46–48). Thus, the number of metastatic sites may be an important indicator for obtaining down-staging by chemotherapy and a good prognosis after conversion surgery. Additionally, rates of relatively severe postoperative complications between 14.2 and 40% (35, 40, 41, 48) make stringent selection of unresectable stage IV GC patients who may benefit from conversion surgery increasingly necessary. Criteria for conversion surgery included: no sign of organ failure, age between 20 and 80 years, Eastern Cooperative Oncology Group scale performance status 0–2, and one single incurable factor (41, 45). Moreover, modern diagnostic tools, such as computed tomography (CT), magnetic resonance imaging (MRI), positron emission tomography CT (PET-CT), upper gastrointestinal tract endoscopy, and ultrasonography, may help determine clinical staging before undertaking surgical intervention for GC patients (41, 42, 44). Additionally, staging laparoscopy with or without peritoneal lavage also plays an important role in order to confirm whether the peritoneal deposits disappeared completely or whether positive cytology turned negative (50). Despite recent trials suggesting that candidates for conversion surgery were those for whom R0 resection could be obtained following response to chemotherapy (22, 41), new categories of classification were proposed by Yoshida et al. based on the absence or presence of macroscopic peritoneal dissemination (17) (shown in **Figure 1**). Optimal recommended indications for conversion surgery include marginally resectable metastasis, some incurable and unresectable except certain circumstances of local palliation needs, and a few non-curable metastasis patients with GC. Based on this novel classification, promising results of conversion surgery in unresectable stage IV GC patients have been achieved in three cohort studies (46–48). However, as it is sometimes extremely difficult to determine between marginally resectable or unresectable tumors, it is controversial whether the Yoshida classification can be used as a definite standard (18). Thus, adequate selection of stage IV GC patients for conversion surgery is an important upcoming task for surgical oncologists.

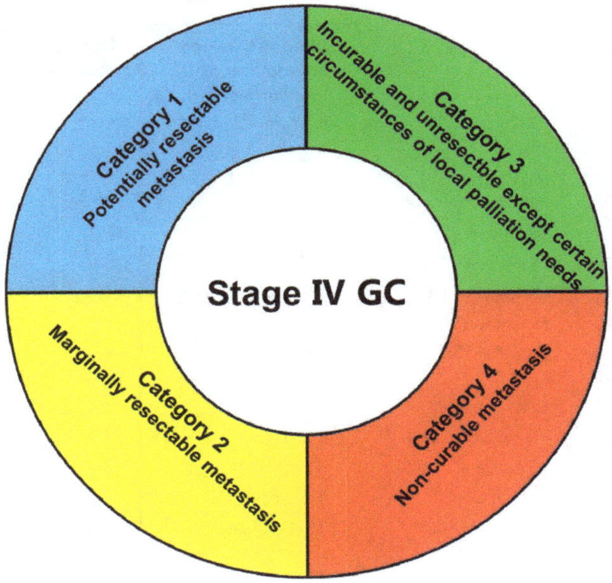

FIGURE 1 | Biological categories for conversion surgery introduced by Yoshida et al. (17).

Selecting the Best Timing for Conversion Surgery

Optimally, surgery is performed when the tumor has decreased most in size in response to chemotherapy and before chemotherapy resistance allows it to grow again (17, 22, 78). This literature review found interval times between chemotherapy and surgery ranging from 4 to 391 days (**Table 2**). Yoshida et al. estimated the optimal operation opportunity to be after a CR or PR response is determined following chemotherapy (17), with a mean interval time for resection after chemotherapy of approximately 126 days (**Table 2**). However, a randomized phase II study (COMPASS trial) by Yoshikawa et al. reported that 2–6 weeks after completion of neoadjuvant chemotherapy might be adequate (79). This is consistent with results from many studies listed in **Table 2**. Thus, there are currently two perspectives for optimal surgery time among surgical oncologists: (1) patients who have achieved the indications of surgical treatment after definitive chemotherapy should have conversion surgery performed, or (2) the chemotherapy duration could be extended to 6 months or even 1 year. After the disease condition is stable, conversion surgery could then be carried out, possibly increasing patient benefits and safety. Both views are reasonable, however whether one is superior remains to be further explored with additional evidence needed.

Selecting Preoperative Drug Therapeutic Strategies to Achieve Conversion

Based on good response to S-1/cisplatin (SP)(52), S-1/docetaxel (DS) (80), capecitabine plus cisplatin (XP) with or without trastuzumab (11), S-1 plus irinotecan (IRI-S) (81) and S-1 plus docetaxel, cisplatin (DCS) (68), and cisplatin/paclitaxel

TABLE 2 | Time of interval to surgery, postoperative chemotherapy, overall survival, and median survival time.

Year	References	Interval between chemotherapy and surgery	Postoperative chemotherapy	OS (rate)			MST (months)		
				CHT	CHT + surgery		CHT	CHT + surgery	
					R1/R2	R0		R1/R2	R0
1997	Nakajima et al. (35)	NS	NS			5-yr (55.6%)	4.7	6.5	
2002	Yano et al. (36)	NS	NS						
2012	Satoh et al. (15)	2–4 weeks	Yes	2-yr (12%)		2-yr (75.0%)*			19.2
2012	Kanda et al. (16)	130 (59–391) days	Yes		3-yr (0%)	3-yr (49.5%)			29
2013	Han et al. (37)	1.3 (0.3–2.3) months	Yes			3-yr (41.4%)		7.8	22.9
2014	Kim et al. (38)	5.6 (2–12) months	Yes	3-yr (0%)	3-yr (0%)	3-yr (50%) 5-yr (40%)	8	18	37
2014	Saito et al. (39)	4–6 weeks	Yes			3-yr (53.8%)			53
2015	Fukuchi et al. (22)	6 weeks	Yes	5-yr (1%)	5-yr (15%)	5-yr (49%)	14	30	62
2015	Kinoshita et al. (40)	85 (43–414) days	Yes	3-yr (0%)	3-yr (16%)	3-yr (50.1%)	9.6	15.6	29.9
2017	Sato et al. (41)	5–6 weeks	Yes	5-yr (0%)	5-yr (0%)	5-yr (48.6%)	15.7	21.7	47.9
2017	Mieno et al. (42)	36 (4–70)days	Yes			3-yr (73.1%)			
2017	Uemura (43)	NS	NS				13.7		24
2017	Einama et al. (44)	5–6 weeks	Yes						29
2017	Maeda et al. (45)	NS	Yes			2-yr (100%)			
2017	Yamaguchi et al. (46)	126 days*	Yes				11.3	21.2	41.3
2017	AIO-FLOT3 (29)	3 weeks	Yes				15.9		
2018	Morgagni et al. (47)	NS	NS	3-yr (0%)		3-yr (39.4%)			38
2018	Beom et al. (32)	24 weeks	Yes						
2019	Solaini et al. (48)	3–6 months	Yes						
2019	Li et al. (49)	NS	Yes				10.9		

*OS, Overall survival; MST, Median survival time; CHT, Chemotherapy; *R0 in only pre-Cy1 patients; **Data from consultation with authors by email.*

(82) in advanced unresectable GC, preoperative S-1 based chemotherapies are considered as main therapeutic options for conversion therapy. Additionally, clinical targeted drugs have been developing quickly, especially in the fields of lung cancer, breast cancer and soft tissue tumor. For GC, the ToGA study gives hope that HER2 positive advanced GC patients undergoing chemotherapy combined with trastuzumab can significantly prolong their OS compared with chemotherapy alone, and this regimen has become a standard treatment for HER2 positive advanced GC patients (11, 56). Additionally, ramucirumab, an anti-angiogenesis drug, has been well-verified in clinical practice for treating advanced GC (12, 13), indicating that targeted drugs for conversion surgery in unresectable stage IV GC patients may serve as promising therapeutic options to improve clinical outcomes. Furthermore, combination immunotherapy for conversion therapy in unresectable advanced colorectal cancer or inoperable advanced lung cancer has achieved broad prospects with a good rate of conversion or high rate of R0 resection (83, 84). Although several clinical trials examining PD-1/PD-L blockade combination treatments in advanced GC were identified (NCT01848834, NCT01928394, NCT02335411, NCT02340975), studies of immunotherapy for conversion surgery in unresectable stage IV GC are still scarce. Thus, combination immunotherapy for conversion surgery in unresectable stage IV GC is expected to prolong survival of this cohort with a high rate of conversion, and further studies are necessary to determine its feasibility and safety.

In conclusion, conversion surgery for unresectable stage IV gastric cancer was associated with longer survival over chemotherapy alone. GC patients with a single incurable factor who experienced a favorable response to combination chemotherapy achieved better survival outcomes than those with multiple metastatic organs. Additionally, patients undergoing R0 resection had better prognosis than those with R1 or R2 resection. Common definitions remain to be clarified regarding the selection of initial combination chemotherapy, the timing of conversion surgery, and indications for postoperative chemotherapy. Additional trials are imperative to address these important issues and to confirm their feasibility and validity to further improve the prognosis of unresectable stage IV GC patients.

AUTHOR CONTRIBUTIONS

FZ played a major role in writing the manuscript. XH and PG provided important feedback and helped in editing the manuscript. YS, ZWa, and PG participated in studies selection. CZ, ZG, JS, and ZWu contributed to the literature search. All authors have approved the final version of the manuscript.

REFERENCES

1. Bray F, Ferlay J, Soerjomataram I, Siegel R, Torre L, Jemal A. Global Cancer Statistics 2018: GLOBOCAN Estimates of Incidence and Mortality Worldwide for 36 Cancers in 185 Countries. *CA Cancer J Clin.* (2018) 68:394–24. doi: 10.3322/caac.21492
2. Fitzmaurice C, Akinyemiju TF, Al Lami FH, Alam T, Alizadeh-Navaei R, Allen C, et al. Global, regional, and national cancer incidence, mortality, years of life lost, years lived with disability, and disability-adjusted life-years for 29 cancer groups, 1990 to 2016: a systematic analysis for the global burden of disease study. *JAMA Oncol.* (2018) 4:1553–68. doi: 10.1200/JCO.2018.36.15_suppl.1568
3. Sano T, Aiko T. New Japanese classifications and treatment guidelines for gastric cancer: revision concepts and major revised points. *Gastric Cancer.* (2011) 14:97–100. doi: 10.1007/s10120-011-0040-6
4. Dittmar Y, Rauchfuss F, Goetz M, Jandt K, Scheuerlein H, Heise M, et al. Non-curative gastric resection for patients with stage 4 gastric cancer–a single center experience and current review of literature. *Langenbeck's Arch Surg.* (2012) 397:745–53. doi: 10 1007/s00423-012-0902-3
5. Van Cutsem E, Moiseyenko VM, Tjulandin S, Majlis A, Constenla M, Boni C, et al. Phase III study of docetaxel and cisplatin plus fluorouracil compared with cisplatin and fluorouracil as first-line therapy for advanced gastric cancer: a report of the V325 Study Group. *J Clin Oncol.* (2006) 24:4991–7. doi: 10.1200/JCO.2006.06.8429
6. Boku N, Yamamoto S, Fukuda H, Shirao K, Doi T, Sawaki A, et al. Fluorouracil versus combination of irinotecan plus cisplatin versus S-1 in metastatic gastric cancer: a randomised phase 3 study. *Lancet Oncol.* (2009) 10:1063–9. doi: 10.1016/S1470-2045(09)70259-1
7. Lordick F, Siewert JR. Recent advances in multimodal treatment for gastric cancer: a review. *Gastric Cancer.* (2005) 8:78–85. doi: 10.1007/s10120-005-0321-z
8. Mahar AL, Coburn NG, Karanicolas PJ, Viola R, Helyer LK. Effective palliation and quality of life outcomes in studies of surgery for advanced, non-curative gastric cancer: a systematic review. *Gastric Cancer.* (2012) 15 (Suppl. 1):S138–45. doi: 10.1007/s10120-011-0070-0
9. Shen L, Shan YS, Hu HM, Price TJ, Sirohi B, Yeh KH, et al. Management of gastric cancer in Asia: resource-stratified guidelines. *Lancet Oncol.* (2013) 14:e535–47. doi: 10.1016/S1470-2045(13)70436-4
10. Fujitani K, Yang H-K, Mizusawa J, Kim Y-W, Terashima M, Han S-U, et al. Gastrectomy plus chemotherapy versus chemotherapy alone for advanced gastric cancer with a single non-curable factor (REGATTA): a phase 3, randomised controlled trial. *Lancet Oncol.* (2016) 17:309–18. doi: 10.1016/S1470-2045(15)00553-7
11. Bang Y-J, Van Cutsem E, Feyereislova A, Chung HC, Shen L, Sawaki A, et al. Trastuzumab in combination with chemotherapy versus chemotherapy alone for treatment of HER2-positive advanced gastric or gastro-oesophageal junction cancer (ToGA): a phase 3, open-label, randomised controlled trial. *Lancet.* (2010) 376:687–97. doi: 10.1016/S0140-6736(10)61121-X
12. Wilke H, Muro K, Van Cutsem E, Oh SC, Bodoky G, Shimada Y, et al. Ramucirumab plus paclitaxel versus placebo plus paclitaxel in patients with previously treated advanced gastric or gastro-oesophageal junction adenocarcinoma (RAINBOW): a double-blind, randomised phase 3 trial. *Lancet Oncol.* (2014) 15:1224–35. doi: 10.1016/S1470-2045(14)70420-6
13. Fuchs CS, Tomasek J, Yong CJ, Dumitru F, Passalacqua R, Goswami C, et al. Ramucirumab monotherapy for previously treated advanced gastric or gastro-oesophageal junction adenocarcinoma (REGARD): an international, randomised, multicentre, placebo-controlled, phase 3 trial. *Lancet.* (2014) 383:31–9. doi: 10.1016/S0140-6736(13)61719-5
14. Ito S, Oki E, Nakashima Y, Ando K, Hiyoshi Y, Ohgaki K, et al. Clinical significance of adjuvant surgery following chemotherapy for patients with initially unresectable stage IV gastric cancer. *Anticancer Res.* (2015) 35:401–6.
15. Satoh S, Okabe H, Teramukai S, Hasegawa S, Ozaki N, Ueda S, et al. Phase II trial of combined treatment consisting of preoperative S-1 plus cisplatin followed by gastrectomy and postoperative S-1 for stage IV gastric cancer. *Gastric Cancer.* (2012) 15:61–9. doi: 10.1007/s10120-011-0066-9
16. Kanda T, Yajima K, Kosugi S, Ishikawa T, Ajioka Y, Hatakeyama K. Gastrectomy as a secondary surgery for stage IV gastric cancer patients who underwent S-1-based chemotherapy: a multi-institute retrospective study. *Gastric Cancer.* (2012) 15:235–44. doi: 10.1007/s10120-011-0100-y
17. Yoshida K, Yamaguchi K, Okumura N, Tanahashi T, Kodera Y. Is conversion therapy possible in stage IV gastric cancer: the proposal of new biological categories of classification. *Gastric Cancer.* (2016) 19:329–38. doi: 10.1007/s10120-015-0575-z
18. Zurleni T, Gjoni E, Altomare M, Rausei S. Conversion surgery for gastric cancer patients: a review. *World J Gastrointestinal Oncol.* (2018) 10:398–409. doi: 10.4251/wjgo.v10.i11.398
19. Yoshida M, Ohtsu A, Boku N, Miyata Y, Shirao K, Shimada Y, et al. Long-term survival and prognostic factors in patients with metastatic gastric cancers treated with chemotherapy in the Japan Clinical Oncology Group (JCOG) study. *Jpn J Clin Oncol.* (2004) 34:654–9. doi: 10.1093/jjco/hyh120
20. Lee JH, Paik YH, Lee JS, Song HJ, Ryu KW, Kim CG, et al. Candidates for curative resection in advanced gastric cancer patients who had equivocal para-aortic lymph node metastasis on computed tomographic scan. *Ann Surg Oncol.* (2006) 13:1163–7. doi: 10.1245/s10434-006-9002-3
21. Terashima M. Conversion therapy for gastric cancer: who can make conversion as successful as Goromaru? *Gastric Cancer.* (2016) 19:685–6. doi: 10.1007/s10120-016-0609-1
22. Fukuchi M, Ishiguro T, Ogata K, Suzuki O, Kumagai Y, Ishibashi K, et al. Prognostic role of conversion surgery for unresectable gastric cancer. *Ann Surg Oncol.* (2015) 22:3618–24. doi: 10.1245/s10434-015-4422-6
23. Muto O, Kotanagi H. Palliative resection for stage IV gastric cancer. *J Clin Oncol.* (2011) 29(4 Suppl):148. doi: 10.1200/jco.2011.29.4_suppl.148
24. Muto O, Kotanagi H. The efficacy of gastrectomy plus chemotherapy for stage IV gastric cancer. *J Clin Oncol.* (2012) 30(4 Suppl):132. doi: 10.1200/jco.2012.30.4_suppl.132
25. Sun J, Song Y, Wang Z, Chen X, Gao P, Xu Y, et al. Clinical significance of palliative gastrectomy on the survival of patients with incurable advanced gastric cancer: a systematic review and meta-analysis. *BMC Cancer.* (2013) 13:577. doi: 10.1186/1471-2407-13-577
26. Markar S, Gronnier C, Duhamel A, Pasquer A, Théreaux J, Rieu MCd, et al. Salvage surgery after chemoradiotherapy in the management of esophageal cancer: is it a viable therapeutic option? *J Clin Oncol.* (2015) 33:3866–73. doi: 10.1200/JCO.2014.59.9092
27. Suzuki T, Tanabe K, Taomoto J, Yamamoto H, Tokumoto N, Yoshida K, et al. Preliminary trial of adjuvant surgery for advanced gastric cancer. *Oncol Lett.* (2010) 1:743–7. doi: 10.3892/ol_00000130
28. Ramos M, Pereira MA, Charruf AZ, Dias AR, Castria TB, Barchi LC, et al. Conversion therapy for gastric cancer: expanding the treatment possibilities. *Arquivos Brasileiros de Cirurgia Digestiva.* (2019) 32:e1435. doi: 10.1590/0102-672020190001e1435
29. Al-Batran SE, Homann N, Pauligk C, Illerhaus G, Martens UM, Stoehlmacher J, et al. Effect of neoadjuvant chemotherapy followed by surgical resection on survival in patients with limited metastatic gastric or gastroesophageal junction cancer: the AIO-FLOT3 Trial. *JAMA Oncol.* (2017) 3:1237–44. doi: 10.1001/jamaoncol.2017.0515
30. Kodera Y. Neoadjuvant chemotherapy for gastric adenocarcinoma in Japan. *Surg Today.* (2017) 47:899–907. doi: 10.1007/s00595-017-1473-2
31. Hu S-B, Liu C-H, Wang X, Dong Y-W, Zhao L, Liu H-F, et al. Pathological evaluation of neoadjuvant chemotherapy in advanced gastric cancer. *World J Surg Oncol.* (2019) 17:3. doi: 10.1186/s12957-018-1534-z
32. Beom SH, Choi YY, Baek SE, Li SX, Lim JS, Son T, et al. Multidisciplinary treatment for patients with stage IV gastric cancer: the role of conversion surgery following chemotherapy. *BMC Cancer.* (2018) 18:1116. doi: 10.1186/s12885-018-4998-x
33. Kodera Y. Surgery with curative intent for stage IV gastric cancer: is it a reality of illusion? *Ann Gastroenterol Surg.* (2018) 2:339–47. doi: 10.1002/ags3.12191
34. Du R, Hu P, Liu Q, Zhang J. Conversion surgery for unresectable advanced gastric cancer: a systematic review and meta-analysis. *Cancer Investig.* (2019) 37:16–28. doi: 10.1080/07357907.2018.1551898
35. Nakajima T, Ota K, Ishihara S, Oyama S, Nishi M, Ohashi Y, et al. Combined intensive chemotherapy and radical surgery for incurable gastric cancer. *Ann Surg Oncol.* (1997) 4:203–8. doi: 10.1007/BF02306611
36. Yano M, Shiozaki H, Inoue M, Tamura S, Doki Y, Yasuda T, et al. Neoadjuvant chemotherapy followed by salvage surgery: effect on survival of patients

with primary noncurative gastric cancer. *World J Surg.* (2002) 26:1155–9. doi: 10.1007/s00268-002-6362-0
37. Han DS, Suh YS, Kong SH, Lee HJ, Im SA, Bang YJ, et al. Outcomes of surgery aiming at curative resection in good responder to induction chemotherapy for gastric cancer with distant metastases. *J Surg Oncol.* (2013) 107:511–6. doi: 10.1002/jso.23284
38. Kim SW. The result of conversion surgery in gastric cancer patients with peritoneal seeding. *J Gastr Cancer.* (2014) 14:266–70. doi: 10.5230/jgc.2014.14.4.266
39. Saito M, Kiyozaki H, Takata O, Suzuki K, Rikiyama T. Treatment of stage IV gastric cancer with induction chemotherapy using S-1 and cisplatin followed by curative resection in selected patients. *World J Surg Oncol.* (2014) 12:406. doi: 10.1186/1477-7819-12-406
40. Kinoshita J, Fushida S, Tsukada T, Oyama K, Okamoto K, Makino I, et al. Efficacy of conversion gastrectomy following docetaxel, cisplatin, and S-1 therapy in potentially resectable stage IV gastric cancer. *Eur J Surg Oncol.* (2015) 41:1354–60. doi: 10.1016/j.ejso.2015.04.021
41. Sato Y, Ohnuma H, Nobuoka T, Hirakawa M, Sagawa T, Fujikawa K, et al. Conversion therapy for inoperable advanced gastric cancer patients by docetaxel, cisplatin, and S-1 (DCS) chemotherapy: a multi-institutional retrospective study. *Gastric Cancer.* (2017) 20:517–26. doi: 10.1007/s10120-016-0633-1
42. Mieno H, Yamashita K, Hosoda K, Moriya H, Higuchi K, Azuma M, et al. Conversion surgery after combination chemotherapy of docetaxel, cisplatin and S-1 (DCS) for far-advanced gastric cancer. *Surgery Today.* (2017) 47:1249–58. doi: 10.1007/s00595-017-1512-z
43. Uemura N, Kikuchi S, Sato Y, Ohnuma H, Okamoto K, Miyamoto H, et al. A phase II study of modified docetaxel, cisplatin, and S-1 (mDCS) chemotherapy for unresectable advanced gastric cancer. *Cancer Chemotherap Pharmacol.* (2017) 80:707–13. doi: 10.1007/s00280-017-3404-8
44. Einama T, Abe H, Shichi S, Matsui H, Kanazawa R, Shibuya K, et al. Long-term survival and prognosis associated with conversion surgery in patients with metastatic gastric cancer. *Mol Clin Oncol.* (2017) 6:163–6. doi: 10.3892/mco.2017.1128
45. Maeda O, Matsuoka A, Miyahara R, Funasaka K, Hirooka Y, Fukaya M, et al. Modified docetaxel, cisplatin and capecitabine for stage IV gastric cancer in Japanese patients: a feasibility study. *World J Gastroenterol.* (2017) 23:1090–7. doi: 10.3748/wjg.v23.i6.1090
46. Yamaguchi K, Yoshida K, Tanahashi T, Takahashi T, Matsuhashi N, Tanaka Y, et al. The long-term survival of stage IV gastric cancer patients with conversion therapy. *Gastric Cancer.* (2018) 21:315–23. doi: 10.1007/s10120-017-0738-1
47. Morgagni P, Solaini L, Framarini M, Vittimberga G, Gardini A, Tringali D, et al. Conversion surgery for gastric cancer: a cohort study from a western center. *Int J Surg.* (2018) 53:360–5. doi: 10.1016/j.ijsu.2018.04.016
48. Solaini L, Ministrini S, Bencivenga M, D'Ignazio A, Marino E, Cipollari C, et al. Conversion gastrectomy for stage IV unresectable gastric cancer: a GIRCG retrospective cohort study. *Gastric Cancer.* (2019) 22:1285–93. doi: 10.1007/s10120-019-00968-2
49. Li W, Jiang H, Yu Y, Wang Y, Wang Z, Cui Y, et al. Outcomes of gastrectomy following upfront chemotherapy in advanced gastric cancer patients with a single noncurable factor: a cohort study. *Cancer Manage Res.* (2019) 11:2007–13. doi: 10.2147/CMAR.S192570
50. Chan DY, Syn NL, Yap R, Phua JN, Soh TI, Chee CE, et al. Conversion surgery post-intraperitoneal paclitaxel and systemic chemotherapy for gastric cancer carcinomatosis peritonei. are we ready? *J Gastrointest Surg.* (2017) 21:425–33. doi: 10.1007/s11605-016-3336-3
51. Thomassen I, van Gestel YR, van Ramshorst B, Luyer MD, Bosscha K, Nienhuijs SW, et al. Peritoneal carcinomatosis of gastric origin: a population-based study on incidence, survival and risk factors. *Int J Cancer.* (2014) 134:622–8. doi: 10.1002/ijc.28373
52. Koizumi W, Narahara H, Hara T, Takagane A, Akiya T, Takagi M, et al. S-1 plus cisplatin versus S-1 alone for first-line treatment of advanced gastric cancer (SPIRITS trial): a phase III trial. *Lancet Oncol.* (2008) 9:215–21. doi: 10.1016/S1470-2045(08)70035-4
53. Nakayama N, Koizumi W, Sasaki T, Higuchi K, Tanabe S, Nishimura K, et al. A multicenter, phase I dose-escalating study of docetaxel, cisplatin and S-1 for advanced gastric cancer (KDOG0601). *Oncology.* (2008) 75(1–2):1–7. doi: 10.1159/000151613
54. Fushida S, Fujimura T, Oyama K, Yagi Y, Kinoshita J, Ohta T. Feasibility and efficacy of preoperative chemotherapy with docetaxel, cisplatin and S-1 in gastric cancer patients with para-aortic lymph node metastases. *Anti-cancer Drugs.* (2009) 20:752–6. doi: 10.1097/CAD.0b013e32832ec02b
55. Sato Y, Takayama T, Sagawa T, Takahashi Y, Ohnuma H, Okubo S, et al. Phase II study of S-1, docetaxel and cisplatin combination chemotherapy in patients with unresectable metastatic gastric cancer. *Cancer Chemotherap Pharmacol.* (2010) 66:721–8. doi: 10.1007/s00280-009-1215-2
56. Shitara K, Ohtsu A. Advances in systemic therapy for metastatic or advanced gastric cancer. *J Natl Comp Cancer Netw.* (2016) 14:1313–20. doi: 10.6004/jnccn.2016.0138
57. Sautner T, Hofbauer F, Depisch D, Schiessel R, Jakesz R. Adjuvant intraperitoneal cisplatin chemotherapy does not improve long-term survival after surgery for advanced gastric cancer. *J Clin Oncol.* (1994) 12:970–4. doi: 10.1200/JCO.1994.12.5.970
58. Shitara K. Chemotherapy for advanced gastric cancer: future perspective in Japan. *Gastric Cancer.* (2017) 20(Suppl 1):102–10. doi: 10.1007/s10120-016-0648-7
59. Yamaguchi H, Kitayama J, Ishigami H, Emoto S, Yamashita H, Watanabe T. A phase 2 trial of intravenous and intraperitoneal paclitaxel combined with S-1 for treatment of gastric cancer with macroscopic peritoneal metastasis. *Cancer.* (2013) 119:3354–8. doi: 10.1002/cncr.28204
60. Kitayama J, Ishigami H, Yamaguchi H, Yamashita H, Emoto S, Kaisaki S, et al. Salvage gastrectomy after intravenous and intraperitoneal paclitaxel (PTX) administration with oral S-1 for peritoneal dissemination of advanced gastric cancer with malignant ascites. *Ann Surg Oncol.* (2014) 21:539–46. doi: 10.1245/s10434-013-3208-y
61. Desiderio J, Chao J, Melstrom L, Warner S, Tozzi F, Fong Y, et al. The 30-year experience-A meta-analysis of randomised and high-quality non-randomised studies of hyperthermic intraperitoneal chemotherapy in the treatment of gastric cancer. *Eur J Cancer.* (2017) 79:1–14. doi: 10.1016/j.ejca.2017.03.030
62. Ishigami H, Fujiwara Y, Fukushima R, Nashimoto A, Yabusaki H, Imano M, et al. Phase III Trial Comparing intraperitoneal and intravenous paclitaxel plus S-1 versus cisplatin Plus S-1 in patients with gastric cancer with peritoneal metastasis: PHOENIX-GC Trial. *J Clin Oncol.* (2018) 36:1922–9. doi: 10.1200/JCO.2018.77.8613
63. Glehen O, Gilly FN, Arvieux C, Cotte E, Boutitie F, Mansvelt B, et al. Peritoneal carcinomatosis from gastric cancer: a multi-institutional study of 159 patients treated by cytoreductive surgery combined with perioperative intraperitoneal chemotherapy. *Ann Surg Oncol.* (2010) 17:2370–7. doi: 10.1245/s10434-010-1039-7
64. Sugarbaker PH. Cytoreductive surgery and hyperthermic intraperitoneal chemotherapy in the management of gastrointestinal cancers with peritoneal metastases: progress toward a new standard of care. *Cancer Treat Rev.* (2016) 48:42–9. doi: 10.1016/j.ctrv.2016.06.007
65. Cheon SH, Rha SY, Jeung HC, Im CK, Kim SH, Kim HR, et al. Survival benefit of combined curative resection of the stomach (D2 resection) and liver in gastric cancer patients with liver metastases. *Ann Oncol.* (2008) 19:1146–53. doi: 10.1093/annonc/mdn026
66. Sakamoto Y, Sano T, Shimada K, Esaki M, Saka M, Fukagawa T, et al. Favorable indications for hepatectomy in patients with liver metastasis from gastric cancer. *J Surg Oncol.* (2007) 95:534–9. doi: 10.1002/jso.20739
67. Guner A, Son T, Cho I, Kwon IG, An JY, Kim H-I, et al. Liver-directed treatments for liver metastasis from gastric adenocarcinoma: comparison between liver resection and radiofrequency ablation. *Gastric Cancer.* (2016) 19:951–60. doi: 10.1007/s10120-015-0522-z
68. Ito S, Sano T, Mizusawa J, Takahari D, Katayama H, Katai H, et al. A phase II study of preoperative chemotherapy with docetaxel, cisplatin, and S-1 followed by gastrectomy with D2 plus para-aortic lymph node dissection for gastric cancer with extensive lymph node metastasis: JCOG1002. *Gastric Cancer.* (2017) 20:322–31. doi: 10.1007/s10120-016-0619-z
69. Park IH, Kim SY, Kim YW, Ryu KW, Lee JH, Lee JS, et al. Clinical characteristics and treatment outcomes of gastric cancer patients with isolated para-aortic lymph node involvement. *Cancer Chemotherap Pharmacol.* (2011) 67:127–36. doi: 10.1007/s00280-010-1296-y

70. Nomura E, Sasako M, Yamamoto S, Sano T, Tsujinaka T, Kinoshita T, et al. Risk factors for para-aortic lymph node metastasis of gastric cancer from a randomized controlled trial of JCOG9501. *Jpn J Clin Oncol.* (2007) 37:429–33. doi: 10.1093/jjco/hym067
71. Roviello F, Pedrazzani C, Marrelli D, Di Leo A, Caruso S, Giacopuzzi S, et al. Super-extended (D3) lymphadenectomy in advanced gastric cancer. *Eur J Surg Oncol.* (2010) 36:439–46. doi: 10.1016/j.ejso.2010.03.008
72. Yoshikawa T, Sasako M, Yamamoto S, Sano T, Imamura H, Fujitani K, et al. Phase II study of neoadjuvant chemotherapy and extended surgery for locally advanced gastric cancer. *Br J Surg.* (2009) 96:1015–22. doi: 10.1002/bjs.6665
73. Tsuburaya A, Mizusawa J, Tanaka Y, Fukushima N, Nashimoto A, Sasako M. Neoadjuvant chemotherapy with S-1 and cisplatin followed by D2 gastrectomy with para-aortic lymph node dissection for gastric cancer with extensive lymph node metastasis. *Br J Surg.* (2014) 101:653–60. doi: 10.1002/bjs.9484
74. Koizumi W, Nakayama N, Tanabe S, Sasaki T, Higuchi K, Nishimura K, et al. A multicenter phase II study of combined chemotherapy with docetaxel, cisplatin, and S-1 in patients with unresectable or recurrent gastric cancer (KDOG 0601). *Cancer Chemotherap Pharmacol.* (2012) 69:407–13. doi: 10.1007/s00280-011-1701-1
75. Martin-Romano P, Sola JJ, Diaz-Gonzalez JA, Chopitea A, Iragorri Y, Martinez-Regueira F, et al. Role of histological regression grade after two neoadjuvant approaches with or without radiotherapy in locally advanced gastric cancer. *Br J Cancer.* (2016) 115:655–63. doi: 10.1038/bjc.2016.252
76. Dong HM, Wang Q, Wang WL, Wang G, Li XK, Li GD, et al. A clinical analysis of systemic chemotherapy combined with radiotherapy for advanced gastric cancer. *Medicine.* (2018) 97:e10786. doi: 10.1097/MD.0000000000010786
77. Ustaalioglu BBO, Bilici A, Tilki M, Surmelioglu A, Erkol B, Figen M, et al. Capecitabine-cisplatin versus 5-fluorouracil/leucovorin in combination with radiotherapy for adjuvant therapy of lymph node positive locally advanced gastric cancer. *J Cancer Res Therap.* (2018) 14(Supplement):S736–41. doi: 10.4103/0973-1482.183548
78. Raut CP, Posner M, Desai J, Morgan JA, George S, Zahrieh D, et al. Surgical management of advanced gastrointestinal stromal tumors after treatment with targeted systemic therapy using kinase inhibitors. *J Clin Oncol.* (2006) 24:2325–31. doi: 10.1200/JCO.2005.05.3439
79. Yoshikawa T, Tanabe K, Nishikawa K, Ito Y, Matsui T, Kimura Y, et al. Induction of a pathological complete response by four courses of neoadjuvant chemotherapy for gastric cancer: early results of the randomized phase II COMPASS trial. *Ann Surg Oncol.* (2014) 21:213–9. doi: 10.1245/s10434-013-3055-x
80. Koizumi W, Kim YH, Fujii M, Kim HK, Imamura H, Lee KH, et al. Addition of docetaxel to S-1 without platinum prolongs survival of patients with advanced gastric cancer: a randomized study (START). *J Cancer Res Clin Oncol.* (2014) 140:319–28. doi: 10.1007/s00432-013-1563-5
81. Kodera Y, Ito S, Mochizuki Y, Ohashi N, Tanaka C, Kobayashi D, et al. Long-term follow up of patients who were positive for peritoneal lavage cytology: final report from the CCOG0301 study. *Gastric Cancer.* (2012) 15:335–7. doi: 10.1007/s10120-012-0156-3
82. Shin SJ, Chun SH, Kim KO, Kim MK, Lee KH, Hyun MS, et al. The efficacy of paclitaxel and cisplatin combination chemotherapy for the treatment of metastatic or recurrent gastric cancer: a multicenter phase II study. *Korean J Int Med.* (2005) 20:135–40. doi: 10.3904/kjim.2005.20.2.135
83. Nakai T, Okuno K, Kitaguchi H, Ishikawa H, Yamasaki M. Unresectable colorectal liver metastases: the safety and efficacy of conversion therapy using hepatic arterial infusion immunochemotherapy with 5-fluorouracil and polyethylene glycol-interferon alpha-2a. *World J Surg.* (2013) 37:1919–26. doi: 10.1007/s00268-013-2043-4
84. Bott MJ, Cools-Lartigue J, Tan KS, Dycoco J, Bains MS, Downey RJ, et al. Safety and feasibility of lung resection after immunotherapy for metastatic or unresectable tumors. *Ann Thorac Surg.* (2018) 106:178–83. doi: 10.1016/j.athoracsur.2018.02.030

14

m^{6}A RNA Methylation Regulators Contribute to Malignant Progression and have Clinical Prognostic Impact in Gastric Cancer

Yunshu Su [1], Jinqi Huang [2] and Jichang Hu [3]*

[1] Department of Thoracic Surgery, Renmin Hospital of Wuhan University, Wuhan, China, [2] Division of Cardiothoracic Surgery, Central Hospital of EnShi Tujia and Miao Autonomous Prefecture, EnShi Clinical College of Wuhan University, EnShi, China, [3] Department of Pathology, Renmin Hospital of Wuhan University, Wuhan, China

***Correspondence:**
Jichang Hu
hujichang@whu.edu.cn

N6-methyladenosine (m^{6}A) is the most common form of mRNA modification, and is dynamically regulated by the m^{6}A RNA methylation regulators. However, little is known about m^{6}A in gastric cancer. The aim of this work is to investigate the effects of m^{6}A RNA methylation regulators in gastric cancer. Here, we found that most of the 13 main m^{6}A RNA methylation regulators are higher expressed in 375 patients with gastric cancer. We identified two subgroups of gastric cancer (cluster1 and 2) by applying consensus clustering to m^{6}A RNA methylation regulators. Compared with the cluster1 subgroup, the cluster2 subgroup correlates with a poorer prognosis, and most of the 13 main m^{6}A RNA methylation regulators are higher expressed in cluster2. Moreover, the cancer-specific pathways are also significantly enriched in the cluster2 subgroup. This finding indicates that m^{6}A RNA methylation regulators are closely associated with gastric cancer. Based on this finding, we derived a risk signature, using 3 m^{6}A RNA methylation regulators (FTO, RBM15, ALKBH5), that is not only an independent prognostic marker but can also predict the clinicopathological features of gastric cancer. Moreover, FTO is higher expressed in high risk scores subtype in gastric cancer. Thus, this first finding provide us clues to understand epigenetic modification of RNA in gastric cancer.

Keywords: gastric cancer, m^{6}A, TCGA, epigenetic modification, FTO

INTRODUCTION

N6-methyladenosine (m^{6}A) is a methylation modification that can occur on RNA adenine (A) (1). Of the 171 known RNA post-transcriptional modifications (2), m^{6}A is one of the most abundant modifications in most eukaryotic mRNA and lncRNA, accounting for 0.1–0.4% of adenylate and 50% of total ribonucleotides in mammalian RNA (3, 4). In addition to the extensive m^{6}A modification in plants and vertebrates, this modification has also been found in single-celled organisms such as bacteria and yeast (5, 6). m^{6}A modification mainly occurred in the common sequence of RRACH (R = G or A, H = A, C, or U) (7, 8). Through high throughput sequencing, it was found that m^{6}A was not randomly distributed.

Instead, it was aggregated in the stop codon, 3′ untranslated region (3′UTR), and internal exons (9–11), and more were found in the precursor mRNA (12). More and more studies have shown that m^6A modification plays an important role in the occurrence and development of human complex diseases, especially in the occurrence and development of cancer (13–15).

Through the study of m^6A related proteins, it is found that m^6A methylation is a dynamic reversible process (16), which is composed of methyltransferase complex (writers), demethylase (erasers), and function manager (readers) (17). Writers is a process of "writing" methylated modifications into RNA, that is, mediating the process of methylated modification of RNA, including METTL3, METTL14, KIAA1429, WTAP, RBM15, and ZC3H13 (18).Erasers can "erase" the RNA methylation modification signal, that is, mediating the demethylation process of RNA, including FTO and ALKBH5 (19, 20). Readers is responsible for "reading" RNA methylated information and participating in the translation and degradation of downstream RNA, including YTHDC1, YTHDC2, YTHDF1, YTHDF2, and HNRNPC (21). m^6A, under the influence of the "writer," adds methyl groups to RNA, and recognizes those m^6A-modified RNAs through different "readers" to produce different functions, including RNA processing, nuclear export, translation, and decay. Finally, relying on the role of "Erasers," the process of m^6A modification becomes dynamic and reversible, thereby functioning to regulate the expression of various genes (14).

Due to RNA regulation is closely related to human diseases, as one of the most abundant internal modifications in mammalian cells, m^6A methylation modification has been confirmed with various diseases such as obesity (22), diabetes (23), infertility (24), tumor (25), and neuronal diseases (26). However, little is known about m^6A in gastric cancer. In this study, we systematically analyzed the expression of 13 widely reported m^6A RNA regulators in 375 gastric cancer with RNA sequencing data from The Cancer Genome Atlas (TCGA) datasets, as well as the association between clinicopathological characteristics.

MATERIALS AND METHODS

Data Acquisition

The RNA-seq transcriptome data and corresponding clinical information of STAD cohort were downloaded from TCGA (https://cancergenome.nih.gov/) data portal (level 3). All mRNASeq gene expression data are downloaded through the R package "TCGA-Assembler."

Selection of m^6A RNA Methylation Regulators

There are 13 genes in the m^6A RNA methylation regulator. We extracted the expression matrix of these 13 genes and the clinical information of the sample. The extracted information is used for subsequent bioinformatics analysis.

Bioinformatic Analysis

To investigate the function of m^6A RNA methylation regulators in gastric cancer, we used Limma package to analyze the expression of 13 genes in 375 tumor patients and 32 normal gastric tissue. The upper tree diagram represents clustering results for different samples from different experimental groups, and the left tree shows cluster analysis results for different genes from different samples. Next, we used a vioplot to visualize the expression of 13 genes in 375 tumor patients and 32 normal gastric tissue. The white point represents the median Q2 (half of the data is greater than the median, above it, and the other half is less than the median, below it). The black rectangle is the range from the lower quartile to the upper quartile. The upper edge of the rectangle is the upper quartile Q3, which means that one quarter of the data is larger than the upper quartile, and the lower edge is the lower quad. The quantile Q1 represents that one quarter of the data is less than the lower quartile. The length of the interquartile range IQR (the upper quartile and the lower quadrant) represents the dispersion and symmetry of the non-abnormal data. The length is scattered and the short is concentrated. The black line running through the violin map represents the minimum non-abnormal value min. To the interval of the maximum non-outlier max, the lower and upper limits represent the upper and lower limits, respectively, and the range is beyond the abnormal data; the outer shape of the black rectangle is the kernel density estimation, the length of the vertical axis of the graph represents the degree of data dispersion, and the length of the horizontal axis represents the Data distribution of an ordinate position.

Next, we removed 32 normal tissue samples and grouped 375 cancer tissues using the ConsensusClusterPlus package, using PCA to verify the results of the grouping. GO and KEGG analysis of genes with different expression of cluster2 relative to cluster1 using GOplot package. Finally, we use the survival package to analyze the survival of the cluster, and we performed univariate Cox regression analyses of their expression in the TCGA dataset.

Statistical Analyses

One-way ANOVA was used to compare the expression level of 13 genes in 375 tumor patients and 32 normal gastric tissue in TCGA dataset, and *t*-tests were used to compare the expression levels in gastric cancer for age, gender, stage, T status, M status, and N status. Overall survival (OS) is defined as the interval from the date of diagnosis to the date of death. Before constructing the scoring model, we first obtain the optimal cut-off value of each risk score in the training group through the "survminer" package in the software, and divide the cells into high and low groups according to the best cutoff value, and was represented by 1.0. Cox regression analysis was used to evaluate the association between risk score and OS, in which age and sex were used as covariates. The missing data is processed by list deletion, and if any single value is missing, the entire sample is excluded from the analysis. Using R version 3.5 for all statistical analysis, $P < 0.05$ was statistically significant.

RESULTS

The Landscape of m^6A RNA Methylation Regulators in Gastric Cancer

Considering the important biological functions of each m^6A RNA methylation regulator in tumorigenesis and development.

We first compare the expression level of 13 m^{6}A RNA methylation regulators in 375 gastric cancer tissues and 32 normal gastric tissue in TCGA dataset. Compared with normal gastric tissue, gastric cancer patients generally contain a higher proportion of METTL3, METTL14, WTAP, KIAA1429, RBM15, ZC3H13, YTHDC1, YTHDC2, YTHDF1, YTHDF2, HNRNPC, and FTO (**Figures 1A,B**). We speculate that the change of m^{6}A RNA methylation regulators ratio may be an intrinsic feature that can characterize individual differences, **Figure 1C** showed the proportion of different m^{6}A RNA methylation regulators is weakly to moderately correlated. The relationship between the 13 m^{6}A RNA methylation regulators is positively correlated, and the YTHDF2 gene and the RBM15 gene are most relevant. When the YTHDF2 gene is up-regulated, the RBM15 gene is most likely to be up-regulated (**Figure 1C**). We also systematically investigated the relationships between each individual m^{6}A RNA methylation regulator and the pathological features of gastric cancer, including age, gender, grades, stage status, T status, M status, and N status, and found there is relationship between m^{6}A RNA methylation regulator and pathological features of gastric cancer (**Figure 1D**).

Consensus Clustering of m^{6}A RNA Methylation Regulators Identified Two Clusters of Gastric Cancer

Next, we removed 32 normal gastric tissue samples and grouped 375 cancer tissues using the ConsensusClusterPlus package. Based on the expression similarity of m^{6}A RNA methylation regulators, $k = 3$ seemed has smaller CDF value in the TCGA datasets (**Figures 2B,C**), however, after being divided into three groups, the correlation between the groups is high, and there is a small number of samples. Therefore, we are divided into two groups (**Figure 2A**). In order to judge whether our classification is correct, we will analyze the two subclasses by PCA, and the results show cluster 1 can gathered together and cluster 2 can also be gathered together (**Figure 2D**). These results indicate that the results of our classification by m^{6}A RNA methylation regulators are correct.

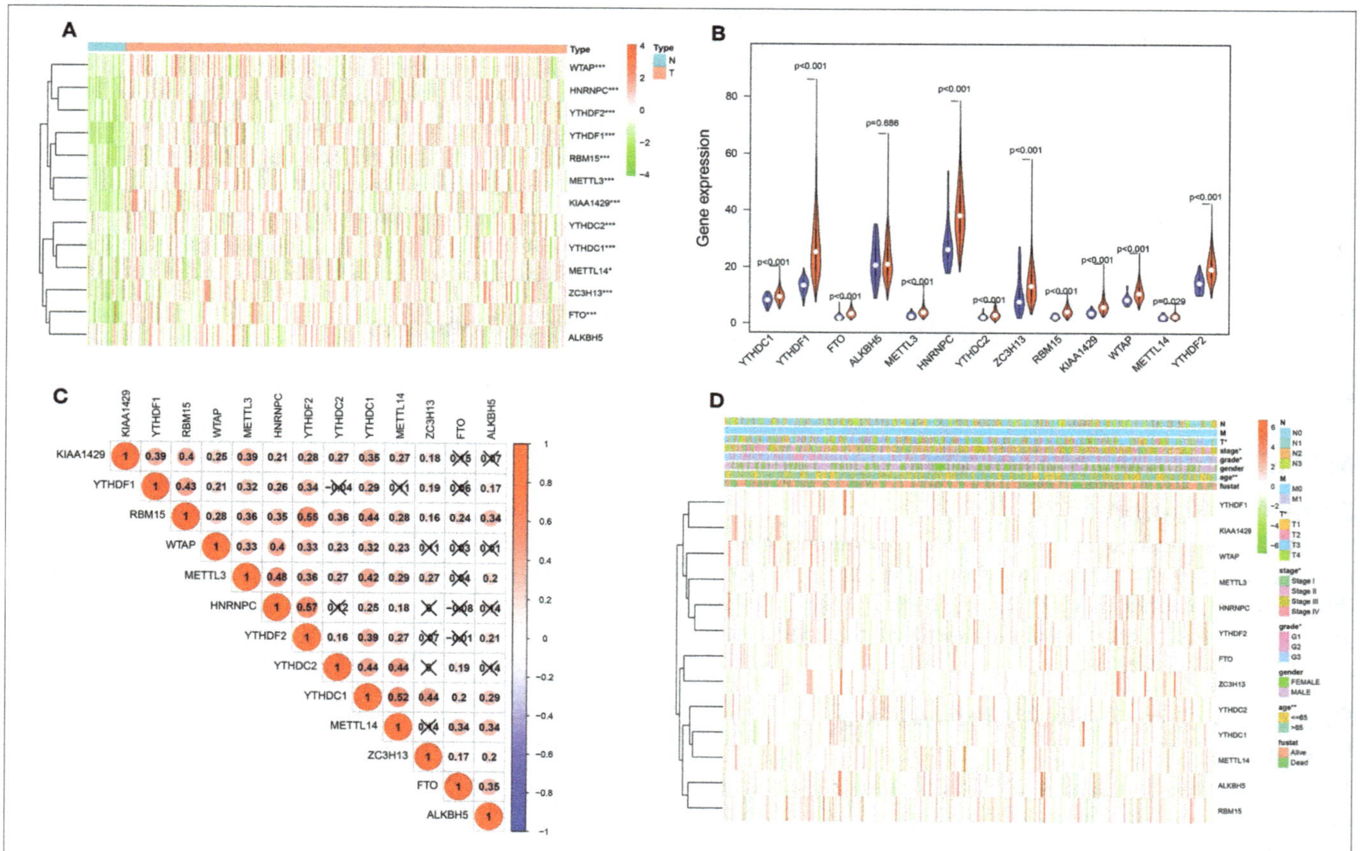

FIGURE 1 | The landscape of m^{6}A RNA methylation regulators in gastric cancer. **(A)** The expression levels of 13 m^{6}A RNA methylation regulators in gastric cancer. The higher or lower the expression, the darker the color (red is up-regulated and green is down-regulated). The upper tree diagram represents clustering results for different samples from different experimental groups, and the left tree shows cluster analysis results for different genes from different samples. **(B)** Vioplot visualizing the differentially m^{6}A RNA methylation regulators in gastric cancer (assume blue is normal and red is gastric cancer). **(C)** Spearman correlation analysis of the 13 m^{6}A modification regulators in gastric cancer. **(D)** Expression of m^{6}A modification regulators in gastric cancer with different clinicopathological features. $^*P < 0.05$, $^{**}P < 0.01$, and $^{***}P < 0.001$.

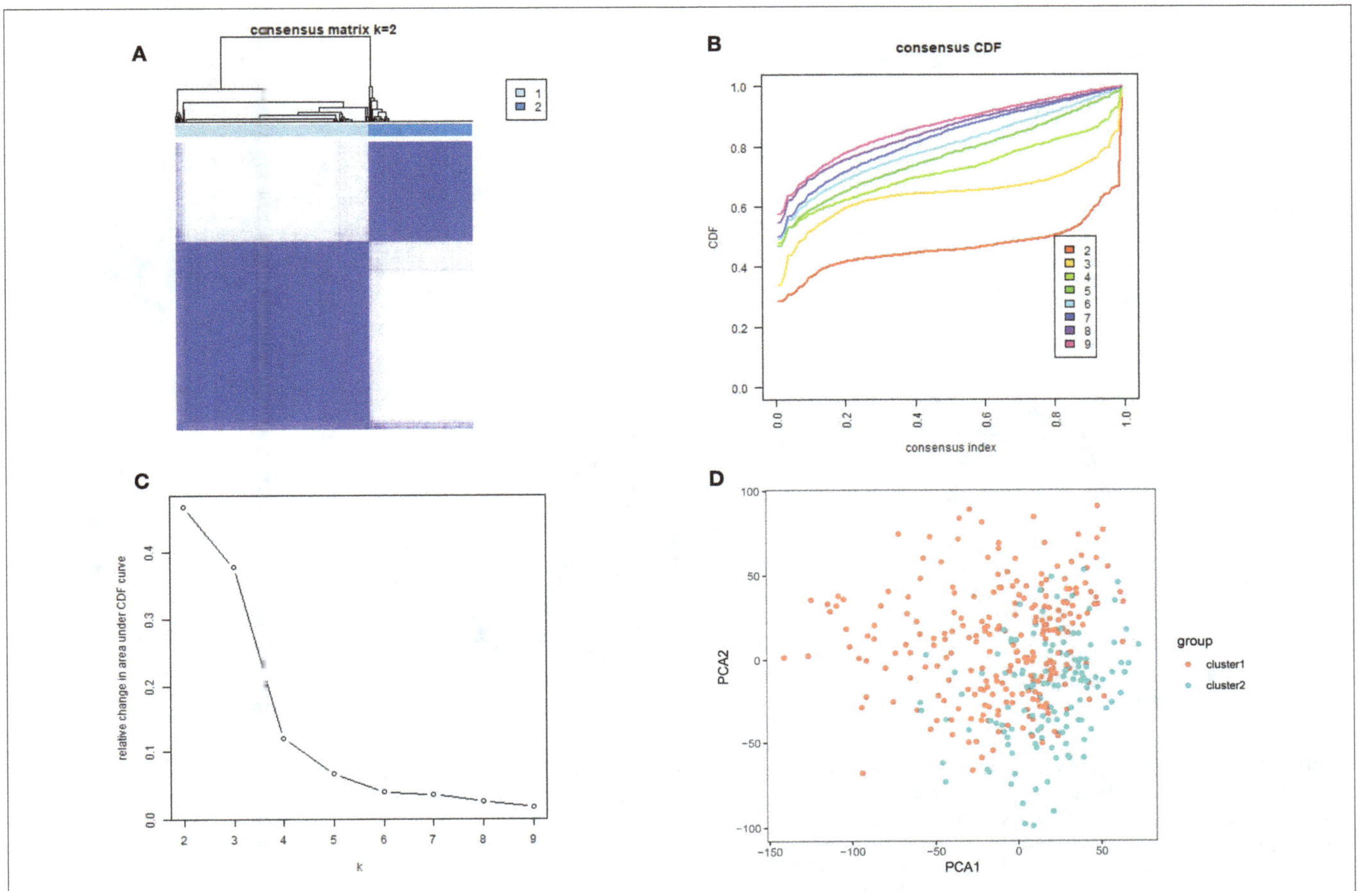

FIGURE 2 | Identification of consensus clusters by m^{6}A RNA methylation regulators. **(A)** Consensus clustering matrix for $k = 2$; **(B)** consensus clustering cumulative distribution function (CDF) for $k = 2$–9; **(C)** relative change in area under CDF curve for $k = 2$–9; **(D)** principal component analysis of the total RNA expression profile in the TCGA dataset. Gastric cancer in the cluster1 subgroup are marked with red, and the cluster2 subgroup are marked with blue.

Categories Identified by Consensus Clustering Are Closely Correlated to Clinical Outcomes and Clinicopathological Features

To better understand the clustering result and clinical outcomes and clinicopathological features, we analyzed the clustering result and OS curves for 375 gastric cancer patients. We found the cluster 2 subgroup has a significantly shorter OS than the cluster 1 subgroup (**Figure 3A**). Moreover, we found that most of m^{6}A RNA methylation regulators have high expression in cluster 2 subgroup. Compare with the cluster 1 subgroup, the cluster 2 subgroup is significantly correlated with older age at diagnosis at diagnosis, higher grade, higher stage, higher T status, higher M status, and higher N status (**Figure 3B**). According to the evidence, the clustering result was closely correlated to the malignancy of the gastric cancer. To better understand the clustering result and their function, we analyzed GO and KEGG analysis of genes with different expression of cluster2 relative to cluster1 using GOplot package. Go results indicated that upregulated genes are enriched in malignancy-related biological processes, including extracellular structure organization, extracellular matrix organization, humoral immune response, humoral immune response mediated by circulating immunoglobulin, and complement activation, classical pathway (**Figures 3C,D**). KEGG results indicated that upregulated genes are enriched in cell cycle, ras signaling pathway and platinum drug resistance (**Figures 3E,F**).

Prognostic Value of Risk Signature and m^{6}A RNA Methylation Regulators

To better understand the prognostic role of m^{6}A RNA methylation regulators in gastric cancer, we performed a univariate Cox regression analysis on the expression levels in the TCGA dataset. The results indicated that high expression of FTO (HR = 1.15, 95% CI = 1.02–1.29), HNRNPC (HR = 1.09, 95% CI = 1.02–1.18), YTHDC2 (HR = 1.22, 95% CI = 1.07–1.42), and WTAP (HR = 1.18, 95% CI = 1.02–1.33) have a worse survival in patients with gastric cancer. In contrast, high expression of ALKBH5 (HR = 0.94, 95% CI = 0.89–0.98) and RBM15 (HR =

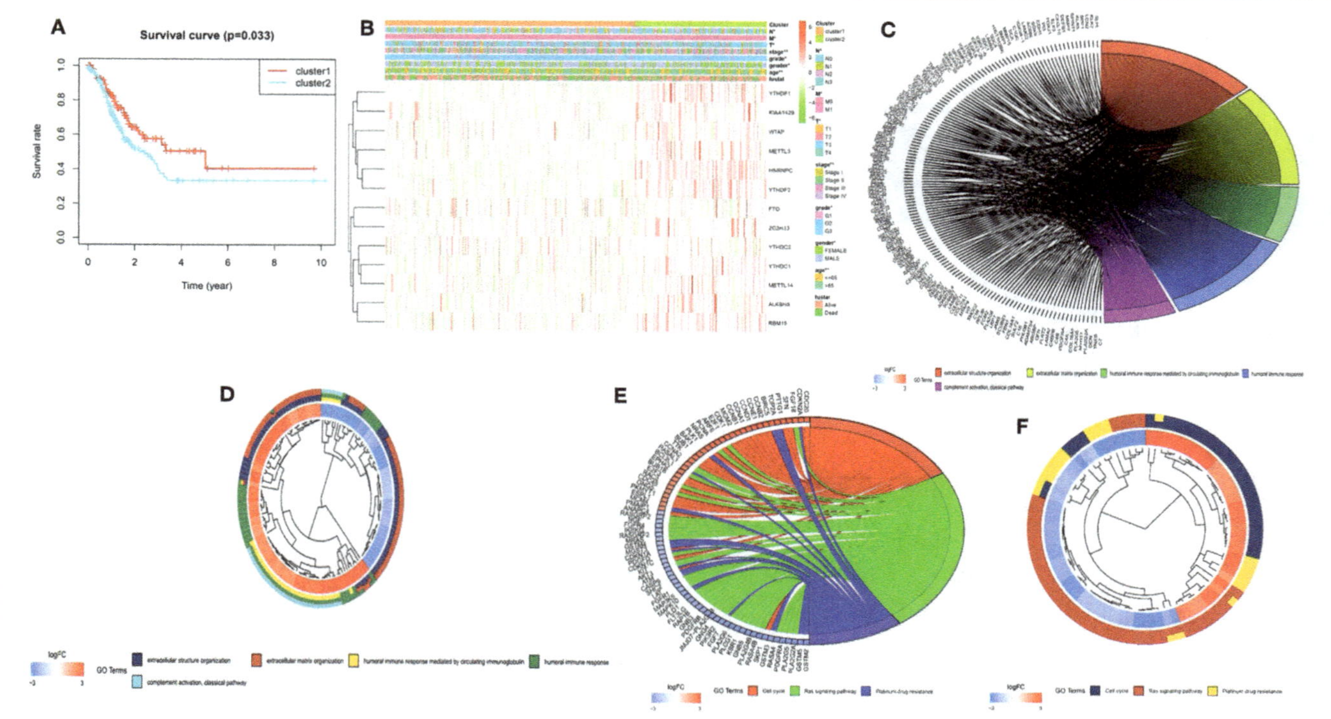

FIGURE 3 | Differential clinicopathological features and overall survival of gastric cancer in the cluster 1/2 subgroups. **(A)** Kaplan–Meier overall survival (OS) curves for 375 TCGA gastric cancer patients. Gastric cancer patients in the cluster1 subgroup are marked with red, and the cluster2 subgroup are marked with blue. **(B)** Heatmap and clinicopathologic features of the two clusters (cluster1/2) defined by the m^{6}A RNA methylation regulators consensus expression. The higher or lower the expression, the darker the color (red is up-regulated and green is down-regulated). The upper tree diagram represents clustering results for different samples from different experimental groups, and the left tree shows cluster analysis results for different genes from different samples. **(C–F)** Functional annotation of the genes with higher expression in the clusters 2 subgroup using GO terms of biological processes **(C,D)** and KEGG pathway **(E,F)**. $^*P < 0.05$, $^{**}P < 0.01$.

0.83, 95% CI = 0.74–0.93), have a better survival in patients with gastric cancer (**Figure 4A**).

In order to predict the clinical outcomes of gastric cancer with m^{6}A RNA methylation regulators, we applied the least absolute shrinkage and selection operator (LASSO) Cox regression algorithm to the 13 genes in the TCGA dataset. Three genes (FTO, ALKBH5, and RBM15) were selected to build the risk signature based on the minimum criteria, and the coefficients obtained from the LASSO algorithm were used to calculate the risk score for TCGA dataset (**Figures 4B,C**). To investigate the prognostic role of the three-gene risk signature, we separated the gastric cancer patients in TCGA dataset into low and high-risk groups based on the median risk score, the results indicated that high-risk group have a worse survival in patients with gastric cancer (**Figure 4D**).

Prognostic Risk Scores Showed Strong Associations With Clinicopathological Features in Gastric Cancer

In order to better understand the clinical outcomes of gastric cancer with high-risk groups, we systematically investigated the relationships between the three selected m^{6}A RNA methylation regulators in high risk group and low risk group patients in the TCGA dataset and the pathological features of gastric cancer, including age, stage status, T status, M status, and N status, and found there is relationship between three selected m^{6}A RNA methylation regulators in high risk group and low risk group patients and pathological features of gastric cancer (**Figure 5A**). Moreover, compare with low risk group patients, gastric cancer patients generally contain a higher proportion of FTO, lower proportion of ALKBH5 and RBM15 in the high risk group (**Figure 5A**).

To better understand the relationships between risk scores and gastric cancer patients, firstly, we do a ROC curve to predict risk scores and 3-year survival rates for gastric cancer patients, the results indicated that the risk score can predict 3-year survival rates for gastric cancer patients (AUC = 0.781) (**Figure 5B**). Next, we performed univariate and multivariate Cox regression analyses for the TCGA dataset to determine whether the risk signature is an independent prognostic indicator. Both the univariate and multivariate Cox regression analyses results indicated that the risk score, age, stage status, T status, M status, and N status were all correlated with the OS. As the risk score, age, stage status, T status, M status, and N status increases, the risk increases (**Figures 5C,D**). According to the evidence, prognostic risk scores showed strong associations with clinicopathological features in gastric cancer, and FTO was correlated with the malignancy of gastric cancer.

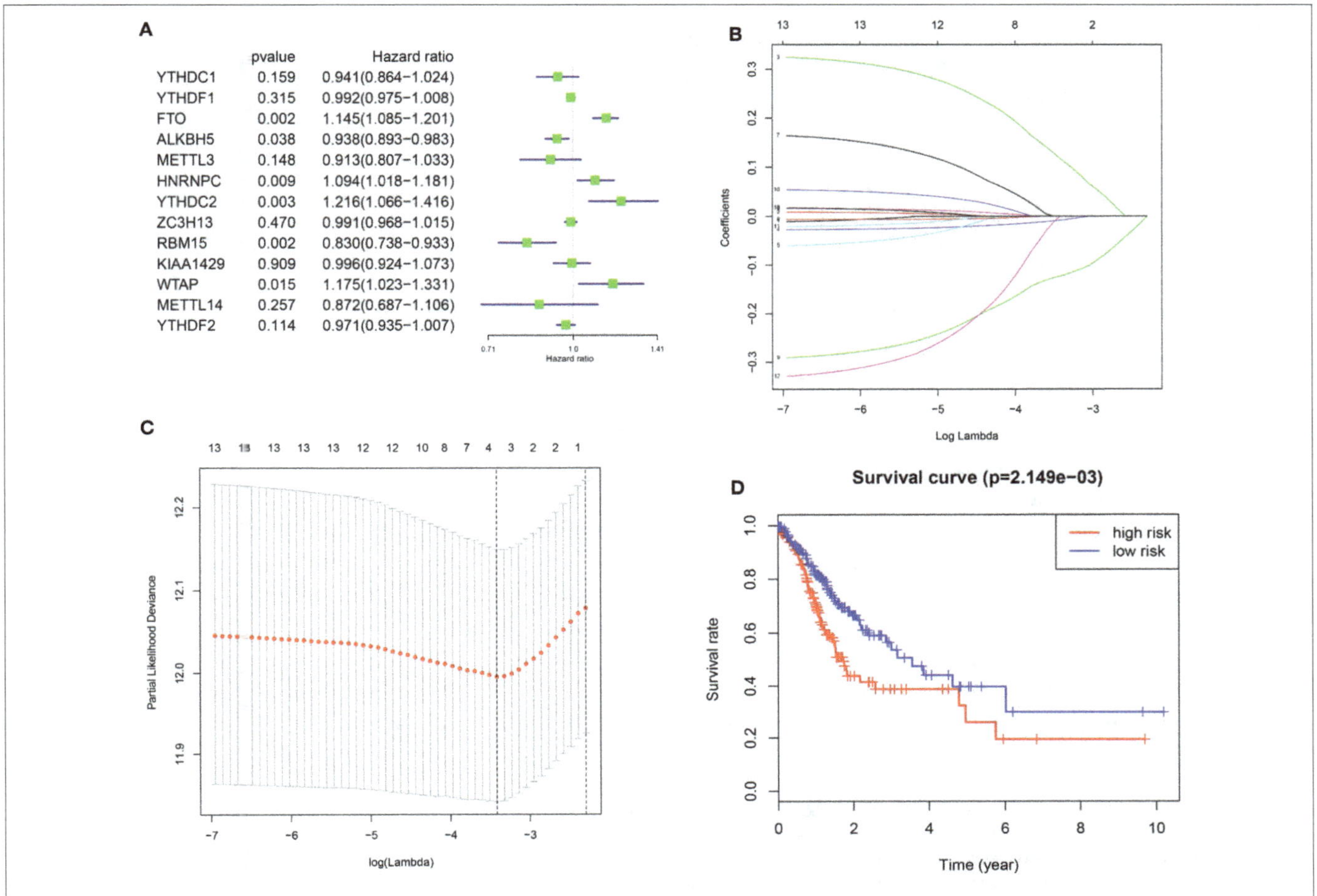

FIGURE 4 | Risk signature with three m^{6}A RNA methylation regulators. **(A)** The process of building the signature containing 13 m^{6}A RNA methylation regulators. The hazard ratios (HR), 95% confidence intervals (CI) calculated by univariate Cox regression. **(B,C)** The coefficients calculated by multivariate Cox regression using LASSO are shown. **(D)** Kaplan–Meier overall survival (OS) curves for patients in the TCGA datasets assigned to high and low risk groups based on the risk score.

FTO Showed High Expression in Human Tissues

To better understand FTO in human tissues, we used GTEx (Genotype-tissue expression) dataset to know FTO expression differs among different tissues and individuals. The GTEx database contains more than 7,000 autopsy samples from 449 pre-healthy human donors, covering 44 organizations (42 different tissue types), including 31 solid organ tissues, 10 brain regions, whole blood, and 2 from donor blood and skin cell lines. The results indicated higher of FTO expression was found in the 31 solid organ tissues (**Figure 6D**) and in female and male (**Figures 6A,B**). In most female and male tissues, there is no difference in the expression of FTO, and there were significantly differences in breast, colon, spleen, and thyroid (**Figure 6C**).

DISCUSSION

Gastric cancer is the fifth largest malignant tumor in the world, which is a serious threat to human health and life safety (27). Surgery is the first choice for the treatment of gastric cancer, combined with adjuvant chemotherapy, radiotherapy, targeted drugs, and immunotherapy (28). Although, the global incidence of gastric cancer has declined significantly over the past few decades, the 5-year survival rate of gastric cancer is usually <30%, and there are still many key issues that remain unresolved (29). The occurrence and development of gastric cancer is very complicated. It is a multi-factor, multi-step complex process involving external environmental factors, diet, living habits, and also involves tissue cell differentiation, genetic changes, cell cycle changes, metabolism, gene expression, molecular interaction, signal transduction pathway changes, it is also related to host immune status, homeostasis and other factors (30). Although targeted therapy can prolong the survival of patients, tumor drug resistance and economic burden are considerable problems in clinical practice (31). Therefore, exploring the molecular mechanisms of gastric cancer pathogenesis and new therapeutic targets remains a challenging issue.

m^{6}A, as a member of RNA epigenetic modification families, is not "good or bad" based on the current understanding of m^{6}A and tumor. It can promote or inhibit tumor cells mainly

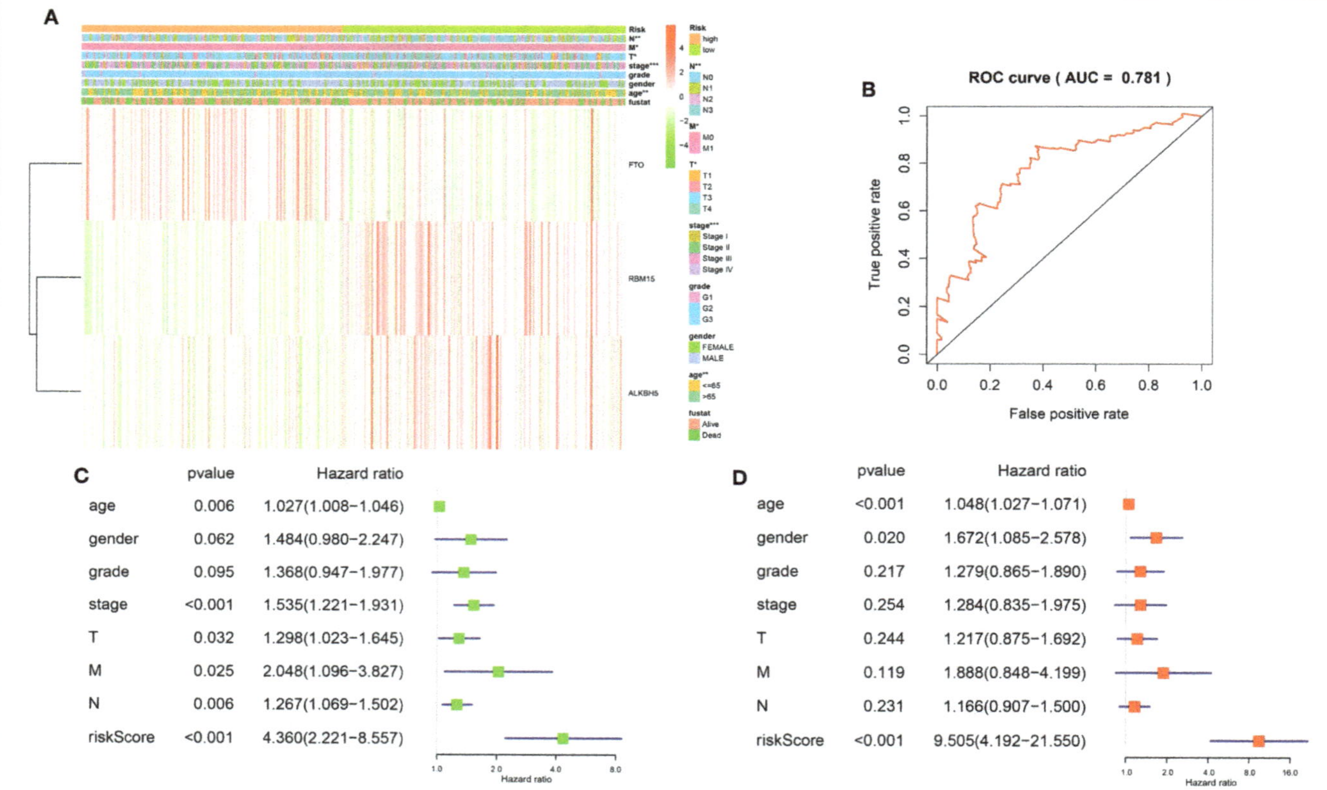

FIGURE 5 | Relationship between the risk score, clinicopathological features, and clusters subgroups. **(A)** The heatmap shows the expression levels of the three m^{6}A RNA methylation regulators in low and high risk gastric cancer patients. The distribution of clinicopathological features was compared between the low- and high-risk groups. **(B)** ROC curves showed the predictive efficiency of the risk signature. **(C)** Univariate Cox regression analyses of the association between clinicopathological factors (including the risk score) and overall survival of patients in the TCGA datasets. **(D)** Multivariate Cox regression analyses of the association between clinicopathological factors (including the risk score) and overall survival of patients in the TCGA datasets. **P* < 0.05, ***P* < 0.01, and ****P* < 0.001.

by regulating the mRNA expression of related oncogenes or tumor suppressor genes. The m^{6}A methylation site appeared in the nuclear RNA under the action of Writers. The m^{6}A methylation site of RNA in the nucleus can also be erased under the action of erasers. Subsequently, in the further processing of the nuclear RNA, the readers (reading protein) in the nucleus will bind to the m^{6}A methylated site; when the mature RNA comes out of the nucleus, there will still be some readers outside the nucleus will bind to its m^{6}A site. It is worth noting that different Reader binding to m^{6}A will produce different biological effects (14). The methylation level of m^{6}A is closely related to the expression level of intracellular writing and erasing genes, while the protein molecules that read gene expression are combined with the m^{6}A methylation site to perform a series of biological functions (32). Therefore, in tumors, both m^{6}A-related genes and protein expression levels may become potential markers for tumor molecular diagnosis, and will also provide new targets for the development of clinical molecular targeted therapeutic drugs.

This study attempted to the effects of m^{6}A RNA methylation regulators in gastric cancer, and found m^{6}A RNA methylation regulators was closely associated with pathological features of gastric cancer. We identified two subgroups of gastric cancer by applying consensus clustering to m^{6}A RNA methylation regulators, and the cluster 2 subgroup correlates with a poorer prognosis. In addition, we derived a risk signature by using 3 m^{6}A RNA methylation regulators. The risk score is not only an independent prognostic marker but can also predict the clinicopathological features of gastric cancer. Moreover, FTO is higher expressed in high risk scores subtype in gastric cancer. According to the evidence, FTO was correlated with the malignancy of gastric cancer.

FTO was originally reported as a demethylase for N3-methylthymidine in single-stranded DNA and for N3-methyluridine in single-stranded RNA *in vitro*. Depletion of FTO induces significant increase in total m6A levels of polyadenylated RNA. As FTO oxidizes m6A to A, it generates N6-hydroxymethyladenosine (hm6A) as an intermediate product, and N6-formyladenosine (f6A) as a further oxidized product. The potential function of these oxidized labile intermediates needs further exploration (17). Li et al. found that in acute myeloid leukemia (AML), high expression of FTO can reduce the level of m^{6}A methylation in the mRNA of ASB2 and RARA genes, which leads to the occurrence and development of AML, and it was found that high expression of FTO could

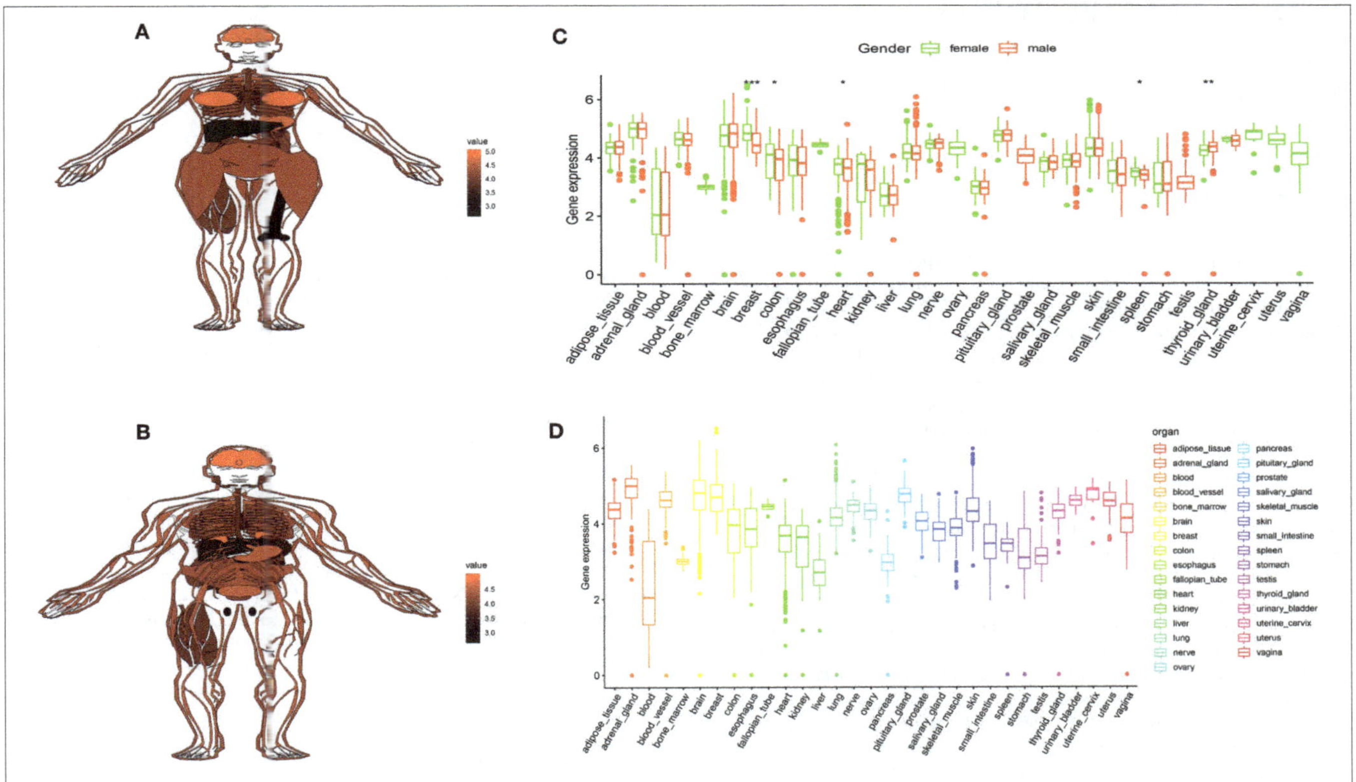

FIGURE 6 | FTO showed high expression in human tissues. **(A,B)** The map shows the expression levels of the FTO in the 31 solid organ tissues in female and male. **(C)** Histogram visualizing the differentially FTO in the 31 solid organ tissues in female and male. **(D)** Histogram visualizing the differentially FTO in the 31 solid organ tissues. *$P < 0.05$, **$P < 0.01$, and ***$P < 0.001$.

inhibit the differentiation of AML cells into normal blood cells mediated by all-trans-retinoic acid (33). This makes the FTO demethylation gene an oncogene for AML. Zhou et al. found a significant increase in the expression of FTO in tumor tissues of patients with cervical squamous cell carcinoma (CSCC), and found that these patients developed tolerance to radiotherapy and chemotherapy. This may be due to the fact that FTO reduces the m^{6}A methylation level of certain genes, thereby activating the β-catenin pathway and affecting the expression of ERCC1 genes. In addition, it was also found that both FTO and β-catenin expression in CSCC patients showed a worse prognosis than patients who were elevated alone ($P = 0.041$). Thus, the expression of FTO and β-catenin has certain value in evaluating the clinical prognosis of CSCC (34).

Tumor stem cells are a kind of pluripotent tumor cells, which are highly malignant and have the ability of self-renewal to mutate more quickly to produce drug resistance or adapt to changes in the microenvironment. It has been found that a certain number of m^{6}A methylation and tumor studies are related to tumor stem cells (35–37). Cui et al. found that the use of FTO inhibitors can significantly inhibit the growth of glioblastoma stem cells (GSC) and reduce the frequency of transformation of GSC cells into tumor stem cells. Moreover, the use of MA2 in glioblastoma can effectively inhibit FTO expression and inhibit tumor progression. This also provides guidance for people looking for new targeted drugs (38). The above studies emphasize the importance of FTO and provide evidence for exploring the pathogenesis of some tumors and seeking new potential therapeutic targets by revealing the previously unconfirmed mechanism of tumor gene regulation. It also provides a new idea for the mechanism of tumor epigenetic modification and tumor gene targeting therapy.

However, to date, many FTO inhibitors (rheumine, IOX3, and meclofenamic acid) have been reported, most of which are not specific. Meclofenamic acid can stably bind to FTO, but the effect on ALKBH5 is still in the research stage (39). IOX3 is a HIF proline hydroxylase inhibitor, which can bind to the active site of FTO and reduce the expression level of FTO, but the inhibitor failed to alter the level of intracellular m^{6}A (40). So far, the role and specific mechanism of m6A demethylase inhibitors found in *in vitro* and *in vivo* studies are not fully understood and lack specificity. Therefore, researchers are expecting more inhibitors against m^{6}A-related factors, especially more specific inhibitors, to bring new dawn to guide tumor gene targeting therapy.

In conclusion, our results systematically demonstrate the expression, potential function, and prognostic value of m^{6}A RNA methylation regulators in gastric cancer. The expression of m^{6}A RNA methylation regulator is highly correlated with the malignant clinicopathological features of gastric cancer. Our study provides important evidence for future detection of the role of m^{6}A methylation in gastric cancer.

AUTHOR CONTRIBUTIONS

JicH designed the research, analyzed the data and wrote the paper. YS performed the data analysis and interpreted the data. JinH help to revised manuscript the article. All authors read and approved the final manuscript.

REFERENCES

1. Dubin DT, Taylor RH. The methylation state of poly A-containing messenger RNA from cultured hamster cells. *Nucleic Acids Res.* (1975) 2:1653–68. doi: 10.1093/nar/2.10.1653
2. Boccaletto P, Machnicka MA, Purta E, Piatkowski P, Baginski B, Wirecki TK, et al. MODOMICS: a database of RNA modification pathways. 2017 update. *Nucleic Acids Res.* (2018) 46:D303–d7. doi: 10.1093/nar/gkx1030
3. Desrosiers R, Friderici K, Rottman F. Identification of methylated nucleosides in messenger RNA from Novikoff hepatoma cells. *Proc Natl Acad Sci USA.* (1974) 71:3971–5. doi: 10.1073/pnas.71.10.3971
4. Wei CM, Gershowitz A, Moss B. Methylated nucleotides block 5' terminus of HeLa cell messenger RNA. *Cell.* (1975) 4:379–86. doi: 10.1016/0092-8674(75)90158-0
5. Deng X, Chen K, Luo GZ, Weng X, Ji Q, Zhou T, et al. Widespread occurrence of N6-methyladenosine in bacterial mRNA. *Nucleic Acids Res.* (2015) 43:6557–67. doi: 10.1093/nar/gkv596
6. Kennedy TD, Lane BG. Wheat embryo ribonucleates. XIII. Methyl-substituted nucleoside constituents and 5'-terminal dinucleotide sequences in bulk poly(AR)-rich RNA from imbibing wheat embryos. *Can J Biochem.* (1979) 57:927–31. doi: 10.1139/o79-112
7. Csepany T, Lin A, Baldick CJ Jr, Beemon K. Sequence specificity of mRNA N6-adenosine methyltransferase. *J Biol Chem.* (1990) 265:20117–22.
8. Narayan P, Ludwiczak RL, Goodwin EC, Rottman FM. Context effects on N6-adenosine methylation sites in prolactin mRNA. *Nucleic Acids Res.* (1994) 22:419–26. doi: 10.1093/nar/22.3.419
9. Dominissini D, Moshitch-Moshkovitz S, Schwartz S, Salmon-Divon M, Ungar L, Osenberg S, et al. Topology of the human and mouse m6A RNA methylomes revealed by m6A-seq. *Nature.* (2012) 485:201–6. doi: 10.1038/nature11112
10. Meyer KD, Saletore Y, Zumbo P, Elemento O, Mason CE, Jaffrey SR. Comprehensive analysis of mRNA methylation reveals enrichment in 3' UTRs and near stop codons. *Cell.* (2012) 149:1635–46. doi: 10.1016/j.cell.2012.05.003
11. Bodi Z, Bottley A, Archer N, May ST, Fray RG. Yeast m6A methylated mRNAs are enriched on translating ribosomes during meiosis, and under rapamycin treatment. *PLoS ONE.* (2015) 10:e0132090. doi: 10.1371/journal.pone.0132090
12. Carroll SM, Narayan P, Rottman FM. N6-methyladenosine residues in an intron-specific region of prolactin pre-mRNA. *Mol Cell Biol.* (1990) 10:4456–65. doi: 10.1128/MCB.10.9.4456
13. Wang S, Sun C, Li J, Zhang E, Ma Z, Xu W, et al. Roles of RNA methylation by means of N(6)-methyladenosine (m(6)A) in human cancers. *Cancer Lett.* (2017) 408:112–20. doi: 10.1016/j.canlet.2017.08.030
14. Chen XY, Zhang J, Zhu JS. The role of m(6)A RNA methylation in human cancer. *Mol Cancer.* (2019) 18:103. doi: 10.1186/s12943-019-1033-z
15. Chen B, Li Y, Song R, Xue C, Xu F. Functions of RNA N6-methyladenosine modification in cancer progression. *Mol Biol Rep.* (2019) 46:2567–75. doi: 10.1007/s11033-019-04655-4
16. Jia G, Fu Y, Zhao X, Dai Q, Zheng G, Yang Y, et al. N6-methyladenosine in nuclear RNA is a major substrate of the obesity-associated FTO. *Nat Chem Biol.* (2011) 7:885–7. doi: 10.1038/nchembio.687
17. Yang Y, Hsu PJ, Chen YS, Yang YG. Dynamic transcriptomic m(6)A decoration: writers, erasers, readers and functions in RNA metabolism. *Cell Res.* (2018) 28:616–24. doi: 10.1038/s41422-018-0040-8
18. Scholler E, Weichmann F, Treiber T, Ringle S, Treiber N, Flatley A, et al. Interactions, localization, and phosphorylation of the m(6)A generating METTL3-METTL14-WTAP complex. *RNA.* (2018) 24:499–512. doi: 10.1261/rna.064063.117
19. Tang C, Klukovich R, Peng H, Wang Z, Yu T, Zhang Y, et al. ALKBH5-dependent m6A demethylation controls splicing and stability of long 3'-UTR mRNAs in male germ cells. *Proc Natl Acad Sci USA.* (2018) 115:E325–e33. doi: 10.1073/pnas.1717794115
20. Ding C, Zou Q, Ding J, Ling M, Wang W, Li H, et al. Increased N6-methyladenosine causes infertility is associated with FTO expression. *J Cell Physiol.* (2018) 233:7055–66. doi: 10.1002/jcp.26507
21. Wojtas MN, Pandey RR, Mendel M, Homolka D, Sachidanandam R, Pillai RS. Regulation of m(6)A transcripts by the 3'->5' RNA helicase YTHDC2 is essential for a successful meiotic program in the mammalian germline. *Mol Cell.* (2017) 68:374–87.e12. doi: 10.1016/j.molcel.2017.09.021
22. Ben-Haim MS, Moshitch-Moshkovitz S, Rechavi G. FTO: linking m6A demethylation to adipogenesis. *Cell Res.* (2015) 25:3–4. doi: 10.1038/cr.2014.162
23. Shen F, Huang W, Huang JT, Xiong J, Yang Y, Wu K, et al. Decreased N(6)-methyladenosine in peripheral blood RNA from diabetic patients is associated with FTO expression rather than ALKBH5. *J Clin Endocrinol Metab.* (2015) 100:E148–54. doi: 10.1210/jc.2014-1893
24. Zheng G, Dahl JA, Niu Y, Fedorcsak P, Huang CM, Li CJ, et al. ALKBH5 is a mammalian RNA demethylase that impacts RNA metabolism and mouse fertility. *Mol Cell.* (2013) 49:18–29. doi: 10.1016/j.molcel.2012.10.015
25. Chen J, Du B. Novel positioning from obesity to cancer: FTO, an m(6)A RNA demethylase, regulates tumour progression. *J Cancer Res Clin Oncol.* (2019) 145:19–29. doi: 10.1007/s00432-018-2796-0
26. Angelova MT, Dimitrova DG, Dinges N, Lence T, Worpenberg L, Carre C, et al. The Emerging field of epitranscriptomics in neurodevelopmental and neuronal disorders. *Front Bioeng Biotechnol.* (2018) 6:46. doi: 10.3389/fbioe.2018.00046
27. Siegel RL, Miller KD, Jemal A. Cancer statistics, 2019. *CA Cancer J Clin.* (2019) 69:7–34. doi: 10.3322/caac.21551
28. Johnston FM, Beckman M. Updates on management of gastric cancer. *Curr Oncol Rep.* (2019) 21:67. doi: 10.1007/s11912-019-0820-4
29. Hironaka S. Anti-angiogenic therapies for gastric cancer. *Asia Pac J Clin Oncol.* (2019) 15:208–17. doi: 10.1111/ajco.13174
30. Necula L, Matei L, Dragu D, Neagu AI, Mambet C, Nedeianu S, et al. Recent advances in gastric cancer early diagnosis. *World J Gastroenterol.* (2019) 25:2029–44. doi: 10.3748/wjg.v25.i17.2029
31. Coutzac C, Pernot S, Chaput N, Zaanan A. Immunotherapy in advanced gastric cancer, is it the future? *Crit Rev Oncol Hematol.* (2019) 133:25–32. doi: 10.1016/j.critrevonc.2018.10.007
32. Sun T, Wu R, Ming L. The role of m6A RNA methylation in cancer. *Biomed Pharmacother.* (2019) 112:108613. doi: 10.1016/j.biopha.2019.108613
33. Li Z, Weng H, Su R, Weng X, Zuo Z, Li C, et al. FTO plays an oncogenic role in acute myeloid leukemia as a N(6)-methyladenosine RNA demethylase. *Cancer Cell.* (2017) 31:127–41. doi: 10.1016/j.ccell.2016.11.017
34. Zhou S, Bai ZL, Xia D, Zhao ZJ, Zhao R, Wang YY, et al. FTO regulates the chemo-radiotherapy resistance of cervical squamous cell carcinoma (CSCC) by targeting beta-catenin through mRNA demethylation. *Mol Carcinogen.* (2018) 57:590–7. doi: 10.1002/mc.22782
35. Bai Y, Yang C, Wu R, Huang L, Song S, Li W, et al. YTHDF1 regulates tumorigenicity and cancer stem cell-like activity in human colorectal carcinoma. *Front Oncol.* (2019) 9:332. doi: 10.3389/fonc.2019.00332
36. Weng H, Huang H, Wu H, Qin X, Zhao BS, Dong L, et al. METTL14 inhibits hematopoietic stem/progenitor differentiation and promotes leukemogenesis via mRNA m(6)A modification. *Cell Stem Cell.* (2018) 22:191–205.e9. doi: 10.1016/j.stem.2017.11.016
37. Visvanathan A, Patil V, Arora A, Hegde AS, Arivazhagan A, Santosh V, et al. Essential role of METTL3-mediated m(6)A modification in glioma stem-like cells maintenance and radioresistance. *Oncogene.* (2018) 37:522–33. doi: 10.1038/onc.2017.351
38. Cui Q, Shi H, Ye P, Li L, Qu Q, Sun G, et al. m(6)A RNA methylation regulates

the self-renewal and tumorgenesis of glioblastoma stem cells. *Cell Rep*. (2017) 18:2622–34. doi: 10.1016/j.celrep.2017.02.059

39. Huang Y, Yan J, Li Q, Li J, Gong S, Zhou H, et al. Meclofenamic acid selectively inhibits FTO demethylation of m6A over ALKBH5. *Nucleic Acids Res*. (2015) 43:373–84. doi: 10.1093/nar/gku1276

40. McMurray F, Demetriades M, Aik W, Merkestein M, Kramer H, Andrew DS, et al. Pharmacological inhibition of FTO. *PLoS ONE*. (2015) 10:e0121829. doi: 10.1371/journal.pone.0121829

15

Prognostic Biomarkers for Gastric Cancer: An Umbrella Review of the Evidence

*Cen Zhou†, Xi Zhong†, Yongxi Song, Jinxin Shi, Zhonghua Wu, Zhexu Guo, Jie Sun and Zhenning Wang**

Department of Surgical Oncology and General Surgery, Key Laboratory of Precision Diagnosis and Treatment of Gastrointestinal Tumors, Ministry of Education, The First Affiliated Hospital of China Medical University, Shenyang, China

***Correspondence:**
Zhenning Wang
josieon826@sina.cn

† These authors have contributed equally to this work

Introduction: Biomarkers are biological molecules entirely or partially participating in cancerous processes that function as measurable indicators of abnormal changes in the human body microenvironment. Aiming to provide an overview of associations between prognostic biomarkers and gastric cancer (GC), we performed this umbrella review analyzing currently available meta-analyses and grading the evidence depending on the credibility of their associations.

Methods: A systematic literature search was conducted by two independent investigators of the PubMed, Embase, Web of Science, and Cochrane Databases to identify meta-analyses investigating associations between prognostic biomarkers and GC. The strength of evidence for prognostic biomarkers for GC were categorized into four grades: strong, highly suggestive, suggestive, and weak.

Results: Among 120 associations between prognostic biomarkers and GC survival outcomes, only one association, namely the association between platelet count and GC OS, was supported by strong evidence. Associations between FITC, CEA, NLR, foxp3+ Treg lymphocytes (both 1- and 3-year OS), CA 19-9, or VEGF and GC OS were supported by highly suggestive evidence. Four associations were considered suggestive and the remaining 108 associations were supported by weak or not suggestive evidence.

Discussion: The association between platelet count and GC OS was supported by strong evidence. Associations between FITC, CEA, NLR, foxp3+ Treg lymphocytes (both 1- and 3-year OS), CA 19-9, or VEGF and GC OS were supported by highly suggestive evidence, however, the results should be interpreted cautiously due to inadequate methodological quality as deemed by AMSTAR 2.0.

Keywords: biomarkers, gastric cancer, umbrella review, prognostic, survival

INTRODUCTION

Gastric cancer (GC) was the most common cancer worldwide less than a century ago (1). Despite a decreasing incidence in recent decades, GC remains the most commonly diagnosed cancer in Eastern Asia (2). According to the National Central Cancer Registry in China, GC is the second most common cancer in china, with 298,800 cases in 2013 alone, which means that approximately 42 individuals suffer GC in every 100,000 people (3). The best options to reduce mortality are treatments aimed at early detection, systematic prevention and personalized therapy. Meanwhile, traditional treatment strategies such as surgery have potentially reached a ceiling regarding locoregional control and mortality reduction, reflecting the dilemma that GC remains unsatisfactorily incurable worldwide (4).

Biomarkers are biological molecules entirely or partially participating in cancerous processes that function as measurable indicators of abnormal changes in the human body microenvironment (5, 6). Many studies have reported the importance of biomarkers in clinical GC applications including diagnosis, treatments and prognosis. There are currently three main types of cancer biomarkers distinguished by clinical use: predictive, prognostic, and pharmacodynamic markers (7–10). Countries with high GC incidence, such as Japan, have established adequate tumor monitoring systems to detect and diagnose GC at early stages, greatly improving survival (4). Prognostic biomarkers play essential roles in distinguishing between benign and malignant tumors, monitoring progress of advanced GCs, and predicting survival outcomes. Several protein cancer biomarkers are widely used and have become routine in clinical practice, especially α-fetoprotein (AFP) which has been proven to improve early diagnosis of hepatocellular cancer, resulting in more superior survival outcomes (11, 12). Many cohort and case-control studies have explored biomarkers associated with GC, and several meta-analyses have been published to systematically analyze these results. Aiming to provide an overview of associations between prognostic biomarkers and GC, we performed this umbrella review analyzing currently available meta-analyses and grading the evidence depending on the credibility of their associations.

METHODS

Search Strategy and Eligibility Criteria

A systematic literature search was conducted by two independent investigators of the PubMed, Embase, Web of Science, and Cochrane Databases to identify meta-analyses investigating associations between prognostic biomarkers and GC published from inception through April 11, 2019. The following relevant keywords were used to conduct our electronic database search: (risk factors OR Helicobacter pylori OR H. pylori OR peptic ulcer disease OR gastritis OR inflammation OR IL-7 OR IL-10 OR gastric ulcer OR gastroesophageal reflux disease OR GERD OR esophagogastric junction OR dysplastic intestinal metaplasia OR cardia OR smoking OR smoker OR alcohol OR chemical exposure OR occupational exposure OR high temperature OR particulates OR metal OR chromium OR asbestos OR talc OR crystalline silica OR diet OR salt OR preserved meat OR red meat OR coffee OR caffeinated intake OR caffeine intake OR caffeine OR decaffeinated OR decaffeinated intake OR fruits OR vegetables OR obesity OR obese OR BMI OR body mass index OR anemia OR gastric surgery OR radiation OR Epstein-Barr virus OR EBV OR socioeconomic status OR poverty OR wealth OR education OR level of education OR educational level OR schooling OR blood group OR blood type OR sex OR gender OR sexuality OR man OR male OR woman OR female OR anti-estrogen drugs OR tamoxifen OR hormone replacement therapy OR HRT OR parity OR pregnancy OR menopause OR premenopausal OR post-menopausal OR ethnic origin OR ethnicity OR race OR screening programs OR radiography OR endoscopy OR serum pepsinogen level OR exercise OR physical activity OR family history OR familial OR radiation OR radiotherapy OR cohabiting OR living together OR partner OR partnered OR insulin OR metformin OR aspirin OR aspirin containing medications OR drugs OR medicine) AND (gastric cancer OR gastric carcinoma OR gastric neoplasia OR gastric tumor OR gastric neoplasm OR gastric maligna* OR GC OR stomach carcinoma OR stomach neoplasia OR stomach tumor OR stomach neoplasm OR stomach maligna*) AND (systematic review OR meta-analysis OR metaanalysis). Only meta-analyses were included in this umbrella review, irrespective of publication year or language; case reports, commentaries, editorials, conference abstracts and letters were excluded. We also manually reviewed the reference lists in the retrieved meta-analyses to include any related studies.

A detailed eligibility criterion was formulated for study inclusion: (1) we included studies clearly examining associations between prognostic biomarkers, rather than predictive or pharmacodynamic markers, and GC survival outcomes including but not limited to overall survival (OS), disease-free survival (DFS), progression-free survival (PFS) and cancer-specific survival (CSS). (2) We excluded studies investigating genetic polymorphism and GC incidence. Studies focusing on benign gastric tumors such as leiomyoma, neurofibroma and gastrointestinal stromal tumors were also excluded (3). We excluded meta-analyses containing less than three original studies or not providing sufficient data from each individual study. When two or more meta-analyses focused on one specific association, we included the meta-analysis with largest sample size.

Data Extraction

Two investigators independently performed data extraction from included meta-analyses and resolved differences through discussion. The following values were retrieved from each included study: first author name, publication year; country, name and classification of biomarker and its associations with GC, relative risk estimates, including risk ratio (RR), odds ratio (OR), hazard ratio (HR) and the corresponding 95% confidence interval (CI), number of include studies, number of cases, and population size.

Quality Assessment

The methodological quality of included meta-analyses was evaluated through AMSTAR (A MeaSurement Tool to Assess systematic Reviews) version 2.0 (2017) (13), a vital appraisal tool for umbrella reviews to assess involved randomized trials with high efficiency. The revised version simplifies response categories and contains 16 items in all which provide a more comprehensive appraisal compared with the original AMSTAR. Rather than outputting an overall score, AMSTAR 2 evaluates single study quality by calculating scores in specific items and then describes results as either high, moderate, low, or critically low grade.

Statistical Analysis

Statistical analyses were conducted using STATA version 12.0 (StataCorp. LLC, College Station, TX, USA). Random-effect models were used to estimate summary effects for included studies considering the inevitable heterogeneity caused by multiple sources. Relative risk estimates, 95% confidence interval (CI) and corresponding *P*-values were calculated. The significance level was set to $P < 0.05$ (14).

Interstudy heterogeneity was analyzed through Cochran's Q test and the I^2 statistic was calculated. Ranging from 0 to 100%, I^2 quantitatively demonstrates variability among risk estimates, with $I^2 > 50\%$ indicating great heterogeneity (15). Interstudy heterogeneity was also analyzed using 95% prediction intervals (PI), assessing the impact of uncertainty in individual studies and prone to be more conservative (16, 17).

Several methods were used to evaluate bias in associations between prognostic biomarkers and GC. Egger's regression

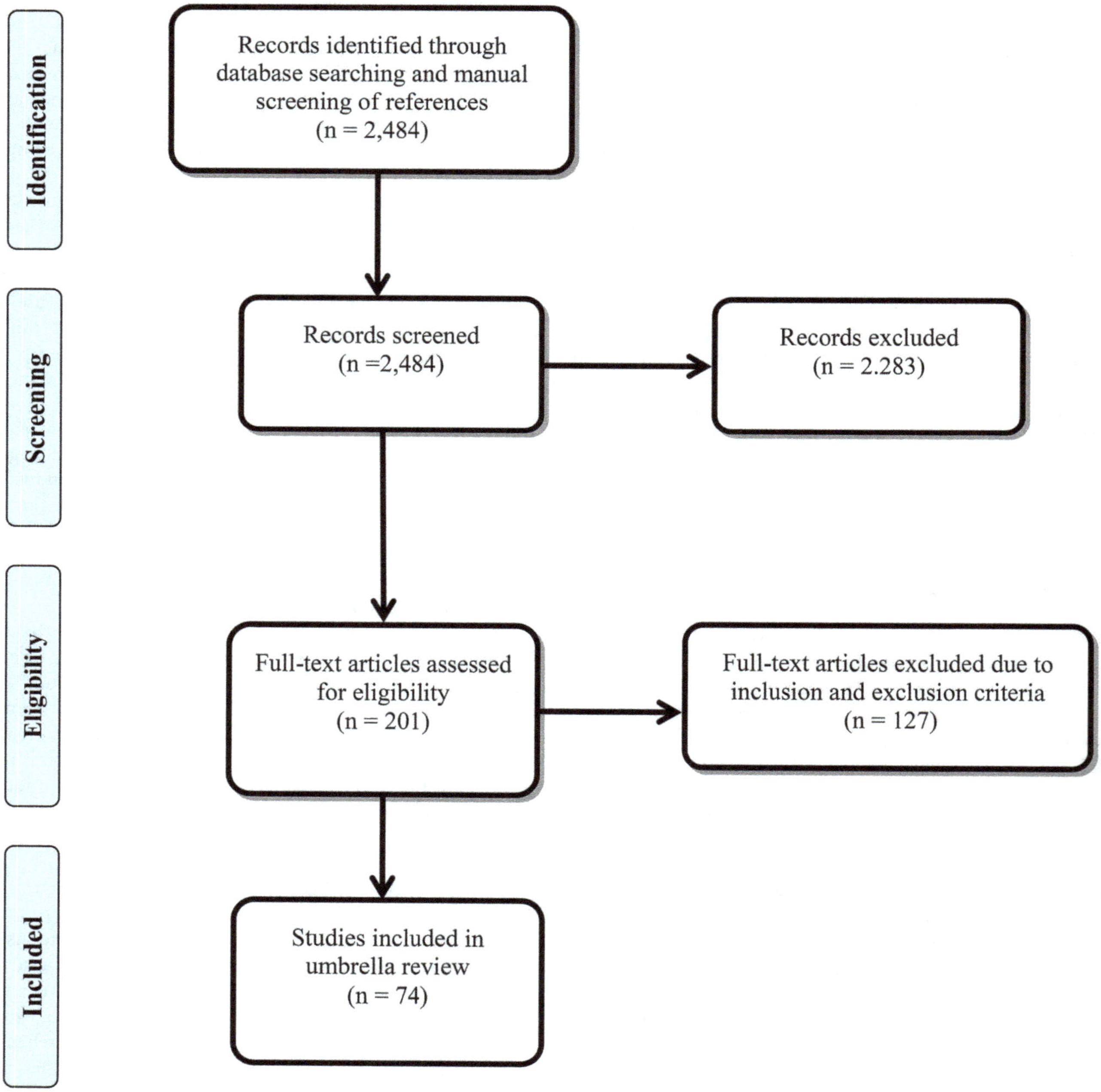

FIGURE 1 | Flow diagram.

asymmetry test was performed to assess whether small-study effects existed (17), with a $P < 0.01$ considered statistically significant with more conservative results in the largest study.

Excess significance bias was applied to avoid potential biases such as selective reporting biases or publication biases. To assess whether the number of expected studies (E) was in accordance with the observed number (O) with nominally significant results or less, chi-square statistics were performed (18) with a two-tailed $P < 0.10$ as the statistical significance threshold. The number of studies expected to be statistically significant was calculated by summing up statistical power estimates extracted from each component using an algorithm from a non-central t distribution. The observed number was extracted from the relative risk estimate of the largest study. In cases where O > E and $P < 0.10$, excess significance was considered positive.

Credibility ceiling sensitivity analyses were performed for weak evidence to skeptically analyze precise results provided by included meta-analyses. The credibility ceiling was set at 10% for this study, based on the assumption that the likelihood of a specific effect always has a limitation, in other words, no matter how well-designed a study was, its effect in this particular aspect is restricted and impossible to exceed maximum value (19).

Strength of Existing Evidence

The strength of evidence for prognostic biomarkers for GC were categorized into four grades in accordance with previous studies (20, 21): strong, highly suggestive, suggestive, and weak. Categorization criteria are as follow: (1) a study was considered as strong evidence if it presented a $P < 10^{-6}$, $I^2 < 50\%$, calculated 95% PI excluding the null value, a sample size >1,000 cases, was absent evidence of small-study effects and excess significance and survived the 10% credibility ceiling ($P > 0.05$); (2) a study would be rated as highly suggestive evidence if it presented a $P < 10^{-6}$ with a sample size >1,000 cases; (3) a study would be categorized as suggestive evidence if it presented a $P < 10^{-3}$ with a sample size >1,000 cases; (4) a study would be assessed as weak evidence if it presented a $P < 0.05$

RESULTS

Characteristics of the Included Systematic Reviews and Meta-Analyses

A total of 2,484 records were identified from the literature search and manual screening of references, of which 2,283 were excluded after title and abstract screening. Ultimately, 74 of the remaining 201 studies met the inclusion criteria after full-text review (22–97). The search flowchart is shown in **Figure 1**, and the full list of the 201 studies and exclusion reasons for 127 of them are shown in **Supplementary Table S1**. Of note, we selected the most recent systematic review and meta-analysis investigating the association between HER2 and GC mortality (96) rather than the study with the largest number of primary studies (98) for inclusion because the latter searched for studies published in 2015 while the former was published in 2017 and the included studies needed to be updated. The included studies covered 120 different associations between prognostic biomarkers and GC survival outcomes, more than 79,000 subjects, and over 1,000 studies. Characteristics of the 120 associations in the included systematic reviews and meta-analyses are shown in **Table 1**. Data on the primary studies included in the 74 systematic reviews and meta-analyses were also extracted, processed, and coded to perform various analyses.

Methodological Quality Assessment Using AMSTAR 2.0

The methodological quality of all included systematic reviews and meta-analyses was deemed critically low using the 16-item AMSTAR 2.0. Detailed results, scoring criteria, and rating criteria are shown in **Supplementary Table S2**. All included studies had more than two critical flaws [usually in items 2 (74/74, 100%), 7 (74/74, 100%), and 13 (74/74, 100%)] and several non-critical flaws [usually in items 3 (74/74, 100%), 10 (74/74, 100%), and 12 (74/74, 100%)]. Of note, studies with at least two critical flaws with or without non-critical flaws were considered as having critically low methodological quality.

Summary Effect Size

The quantitative syntheses of the 120 associations were re-performed using a random-effect model to provide more conservative estimates. Forty-seven associations reached $P < 10^{-6}$ (**Table 2** and **Supplementary Table S3**). Twenty-one associations had moderate statistical significance ($P < 10^{-3}$). The remaining 52 associations presented either $P < 0.05$ or no statistical significance. Most associations that reached statistical significance reported an increased risk of mortality of GC, indicating the potential prognostic effect of biomarkers for GC. Associations between Foxp3+ Treg lymphocytes and 1-, 3-, and 5-year survival of GC, between intraperitoneal free cancer cell (IFCC) and OS of GC, between Forkhead Box M1 (FOXM1) and 1- and 5-year survival of GC, between Silent information regulator 1 (Sirt1) and 3-year survival of GC, and between CC chemokine receptor type 7 (CCR7) and 5-year survival of GC all reported a decreased risk of mortality of GC.

Heterogeneity

Seventy-six of the 120 (63.3%) associations demonstrated significant heterogeneity ($P < 0.1$), of which 54 showed high heterogeneity and 23 presented moderate to high heterogeneity. The 95% PI was also calculated to further assess inter-study heterogeneity. The 95% PIs of 38 associations excluded the null value (**Table 2** and **Supplementary Table S3**).

Small-Study Effects

Small study effects were found in fifteen associations: FITCs and GC OS, tissue VEGF and GC OS, β-catenin and GC OS, p53 and GC OS, MAPF and GC OS, uPAR and GC OS, MET and GC OS, CD133 and 5-year-survival of GC, PTEN and 5-year-survival of GC, FOXM1 and 5-year-survival of GC, Sirt1 and 3-year-survival of GC, MMP9 and 5-year-survival of GC, SOX2 and GC OS, S100A4 and GC OS, NME1 and GC OS all had $P < 0.1$ for Egger's test (**Table 2** and **Supplementary Table S3**). Only one of the 120 associations contained an inadequate number of studies (<10) and failed to empower Egger's test to identify small-study effects: CD44v6 and GC OS.

TABLE 1 | Characteristics of the 120 associations in the included systematic reviews and meta-analyses.

References	Biomarker	Association between biomarker and gastric cancer	Effect metrics	Country	No. of study estimates	No. of cases/total population	Summary relative risk estimate (95% CI)
Kim et al. (25)	ARID1A	OS	HR	Korea	4	344/1,316	1.51 (1.25–1.82)
Liu et al. (88)	BIRC5	OS	HR	China	18	492#/1,528#	1.15 (0.82–1.61)
Chen et al. (82)	BIRC5	5-year OS	OR	China	6	230#/634	1.61 (1.41–1.85)
	PTEN	5-year OS	OR	China	9	639#/1,548	1.59 (1.38–1.84)
	HIF-1α	5-year OS	OR	China	10	454/1,400	1.52 (1.28–1.81)
Shao et al. (75)	Bmi-1	OS	HR	China	3	396#/633	1.50 (1.22–1.85)
Song et al. (57)	CA 19-9	OS	HR	China	29	2609#/8882	1.83 (1.56–2.15)
		DFS	HR	China	7	497#/2037	1.86 (1.17–2.96)
		DSS	HR	China	6	473#/1304	1.30 (1.04–1.61)
Du et al. (37)	CCR7	5-year OS	HR	China	4	94#/569	0.47 (0.31–0.70)
Lu et al. (41)	CD44	5-year OS	HR	China	9	653/1234	1.87 (1.55–2.26)
	CD133	5-year OS	HR	China	8	901/1424	2.15 (1.71–2.70)
Jiang et al. (26)	CD3+ T lymphocytes	OS	HR	China	11	826#/1851	0.66 (0.54–0.80)
	CD4+ T lymphocytes	OS	HR	China	9	655#/1762	0.80 (0.64–1.00)
	CD8+ T lymphocytes	OS	HR	China	13	1012/2185	0.83 (0.70–0.99)
	Foxp3+ Treg lymphocytes	OS	HR	China	20	1147/2725	0.97 (0.74–1.28)
	Dendritic cells	OS	HR	China	3	149/402	0.62 (0.15–2.51)
Wu et al. (54)	CD44	OS	HR	China	9	594/1210	0.91 (0.59–1.41)
		DFS	HR	China	3	121/286	1.68 (1.14–2.49)
	CD44v6	OS	HR	China	5	154#/441	1.26 (0.33–4.84)
Lu et al. (42)	CD44v6	5-year OS	OR	China	5	394/796	1.41 (0.80–2.49)
Meng et al. (60)	CDH17	5-year OS	RR	China	6	456#/1716	0.87 (0.67–1.14)
Wang et al. (92)	Cdx2	5-year OS	HR	China	4	199/475	2.21 (1.78–2.74)
Deng et al. (65)	CEA	OS	HR	China	51	3491#/8519	1.73 (1.57–1.90)
		DFS	HR	China	6	295#/1535	2.27 (1.72–3.01)
		DSS	HR	China	7	542/1227	1.95 (1.50–2.54)
Liu et al. (94)	Tissue VEGF	OS	HR	China	21	1056#/2691	2.13 (1.71–2.64)
		DFS	HR	China	7	465/1114	2.03 (1.57–2.62)
		DSS	HR	China	3	190/381	2.59 (1.33–5.06)
	Circulating VEGF	OS	HR	China	3	105/209	4.22 (2.47–7.18)
	Tissue VEGF-D	OS	HR	China	4	99#/282	1.73 (1.25–2.40)
Liu et al. (62)	CLDN4	OS	HR	China	7	378#/1030	2.01 (1.62–2.50)
Yu et al. (85)	c-Met	OS	HR	China	16	770#/1789	2.11 (1.62–2.75)
Yu et al. (86)	CRP	OS	HR	China	12	996#/2597	1.77 (1.56–2.00)
Zhang et al. (68)	CTCs	OS	HR	China	30	698#/2090	1.79 (1.49–2.15)
		RFS	HR	China	10	201#/781	2.91 (1.83–4.62)
Wang et al. (72)	CTCs	RFS*	HR	China	11	259#/1538	2.41 (1.93–3.01)
Liu et al. (43)	DKK1	OS	RR	China	3	209/616	2.67 (2.05–3.48)
Li et al. (78)	E-cadherin	5-year OS	RR	China	8	584#/1265#	1.61 (1.37–1.88)
Chen et al. (90)	EGFR	OS	HR	China	7	613/1289	1.66 (1.35–2.03)
Song et al. (58)	ERCC1	OS	HR	China	15	869#/1594	1.48 (1.02–2.13)
Guo et al. (80)	EZH2	OS	HR	China	4	282/496	1.20 (0.51–2.81)
Zeng et al. (34)	FAK	OS	HR	China	7	750#/2408	2.65 (1.74–4.02)
Tan et al. (87)	Fascin-1	OS	HR	UK	3	273#/750	1.15 (0.83–1.57)
Liu et al. (24)	FGFR2	3-year OS	OR	China	10	1154/2093	1.90 (1.17–3.07)
	FGFR2	5-year OS	OR	China	8	973/1922	1.77 (1.04–3.02)
Wang et al. (73)	FHIT	OS	HR	China	8	855#/1361	1.27 (1.07–1.51)

(Continued)

TABLE 1 | Continued

References	Biomarker	Association between biomarker and gastric cancer	Effect metrics	Country	No. of study estimates	No. of cases/total population	Summary relative risk estimate (95% CI)
Pecqueux et al. (59)	FITC	OS	HR	Germany	51	5567#/11540	3.23 (2.79–3.73)
Dai et al. (66)	FOXM1	OS	HR	China	3	41#/220	2.27 (1.13–4.58)
Jiang et al. (26)	FOXM1	1-year OS	OR	China	6	46#/419	0.23 (0.11–0.48)
		3-year OS	OR	China	4	35#/282	0.14 (0.04–0.56)
		5-year OS	OR	China	4	38#/282	0.16 (0.07–0.38)
Huang et al. (97)	Foxp3+ Treg lymphocytes	1-year OS	OR	China	12	1672/1901	0.39 (0.29–0.54)
		3-year OS	OR	China	11	1167/1825	0.28 (0.21–0.38)
		5-year OS	OR	China	12	964/1888	0.31 (0.21–0.44)
Lei et al. (96)	HER2	OS	RR	China	10	2170#/3913	1.47 (1.09–1.98)
Gu et al. (81)	HER2	RFS	HR	China	4	701/3054	1.07 (0.84–1.37)
Cao et al. (51)	HER4	3-year OS	OR	China	3	27#/415	1.00 (0.85–1.18)
Zhang et al. (84)	HIF-1α	OS	HR	China	10	533/1252	1.34 (1.13–1.58)
		DFS	HR	China	5	266/403	1.67 (0.99–2.82)
Ma et al. (61)	HOTAIR	OS	HR	China	4	239/396	1.55 (0.84–2.88)
Tustumi et al. (39)	IFCC	OS	RD	Brazil	11	984#/2520	0.37 (0.31–0.44)
Gao et al. (63)	IGF-1R	OS	HR	China	4	373#/1289	2.63 (1.29–5.40)
Luo et al. (22)	Ki-67	OS	HR	China	22	1741#/3197	1.23 (1.06–1.42)
		DFS	HR	China	5	217/464	1.87 (1.30–2.69)
Huang et al. (46)	LGR5	OS	HR	China	4	39/359	1.66 (1.02–2.69)
Wang et al. (38)	TAMs	OS	HR	China	7	462#/771	1.71 (1.35–2.15)
	M2 TAM	OS	HR	China	4	537/886	1.71 (1.19–2.45)
Deng et al. (50)	MAPF	OS	HR	China	7	348#/871	2.74 (2.20–3.42)
		DFS	HR	China	6	381#/750	3.28 (1.93–5.59)
		Peritoneal RFS	HR	China	6	323/822	4.95 (3.23–7.57)
Peng et al. (76)	MET (HGFR)	OS	HR	China	16	749/2302	2.57 (1.97–3.35)
Dong et al. (64)	MMP14	OS	HR	China	3	360594	2.17 (1.64–2.86)
Shen et al. (74)	MMP2	OS	HR	China	10	1020/1514	1.92 (1.48–2.48)
Zhang et al. (91)	MMP9	OS	HR	China	11	790#/1611	1.25 (1.11–1.40)
Chen et al. (67)	MMP9	5-year OS	RR	China	8	328#/1090	1.51 (1.24–1.84)
Wang et al. (37)	MUC1	5-year OS	HR	China	4	423/758	0.28 (0.12–0.66)
Zhang et al. (52)	MUC5AC	OS	HR	China	6	422#/1384	1.34 (1.00–1.81)
Sun et al. (40)	NLR	OS	HR	China	19	2926#/5431	1.98 (1.75–2.25)
		DFS	HR	China	3	382/488	1.48 (1.05–2.09)
		PFS	HR	China	4	452/488	1.62 (1.32–1.98)
Fang et al. (29)	NM23	5-year OS	OR	China	9	732/1685	0.60 (0.24–1.46)
Han et al. (47)	NME1	OS	HR	China	5	444/960	0.75 (0.35–1.63)
Gu et al. (48)	OPN	OS	HR	China	8	879/1633	1.59 (1.15–2.22)
Wei et al. (56)	P53	OS	HR	China	21	2487#/4670	1.56 (1.23–1.98)
		DSS	HR	China	14	1015#/2053	1.59 (1.34–1.88)
Brungs et al. (33)	uPA	OS	HR	Australia	12	537#/1130	2.21 (1.74–2.8)
		RFS	HR	Australia	3	287/468	1.90 (1.17–1.98)
	uPAR	OS	HR	Australia	11	459#/1016	2.19 (1.80–2.66)
	PAI-1	OS	HR	Australia	9	407#/798	1.80 (1.25–2.60)
		RFS	HR	Australia	3	161/465	1.96 (1.07–3.57)
Cao et al. (32)	p-Akt	OS	HR	China	11	615#/1737	1.41 (1.01–1.97)
Gu et al. (27)	PD-L1	OS	HR	China	15	1312#/3291	1.46 (1.08–1.98)
Wu et al. (55)	PD-L1	3-year OS	OR	China	3	161/313	4.13 (1.84–9.21)

(Continued)

TABLE 1 | Continued

References	Biomarker	Association between biomarker and gastric cancer	Effect metrics	Country	No. of study estimates	No. of cases/total population	Summary relative risk estimate (95% CI)
Xin-Ji et al. (53)	Platelet count	OS	HR	China	7	1132#/5515	1.74 (1.41–2.13)
Xu et al. (35)	PLR	OS	HR	China	7	1290#/4121	0.99 (0.89–1.10)
Hu et al. (89)	PRL-3	OS	HR	China	6	756#/1249	1.90 (1.38–2.60)
Ji et al. (45)	pSTAT3	OS	HR	China	11	815#/1547	1.97 (1.49–2.63)
Wang et al. (71)	S100A4	OS	HR	China	7	500#/866#	1.47 (0.77–2.81)
Jiang et al. (44)	Sirt1	3-year OS	OR	China	5	618/987	0.32 (0.19–0.55)
		5-year OS	OR	China	4	785/1264	0.44 (0.15–1.29)
Zhang et al. (69)	SK1	5-year OS	HR	China	3	597/677	1.58 (1.08–2.30)
Lin et al. (77)	SOX2	OS	HR	China	8	415/875	1.46 (0.84–2.54)
Wang et al. (70)	SPARC	OS	RR	China	6	458/851	1.67 (1.44–1.93)
Wu et al. (36)	STAT3	3-year OS	OR	China	10	960/1647	4.08 (1.81–9.21)
		5-year OS	OR	China	10	768/1647	5.47 (2.16–13.86)
Gao et al. (49)	TS	OS	HR	China	12	735#/2174	1.07 (0.75–1.52)
		EFS	HR	China	10	667#/2072	1.16 (0.84–1.61)
Chen et al. (95)	VEGF	5-year OS	RR	China	11	468#/1195#	2.43 (1.95–3.03)
Peng et al. (93)	VEGF-A	OS	HR	China	15	657#/2166	1.96 (1.56–2.45)
		DFS	HR	China	7	370#/1233	2.10 (1.57–2.81)
	VEGF-D	DFS	HR	China	5	138#/536	2.54 (1.58–4.07)
Cao et al. (83)	VEGF-C	OS	HR	China	11	520#/1594	1.67 (1.26–2.21)
		DFS	HR	China	5	217#/1020	1.53 (0.92–2.57)
Ge et al. (28)	VEGFR-3	3-year OS	HR	China	6	334/699	1.38 (0.93–2.04)
		5-year OS	HR	China	6	373/511	1.45 (1.06–1.97)
Chen et al. (31)	ZEB1	OS	HR	China	3	373/511	2.06 (1.49–2.84)
	ZEB2	OS	HR	China	3	309/481	2.06 (1.57–2.62)
Li et al. (79)	β-catenin	OS	HR	China	15	1215#/2261	1.85 (1.39–2.46)

CI, confidence interval; OS, overall survival; DFS, disease free survival; RFS, recurrence free survival; PFS, progression free survival; EFS, event-free survival; peritoneal RFS, peritoneal recurrence-free survival; DSS, disease-specifc survival; RFS, relapse free survival; ARID1A, AT-rich interactive domain-containing 1A protein; BIRC5, (Survivin); PTEN, Phosphatase and tensin homolog; HIF-1α, Hypoxia inducible factor-1α; Bmi-1, B-cell-specific moloney leukemia virus insertion site 1; CA 19-9, serum carbohydrate antigen 19; CCR7, CC chemokine receptor type 7; CDH17, cadherin-17; CEA, carcinoembryonic antigen; Tissue VEGF, tissue vascular endothelial growth factor; Circulating VEGF, circulating vascular endothelial growth factor; Tissue VEGF-D, tissue vascular endothelial growth factor D; CLDN4, claudin 4; CRP, C-reactive protein; CTCs, circulating tumor cells; DKK1, Dickkopf-1; EGFR, human epidermal growth factor receptor; ERCC1, excision repair cross-complementing group 1; EZH2, Zeste homolog 2; FAK, focal adhesion kinase; FGFR2, fibroblast growth factor receptors; FHIT (bis(5′-adenosyl)-triphosphatase), fragile histidine triad protein; FITC, free intraperitoneal tumor cells; FOXM1, forkhead Box M1; HER2, human epidermal growth factor receptor-2; HOTAIR, HOX transcript antisense intergenic RNA; IFCC, intraperitoneal free cancer cell; IGF-1R, insulin-like growth factor receptor type I; LGR5, leucinerich repeat-containing G-protein-coupled receptor 5; TAMs, Tumor-associated macrophages; MAPF, molecular analysis of peritoneal fluid; MET (HGFR), hepatocyte growth factor receptor; MMP14, matrix metalloproteinase 14; MMP2, matrix metalloproteinase 2; MMP9, matrix metalloproteinase 9; MUC1, mucin 1; MUC5AC, mucin 5AC; NLR, neutrophil-to-lymphocyte ratio; NM23, non-metastatic protein 23; NME1 (NM23-H1 or NDPK-A); OPN, osteopontin; uPA, the urokinase plasminogen activation; uPAR, urokinase plasminogen activator receptor; PAI-1, plasminogen activator inhibitor-1; p-Akt, phosphorylated protein kinase B; PD-L1, programmed cell death ligand 1; PLR, platelet-lymphocyte ratio; PRL-3, phosphatase of regenerating liver 3; pSTAT3, phosphorylated signal transducer and activator of transcription proteins 3; Sirt1, silent information regulator 1; SOX2, Sex-determining region Y-box 2; SPARC (osteonectin or BM-40), secreted protein acidic and rich in cysteine; STAT3, signal transducer and activator of transcription proteins 3; TS, thymidylate synthase; VEGF, vascular endothelial growth factor; VEGF, vascular endothelial growth factor; VEGF-C, vascular endothelial growth factor-C; VEGFR-3, vascular endothelial growth factor receptors 3; ZEB1, (TCF8, AREB6 or Zfhx1a) zinc fnger E-box binding homeobox 1; ZEB2, (SIP1, HSPC082 and Zfhx1b) zinc fnger E-box binding homeobox 2. #Contain missing values.*

EXCESS SIGNIFICANCE

Excess significance was significant (O>E and $P < 0.1$) in 45 associations (**Table 2** and **Supplementary Table S3**).

10% Credibility Ceiling

Seventy-seven of the 120 associations survived the 10% credibility ceiling, including all associations graded as strong, highly suggestive, or suggestive and most of the associations classified as weak evidence. Details can be found in **Table 2** and **Supplementary Table S3**.

Robustness of Evidence

None of the 120 associations between prognostic biomarkers and GC survival outcomes were considered strong evidence. Only one association, namely the association between platelet count and GC OS, was supported by strong evidence. Seven associations were supported by highly suggestive evidence, including associations between free intraperitoneal tumor cells (FITCs) and GC OS, between CEA and GC OS, between neutrophils to lymphocytes ratio (NLR) and GC OS, between foxp3+ Treg lymphocytes and 1- and 3-year-OS of GC, between serum carbohydrate

TABLE 2 | Evidence-rating results based on the results of statistical analyses of the 120 associations.

Study	Association between biomarkers and gastric cancer	Summary relative risk estimate (random-effect *P*)*	Cases >1000	Largest study relative risk estimate *P*<0.05	I^2 < 50%	Small study effects	95% prediction interval exclude the null value	Excess significance	10% credibility ceiling survival
Associations supported by strong evidence (1)									
Zhang et al. (52)	platelet count OS	+++	+	+	−	−	+	−	+
Associations supported by highly suggestive evidence (7)									
Song et al. (57)	CA 19-9 OS	+++	+	+	−	−	−	+	+
Deng et al. (65)	CEA OS	+++	+	+	+	−	+	−	+
Pecqueux et al. (59)	FITC OS	+++	+	+	−	+	+	+	+
Huang et al. (97)	Foxp3+ Treg lymphocytes 1-year OS	+++	+	+	+	−	+	−	+
Huang et al. (97)	Foxp3+ Treg lymphocytes 3-year OS	+++	+	+	+	−	+	+	+
Sun et al. (40)	NLR OS	+++	+	+	−	−	+	+	+
Liu et al. (94)	Tissue VEGF OS	+++	+	+	−	+	−	+	+
Associations supported by suggestive evidence (4)									
Shen et al. (74)	MMP2 OS	+++	+	−	−	−	−	+	+
Wei et al. (56)	p53 OS	++	+	−	−	+	−	+	+
Wei et al. (56)	p53 DSS	+++	+	−	+	−	+	+	+
Li et al. (79)	β-catenin OS	++	+	−	−	+	−	−	+
Associations supported by weak evidence (84)									
Kim et al. (25)	ARID1A OS	++	−	+	+	−	+	+	+
Chen et al. (82)	BIRC5 5-year OS	+++	−	+	+	−	+	−	+
Shao et al. (75)	Bmi-1 OS	++	−	+	+	−	−	−	+
Song et al. (57)	CA 19-9 DFS	+	−	+	−	−	−	−	+
Song et al. (57)	CA 19-9 DSS	+	−	+	+	−	−	−	−
Du et al. (37)	CCR7 5-year OS	++	−	+	+	−	−	−	−
Lu et al. (41)	CD133 5-year OS	+++	−	+	+	+	+	−	+
Jiang et al. (26)	CD3+ T lymphocytes OS	++	−	+	+	−	−	−	+
Jiang et al. (26)	CD4+ T lymphocytes OS	+	−	+	−	−	−	−	−
Lu et al. (41)	CD44 5-year OS	+++	−	−	+	−	+	+	+
Wu et al. (54)	CD44 DFS	+	−	−	+	−	−	−	−
Jiang et al. (26)	CD8+ T lymphocytes OS	+	+	+	+	−	−	+	−
Wang et al. (92)	Cdx2 5-year OS	+++	−	+	+	−	+	−	+
Deng et al. (65)	CEA DFS	+++	−	+	+	−	+	−	+
Deng et al. (65)	CEA DSS	+++	−	+	+	−	+	−	+
Liu et al. (94)	Circulating VEGF OS	+++	−	+	+	−	−	−	+
Liu et al. (62)	CLDN4 OS	+++	−	+	+	−	+	−	+
Yu et al. (85)	c-MET OS	+++	−	−	−	−	−	+	+
Yu et al. (86)	CRP OS	+++	−	+	+	−	+	+	+
Zhang et al. (68)	CTCs OS	+++	−	+	+	−	+	−	+
Zhang et al. (68)	CTCs RFS	+++	−	+	−	−	−	−	+
Wang et al. (72)	CTCs RFS*	+++	−	+	+	−	+	+	+
Liu et al. (43)	DKK1 OS	+++	−	+	+	−	−	−	+
Li et al. (78)	E-cadherin 5-year OS	+++	−	+	+	−	+	−	+
Chen et al. (90)	EGFR OS	+++	−	+	+	−	+	+	+

(Continued)

TABLE 2 | Continued

Study	Association between biomarkers and gastric cancer	Summary relative risk estimate (random-effect *P*)*	Cases >1000	Largest study relative risk estimate *P*<0.05	I^2 < 50%	Small study effects	95% prediction interval exclude the null value	Excess significance	10% credibility ceiling survival
Song et al. (58)	ERCC1 OS	+	−	+	−	−	−	+	−
Zeng et al. (34)	FAK OS	+++	−	+	−	−	−	−	+
Liu et al. (24)	FGFR2 3-year OS	+	+	+	−	−	−	−	+
Liu et al. (24)	FGFR2 5-year OS	+	−	−	−	−	−	−	−
Wang et al. (73)	FHIT OS	+	−	−	+	−	+	−	+
Dai et al. (66)	FOXM1 OS	+	−	−	+	−	−	−	−
Jiang et al. (26)	FOXM1 1-year OS	++	−	+	+	−	+	−	+
Jiang et al. (26)	FOXM1 3-year OS	+	−	+	−	−	−	−	+
Jiang et al. (26)	FOXM1 5-year OS	++	−	+	+	+	−	−	+
Huang et al. (97)	Foxp3+ Treg lymphocytes 5-year OS	+++	−	+	−	−	−	+	+
Lei et al. (96)	HER2 OS	+	+	+	−	−	−	−	−
Zhang et al. (84)	HIF-1α OS	++	−	−	+	−	+	+	+
Chen et al. (82)	HIF-1α 5-year OS	+++	−	+	+	−	+	−	+
Tustumi et al. (39)	IFCC OS	+++	−	+	+	−	+	+	+
Gao et al. (63)	IGF-1R OS	+	−	+	−	−	−	−	+
Luo et al. (22)	Ki-67 OS	+	+	−	−	+	−	+	−
Luo et al. (22)	Ki-67 DFS	++	−	−	+	−	−	+	+
Huang et al. (46)	LGR5 OS	+	−	+	−	−	−	+	−
Wang et al. (38)	M2 TAM OS	+	−	+	−	−	−	−	+
Deng et al. (50)	MAPF OS	+++	−	+	+	+	+	−	+
Deng et al. (50)	MAPF DFS	++	−	+	−	−	−	+	+
Deng et al. (50)	MAPF peritoneal RFS	+++	−	+	+	−	+	+	+
Peng et al. (76)	MET OS	+++	−	−	+	+	+	−	+
Dong et al. (64)	MMP14 OS	+++	−	+	+	−	−	−	+
Zhang et al. (91)	MMP9 OS	++	−	−	−	−	−	+	+
Chen et al. (67)	MMP9 5-year OS	++	−	+	−	+	−	−	+
Wang et al. (37)	MUC1 5-year OS	+	−	+	−	−	−	−	+
Sun et al. (40)	NLR DFS	+	−	+	+	−	+	−	−
Sun et al. (40)	NLR PFS	+++	−	+	+	−	+	+	+
Gu et al. (48)	OPN OS	+	−	+	−	−	−	+	−
Brungs et al. (33)	PAI-1 OS	+	−	+	−	−	−	+	−
Brungs et al. (33)	PAI-1 RFS	+	−	−	−	−	−	+	−
Cao et al. (32)	p-Akt OS	+	−	+	−	−	−	−	+
Gu et al. (27)	PD-L1 OS	+	+	−	−	−	−	+	−
Wu et al. (55)	PD-L1 3-year OS	++	−	+	−	−	−	−	+
Hu et al. (89)	PRL-3 OS	++	−	+	−	−	−	+	+
Ji et al. (45)	pSTAT3 OS	+++	−	+	−	−	−	−	+
Chen et al. (82)	PTEN 5-year OS	+++	−	−	+	+	+	+	+
Jiang et al. (44)	Sirt1 3-year OS	++	−	+	−	+	−	+	+
Zhang et al. (69)	SK1 5-year OS	+	−	−	+	−	−	−	−
Wang et al. (70)	SPARC OS	+++	−	+	+	−	+	+	+

(Continued)

TABLE 2 | Continued

Study	Association between biomarkers and gastric cancer	Summary relative risk estimate (random-effect *P*)*	Cases >1000	Largest study relative risk estimate *P*<0.05	I^2 < 50%	Small study effects	95% prediction interval exclude the null value	Excess significance	10% credibility ceiling survival
Wu et al. (36)	STAT3 3-year OS	++	−	+	−	−	−	−	+
Wu et al. (36)	STAT3 5-year OS	++	−	−	−	−	−	−	+
Wang et al. (38)	TAMs OS	+++	−	−	+	−	+	+	+
Liu et al. (94)	Tissue VEGF DFS	+++	−	+	+	−	+	−	+
Liu et al. (94)	Tissue VEGF DSS	+	−	−	−	−	−	+	−
Brungs et al. (33)	uPA OS	+++	−	+	+	−	+	+	+
Brungs et al. (33)	uPA RFS	+	−	−	−	−	−	+	−
Brungs et al. (33)	uPAR OS	+++	−	+	+	+	+	−	+
Chen et al. (95)	VEGF 5-year OS	+++	−	+	−	−	+	−	+
Peng et al. (93)	VEGF-A OS	+++	−	+	+	−	+	−	+
Peng et al. (93)	VEGF-A DFS	+++	−	+	+	−	+	−	+
Cao et al. (83)	VEGF-C OS	++	−	+	+	−	−	−	+
Liu et al. (94)	VEGF-D OS	++	−	−	+	−	−	−	+
Peng et al. (93)	VEGF-D DFS	++	−	+	+	−	−	−	+
Ge et al. (28)	VEGFR-3 5-year OS	+	−	−	+	−	−	−	−
Chen et al. (31)	ZEB1 OS	+++	−	+	+	−	−	+	+
Chen et al. (31)	ZEB2 OS	+++	−	+	+	−	−	+	+
Associations supported by not suggestive evidence (24)									
Liu et al. (88)	BIRC5 OS	−	−	+	−	−	−	+	+
Wu et al. (54)	CD44 OS	−	−	−	+	−	−	−	−
Wu et al. (54)	CD44v6 OS	−	−	−		−	−	−	−
Lu et al. (41)	CD44v6 5-year OS	−	−	+	−	−	−	−	−
Meng et al. (60)	CDH17 5-year OS	−	−	+	−	−	−	+	−
Jiang et al. (26)	Dendritic cells OS	−	−	+	−	−	−	−	−
Guo et al. (80)	EZH2 OS	−	−	+	+	−	−	−	−
Tan et al. (87)	Fascin-1 OS	−	−	−	+	−	−	−	−
Jiang et al. (26)	Foxp3+ Treg lymphocytes OS	−	+	−	−	−	−	+	−
Gu et al. (81)	HER2 RFS	−	−	−	+	−	−	−	−
Cao et al. (51)	HER4 3-year OS	−	−	−	+	−	−	−	−
Zhang et al. (84)	HIF-1α DFS	−	−	−	−	−	−	+	−
Ma et al. (61)	HOTAIR OS	−	−	+	+	−	−	−	−
Zhang et al. (52)	MUC5AC OS	−	−	+	+	−	−	−	−
Fang et al. (29)	NM23 OS	−	−	+	−	−	−	−	−
Han et al. (47)	NME1 OS	−	−	+	−	+	+	−	−
Xu et al. (35)	PLR OS	−	+	−	+	−	−	−	−
Wang et al. (71)	S100A4 OS	−	−	−	+	+	−	+	−
Jiang et al. (44)	Sirt1 5-year OS	−	−	+	−	−	−	+	−
Lin et al. (77)	SOX2 OS	−	−	+	−	−	−	−	−
Gao et al. (49)	TS OS	−	−	−	−	−	−	−	−
Gao et al. (49)	TS EFS	−	−	−	−	−	−	−	−

(Continued)

TABLE 2 | Continued

Study	Association between biomarkers and gastric cancer	Summary relative risk estimate (random-effect *P*)*	Cases >1000	Largest study relative risk estimate *P*<0.05	$I^2 < 50\%$	Small study effects	95% prediction interval exclude the null value	Excess significance	10% credibility ceiling survival
Cao et al. (83)	VEGF-C DFS	–	–	–	–	–	–	–	–
Ge et al. (28)	VEGFR-3 3-year OS	–	–	–	+	–	–	–	–

P-value calculated using random-effect model: $+++P < 10^{-6}$; $++P < 10^{-3}$; $+P < 0.05$; $-P > 0.05$. For other items, + = yes, − = no. CI, confidence interval; OS, overall survival; DFS, disease free survival; RFS, recurrence free survival; PFS, progression free survival; EFS, event-free survival; peritoneal RFS, peritoneal recurrence-free survival; DSS, disease-specifc survival; RFS, relapse free survival; ARID1A, AT-rich interactive domain-containing 1A protein; BIRC5, (Survivin); PTEN, phosphatase and tensin homolog; HIF-1α, hypoxia inducible factor-1α; Bmi-1, B-cell-specific moloney leukemia virus insertion site 1; CA 19-9, serum carbohydrate antigen 19; CCR7, CC chemokine receptor type 7; CDH17, cadherin-17; CEA, carcinoembryonic antigen; Tissue VEGF, tissue vascular endothelial growth factor; Circulating VEGF, circulating vascular endothelial growth factor; Tissue VEGF-D, tissue vascular endothelial growth factor D; CLDN4, claudin 4; CRP, C-reactive protein; CTCs, circulating tumor cells; DKK1, dickkopf-1; EGFR, human epidermal growth factor receptor; ERCC1, excision repair cross-complementing group 1; EZH2, zeste homolog 2; FAK, focal adhesion kinase; FGFR2, fibroblast growth factor receptors; FHIT (bis(5′-adenosyl)-triphosphatase), fragile histidine triad protein; FITC, free intraperitoneal tumor cells; FOXM1, forkhead box M1; HER2, human epidermal growth factor receptor-2; HOTAIR, HOX transcript antisense intergenic RNA; IFCC, intraperitoneal free cancer cell; IGF-1R, insulin-like growth factor receptor type I; LGR5, leucinerich repeat-containing G-protein-coupled receptor 5; TAMs, tumor-associated macrophages; MAPF, molecular analysis of peritoneal fluid; MET (HGFR), hepatocyte growth factor receptor; MMP14, matrix metalloproteinase 14; MMP2, matrix metalloproteinase 2; MMP9, matrix metalloproteinase 9; MUC1, mucin 1; MUC5AC, mucin 5AC; NLR, neutrophil-to-lymphocyte ratio; NM23, non-metastatic protein 23; NME1 (NM23-H1 or NDPK-A); OPN, osteopontin; uPA, the urokinase plasminogen activation; uPAR, urokinase plasminogen activator receptor; PAI-1, plasminogen activator inhibitor-1; p-Akt, phosphorylated protein kinase B; PD-L1, programmed cell death ligand 1; PLR, platelet-lymphocyte ratio; PRL-3, phosphatase of regenerating liver 3; pSTAT3, phosphorylated signal transducer and activator of transcription proteins 3; Sirt1, Silent information regulator 1; SOX2, Sex-determining region Y-box 2; SPARC (osteonectin or BM-40), secreted protein acidic and rich in cysteine; STAT3, signal transducer and activator of transcription proteins 3; TS, thymidylate synthase; VEGF, vascular endothelial growth factor; VEGF, vascular endothelial growth factor; VEGF-C, vascular endothelial growth factor-C; VEGFR-3, vascular endothelial growth factor receptors 3; ZEB1, (TCF8, AREB6 or Zfhx1a) zinc fnger E-box binding homeobox 1; ZEB2, (SIP1, HSPC082 and Zfhx1b) zinc fnger E-box binding homeobox 2.

antigen 19-9 (CA 19-9) and GC OS, and between tissue vascular endothelial growth factor (VEGF) and GC OS (**Table 2**). Evidence supporting associations between p53 and OS or disease-specific survival of GC, between matrix metalloproteinase 2 (MMP2) and GC OS, and between β-catenin and GC OS were considered suggestive. The remaining 108 associations were supported by weak or not suggestive evidence. Detailed results of these analyses are shown in **Supplementary Table S3**.

DISCUSSION

Principal Finding

Biomarkers play essential role in clinical applications during several procedures in cancers including diagnosis, treatment, and prognosis. Cancer diagnosis based on biomarkers may improve the accuracy of early diagnosis and facilitate efficient subsequent treatment. Quite a few biomarkers have been identified in clinical trials, which show promises in the benefit of cancer patients, yet limitations exist. Some appear to be predictive biomarkers and their potential of indicating cancer developments remains to be seen. Others are restricted in clinical application due to the poor efficiency of traditional detection methods such as enzyme-linked immunosorbent assay (ELISA) and polymerase chain reaction (PCR). As novel biosensing approaches sprang up, the predictive and prognostic value of the biomarker has been widely tested in clinical trials. Since clinical practitioners can hardly perform intervention in cancer patients before diagnosis, we focused more on prognostic biomarkers instead of predictive biomarkers. To evaluate the prognostic potential of existing biomarkers and to facilitate the clinical application of more robust prognostic biomarkers, we performed this umbrella review.

This umbrella review was the first to comprehensively collect existing meta-analyses and systematically appraise the robustness of evidence to provide an overview of associations between prognostic biomarkers and GC. Overall, 74 meta-analyses comprising 80 different kinds of biomarkers were included in our umbrella review, only one association (the association between platelet count and GC OS) was supported by strong evidence. Several associations were supported by highly suggestive evidence, namely associations between GC OS and free intraperitoneal tumor cells (FITC), CEA, neutrophils to lymphocytes ratio (NLR), foxp3+ Treg lymphocytes (1- and 3-year OS), serum carbohydrate antigen 19-9 (CA 19-9), and tissue vascular endothelial growth factor (VEGF). Associations between p53, matrix metalloproteinase 2 (MMP2), β-catenin and GC OS were graded as suggestive and the remaining were graded as weak evidence. These results should be interpreted cautiously considering the poor methodological quality of the included meta-analyses as ascribed by AMSTAR 2.0.

Comparison With Other Studies and Possible Explanations

Classical Biomarkers and GC

CEA and CA 19-9 are two classical biomarkers detected in the last century and their predictive value for several cancers have been clinically confirmed (99, 100). However, the prognostic value of these two blood group antigens remains controversial. After systematically assessing the methodological quality and robustness of the pooled meta-analysis of 41 studies covering 14,651 participants, we found that CEA overexpression may relate to reduced OS for GC patients. However, associations between elevated CEA and GC DFS and GC disease specific survival (DSS) were found to be supported by weak evidence. These results might be explained by the low numbers of included studies and subjects: 29/3,491 for OS, 6/295 for DFS, and 7/542 for DSS. Another possible explanation is that elevated CEA is often detected in patients with GC of later stage, meaning the cause of death is not necessarily GC itself, considering severe complications. Of note, this pattern also holds for associations between CA19-9 and GC survival outcomes.

Novel Biomarkers and GC

Blood contains rich sources of tumor-associated biomarkers and is one of the human fluids that are easily accessible and can be analyzed in anytime and anywhere. These biomolecules are considered to be part of primary tumors, products of passive release during apoptosis and necrosis of tumor cells or biomolecules affected by tumor microenvironment (101).

In our research, we found that several biomolecules in blood may be considered as candidate prognostic biomarkers for GC patients. The association between platelet count and GC OS was the only one association that was supported by strong evidence. Platelet was previously reported to extensively interact with tumor cells, promoting tumor chemotaxis, adhesion, proliferation, and metastasis, which reasonably accounts for the robust indicative role of platelet in GC prognosis (102). High platelet count has proven to be associated with increased mortality in several cancers such as gynecologic malignancies, breast cancer, and lung cancer (103–105). Platelet count may also serve as an indicator of worse prognosis in GC based on the meta-analysis covering 5,515 subjects.

The prognosis indicative role of another inflammatory marker, NLR, is supported by highly suggestive evidence. Convincing evidence have been found between systematic inflammatory and tumor development. On one hand, myeloid growth factors secreted by cancer cells can upregulate production of neutrophils, on the other hand, immune cytokines provided by cancer cells downregulate function of lymphocyte (106). Elevated neutrophil stimulates angiogenesis and aids tumor progression while relative lymphocytopenia depresses innate anti-tumor cellular immunity, which explains why elevated NLR indicates poor OS in GC patients (107).

The other two highly suggestive evidences are that Foxp3+ Treg lymphocytes contribute to significantly poorer 1- and 3-year OS, while inconsistent result was found in 5-year OS. As a subgroup of CD4+ T help cells, Foxp3+ Treg lymphocytes play a critical role in suppressed T-cell immunity. Foxp3+ Treg lymphocytes turned out to be an unfavorable indicator of poor prognosis in GC.

Peritoneal dissemination is one of the most common and severe complications for GC. Detection of ascitic fluids and blood samples is frequently used clinically for easy accessibility and enhanced modern technologies. Evidence supporting the association between FITC and GC OS was graded as highly suggestive while the associations between circulating tumor cells (CTCs) and several GC survival outcomes were deemed to be supported by weak evidence. These results demonstrate that the role of FITC as a specific prognostic indicator of GC is more certain than that of CTC. Previous studies also suggest that FITC is a convincing predictive and prognostic biomarker for GC (108, 109) while the prognostic role of CTCs still need further confirmation.

Angiogenesis, the formation of new vascular network, plays an essential role in tumorigenesis and metastasis. As a vital target for prognosis evaluation, indicators to assess disease severity qualitatively and quantitatively are urgently needed. The vascular endothelial growth factor (VEGF) and its receptors (VEGFRs), which may modulate angiogenesis, show promises in this regard. Numerous studies report increased VEGFs and VEGFRs in both resectable and advanced GC patients. Five relevant meta-analyses of more than 11,307 participants were included in our umbrella review. The association between tissue VEGF and GC OS was supported by highly suggestive evidence while the association between tissue VEGF and GC DFS and other associations concerning VEGF, circulating VEGF, VEGF-A, VEGF-C, VEGF-D, VEGFR-3, and GC survival outcomes were supported by weak evidence. These differences can be explained by inadequate data and data quality as almost all relevant meta-analyses included less than five studies, covered fewer than 1,000 cases, or had high heterogeneity. The results concerning VEGF-C, VEGF-D are basically consistent with those concerning VEGFR-3, as the former two are essential factors in combination with the latter.

LIMITATIONS

This umbrella review was the first to provide an overview of associations between prognostic biomarkers and GC, and several limitations exist in this work. First, the umbrella review included published meta-analyses, meaning that studies that had not been systematically evaluated were unintentionally excluded, leading to unreliable results. Second, we only focused on associations between prognostic biomarkers and GC survival outcomes, while predictive biomarkers, mostly genetic markers comprising essential component of biomarkers, were not taken into consideration. Third, the majority of cases included in these meta-analyses are from Eastern countries and in this regard, we should interpret the findings with caution when it comes to population of Western origin. Fourth, subgroup analysis was not performed due to insufficient data provided by the included meta-analyses. Future work is required to establish a more comprehensive review to assess the true associations between prognostic biomarkers and GC survival and translate these associations into clinical practice to the utmost extent.

In conclusion, the association between platelet count and GC OS was supported by strong evidence. Associations between FITC, CEA, NLR, foxp3+ Treg lymphocytes (both 1- and 3-year OS), CA 19-9, or VEGF and GC OS were supported by highly suggestive evidence, however, the results should be interpreted cautiously due to inadequate methodological quality as deemed by AMSTAR 2.0.

AUTHOR CONTRIBUTIONS

ZWa and XZ conceived and designed the study. CZ and XZ performed the literature search, acquired, and collated the data, which were analyzed by YS, ZWu, JSh, ZG, and JSu. ZWa was guarantor. ZWa attests that all listed authors meet authorship criteria and that no others meeting the criteria have been omitted. All authors drafted and critically revised the manuscript for important intellectual content, and gave final approval of the version to be published and contributed to the manuscript.

REFERENCES

1. Karimi P, Islami F, Anandasabapathy S, Freedman ND, Kamangar F. Gastric cancer: descriptive epidemiology, risk factors, screening, and prevention. *Cancer Epidemiol Biomark Prev.* (2014) 23:700–13. doi: 10.1158/1055-9965.EPI-13-1057
2. Bray F, Ren JS, Masuyer E, Ferlay J. Global estimates of cancer prevalence for 27 sites in the adult population in 2008. *Int J Cancer.* (2013) 132:1133–45. doi: 10.1002/ijc.27711
3. Zheng R, Zeng H, Zhang S, Chen W. Estimates of cancer incidence and mortality in China, 2013. *Chin J Cancer.* (2017) 36:66. doi: 10.1186/s40880-017-0234-3
4. Hartgrink HH, Jansen EP, van Grieken NC, van de Velde CJ. Gastric cancer. *Lancet.* (2009) 374:477–90. doi: 10.1016/S0140-6736(09)60617-6
5. Biomarkers Definitions Working Group. Biomarkers and surrogate endpoints: preferred definitions and conceptual framework. *Clin Pharmacol Therapeut.* (2001) 69:89–95. doi: 10.1067/mcp.2001.113989
6. Fuzery AK, Levin J, Chan MM, Chan DW. Translation of proteomic biomarkers into FDA approved cancer diagnostics: issues and challenges. *Clin Proteom.* (2013) 10:13. doi: 10.1186/1559-0275-10-13
7. La Thangue NB, Kerr DJ. Predictive biomarkers: a paradigm shift towards personalized cancer medicine. *Nat Rev Clin Oncol.* (2011) 8:587–96. doi: 10.1038/nrclinonc.2011.121
8. Duffy MJ, Crown J. A personalized approach to cancer treatment: how biomarkers can help. *Clin Chem.* (2008) 54:1770–9. doi: 10.1373/clinchem.2008.110056
9. Sawyers CL. The cancer biomarker problem. *Nature.* (2008) 452:548–52. doi: 10.1038/nature06913
10. Simon R, Roychowdhury S. Implementing personalized cancer genomics in clinical trials. *Nat Rev Drug Discov.* (2013) 12:358–69. doi: 10.1038/nrd3979
11. Zhang BH, Yang BH, Tang ZY. Randomized controlled trial of screening for hepatocellular carcinoma. *J Cancer Res Clin Oncol.* (2004) 130:417–22. doi: 10.1007/s00432-004-0552-0
12. Chen JG, Parkin DM, Chen QG, Lu JH, Shen QJ, Zhang BC, et al. Screening for liver cancer: results of a randomised controlled trial in Qidong, China. *J Med Screen.* (2003) 10:204–9. doi: 10.1258/096914103771773320
13. Shea BJ, Reeves BC, Wells G, Thuku M, Hamel C, Moran J, et al. AMSTAR 2: a critical appraisal tool for systematic reviews that include randomised or non-randomised studies of healthcare interventions, or both. *BMJ.* (2017) 358:j4008. doi: 10.1136/bmj.j4008
14. Liebig C, Ayala G, Wilks J, Verstovsek G, Liu H, Agarwal N, et al. Perineural invasion is an independent predictor of outcome in colorectal cancer. *J Clin Oncol.* (2009) 27:5131–7. doi: 10.1200/JCO.2009.22.4949
15. Ioannidis JP, Patsopoulos NA, Evangelou E. Uncertainty in heterogeneity estimates in meta-analyses. *BMJ.* (2007) 335:914–6. doi: 10.1136/bmj.39343.408449.80
16. Riley RD, Higgins JP, Deeks JJ. Interpretation of random effects meta-analyses. *BMJ.* (2011) 342:d549. doi: 10.1136/bmj.d549
17. Patsopoulos NA, Evangelou E, Ioannidis JP. Heterogeneous views on heterogeneity. *Int J Epidemiol.* (2009) 38:1740–2. doi: 10.1093/ije/dyn235
18. Ioannidis JP, Trikalinos TA. An exploratory test for an excess of significant findings. *Clin Trials.* (2007) 4:245–53. doi: 10.1177/1740774507079441
19. Salanti G, Ioannidis JP. Synthesis of observational studies should consider credibility ceilings. *J Clin Epidemiol.* (2009) 62:115–22. doi: 10.1016/j.jclinepi.2008.05.014
20. Rezende LFM, Sa TH, Markozannes G, Rey-Lopez JP, Lee IM, Tsilidis KK, et al. Physical activity and cancer: an umbrella review of the literature including 22 major anatomical sites and 770 000 cancer cases. *Br J Sports Med.* (2018) 52:826–33. doi: 10.1136/bjsports-2017-098391
21. Raglan O, Kalliala I, Markozannes G, Cividini S, Gunter MJ, Nautiyal J, et al. Risk factors for endometrial cancer: an umbrella review of the literature. *Int J Cancer.* (2018) 145:1719–30. doi: 10.1002/ijc.31961
22. Luo G, Hu Y, Zhang Z, Wang P, Luo Z, Lin J, et al. Clinicopathologic significance and prognostic value of Ki-67 expression in patients with gastric cancer: a meta-analysis. *Oncotarget.* (2017) 8:50273–83. doi: 10.18632/oncotarget.17305
23. Liu G, Xiong D, Zeng J, Chen B, Huang Z. Clinicopathological and prognostic significance of Ki-67 immunohistochemical expression in gastric cancer: a systematic review and meta-analysis. *OncoTargets Ther.* (2017) 10:4321–8. doi: 10.2147/OTT.S143089
24. Liu G, Xiong D, Xiao R, Huang Z. Prognostic role of fibroblast growth factor receptor 2 in human solid tumors: a systematic review and meta-analysis. *Tumour Biol.* (2017) 39:1010428317707424. doi: 10.1177/1010428317707424
25. Kim YS, Jeong H, Choi JW, Oh HE, Lee JH. Unique characteristics of ARID1A mutation and protein level in gastric and colorectal cancer: a meta-analysis. *Saudi J Gastroenterol.* (2017) 23:268–74. doi: 10.4103/sjg.SJG_184_17
26. Jiang W, Liu K, Guo Q, Cheng J, Shen L, Cao Y, et al. Tumor-infiltrating immune cells and prognosis in gastric cancer: a systematic review and meta-analysis. *Oncotarget.* (2017) 8:62312–29. doi: 10.18632/oncotarget.17602
27. Gu L, Chen M, Guo D, Zhu H, Zhang W, Pan J, et al. PD-L1 and gastric cancer prognosis: a systematic review and meta-analysis. *PLoS ONE.* (2017) 12:e0182692. doi: 10.1371/journal.pone.0182692
28. Ge H, Yan Y, Guo L, He X, Yang X. Prognostic and clinical significance of VEGFR-3 in gastric cancer: a meta-analysis. *Clin Chim Acta.* (2017) 474:114–9. doi: 10.1016/j.cca.2017.09.013
29. Fang M, Tao Y, Liu Z, Huang H, Lao M, Huang L, et al. Meta-analysis of the relationship between NM23 expression to gastric cancer risk and clinical features. *BioMed Res Int.* (2017) 2017:8047183. doi: 10.1155/2017/8047183
30. Du P, Liu Y, Ren H, Zhao J, Zhang X, Patel R, et al. Expression of chemokine receptor CCR7 is a negative prognostic factor for patients with gastric cancer: a meta-analysis. *Gastric Cancer.* (2017) 20:235–45. doi: 10.1007/s10120-016-0602-8
31. Chen H, Lu W, Huang C, Ding K, Xia D, Wu Y, et al. Prognostic significance of ZEB1 and ZEB2 in digestive cancers: a cohort-based analysis and secondary analysis. *Oncotarget.* (2017) 8:31435–48. doi: 10.18632/oncotarget.15634
32. Cao F, Zhang C, Han W, Gao XJ, Ma J, Hu YW, et al. p-Akt as a potential poor prognostic factor for gastric cancer: a systematic review and meta-analysis. *Oncotarget.* (2017) 8:59878–88. doi: 10.18632/oncotarget.17001
33. Brungs D, Chen J, Aghmesheh M, Vine KL, Becker TM, Carolan MG, et al. The urokinase plasminogen activation system in gastroesophageal cancer: a systematic review and meta-analysis. *Oncotarget.* (2017) 8:23099–109. doi: 10.18632/oncotarget.15485
34. Zeng XQ, Li N, Ma LL, Tseng YJ, Zhao NQ, Chen SY. Prognostic value of focal adhesion kinase (FAK) in human solid carcinomas: a meta-analysis. *PLoS ONE.* (2016) 11:e0162666. doi: 10.1371/journal.pone.0162666
35. Xu Z, Xu W, Cheng H, Shen W, Ying J, Cheng F, et al. The prognostic role of the platelet-lymphocytes ratio in gastric cancer: a meta-analysis. *PLoS ONE.* (2016) 11:e0163719. doi: 10.1371/journal.pone.0163719
36. Wu P, Wu D, Zhao L, Huang L, Shen G, Huang J, et al. Prognostic role of STAT3 in solid tumors: a systematic review and meta-analysis. *Oncotarget.* (2016) 7:19863–83. doi: 10.18632/oncotarget.7887

37. Wang XT, Kong FB, Mai W, Li L, Pang LM. MUC1 Immunohistochemical expression as a prognostic factor in gastric cancer: meta-analysis. *Dis Markers.* (2016) 2016:9421571. doi: 10.1155/2016/9421571
38. Wang XL, Jiang JT, Wu CP. Prognostic significance of tumor-associated macrophage infiltration in gastric cancer: a meta-analysis. *Genet Mol Res.* (2016) 15:gmr15049040. doi: 10.4238/gmr15049040
39. Tustumi F, Bernardo WM, Dias AR, Ramos MF, Cecconello I, Zilberstein B, et al. Detection value of free cancer cells in peritoneal washing in gastric cancer: a systematic review and meta-analysis. *Clinics.* (2016) 71:733–45. doi: 10.6061/clinics/2016(12)10
40. Sun J, Chen X, Gao P, Song Y, Huang X, Yang Y, et al. Can the neutrophil to lymphocyte ratio be used to determine gastric cancer treatment outcomes? a systematic review and meta-analysis. *Dis Markers.* (2016) 2016:7862469. doi: 10.1155/2016/7862469
41. Lu L, Wu M, Sun L, Li W, Fu W, Zhang X, et al. Clinicopathological and prognostic significance of cancer stem cell markers CD44 and CD133 in patients with gastric cancer: a comprehensive meta-analysis with 4729 patients involved. *Medicine.* (2016) 95:e5163. doi: 10.1097/MD.0000000000005163
42. Lu L, Huang F, Zhao Z, Li C, Liu T, Li W, et al. CD44v6: a metastasis-associated biomarker in patients with gastric cancer?: a comprehensive meta-analysis with heterogeneity analysis. *Medicine.* (2016) 95:e5603. doi: 10.1097/MD.0000000000005603
43. Liu QR, Li YF, Deng ZQ, Cao JQ. Prognostic significance of dickkopf-1 in gastric cancer survival: a meta-analysis. *Genet Test Mol Biomark.* (2016) 20:170–5. doi: 10.1089/gtmb.2015.0154
44. Jiang B, Chen JH, Yuan WZ, Ji JT, Liu ZY, Wu L, et al. Prognostic and clinical value of Sirt1 expression in gastric cancer: a systematic meta-analysis. *J Huazhong Univ Sci Technol Med Sci.* (2016) 36:278–84. doi: 10.1007/s11596-016-1580-0
45. Ji K, Zhang L, Zhang M, Chu Q, Li X, Wang W. Prognostic value and clinicopathological significance of p-stat3 among gastric carcinoma patients: a systematic review and meta-analysis. *Medicine.* (2016) 95:e2641. doi: 10.1097/MD.0000000000002641
46. Huang T, Qiu X, Xiao J, Wang Q, Wang Y, Zhang Y, et al. The prognostic role of Leucine-rich repeat-containing G-protein-coupled receptor 5 in gastric cancer: a systematic review with meta-analysis. *Clin Res Hepatol Gastroenterol.* (2016) 40:246–53. doi: 10.1016/j.clinre.2015.07.009
47. Han W, Shi CT, Cao FY, Cao F, Chen MB, Lu RZ, et al. Prognostic value of NME1 (NM23-H1) in patients with digestive system neoplasms: a systematic review and meta-analysis. *PLoS ONE.* (2016) 11:e0160547. doi: 10.1371/journal.pone.0160547
48. Gu X, Gao XS, Ma M, Qin S, Qi X, Li X, et al. Prognostic significance of osteopontin expression in gastric cancer: a meta-analysis. *Oncotarget.* (2016) 7:69666–73. doi: 10.18632/oncotarget.11936
49. Gao Y, Cui J, Xi H, Cai A, Shen W, Li J, et al. Association of thymidylate synthase expression and clinical outcomes of gastric cancer patients treated with fluoropyrimidine-based chemotherapy: a meta-analysis. *OncoTargets Ther.* (2016) 9:1339–50. doi: 10.2147/OTT.S98540
50. Deng K, Zhu H, Chen M, Wu J, Hu R, Tang C. Prognostic significance of molecular analysis of peritoneal fluid for patients with gastric cancer: a meta-analysis. *PLoS ONE.* (2016) 11:e0151608. doi: 10.1371/journal.pone.0151608
51. Cao GD, Chen K, Xiong MM, Chen B. HER3, but not HER4, plays an essential role in the clinicopathology and prognosis of gastric cancer: a meta-analysis. *PLoS ONE.* (2016) 11:e0161219. doi: 10.1371/journal.pone.0161219
52. Zhang CT, He KC, Pan F, Li Y, Wu J. Prognostic value of Muc5AC in gastric cancer: a meta-analysis. *World J Gastroenterol.* (2015) 21:10453–60. doi: 10.3748/wjg.v21.i36.10453
53. Xin-Ji Z, Yong-Gang L, Xiao-Jun S, Xiao-Wu C, Dong Z, Da-Jian Z. The prognostic role of neutrophils to lymphocytes ratio and platelet count in gastric cancer: a meta-analysis. *Int J Surg.* (2015) 21:84–91. doi: 10.1016/j.ijsu.2015.07.681
54. Wu Y, Li Z, Zhang C, Yu K, Teng Z, Zheng G, et al. CD44 family proteins in gastric cancer: a meta-analysis and narrative review. *Int J Clin Exp Med.* (2015), 8:3595—3606.
55. Wu P, Wu D, Li L, Chai Y, Huang J: PD-L1 and survival in solid tumors: a meta-analysis. *PLoS ONE.* (2015) 10:e0131403. doi: 10.1371/journal.pone.0131403
56. Wei K, Jiang L, Wei Y, Wang Y, Qian X, Dai Q, et al. The prognostic significance of p53 expression in gastric cancer: a meta-analysis. *J Cancer Res Clin Oncol.* (2015) 141:735–748. doi: 10.1007/s00432-014-1844-7
57. Song YX, Huang XZ, Gao P, Sun JX, Chen XW, Yang YC, et al. Clinicopathologic and prognostic value of serum carbohydrate antigen 19-9 in gastric cancer: a meta-analysis. *Dis Markers.* (2015) 2015:549843. doi: 10.1155/2015/549843
58. Song P, Yin Q, Lu M, Fu BO, Wang B, Zhao Q. Prognostic value of excision repair cross-complementation group 1 expression in gastric cancer: a meta-analysis. *Exp Therapeut Med.* (2015) 9:1393–400. doi: 10.3892/etm.2015.2284
59. Pecqueux M, Fritzmann J, Adamu M, Thorlund K, Kahlert C, Reissfelder C, et al. Free intraperitoneal tumor cells and outcome in gastric cancer patients: a systematic review and meta-analysis. *Oncotarget.* (2015) 6:35564–78. doi: 10.18632/oncotarget.5595
60. Meng W, Gu T, Gao LM, Zong ZG, Meng L, Fu ZZ, et al. Correlation of cadherin-17 protein expression with clinicopathological features and prognosis of patients with sporadic gastric cancer. *Brazil J Med Biol Res.* (2015) 48:1077–86. doi: 10.1590/1414-431x20154645
61. Ma G, Wang Q, Lv C, Qiang F, Hua Q, Chu H, et al. The prognostic significance of HOTAIR for predicting clinical outcome in patients with digestive system tumors. *J Cancer Res Clin Oncol.* (2015) 141:2139–45. doi: 10.1007/s00432-015-1980-8
62. Liu JX, Wei ZY, Chen JS, Lu HC, Hao L, Li WJ. Prognostic and clinical significance of claudin-4 in gastric cancer: a meta-analysis. *World J Surg Oncol.* (2015) 13:207. doi: 10.1186/s12957-015-0626-2
63. Gao Y, Cui J, Xi H, Shen W, Zhang K, Li J, et al. Association of prognosis with insulin-like growth factor receptor type I expression in gastric cancer patients: a meta-analysis. *Zhonghua Wei Chang Wai Ke Za Zhi.* (2015) 18:1051–5. doi: 10.3760/cma.j.issn.1671-0274.2015.10.019
64. Dong Y, Chen G, Gao M, Tian X. Increased expression of MMP14 correlates with the poor prognosis of Chinese patients with gastric cancer. *Gene.* (2015) 563:29–34. doi: 10.1016/j.gene.2015.03.003
65. Deng K, Yang L, Hu B, Wu H, Zhu H, Tang C. The prognostic significance of pretreatment serum CEA levels in gastric cancer: a meta-analysis including 14651 patients. *PLoS ONE.* (2015) 10:e0124151. doi: 10.1371/journal.pone.0124151
66. Dai J, Yang L, Wang J, Xiao Y, Ruan Q. Prognostic value of FOXM1 in patients with malignant solid tumor: a meta-analysis and system review. *Dis Markers.* (2015) 2015:352478. doi: 10.1155/2015/352478
67. Chen J, Liu X, Jiao H, Peng L, Huo Z, Yang W, et al. Prognostic and clinical significance of STAT3 and MMP9 in patients with gastric cancer: a meta-analysis of a Chinese cohort. *Int J Clin Exp Med.* (2015) 8:546–57.
68. Zhang ZY, Dai ZL, Yin XW, Li SH, Li SP, Ge HY. Meta-analysis shows that circulating tumor cells including circulating microRNAs are useful to predict the survival of patients with gastric cancer. *BMC Cancer.* (2014) 14:773. doi: 10.1186/1471-2407-14-773
69. Zhang Y, Wang Y, Wan Z, Liu S, Cao Y, Zeng Z. Sphingosine kinase 1 and cancer: a systematic review and meta-analysis. *PLoS ONE.* (2014) 9:e90362. doi: 10.1371/journal.pone.0090362
70. Wang Z, Hao B, Yang Y, Wang R, Li Y, Wu Q. Prognostic role of SPARC expression in gastric cancer: a meta-analysis. *Archiv Med Sci.* (2014) 10:863–9. doi: 10.5114/aoms.2014.46207
71. Wang Y, Zhou LB, Li XH. S100A4 expression and prognosis of gastric cancer: a meta-analysis. *Genet Mol Res.* (2014) 13:10398–403. doi: 10.4238/2014.December.12.1
72. Wang S, Zheng G, Cheng B, Chen F, Wang Z, Chen Y, et al. Circulating tumor cells (CTCs) detected by RT-PCR and its prognostic role in gastric cancer: a meta-analysis of published literature. *PLoS ONE.* (2014) 9:e99259. doi: 10.1371/journal.pone.0099259
73. Wang HL, Zhou PY, Liu P, Zhang Y. Abnormal FHIT protein expression may be correlated with poor prognosis in gastric cancer: a meta-analysis. *Tumour Biol.* (2014) 35:6815–21. doi: 10.1007/s13277-014-1936-7
74. Shen W, Xi H, Wei B, Chen L. The prognostic role of matrix metalloproteinase 2 in gastric cancer: a systematic review with meta-analysis. *J Cancer Res Clin Oncol.* (2014) 140:1003–9. doi: 10.1007/s00432-014-1630-6
75. Shao Y, Geng Y, Gu W, Ning Z, Jiang J, Pei H. Prognostic role of high Bmi-1 expression in Asian and Caucasian patients with solid tumors: a meta-analysis. *Biomed Pharmacother.* (2014) 68:969–77. doi: 10.1016/j.biopha.2014.10.017

76. Peng Z, Zhu Y, Wang Q, Gao J, Li Y, Li Y, et al. Prognostic significance of MET amplification and expression in gastric cancer: a systematic review with meta-analysis. *PLoS ONE.* (2014) 9:e84502. doi: 10.1371/journal.pone.0084502
77. Lin S, Qi W, Han K, Gan Z, Yao Y, Miu D. Prognostic value of SOX2 in digestive tumors: a meta-analysis. *Hepatogastroenterology.* (2014) 61:1274–78. doi: 10.5754/hge14079
78. Li T, Chen J, Liu QL, Huo ZH, Wang ZW. Meta-analysis: E-cadherin immunoexpression as a potential prognosis biomarker related to gastric cancer metastasis in Asian patients. *Eur Rev Med Pharmacol Sci.* (2014) 18:2693–703.
79. Li LF, Wei ZJ, Sun H, Jiang B. Abnormal beta-catenin immunohistochemical expression as a prognostic factor in gastric cancer: a meta-analysis. *World J Gastroenterol.* (2014) 20:12313–321. doi: 10.3748/wjg.v20.i34.12313
80. Guo L, Yang TF, Liang SC, Guo JX, Wang Q. Role of EZH2 protein expression in gastric carcinogenesis among Asians: a meta-analysis. *Tumour Biology.* (2014) 35:6649–56. doi: 10.1007/s13277-014-1888-y
81. Gu J, Zheng L, Wang Y, Zhu M, Wang Q, Li X. Prognostic significance of HER2 expression based on trastuzumab for gastric cancer (ToGA) criteria in gastric cancer: an updated meta-analysis. *Tumour Biol.* (2014) 35:5315–21. doi: 10.1007/s13277-014-1693-7
82. Chen J, Li T, Liu Q, Jiao H, Yang W, Liu X, et al. Clinical and prognostic significance of HIF-1alpha, PTEN, CD44v6, and survivin for gastric cancer: a meta-analysis. *PLoS ONE.* (2014) 9:e91842. doi: 10.1371/journal.pone.0091842
83. Cao W, Fan R, Yang W, Wu Y. VEGF-C expression is associated with the poor survival in gastric cancer tissue. *Tumour Biol.* (2014) 35:3377–83. doi: 10.1007/s13277-013-1445-0
84. Zhang ZG, Zhang QN, Wang XH, Tian JH. Hypoxia-inducible factor 1 alpha (HIF-1alpha) as a prognostic indicator in patients with gastric tumors: a meta-analysis. *Asian Pacific J Cancer Prev.* (2013) 14:4195–98. doi: 10.7314/APJCP.2013.14.7.4195
85. Yu S, Yu Y, Zhao N, Cui J, Li W, Liu T. C-Met as a prognostic marker in gastric cancer: a systematic review and meta-analysis. *PLoS ONE.* (2013) 8:e79137. doi: 10.1371/journal.pone.0079137
86. Yu Q, Yu XF, Zhang SD, Wang HH, Wang HY, Teng LS. Prognostic role of C-reactive protein in gastric cancer: a meta-analysis. *Asian Pacific J Cancer Prev.* (2013) 14:5735–40. doi: 10.7314/APJCP.2013.14.10.5735
87. Tan VY, Lewis SJ, Adams JC, Martin RM. Association of fascin-1 with mortality, disease progression and metastasis in carcinomas: a systematic review and meta-analysis. *BMC Med.* (2013) 11:52. doi: 10.1186/1741-7015-11-52
88. Liu JL, Gao W, Kang QM, Zhang XJ, Yang SG. Prognostic value of survivin in patients with gastric cancer: a systematic review with meta-analysis. *PLoS ONE.* (2013) 8:e71930. doi: 10.1371/journal.pone.0071930
89. Hu L, Luo H, Wang W, Li H, He T. Poor prognosis of phosphatase of regenerating liver 3 expression in gastric cancer: a meta-analysis. *PLoS ONE.* (2013) 8:e76927. doi: 10.1371/journal.pone.0076927
90. Chen C, Yang JM, Hu TT, Xu TJ, Yan G, Hu SL, et al. Prognostic role of human epidermal growth factor receptor in gastric cancer: a systematic review and meta-analysis. *Archiv Med Res.* (2013) 44:380–9. doi: 10.1016/j.arcmed.2013.07.001
91. Zhang QW, Liu L, Chen R, Wei YQ, Li P, Shi HS, et al. Matrix metalloproteinase-9 as a prognostic factor in gastric cancer: a meta-analysis. *Asian Pacific J Cancer Prev.* (2012) 13:2903–8. doi: 10.7314/APJCP.2012.13.6.2903
92. Wang XT, Wei WY, Kong FB, Lian C, Luo W, Xiao Q, et al. Prognostic significance of Cdx2 immunohistochemical expression in gastric cancer: a meta-analysis of published literatures. *J Exp Clin Cancer Res.* (2012) 31:98. doi: 10.1186/1756-9966-31-98
93. Peng L, Zhan P, Zhou Y, Fang W, Zhao P, Zheng Y, et al. Prognostic significance of vascular endothelial growth factor immunohistochemical expression in gastric cancer: a meta-analysis. *Mol Biol Rep.* (2012) 39:9473–84. doi: 10.1007/s11033-012-1812-8
94. Liu L, Ma XL, Xiao ZL, Li M, Cheng SH, Wei YQ. Prognostic value of vascular endothelial growth factor expression in resected gastric cancer. *Asian Pacific J Cancer Prev.* (2012) 13:3089–97. doi: 10.7314/APJCP.2012.13.7.3089
95. Chen J, Li T, Wu Y, He L, Zhang L, Shi T, et al. Prognostic significance of vascular endothelial growth factor expression in gastric carcinoma: a meta-analysis. *J Cancer Res Clin Oncol.* (2011) 137:1799–812. doi: 10.1007/s00432-011-1057-2
96. Lei YY, Huang JY, Zhao QR, Jiang N, Xu HM, Wang ZN, et al. The clinicopathological parameters and prognostic significance of HER2 expression in gastric cancer patients: a meta-analysis of literature. *World J Surg Oncol.* (2017) 15:68. doi: 10.1186/s12957-017-1132-5
97. Huang Y, Liao H, Zhang Y, Yuan R, Wang F, Gao Y, et al. Prognostic value of tumor-infiltrating FoxP3^{+} T cells in gastrointestinal cancers: a meta analysis. *PloS One.* (2014) 9:e94376. doi: 10.1371/journal.pone.0094376
98. Wang ZQ, Sun BJ. C-erbB-2 expression and prognosis of gastric cancer: a meta-analysis. *Genet Mol Res.* (2015) 14:1782–7. doi: 10.4238/2015.March.13.5
99. Tatsuta M, Itoh T, Okuda S, Yamamura H, Baba M, Tamura H. Carcinoembryonic antigen in gastric juice as an aid in diagnosis of early gastric cancer. *Cancer.* (1980) 46:2686–92. doi: 10.1002/1097-0142(19801215)46:12<2686::AID-CNCR2820461225>3.0.CO;2-E
100. Kim DY, Kim HR, Shim JH, Park CS, Kim SK, Kim YJ. Significance of serum and tissue carcinoembryonic antigen for the prognosis of gastric carcinoma patients. *J Surg Oncol.* (2000) 74:185–92. doi: 10.1002/1096-9098(200007)74:3<185::AID-JSO4>3.0.CO;2-0
101. Best MG, Wesseling P, Wurdinger T. Tumor-educated platelets as a noninvasive biomarker source for cancer detection and progression monitoring. *Cancer Res.* (2018) 78: 3407–12. doi: 10.1158/0008-5472.CAN-18-0887
102. Pinedo HM, Verheul HM, D'Amato RJ, Folkman J. Involvement of platelets in tumour angiogenesis? *Lancet.* (1998) 352:1775–7. doi: 10.1016/S0140-6736(98)05095-8
103. Stone RL, Nick AM, McNeish IA, Balkwill F, Han HD, Bottsford-Miller J, et al. Paraneoplastic thrombocytosis in ovarian cancer. *N Engl J Med.* (2012) 366: 610–8. doi: 10.1056/NEJMoa1110352
104. Graziano V, Grassadonia A, Iezzi L, Vici P, Pizzuti L, Barba M, et al. Combination of peripheral neutrophil-to-lymphocyte ratio and platelet-to-lymphocyte ratio is predictive of pathological complete response after neoadjuvant chemotherapy in breast cancer patients. *Breast.* (2019) 44:33–8. doi: 10.1016/j.breast.2018.12.014
105. Diem S, Schmid S, Krapf M, Flatz L, Born D, Jochum W, et al. Neutrophil-to-Lymphocyte ratio (NLR) and Platelet-to-Lymphocyte ratio (PLR) as prognostic markers in patients with non-small cell lung cancer (NSCLC) treated with nivolumab. *Lung Cancer.* (2017) 111:176–81. doi: 10.1016/j.lungcan.2017.07.024
106. Asaoka T, Miyamoto A, Maeda S, Tsujie M, Hama N, Yamamoto K, et al. Prognostic impact of preoperative NLR and CA19-9 in pancreatic cancer. *Pancreatology.* (2016) 16: 434–40. doi: 10.1016/j.pan.2015.10.006
107. Dolcetti R, Viel A, Doglioni C, Russo A, Guidoboni M, Capozzi E, et al. High prevalence of activated intraepithelial cytotoxic T lymphocytes and increased neoplastic cell apoptosis in colorectal carcinomas with microsatellite instability. *Am J Pathol.* (1999) 154:1805–13. doi: 10.1016/S0002-9440(10)65436-3
108. De Andrade JP, Mezhir JJ. The critical role of peritoneal cytology in the staging of gastric cancer: an evidence-based review. *J Surg Oncol.* (2014) 110:291–7. doi: 10.1002/jso.23632
109. Nieveen van Dijkum EJ, Sturm PD, de Wit LT, Offerhaus J, Obertop H, Gouma DJ. Cytology of peritoneal lavage performed during staging laparoscopy for gastrointestinal malignancies: is it useful? *Ann Surg.* (1998) 228:728–33. doi: 10.1097/00000658-199812000-00002

16

A Contrast-Enhanced Computed Tomography Based Radiomics Approach for Preoperative Differentiation of Pancreatic Cystic Neoplasm Subtypes

Xiaoyong Shen[1†], Fan Yang[2†], Pengfei Yang[3,4,5†], Modan Yang[2], Lei Xu[3,4], Jianyong Zhuo[2], Jianguo Wang[2], Di Lu[2], Zhikun Liu[2], Shu-sen Zheng[2], Tianye Niu[3,4,6] and Xiao Xu[2]**

[1] Department of Radiology, First Affiliated Hospital, Zhejiang University School of Medicine, Hangzhou, China, [2] Department of Hepatobiliary and Pancreatic Surgery, First Affiliated Hospital, Zhejiang University School of Medicine, Hangzhou, China, [3] Sir Run Run Shaw Hospital, Zhejiang University School of Medicine, Hangzhou, China, [4] Institute of Translational Medicine, Zhejiang University, Hangzhou, China, [5] College of Biomedical Engineering & Instrument Science, Zhejiang University, Hangzhou, China, [6] Nuclear & Radiological Engineering and Medical Physics Programs, Woodruff School of Mechanical Engineering, Georgia Institute of Technology, Atlanta, GA, United States

***Correspondence:**
Tianye Niu
tyniu@gatech.edu
Xiao Xu
zjxu@zju.edu.cn

† These authors have contributed equally to this work

Background: Serous cystadenoma (SCA), mucinous cystadenoma (MCN), and intraductal papillary mucinous neoplasm (IPMN) are three subtypes of pancreatic cystic neoplasm (PCN). Due to the potential of malignant-transforming, patients with MCN and IPMN require radical surgery while patients with SCA need periodic surveillance. However, accurate pre-surgery diagnosis between SCA, MCN, and IPMN remains challenging in the clinic.

Methods: This study enrolled 164 patients including 76 with SCA, 40 with MCN and 48 with IPMN. Patients were randomly split into a training cohort ($n = 115$) and validation cohort ($n = 41$). We performed statistical analysis and Boruta method to screen significantly distinct clinical factors and radiomics features extracted on pre-surgery contrast-enhanced computed tomography (CECT) images among three subtypes. Three reliable machine-learning algorithms, support vector machine (SVM), random forest (RF) and artificial neural network (ANN), were utilized to construct classifiers based on important radiomics features and clinical parameters. Precision, recall, and F1-score were calculated to assess the performance of the constructed classifiers.

Results: Nine of 547 radiomics features and eight clinical factors showed a significant difference among SCA, MCN, and IPMN. Five radiomics features (Histogram_Entropy, Histogram_Skeweness, LLL_GLSZM_GLV, Histogram_Uniformity, HHL_Histogram_Kurtosis), and four clinical factors, including serum carbohydrate antigen 19-9, sex, age, and serum carcinoembryonic antigen, were identified important by Boruta method. The SVM classifier achieved an overall accuracy of 73.04% in training cohort and 71.43% in validation cohort, respectively. The RF classifier achieved overall accuracy of 84.35 and 79.59%, respectively. The constructed ANN model showed an overall accuracy of 77.39% in the training dataset and 71.43% in the validation dataset. All the three classifiers showed high F1 score for differentiation among the three subtypes.

Conclusion: Our study proved the feasibility and translational value of CECT-based radiomics classifiers for differentiation among SCA, MCN, and IPMN.

Keywords: pancreatic cystic neoplasm, contrast-enhanced computed tomography, radiomics, differentiation diagnosis, machine learning

INTRODUCTION

Pancreatic cystic neoplasm (PCN) has been estimated to be present in 2–45% of the general population (1, 2). As computed tomography (CT) and magnetic resonance imaging (MRI) become widely used in clinical work, the incidence of PCN has increased to 3–13% for individuals undergoing cross-sectional imaging (3–5). Serous cystadenomas (SCA), mucinous cystic neoplasm (MCN), and intraductal papillary mucinous neoplasm (IPMN) constitute a majority of the PCN subtypes encountered in practice (6, 7). SCA is of benign nature and periodical surveillance is enough (8). MCN, IPMN are with the degree of malignancy, and thus close surveillance and radical surgery are recommended (8–10).

The pre-surgery classification of PCN subtypes is crucial for making personalized treatment strategies. However, it is still challenging to achieve an accurate differential diagnosis (9, 11, 12) preoperatively in the clinic. Till now, no nucleic acid or protein biomarkers in blood are available to precisely differentiate PCN subtypes in clinical work. DNA markers in cyst fluid, like GNAS, show potential in identifying mucin-producing cyst lesions but far from the bench. The differentiating value of RNA or non-carcinoembryonic antigen (CEA) protein markers is still lacking sufficient evidence (10, 13). Brugge et al. claimed cyst fluid CEA level (>192 ng/mL) could differentiate mucinous from non-mucinous lesions with an accuracy of 79%, while cystic fluid carbohydrate antigen (CA 19-9) (>2,900 U/mL) presented a sensitivity of 68% and specificity of 62% (13, 14). As for radiology method, radiological examination (CT/MRI/Magnetic Resonance Cholangiopancreatography) has limited diagnostic accuracy, even by experienced radiologists. Endoscopic ultrasound (EUS)-based diagnosis methods like endoscopic ultrasound (EUS) guided fine needle aspiration (FNA) should be performed only when diagnosis of CT or MRI are unclear (10). The limit of current methods will hamper the making of proper medical decisions, increase the suffering of the patients and waste of limited medical resources. Thus, a reliable approach for classifying the subtypes of PCN per-surgery is urgently needed to facilitate personalized medicine.

Past decades had witnessed the rapid development of the field of medical image analysis, facilitating the development of the radiomics method which quantifies the tumor heterogeneity into high-dimension features (15). The radiomics approach can help clinicians make individualized decisions based on the quantitative radiomics features and machine-learning-based models (16). Chakraborty et al. investigated the CT based radiomics features as markers for stratifying the high-risk IPMN patients (17). However, the potential of radiomics methods in helping accurate diagnose of subtypes of PCN has yet been fully investigated.

Although MRI is the preferred modality according to the 2018 European evidence-based guideline (10), in developing countries like China, South America, and Africa, MRI is not always accessible. Contrast-enhanced CT (CECT) is the main diagnosis modality for PCN in China. In our center, SCA, MCN, and IPMN are most common subtypes. From retrospective analysis of pre-surgery radiological diagnoses and pathological examination results, we found diagnosis of SCA and MCN were either obscure or wrong. And IPMN was the main misdiagnosed type for both SCA and MCN. Therefore, in this study, we aimed to investigate the feasibility of using CECT based radiomics approach for preoperatively classifying SCA, MCN, and IPMN to facilitate the personalized treatment for patients with PCN.

MATERIALS AND METHODS

Patients

Patients with pancreatic lesions treated from January 2014 to March 2019 in our center were retrospectively evaluated. Patients with pathologically proven SCA, MCN, and IPMN were selected for further analysis. The inclusion criteria were as following: (i) patients had undergone a CECT scan within 2 weeks before surgery; (ii) patients had postoperative pathological diagnosis of SCA, MCN or IPMN. The exclusion criteria were: (i) patients diagnosed with concurrent hepatic-pancreato-biliary malignancies, such as hepatocellular carcinoma; (ii) patients whose CT images were affected by strong imaging artifacts, i.e., artifacts obscuring more than 10% of whole volume of interest; (iii) patients whose clinical data or CT images were missing. Collected clinical data includes patient age, gender, abdominal symptoms (including abdominal pain, diarrhea and obscure abdominal discomfort), tumor location (head and neck, body and tail, both), calcification, tumor maximum diameter, serum platelet count, serum alanine aminotransferase (ALT), serum aspartate aminotransferase (AST), serum albumin (ALB), serum fasting blood glucose (FBG), serum tumor markers [alpha-fetoprotein (AFP), CEA, CA19-9, and serum ferritin (SF)], familial history of pancreatic cancer, chronic pancreatitis history, history of smoking, history of alcoholic consumption, obesity [based on body mass index (BMI), patients with BMI equal to or larger than 25 were identified as obesity], and blood type. The final enrolled patient dataset was randomly split into independent training group (70%) and validation group (30%), using a stratified sampling method (18). Ethical approval was

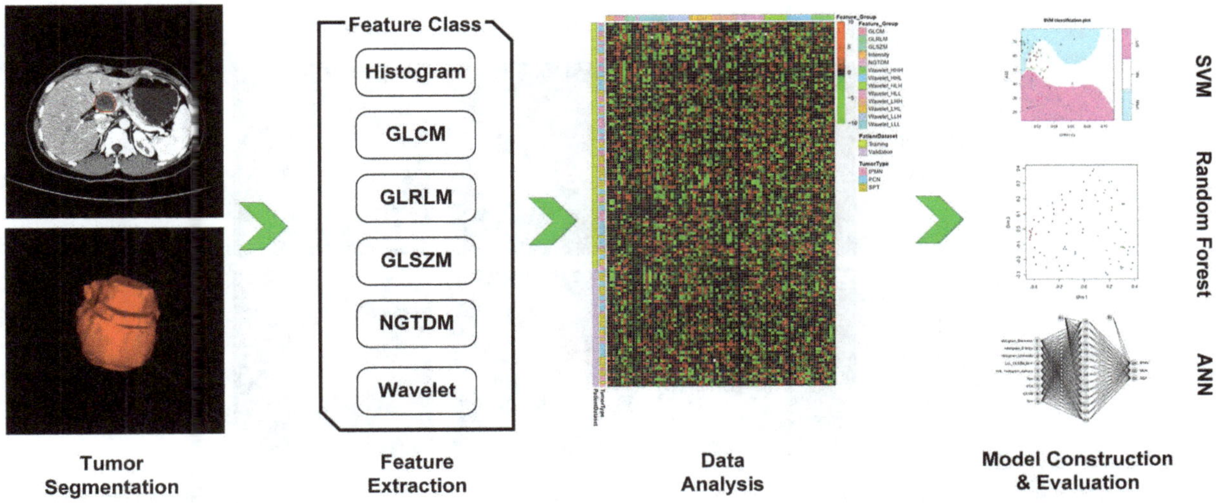

FIGURE 1 | First, we performed delineation of the region of interest and segmentation, then features belong to different categories (Histogram, GLCM, GLRLM, GLSZM, NGTDM, and wavelet) were extracted and further analyzed. According to feature selection algorithm, the most important features were selected for model construction. Then, the performance of constructed model was evaluated in the validation dataset.

obtained from Human Research Ethics Committee (HREC) of our hospital. The patient informed consent was waived by the HREC for the retrospective usage of patients' medical images.

Study Design

The analysis workflow of this study was shown in **Figure 1**. After delineation and segmentation of the region of interest, features belong to different categories [histogram, gray-level co-occurrence matrix (GLCM), gray-level run-length matrix (GLRLM), gray-level size zone matrix (GLSZM), neighborhood gray-tone difference matrix (NGTDM) and wavelet] were extracted and analyzed. Then the most important features were selected for model construction using supporting vector machine (SVM), random forest (RF) and artificial neural network (ANN) algorithm.

Image Acquisition

The preoperative CECT images of patients were retrieved from the Picture Archiving and Communication Systems in our institution. All scans were performed on a 256-Slice CT scanner (Brilliance iCT, Philips, Cleveland, OH, USA) in our hospital. The scan voltage was 100 or 120 kV and the scan current was 110–835 mAs, adjustable for different patient conditions. The CECT images were reconstructed with a standard kernel. The reconstruction slice thickness was 3–5 mm and the pixel spacing of CT images ranged from 0.5 to 1 mm. The scan is performed after a 60 s delay following intravenous administration of 1.5 ml/kg of iodinated contrast medium (Iohexol Injection, 300 mg I/ml, Ousu, Yangtze River Pharmaceutical Group) and 20 ml of saline at a rate of 3 ml/s with an automatic pump injector. Arterial phase was carried out at 25–35 s after contrast injection and CT scans of arterial phase were used for subsequent process.

Tumor Segmentation and Quantification

The arterial phase of the CECT scan showed an enhanced pattern of the tumor region (19) and thus was selected for quantifying the tumor heterogeneity in this study. The delineation of tumor regions was performed, on all 3D CT slices, by a board-certified radiologist using ITK-SNAP [*www.itksnap.org* (20)]. The radiologist was blind to the clinical information before performing segmentation. The final tumor regions of patients were checked and agreed by a senior radiologist. The sample delineation results of SCA, MCN, and IPMN were shown in **Figure 2**. The uncertainty of tumor segmentations contributes to the variation of radiomics feature extraction which is challenging for the reproducibility of radiomics study, as reported in previous studies (21, 22). It is important to screen radiomics features that are robust against tumor segmentation uncertainty. In this study, we conducted a random expansion and corrosion process on the initial tumor region to mimic the uncertainty of manual tumor segmentation. Each slice of the initial tumor segmentation was controlled by a random seed to expand, corrode or keep unchanged. The range of expansion and erosion was 1–4 pixels, controlled by a random seed. By mimicking the tumor segmentation uncertainty, another two sets of tumor regions were generated.

The tumor region on CT images was quantified as quantitative features, namely radiomics features, for building classifier purposes. To eliminate the effect of different voxel spaces on feature extraction, the voxel size of images was resampled into a normalized, $1*1*5$ mm^3, voxel size and all the tumor regions were quantified as 64 gray levels (23) to normalize the inhomogeneity of datasets due to variable tube voltages. The histogram of the tumor region was quantified as seven features, which are variance, skewness, kurtosis, mean, energy, entropy, and uniformity. The textures of the tumor region were quantified using the GLCM, GLRLM, GLSZM, NGTDM methods. The

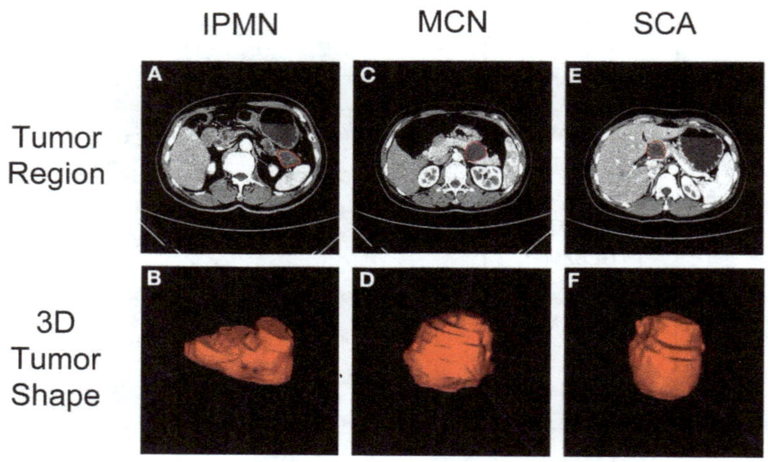

FIGURE 2 | Typical CT imaging (arterial phase) of SCA, MCN, and IPMN were shown in **(A,C,E)**. The region of interest on CT imaging after delineation were shown in **(B,D,F)**.

wavelet transform was used to decompose the images into eight images of different scales to enforce the information in different directions. A total of 547 radiomics features were extracted from the tumor region in this study. The details of the feature quantification method can be found in the study of Vallieres et al. (24). The feature extraction was implanted on the MATLAB 2017b.

Feature Selection and Classifier Construction

Three sets of radiomics features were extracted for robust feature selection, using tumor regions delineated by radiologists and generated using random expansion or corrosion. The radiomics features with an intraclass correlation coefficient of higher than 0.75 were selected for model construction (25). Further, the intercorrelation among radiomics features was assessed to exclude the highly inter-correlated radiomics features (correlation coefficient > 0.75, Pearson) from this study. Only radiomics features and clinical factors that were significantly different among three subtypes were selected.

Then the Boruta algorithm was used for further feature selection (26). Boruta algorithm uses a wrapper method based on the RF classifier for feature selection. A "shadow" attribute was created for each feature in the feature pool by shuffling values of the original feature across all patients. Then the shadow attributes are combined with original features for classification using an RF model. The importance of shadow attribute is used as a reference for selecting truly important features, as determined by RF permutation importance measure.

The multi-class classifiers using the SVM, RF, and ANN models were built based on the final selected features in the training dataset. For SVM modeling, 4 kinds of the kernel were tested, which are "Linear," "Laplacian," "Gaussian,"and "ANOVA RBF." The cost of constraints violation (C-value) ranging from 1 to 10 was tested. For RF modeling, the number of variables randomly sampled as candidates at each split and total tree numbers was tested. For ANN modeling, the number of units in the hidden layer of the network and the parameter for weight decay were optimized using a grid-search strategy. The mean errors for SVM, mean out-of-bag (OOB) errors for RF and accuracy for ANN in 4-fold cross-validation were used to determine the optimal parameters for constructing the SVM, RF, and ANN models. Then the developed models were validated on the independent validation dataset.

For multi-class classification analysis, the precision, recall, and F1-score are suitable to assess the agreement between true class and predicted the result (27). As such, in this study, for characterization of three subtypes of PCNs, the precision, recall and F1 score of each subtype and overall accuracy were used to access the prediction performance of the proposed radiomics SVM and RF models. The precision is used to evaluate the accuracy for users. For example, the precision for IPMN is defined as the rate of truly predicted IPMN patients in all the patients who are predicted as IPMN. The recall is used to evaluate the accuracy of classifier, i.e., the recall for IPMN is defined as the rate of truly predicted IPMN patients in all the IPMN patients. F1 score is an indicator of comprehensively evaluating the performance of a classifier. The F1 score is defined as:

$$F1 = \frac{2 \times Precision \times Recall}{(Precision + Recall)}$$

Statistical Analysis

The Kruskal-Wallis test was performed to evaluate the difference of the radiomics features and continuous clinical factors among three sub-types. The chi-squared test, corrected chi-square test, and Fisher test were performed to find significant different categorical clinical factors among three subtypes, where appropriate. All the statistical analyses and classifier construction were performed with R 3.4.1 (www.R-project.org, 2016). The Boruta feature selection was based on the package "Boruta" in R. The R package "kernlab," "RandomForest," and "nnet"

TABLE 1 | Patient clinical factors in training and validation cohort.

Clinical factors	Training	Validation	*p*-value
Tumor type			0.9914
SCA	53	23	
MCN	28	12	
IPMN	34	14	
Age *median [range]*	[illegible]7 [20–79]	57 [26–79]	0.3844
Maximum Diameter *median [range]*	3[illegible] [0.6–14.8]	3.3 [0.5–11]	0.4936
Serum platelet *median [range]*	1[illegible]9 [46–443]	202 [87–397]	0.8871
Serum ALB *median [range]*	44[illegible] [22.9–54.9]	45 [32.9–52.8]	0.7261
Serum ALT *median [range]*	6 [5–452]	14 [6–134]	0.2255
Serum AST *median [range]*	[illegible]9 [10–280]	19 [11–68]	0.4175
Serum FBG *median [range]*	5.1[illegible] [2.65–15.03]	4.85 [3.98–7.07]	0.1699
Serum AFP *median [range]*	2.3[illegible]0.2 −2374.9]	2.3 [0.7–5.2]	0.2905
Serum CEA *median [range]*	1[illegible] [0.6–682.8]	1.8 [0.6–19.1]	0.3389
Serum CA 19-9 *median [range]*	9[illegible] [1–8170.2]	9.8 [1–128.8]	0.9799
Serum SF *median [range]*	132.4 [[illegible].7–23290.9]	124 [3.8–1547.2]	0.7807
Sex			0.5605
Male	35	12	
Female	80	37	
Location			0.1927
Head and neck	45	21	
Body and tail	62	28	
Other	8	0	
Number of tumors			0.3821
Single	104	47	
Multiple	11	2	
Calcification			1
Without	109	46	
With	6	3	
Chronic Pancreatitis History			1
Without	114	49	
With	1	0	
Abdominal symptom			0.4125
Without	66	24	
With	49	25	
Pancreatic neoplasm family history			1
Without	115	49	
History of smoking			0.6427
Without	101	41	
With	14	8	

(Continued)

TABLE 1 | Continued

Clinical factors	Training	Validation	*p*-value
History of alcoholic consumption			0.4710
Without	94	43	
With	21	6	
Blood type			0.6167
A	34	14	
B	22	6	
AB	9	6	
O	50	23	
Obesity			0.5724
Without	93	37	
With	22	12	

were implanted in the construction of the SVM, RF and ANN model, respectively.

RESULTS

Patient Characteristics

From January 2014 to March 2019, 91 patients were pathologically diagnosed with SCA. Of 91 SCA patients, 15 patients were excluded (one with concurrent malignancy, one patient was sent to our center for emergency exploratory laparotomy, 10 patients' preoperative CT images were missing, three patients' clinical data were missing). Forty-eight patients were pathologically diagnosed with MCN. Of 48 MCN patients, eight patients were excluded (two with concurrent malignancies, four patients' preoperative CT images were missing, two patients' clinical data were incomplete). When we retrospectively analyzed the radiological diagnosis of all 139 patients, the preoperative radiological diagnosis was quite unsatisfying, with only 13.4 and 10.4% were consistent with pathological diagnosis for SCA and MCN, respectively. The most common misdiagnosis for both SCA and MCN was IPMN, indicating difficulty in imaging diagnosis between these three subtypes. Therefore, we randomly enrolled 50 IPMN patients who received surgery in our center between January 2014 and March 2019 based on post-surgery pathology diagnosis, two IPMN patients were excluded for incomplete clinical data. Finally, 164 patients were enrolled (SCA, $n = 76$; MCN, $n = 40$; IPMN, $n = 48$). The patient recruitment process and inclusion/exclusion criteria were shown in **Figure S1**.

The training cohort included 53 SCA patients, 28 MCN patients, and 34 IPMN patients. The validation cohort included 23 SCA patients, 12 MCN patients, and 14 IPMN patients. The patient characteristics in the two cohorts were summarized in **Table 1**. The two datasets showed consistent distribution in all the clinical characteristics.

Feature Selection

A total of 402 radiomics features were robust against the segmentation uncertainties. Among the robust features, 55

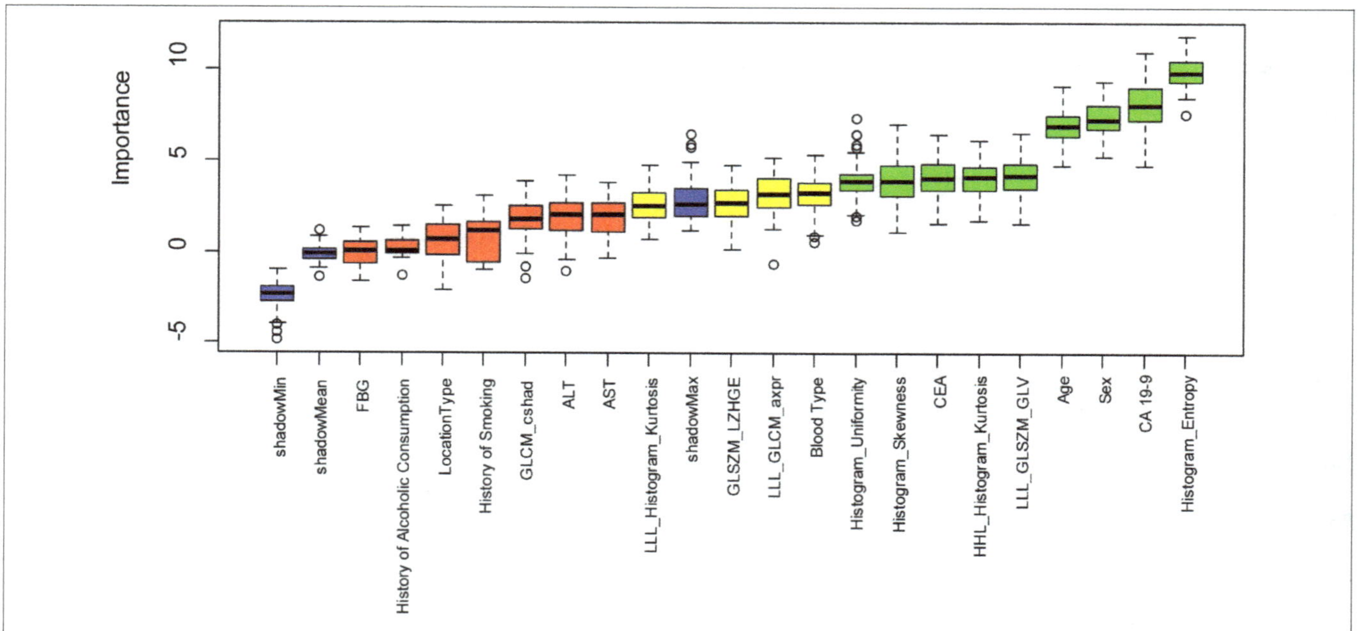

FIGURE 3 | The feature importance in the Boruta feature selection process. The green box showed the features which are confirmed important, the yellow box showed the tentative attributes and the green box showed the unimportant features. Five important radiomics features include Histogram_Entropy, Histogram_Skewness, LLL_GLSZM_GLV, Histogram_Uniformity, HHL_Histogram_Kurtosis. Four important clinical parameters include serum CA 19-9, sex, age, and serum CEA.

TABLE 2 | Diagnosis performance of the constructed SVM model in the training and validation dataset.

	Training dataset						Validation dataset					
TP	**IPMN**	**MCN**	**SCA**	**Pre**	**Rec**	**F1**	**IPMN**	**MCN**	**SCA**	**Pre**	**Rec**	**F1**
IPMN	27	3	5	0.7714	0.7941	0.7826	11	0	4	0.7333	0.7857	0.7586
MCN	2	16	7	0.6400	0.5714	0.6038	0	7	2	0.7778	0.5833	0.6667
SCA	5	9	41	0.7455	0.7736	0.7593	3	5	17	0.6800	0.7391	0.7083
Total	34	28	53	OA	0.7304		14	12	23	OA	0.7143	

T, True type; P, Predicted type; Pre, Precision; Rec, Recall; OA, Overall accuracy.

features with an inter-correlation coefficient of <0.75 were preliminarily selected in the training dataset. Nine radiomics features showed significant differences among the SCA, MCN, and IPMN. Nine radiomics features and eleven significant clinical factors (age, ALT, AST, FBG, CEA, CA 19-9, sex, location, blood type, cigarette history, alcoholic history) were further selected utilizing Boruta feature selection method. In the end, five radiomics features and four clinical parameters were confirmed important. The rank plot of feature importance was shown in **Figure 3**. The radiomics feature, Histogram_Entropy, showed the highest importance. The clinical factor, serum CA 19-9, was the second most important feature. The other 4 radiomics features were the Histogram_Skeweness, LLL_GLSZM_GLV, Histogram_Uniformity and HHL_Histogram_Kurtosis. The detailed formula of the five selected radiomics features was shown in **Table S1**. The other three clinical factors included sex, age, and serum CEA. The radiomics features showed comparable value with clinical factors in these selected features.

Model Construction and Evaluation

The SVM, RF, and ANN models were constructed based on the nine important features. An SVM model with a Gaussian kernel and C-value of 2 showed the least mean error and was selected for classification of SCA, MCN, and IPMN. The detailed parameter optimization process in construction of SVM model was shown in **Table S2**. The constructed SVM model showed an accuracy of 73.04% in the training dataset as shown in **Table 2**. The precision for diagnosis of SCA, MCN, and IPMN was 74.55, 64.00, and 77.14%, respectively. In the validation dataset, the SVM model achieved an overall accuracy of 71.43%, consistent with its performance in the training cohort. The precision for each type was 68.00% for SCA, 77.78% for MCN and 73.33% for IPMN.

The error plot in selecting the tree numbers in the RF model construction was shown in **Figure 4**. When the tree number is more than 3,000, the errors became stable in building RF models. When two variables were randomly sampled as candidates at each split in RF, the mean OOB error was least (**Table S3**. Thus, the RF model with 3,000 trees and two candidate variables was established for tumor diagnosis. In the training dataset, the RF model showed 84.35% overall accuracy in the classification of SCA, MCN, and IPMN. In the validation dataset, the RF model had a precision of 72.41% for SCA, 90.00% for MCN, 90.00% for IPMN (**Table 3**).

The number of hidden units was selected from 10 to 15 and the weight decay was chosen from 2, 1, 0.5, 0.25, 0.125, and 0.0625 in the cross-validation process of ANN structure optimization. The accuracy of ANN in optimizing the number of hidden units and weight decay was shown in **Figure 5A**. When the hidden units are 14 and the weight decay is 1, the mean accuracy in the cross-validation reached the highest and the corresponding ANN structure was shown in **Figure 5B**. The constructed ANN showed an overall accuracy of 77.39% in the training dataset and 71.43% in the validation dataset (**Table 4**). The precision of SCA in the validation dataset was 77.78%. For MCN and IPMN, the precisions were 66.67 and 68.42%, respectively.

The RF model showed the highest overall accuracy in both the training and validation dataset, showing the advantage of RF models in the differential diagnosis of SCA, MCN, and IPMN.

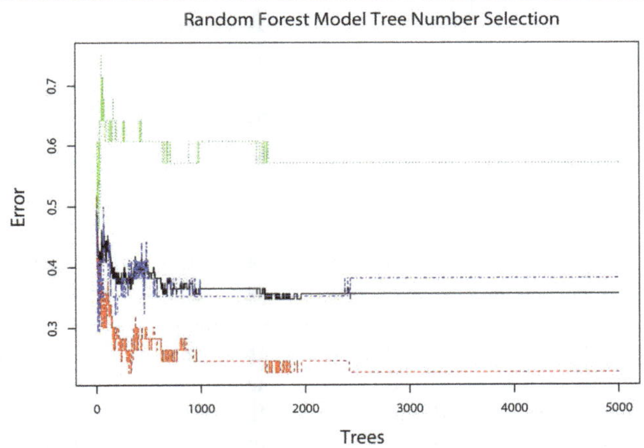

FIGURE 4 | The error plot corresponding different tree numbers in the construction of the RF model. The red line showed the error of "SCA" class; the green line showed the error of "MCN" class; the blue line showed the error of "IPMN" class; the black line showed the OOB error. When tree number is more than 3,000, the errors become stable and thus 3,000 was chosen as the optimal tree number.

As for F1-score, the RF model showed higher F1-score for SCA and MCN, but lower F1-score for IPMN than SVM and ANN model. ANN model showed the highest F1-score for IPMN in the validation dataset. The performance of the three developed models in this study demonstrated the feasibility of models constructed with radiomics and clinical features in the diagnosis of SCA, MCN, and IPMN.

DISCUSSION

In this study, we investigated the potential of the radiomics method for classification of three subtypes of pancreatic cystic neoplasm, i.e., SCA, MCN, and IPMN. All the radiomics features used in the final models developed in this study were robust against tumor segmentation uncertainty. Five radiomics features and four clinical factors were identified important and used for classifier construction.

Three reliable machine learning methods, SVM, RF and ANN methods, were utilized to construct diagnostic classifiers. The built SVM model showed an overall accuracy of 73.04% for training and 71.43% for validation. The RF model showed an overall accuracy of 84.35 and 79.59% in two independent datasets. As for ANN, the overall accuracy in two independent datasets was 77.39 and 71.43%, respectively. All three classifiers present good performance in distinguishing SCA from MCN and IPMN. The result showed that the CECT based radiomics method could classify three subtypes of PCN and may help make personalized treatment decisions preoperatively.

Now the clinical management of patients with pancreatic cystic neoplasm is mainly based on clinical presentation and radiological examinations. EUS-based methods are not routinely performed in every medical center. From the retrospective comparison between preoperative radiology diagnosis and postoperative pathology diagnosis in our center, the pre-surgery accurate diagnosis rate is very low (13.4% for SCA and 10.4% for MCN). Even in Massachusetts General Hospitals, a world-class medical center, over 20% of the cyst lesions resected for concerns about their malignant potential were entirely benign based on histopathologic examination (28). This clinical dilemma reflects the urgent need for an effective and efficient differential method of PCN.

Pancreatic cystic neoplasm is heterogeneous, while the radiologists' diagnosis or cyst fluid examination just reflects a relatively small part of the whole tumor. In this study, the classifiers were constructed by combining radiomics features

TABLE 3 | Diagnosis performance of the constructed RF model in the training and validation dataset.

	Training dataset						Validation dataset					
TP	**IPMN**	**MCN**	**SCA**	**Pre**	**Rec**	**F1**	**IPMN**	**MCN**	**SCA**	**Pre**	**Rec**	**F1**
IPMN	30	4	1	0.8571	0.8824	0.8696	9	0	1	0.9000	0.6429	0.7500
MCN	1	18	3	0.8182	0.6429	0.7200	0	9	1	0.9000	0.7500	0.8182
SCA	3	6	49	0.8448	0.9245	0.8829	5	3	21	0.7241	0.9130	0.8077
Total	34	28	53	OA	0.8435		14	12	23	OA	0.7959	

T, True type; P, Predicted type; Pre, Precision; Rec, Recall; OA, Overall accuracy.

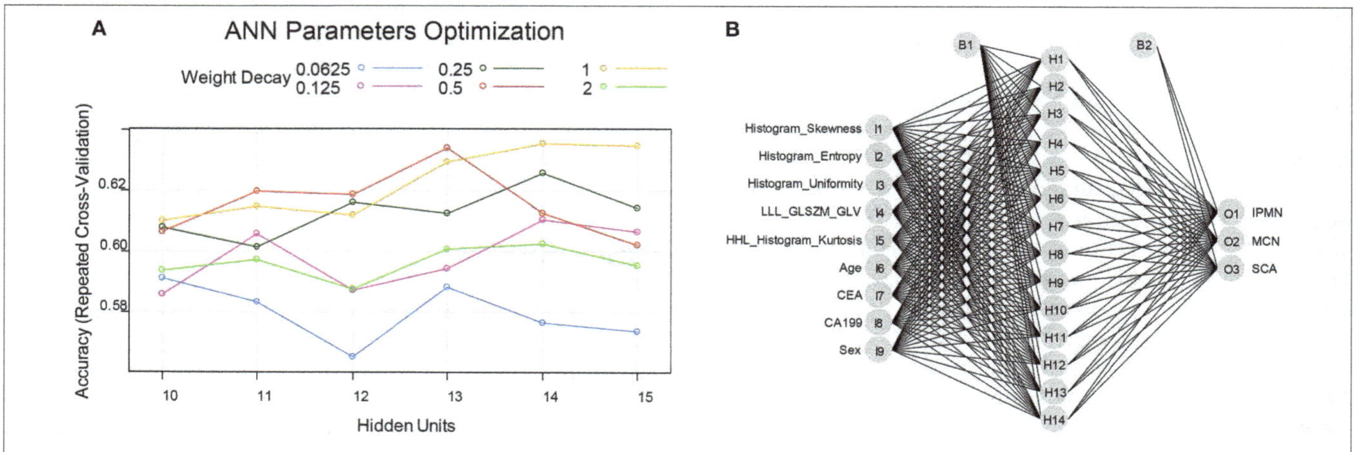

FIGURE 5 | (A) the ANN parameters optimization process: when the hidden units were 14 and the weighted decay was 1, the accuracy reached highest and thus the ANN model was constructed with 14 hidden units and the weighted decay value of 1. **(B)** the final constructed ANN model in this study.

TABLE 4 | Diagnosis performance of the constructed ANN model in the training and validation dataset.

	Training dataset						Validation dataset					
TP	**IPMN**	**MCN**	**SCA**	**Pre**	**Rec**	**F1**	**IPMN**	**MCN**	**SCA**	**Pre**	**Rec**	**F1**
IPMN	31	4	7	0.7381	0.9118	0.8158	13	1	5	0.6842	0.9286	0.7879
MCN	1	15	3	0.7895	0.5357	0.6383	0	8	4	0.6667	0.6667	0.6667
SCA	2	9	43	0.7963	0.8113	0.8037	1	3	14	0.7778	0.6087	0.6829
Total	34	28	53	OA	0.7739		14	12	23	OA	0.7143	

T, True type; P, Predicted type; Pre, Precision; Rec, Recall; OA: Overall accuracy.

with clinical factors (serum CA 19-9, sex, age, serum CEA) and showed promising differential performance. The result was consistent with previous studies. Giuseppe et al. found that age was one of the significant predictors of SCA growth (29). Leung KK et.al found elevated cystic CEA was associated with potentially malignant/malignant cysts (30). Also, Bassi et al. found that positive CEA and/or co-presence of more than two positive serum markers (CEA, CA 19-9, or CA 125) were indicative of presence of mucinous cystic tumors, i.e., MCN and IPMN (31). Our results proved that clinical factors like serum tumor markers together with radiomics features could help differential diagnosis among SCA, MCN, and IPMN.

Treatment choices are sharply different for SCA, MCN, and IPMN. As SCA is a benign entity, periodic surveillance is recommended. MCN had the potential to progress to malignancy. According to current guidelines (10), patients with MCN larger than 4 cm or symptoms should undergo surgery. Ideally, IPMNs with high-grade dysplasia or with invasive adenocarcinoma should undergo resection. But it is still difficult to differentiate low-grade dysplasia in clinical work. Over 20% of the cysts were entirely benign based on histopathologic examination and over 75% of resected IPMNs could have been safely observed (32). With the radiomics approach developed in this study for differentiating SCA, MCN, and IPMN, we might avoid the 20% wrong clinical decision.

There are some limitations to our study. Firstly, as a retrospective study based on single-center data, the sample size of each subtype is relatively small. We take some measures to avoid bias. The training and validation datasets were randomly split (ratio = 7:3) to test the robustness of the results. Multifold cross-validation was carried out in constructing the machine learning classifiers to avoid the over-fitting. However, the bias may still exist due to small sample size. Secondly, there is inevitable subjectivity in the process of manual tumor segmentation. To minimize this bias caused by segmentation uncertainty, all segmentation results were checked and approved by a senior radiologist to ensure the segmentation accuracy. The random expansion and corrosion was also performed to select robust radiomics features. To further improve the performance of CECT based radiomics method, a multicenter-based prospective study with a large study population is needed.

CONCLUSIONS

In conclusion, our study provided preliminary evidence that CECT-based radiomics analysis was feasible and reliable to differentiate SCA, MCN, and IPMN, which is convenient, non-invasive, and repeatable. On the basis of multicenter validation, the present findings may be applicable to clinical routine.

ETHICS STATEMENT

Consent for publication of patients' clinical information (including clinical symptoms, biochemistry examination, and radiology imaging) was obtained from the Human Research Ethics Committee (HREC) of First Affiliated Hospital of Zhejiang University School of Medicine. The written informed consent was obtained from the patient (or in the case of children, their parent or legal guardian).

AUTHOR CONTRIBUTIONS

XS, TN, and XX conceived the project. FY and PY analyzed the data and wrote the paper. MY, JZ, JW, DL, and ZL collected the data. All authors edited the manuscript.

REFERENCES

1. Ip IK, Mortele KJ, Prevedello LM, Khorasani R. Focal cystic pancreatic lesions: assessing variation in radiologists' management recommendations. *Radiology.* (2011) 259:136–41. doi: 10.1148/radiol.10100970
2. Chang YR, Park JK, Jang JY, Kwon W, Yoon JH, Kim SW. Incidental pancreatic cystic neoplasms in an asymptomatic healthy population of 21,745 individuals large-scale, single-center cohort study. *Medicine.* (2016) 95:e5535. doi: 10.1097/MD.0000000000005535
3. Laffan TA, Horton KM, Klein AP, Berlanstein B, Siegelman SS, Kawamoto S, et al. Prevalence of unsuspected pancreatic cysts on MDCT. *Am J Roentgenol.* (2008) 191:802–7. doi: 10.[illegible]214/AJR.07.3340
4. Lee KS, Sekhar A, Rofsky NM, Pedrosa I. Prevalence of incidental pancreatic cysts in the adult population on mr imaging. *Am J Gastroenterol.* (2010) 105:2079–84. doi: 10.1038/ajg.2010.122
5. Shen XY, Lu D, Xu X, Wang JG, Wu J, Yan S, et al. A novel distinguishing system for the diagnosis of malignant pancreatic cystic neoplasm. *Eur J Radiol.* (2013) 82:e648–54. doi: 10.1016/j.ejrad.2013.06.028
6. Lennon AM, Wolfgang C. Cystic neoplasms of the pancreas. *J Gastrointest Surg.* (2013) 17:645–53. doi: 10.1007/s11605-012-2072-6
7. Yamao K, Yanagisawa A, Takahashi K, Kimura W, Doi R, Fukushima N, et al. Clinicopathological features and prognosis of mucinous cystic neoplasm with ovarian-type stroma: a Multi-Institutional Study Of The Japan Pancreas society. *Pancreas.* (2011) [illegible]:67–71. doi: 10.1097/MPA.0b013e3181f749d3
8. Tanaka M, Fernandez-del Castillo C, Adsay V, Chari S, Falconi M, Jang JY, et al. International consensus guidelines 2012 for the management of IPMN and MCN of the pancreas. *Pancreatology.* (2012) 12:183–97. doi: 10.1016/j.pan.2012.0[illegible]004
9. Vege SS, Ziring B, Jain R, Moayyedi P, Clinical Guidelines C. American gastroenterological association institute guideline on the diagnosis and management of asymptomatic neoplastic pancreatic cysts. *Gastroenterology.* (2015) 148:819–22. doi: 10.1053/j.gastro.2015.02.029
10. Del Chiaro M, Besselink MG, Scholten L, Bruno MJ, Cahen DL, Gress TM, et al. European evidence-based guidelines on pancreatic cystic neoplasms. *Gut.* (2018) 67:789–804. doi: 10.1136/gutjnl-2018-316027
11. Del Chiaro M, Segersvard R, Mucelli RP, Rangelova E, Kartalis N, Ansorge C, et al. Comparison of preoperative conference-based diagnosis with histology of cystic tumors of the pancreas. *Ann Surg Oncol.* (2014) 21:1539–44. doi: 10.1245/s10434-013-[illegible]465-9
12. Khashab MA, Shin EJ, Amateau S, Canto MI, Hruban RH, Fishman EK, et al. Tumor size and location correlate with behavior of pancreatic serous cystic neoplasms. *Am J Gastroenterol.* (2011) 106:1521–6. doi: 10.1038/ajg.2011.117
13. Brugge WR, Lewandrowski K, Lee-Lewandrowski E, Centeno BA, Szydlo T, Regan S, et al. Diagnosis of pancreatic cystic neoplasms: a report of the cooperative pancreatic cyst study. *Gastroenterology.* (2004) 126:1330–6. doi: 10.1053/j.gastro.200[illegible]02.013
14. Anand N, Sampath K, Wu BU. Cyst features and risk of malignancy in intraductal papillary mucinous neoplasms of the pancreas: a meta-analysis. *Clin Gastroenterol Hepatol.* (2013) 11:913–21. doi: 10.1016/j.cgh.2013.02.010
15. Lambin P, Leijenaar RTH, Deist TM, Peerlings J, de Jong EEC, van Timmeren J, et al. Radiomics: the bridge between medical imaging and personalized medicine. *Nat Rev Clin Oncol.* (2017) 14:749–62. doi: 10.1038/nrclinonc.2017.141
16. Trebeschi S, Drago SG, Birkbak NJ, Kurilova I, Calin AM, Pizzi AD, et al. Predicting response to cancer immunotherapy using noninvasive radiomic biomarkers. *Ann Oncol.* (2019) 30:998–1004. doi: 10.1093/annonc/mdz108
17. Chakraborty J, Midya A, Gazit L, Attiyeh M, Langdon-Embry L, Allen PJ, et al. CT radiomics to predict high-risk intraductal papillary mucinous neoplasms of the pancreas. *Med Phys.* (2018) 45:5019–29. doi: 10.1002/mp.13159
18. Christman MC, Pontius JS. Bootstrap confidence intervals for adaptive cluster sampling. *Biometrics.* (2000) 56:503–10. doi: 10.1111/j.0006-341X.2000.00503.x
19. Wu SX, Zheng JJ, Li Y, Yu H, Shi SY, Xie WB, et al. A Radiomics Nomogram for the Preoperative Prediction of Lymph Node Metastasis in Bladder Cancer. *Clin Cancer Res.* (2017) 23:6904–11. doi: 10.1158/1078-0432.CCR-17-1510
20. Yushkevich PA, Piven J, Hazlett HC, Smith RG, Ho S, Gee JC, et al. User-guided 3D active contour segmentation of anatomical structures: significantly improved efficiency and reliability. *Neuroimage.* (2006) 31:1116–28. doi: 10.1016/j.neuroimage.2006.01.015
21. Rizzo S, Botta F, Raimondi S, Origgi D, Fanciullo C, Morganti AG, et al. Radiomics: the facts and the challenges of image analysis. *Eur Radiol Exp.* (2018) 2:36. doi: 10.1186/s41747-018-0068-z
22. Qiu QT, Duan JH, Gong GZ, Lu YK, Li DW, Lu J, et al. Reproducibility of radiomic features with GrowCut and GraphCut semiautomatic tumor segmentation in hepatocellular carcinoma. *Transl Cancer Res.* (2017) 6:940–48. doi: 10.21037/tcr.2017.09.47
23. Larue R, van Timmeren JE, de Jong EEC, Feliciani G, Leijenaar RTH, Schreurs WMJ, et al. Influence of gray level discretization on radiomic feature stability for different CT scanners, tube currents and slice thicknesses: a comprehensive phantom study. *Acta Oncol.* (2017) 56:1544–53. doi: 10.1080/0284186X.2017.1351624
24. Vallieres M, Freeman CR, Skamene SR, El Naqa I. A radiomics model from joint FDG-PET and MRI texture features for the prediction of lung metastases in soft-tissue sarcomas of the extremities. *Phys Med Biol.* (2015) 60:5471–96. doi: 10.1088/0031-9155/60/14/5471
25. Qiu QT, Duan JH, Duan ZY, Meng XJ, Ma CS, Zhu J, et al. Reproducibility and non-redundancy of radiomic features extracted from arterial phase CT scans in hepatocellular carcinoma patients: impact of tumor segmentation variability. *Quant Imaging Med Surg.* (2019) 9:453–64. doi: 10.21037/qims.2019.03.02
26. Kursa MB, Rudnicki WR. Feature Selection with the Boruta Package. *J Stat Softw.* (2010) 36:1–13. doi: 10.18637/jss.v036.i11
27. Viani N, Miller TA, Napolitano C, Priori SG, Savova GK, Bellazzi R, et al. Supervised methods to extract clinical events from cardiology reports in Italian. *J Biomed Inform.* (2019) 95:103219. doi: 10.1016/j.jbi.2019.103219
28. Valsangkar NP, Morales-Oyarvide V, Thayer SP, Ferrone CR, Wargo JA, Warshaw AL, et al. 851 resected cystic tumors of the pancreas: a 33-year experience at the Massachusetts General Hospital. *Surgery.* (2012) 152:S4–12. doi: 10.1016/j.surg.2012.05.033
29. Malleo G, Bassi C, Rossini R, Manfredi R, Butturini G, Massignani M, et al. Growth pattern of serous cystic neoplasms of the pancreas: observational study with long-term magnetic resonance surveillance and recommendations for treatment. *Gut.* (2012) 61:746–51. doi: 10.1136/gutjnl-2011-300297
30. Leung KK, Ross WA, Evans D, Fleming J, Lin E, Tamm EP, et al. Pancreatic cystic neoplasm: the role of cyst morphology, cyst fluid analysis, and expectant management. *Ann Surg Oncol.* (2009) 16:2818–24. doi: 10.1245/s10434-009-0502-9

31. Bassi C, Salvia R, Gumbs AA, Butturini G, Falconi M, Pederzoli P. The value of standard serum tumor markers in differentiating mucinous from serous cystic tumors of the pancreas: CEA, Ca 19-9, Ca 125, Ca 15-3. *Langenbecks Arch Surg.* (2002) 387:281–5. doi: 10.1007/s00423-002-0324-8

32. Sahora K, Mino-Kenudson M, Brugge W, Thayer SP, Ferrone CR, Sahani D, et al. Branch duct intraductal papillary mucinous neoplasms does cyst size change the tip of the scale? A critical analysis of the revised international consensus guidelines in a large single-institutional series. *Ann Surg.* (2013) 258:466–75. doi: 10.1097/SLA.0b013e3182a18f48

17

Epidermal Growth Factor Receptor Family and its Role in Gastric Cancer

*Chiara Arienti, Sara Pignatta and Anna Tesei**

Biosciences Laboratory, Istituto Scientifico Romagnolo per lo Studio e la Cura dei Tumori (IRST) IRCCS, Meldola, Italy

***Correspondence:**
Anna Tesei
anna.tesei@irst.emr.it

Despite the gradual decrease in incidence, gastric cancer is still the third leading cause of cancer death worldwide. Although chemotherapy enhances overall survival and quality of life in advanced disease, the median overall survival is < 12 months. In recent years, the human epidermal growth factor receptor (ErbB) family has been extensively investigated in gastric cancer. The ErbB family is composed of four closely-related members: ErbB-1 (HER1 or epidermal growth factor receptor, EGFR), ErbB-2 (HER2), ErbB-3 (HER3), and ErbB-4 (HER4), all of which play a critical role in regulating cell growth, proliferation and migration of tumors. It is well known that gastric cancer overexpresses HER in a heterogeneous pattern, especially EGFR, and HER2. HER3 is another important member of the ErbB family that preferentially activates the phosphatidylinositol 3-kinase (PI3K) pathway. Furthermore, its heterodimerization with HER2 seems fundamental for steering HER2-overexpressing breast cancer tumor growth. Less is known about the impact of HER4 on gastric cancer. Improved survival from the use of trastuzumab has paved the way for ErbB receptor family-targeted treatments in gastric cancer. However, unlike trastuzumab, ErbB receptor-targeted drugs have not consistently maintained the encouraging results obtained in preclinical and early clinical trials. This may be attributable to the intrinsic heterogeneity of gastric cancer and/or to the lack of standardized test quality for established biomarkers used to evaluate these biological targets. This review presents an overview of the most recent clinical studies on agents targeting the ErbB family in gastric cancer.

Keywords: HER2, EGFR, tyrosine kinase inhibitor, targeted therapy, gastric cancer, clinical trial

INTRODUCTION

Gastric cancer is the fifth most common malignancy and the third leading cause of cancer death worldwide (1). In Europe, it is the fifth most common cancer in both sexes, accounting for around 23% of all cancers. The annual incidence is 20/100,000 for men and 9/ 100,000 for women, resulting in ~107,000 deaths annually (2). There is a distinct geographic variability in gastric cancer, the highest rates being observed in East Asia, South America and Eastern Europe, and the lowest rates in the U.S. and Western Europe (3).

TREATMENT OPTIONS FOR GASTRIC CANCER

Surgery

Surgical resection remains the primary treatment for all patients with regionally confined disease, the extent of the intervention depending on the site of the tumor. Total gastrectomy is usually recommended for proximal tumors but is not considered superior to subtotal gastrectomy in terms of survival in distal gastric cancer (4, 5).

Patients with superficial early gastric cancer (T1a) are candidates for endoscopic mucosal resection (EMR). T1a is defined as adenocarcinomas confined to the mucosa, <2 cm in diameter, low-moderate differentiation, no evidence of ulcer, and with no lymphovascular involvement (6, 7). The extent of lymph node dissection is hotly debated and studies have failed to confirm a survival benefit of D1 dissection (dissection of the perigastric nodes) over D2 dissection (dissection of perigastric nodes and nodes along the left gastric, hepatic, celiac, and splenic arteries). D2 dissection is associated with fewer locoregional recurrences and gastric cancer-related death, but also with higher rates of morbidity and mortality. A modified (spleen-preserving) D2 dissection is considered standard treatment in many hospitals. The addition of para-aortic dissection to D2 dissection does not improve survival (8–10).

Surgical resection represents standard curative gastric cancer treatment (11), but around 25% of patients have unresectable tumors at diagnosis due to the presence of metastatic disease.

Chemotherapy or Chemoradiation

Chemotherapy is considered a feasible option in patients with metastases but good functional status and an acceptable life expectancy (12, 13). First-line treatment for metastatic disease includes a combination of a platinum compound and fluorouracil. The addition of another agent such as an anthracycline (e.g., epirubicin) in Europe (ECF = epirubicin, cisplatin, and fluorouracil) or a taxane (e.g., docetaxel) in the U.S. (DCF = docetaxel, cisplatin, and fluorouracil) is common practice (14–16). Other studies have demonstrated that fluorouracil can be substituted by capecitabine, and cisplatin by oxaliplatin (17, 18). Substituting oxaliplatin for cisplatin is associated with lower toxicity (17, 19). Recent trials have used EOX (epirubicin, oxaliplatin, and fluorouracil) and FLO (fluorouracil, calcium folinate [leucovorin], and oxaliplatin) (17, 18).

Overall survival is higher in patients with locally advanced gastric cancer treated with chemoradiation than in those treated with radiation alone (20, 21). Adverse effects of radiation include nausea, vomiting (patients may need to be pre-treated with antiemetics prior to radiation), weight loss, and diarrhea. Less commonly, radiation can cause small bowel obstruction, liver damage, and kidney damage.

Perioperative Chemoradiation or Chemotherapy

In patients with pathologic stage II-IIIC or any T, N+ disease or R1 resection, postoperative radiation combined with adjuvant fluorouracil has been shown to improve overall survival (22, 23). Postoperative chemoradiation consists of one cycle of fluorouracil (with or without calcium folinate) given prior to radiation, followed by two cycles after radiation. During radiation, patients receive fluorouracil on the first 4 and last 3 days of radiation. Preoperative chemoradiation consisting of radiotherapy and fluorouracil (or fluorouracil and paclitaxel) is used to induce tumor downstaging and increase respectability (24). Another option is adjuvant chemotherapy, which improves survival in patients undergoing curative resection (25, 26). In patients with stage II or higher gastric cancer, perioperative chemotherapy with ECF (epirubicin, cisplatin, and fluorouracil) has been shown to improve overall survival (27), although results of trials of postoperative chemotherapy vary substantially. In fact, in the U.S., postoperative studies have failed to demonstrate any benefit, whereas Japanese data favor adjuvant chemotherapy after D2 dissection (28).

Despite the significant improvements obtained from chemotherapy and chemoradiotherapy regimens, the prognosis for patients with advanced gastric cancer remains poor, with a median survival of <12 months, mainly because the disease is already advanced when the initial diagnosis is made. In recent years, substantially longer survival and significantly improved quality of life of gastric cancer patients have been obtained using targeted therapies (29, 30). In particular, molecular drugs targeting the human epidermal growth factor receptor (ErbB) family have been amply investigated and are currently under evaluation in several phase III clinical trials.

ErbB Family

The epidermal growth factor receptor family consists of four related receptor tyrosine kinases: EGFR (ErbB1, HER1), ErbB2 (HER2, *neu* in rodents), ErbB3 (HER3), and ErbB4 (HER4) (31). Although the human ErbB genes are found on four different chromosomes, all members share a common structure, including an extracellular domain, lipophilic transmembrane region, intracellular domain containing tyrosine kinase, and a carboxy-terminal region. EGFR, the first member of this receptor family to be discovered (32), was also the first receptor for which evidence emerged of a relationship between receptor overexpression and cancer (33). Several alterations in ErbB family members were subsequently found to be correlated with the development and progression of numerous human cancers, e.g., non-small cell lung cancer (34), breast (35), colorectal (36), laryngeal (37), esophageal (38), ovarian (39), and prostate cancer (40), and melanoma (41) as a result of their pivotal role in signal transduction. In particular, the ErbB signaling network consists of several overlapping and interconnected modules including the phosphatidylinositol 3-kinase (PI3K)/Akt (PKB) pathway, the Ras/Raf/MEK/ERK1/2 pathway, and the phospholipase C (PLCγ) pathway. The PI3K/Akt pathway plays an important role in mediating cell survival, while the Ras/ERK1/2 and PLCγ pathways are involved in cell proliferation (42). These and other ErbB signaling modules influence angiogenesis, cell adhesion, cell motility, development, and organogenesis (43).

The ligands that bind to each monomeric receptor are shown in **Table 1**. Notably, 7 growth factors bind to EGFR, none binds to HER2, 2 bind to HER3, and 7 bind to HER4. The 4 ErbB family members form 28 homo- and heterodimers. The 11 growth factors in the EGF-like family and the 28 dimers make 614 receptor combinations possible. The binding of ligands to the extracellular domain of EGFR, HER3, and HER4 leads to the formation of kinase-active hetero-oligomers (31). The activation of HER2 and EGFR results in transphosphorylation of the ErbB dimer partner, stimulating intracellular pathways including RAS/RAF/MEK/ ERK, PI3K/AKT/TOR, Src kinases, and STAT transcription factors (42). In particular, HER2 does not bind

TABLE 1 | Pattern of ErbB receptor binding.

Growth factor	Receptor binding			
	EGFR	HER2	HER3	HER4
Epidermal growth factor (EGF)	+	–	–	–
Epiregulin	+	–	–	+
Epigen	+	–	–	–
Betacellulin	+	–	–	+
Heparin-binding epidermal growth factor (HB-EGF)	+	–	–	+
Transforming growth factor-α	+	–	–	–
Amphiregulin	+	–	–	–
Neuregulin 1	–	–	+	+
Neuregulin 2	–	–	+	+
Neuregulin 3	–	–	–	+
Neuregulin 4	–	–	–	+

directly to any ErbB ligand but rather is fixed in a conformation resembling a ligand-activated state, favoring dimerization (44, 45). In fact, although EGFR, HER3, and HER4 are activated by ligand binding, the specific ligands to which HER2 binds have still not been identified (46). However, aberrant HER2 activity and HER2 receptor activation results in receptor dimerization (e.g., HER2/HER3), which triggers a complex signal transduction cascade, modulating survival, proliferation, mobility and cancer cell invasiveness (47).

The HER3 receptor, despite showing weaker kinase activity than that of its ErbB co-receptors, plays a key role in promoting cell survival (48). HER3 binds ATP and catalyzes autophosphorylation. After transphosphorylation by another ErbB family member, HER3 acts as an efficient phosphotyrosine scaffold, leading to strong downstream signaling activation. In particular, HER3 is a powerful inducer of the PI3K/Akt pathway through six consensus phosphor-tyrosine sites on its C-terminal tail which bind the PI3K p85 subunit (49–51). Furthermore, in HER2-driven tumors, the HER2-HER3 dimer has proven essential for tumor formation and maintenance (52, 53). In particular, the role of HER3 in resistance to HER2-targeted therapy in this tumor subtype has been underlined in numerous studies showing that HER3 upregulation may induce resistance to several signaling inhibitors designed to directly or indirectly antagonize activated PI3K signaling. Furthermore, although the HER2-HER3 dimer is the strongest HER family dimer, HER3 has been seen to dimerize with EGFR and with non-ErbB family members, including c-MET (54, 55).

HER4 is a unique cell surface receptor that mediates the activity of transmembrane tyrosine kinase. Unlike other ErbB receptors, there is evidence that HER4 is characterized by antiproliferative and pro-apoptotic activity (56, 57). In cell line experiments when HER2-positive cancer cells were transfected to overexpress HER4, researchers observed reduced proliferation and increased apoptosis (56), suggesting that HER4 antagonizes HER2 signaling activity (58). Four HER4 receptor isoforms resulting from the alternative splicing of *HER4* mRNA have been described (JMa or JMb, Cyt1 or Cyt2) (59). The JMa isoform comprises an extracellular proteolytic site cleaved by the metalloproteinase tumor necrosis factor-alpha converting enzyme (TACE) (60). After cleavage, the transmembrane cleavage product (m80) undergoes a second intramembrane-secretase cleavage that releases a soluble HER4 intracellular domain (4ICD) into the cytoplasm (61). The 4ICD either remains in the cytosol or translocates to the nucleus. The HER4 intracellular domain is characterized by multiple biological activities and cellular responses including differentiation, pro-apoptotic pathway activation, cell cycle arrest, transcription modulation through the formation of complexes with transcription factors, and cell proliferation. These responses are associated with 4ICD localization in different cell compartments (62). Nuclear 4ICD has been found to be a powerful ER co-activator, interacting directly with ligand-associated ER and promoting ER-positive breast tumor cell proliferation (63). It has also been seen that 4ICD accumulates within the mitochondria, promoting tumor cell apoptosis through the activity of the cell-killing BH3 domain (57). The manipulation of 4ICD cell localization is thus a potentially effective therapeutic strategy.

ErbB Expression and Gastric Cancer

EGFR is overexpressed in 27%–64% of gastric tumors (64, 65) and its role as an oncogene in this malignancy is well-known. However, there is no general consensus on the prognostic value of EGFR status in gastric cancer patients. Some authors suggest that high gene amplification is associated with poor outcome (66, 67), while others sustain the opposite (68). Moreover, a 2013 meta-analysis comparing the results obtained in 5 different studies on a total of 1,600 patients concluded that EGFR expression is not an independent predictor of survival in gastric cancer (69).

HER2 overexpression/amplification varies considerably among studies (6 to 30%) and is partly attributable to variability in histologic subtype and primary tumor localization (70). The highest expression rates have been seen in intestinal type tumors located proximally to the gastroesophageal junction (71). Studies on gastric cancer have obtained inconsistent results on the prognostic role of HER2. Although the majority reported that positivity to HER2 is associated with a poor prognosis (72, 73), some did not observe an association between HER2 status and outcome (74) or a longer median overall survival in patients with HER2-positive gastric cancer compared with those with HER2-negative tumors (74, 75). Although the correlation between HER2 status and gastric cancer prognosis is still open to debate, HER2 protein expression or gene amplification is currently used as a biomarker for targeted therapy in this tumor (71–76).

HER3 and HER4, like EGFR and HER2, have also been found to be expressed in 20.7% and 13.3% of gastric cancers, respectively (77). A correlation between high HER3 expression and poor survival has been described in several studies (78–80). Conversely, the few studies performed to date on HER4 in gastric cancer have not clarified its role as a prognostic marker. A recent work by He et al. highlighted an association between high HER4

TABLE 2 | Evaluation of immunostaining for EGFR and HER2.

Classification	IHC Score	EGFR	HER2
Negative	0	No staining or background type staining	No staining or <10%
Negative	1+	Discontinuous membrane staining; >10%	Faint/barely perceptible >10%
Equivocal	2+	–	Weak to moderate; complete or basolateral membrane staining; >10%
Positive	2+	Weak to moderate; >10%	IHC2+ and FISH+
Positive	3+	Moderate to strong; complete membrane staining; >10%	Moderate to strong; complete or basolateral membrane staining; >10%

IHC, immunohistochemistry; FISH, fluorescence in situ hybridization.

expression and TNM (Tumor-Nodes-Metastasis) but not HER4 overexpression and survival (77).

ErbB Testing in Gastric Cancer

Several studies have been conducted on EGFR expression in gastric cancer, and variations in the reported expression of the receptor may be due to differences in sample size, detection methods or evaluation standards used. Some authors observed that EGFR was not expressed in normal gastric mucosa but highly expressed in gastric cancer tissue, concluding that EGFR expression could be related to *EGFR* gene amplification and mutation, continuous EGFR activation, and activation of an abnormal signal transduction pathway. However, it has yet to be proven that high *EGFR* expression in gastric cancer is a result of gene amplification or mutation.

EGFR expression can be detected in several ways, e.g., by genomic assays that quantify the number of *EGFR* gene copies or number of cell surface receptors (**Table 2**). Genomic assays include:

1. Fluorescence *in situ* hybridization (FISH) and chromogenic *in situ* hybridization (CISH), both of which measure *EGFR* gene amplification by quantifying gene copy number (66);
2. Immunohistochemistry (IHC), which measures the number of cell receptors, thus enabling quantification of receptor overexpression (81).

The widespread use of trastuzumab in breast cancer underlines the importance of high-quality HER2 testing and scoring to ensure the accurate identification of patients most likely to benefit from this targeted therapy. HER2 testing in gastric cancer differs from that of breast cancer because of the inherent differences in tumor biology, i.e., HER2 heterogeneity (focal staining) and incomplete membrane staining are more frequent in gastric cancer. These observations have led to the development and standardization of gastric cancer-specific HER2 testing protocols which must be adhered. HER2 status is mainly assessed by IHC (which measures the number of HER2 receptors on the cell surface, thus detecting receptor overexpression) or FISH (which detects gene amplification by measuring the number of *HER2* gene copies in tumor cell nuclei) using biopsy or surgical specimens (82). However, following the results obtained in the ToGA trial, trastuzumab was approved for use in HER2-positive gastric cancer defined as IHC 3+ or, alternatively, in FISH-positive gastric cancer in the USA and Japan. Of note, in Europe HER2-positive gastric cancer is defined as IHC 3+ or IHC 2 + plus positive FISH (83) (**Table 2**).

Unlike EGFR and HER2, there is no standardized method for assessing HER3 status. The most widely used methods are IHC, FISH and quantitative reverse transcription polymerase chain reaction (RT-PCR), which evaluates *HER3* on the basis of messenger RNA levels (79, 84). Finally, as HER4 testing is not routinely performed in clinical practice, there is no standard method for its assessment. However, the method most widely used in clinical trials is IHC (77).

Agents Targeting the ErbB Family in Advanced Gastroesophageal Cancers

Chemotherapy is the cornerstone of treatment for locally advanced and metastatic gastroesophageal cancer. Targeted therapies, in particular those directed against ErbB family receptors, have been investigated in the preclinical setting and some are currently undergoing assessment in clinical trials (**Figure 1**). However, unlike EGFR and HER2, relatively little is known about the role of HER3 and HER4 in gastric carcinogenesis or about the relationship between HER3 and HER4 and clinical pathological features, including overall survival. In particular, a better understanding of HER3 receptor functionality has unveiled the molecular cornerstones of its complex mechanism of action that are targetable through multiple pharmacological strategies, i.e., inhibition of ligand binding to the extracellular domain, receptor dimerization inhibition, and inhibition of the partner tyrosine kinase activity, all of which have the potential to benefit patients with HER3 overexpressing tumors. A lasting response was obtained in a phase I trial of anti-ERBB3 mAb therapy (GSK2849330) in individuals with advanced HER3-positive solid tumors (http://www.clinicaltrials.gov/show/NCT01966445). Moreover, a phase III clinical trial (http://www.clinicaltrials.gov/show/NCT02134015) focusing on new HER3-targeted antibodies was recently concluded and results are eagerly awaited.

A phase I clinical trial (http://www.clinicaltrials.gov/show/NCT03552406) and a phase I/II clinical trial (http://www.clinicaltrials.gov/show/NCT02980341) focusing on new HER3-targeted antibodies are currently recruiting patients with different solid tumors. Furthermore, 2 phase II clinical trials (http://www.clinicaltrials.gov/show/NCT03810872 and http://www.clinicaltrials.gov/show/NCT02501603), both focusing on afatinib, are currently recruiting patients with different solid tumors. Afatinib is a promising novel small ErbB family blocker that covalently binds and irreversibly blocks signaling mediated by activated EGFR, HER2, and HER4 receptors, and also HER3

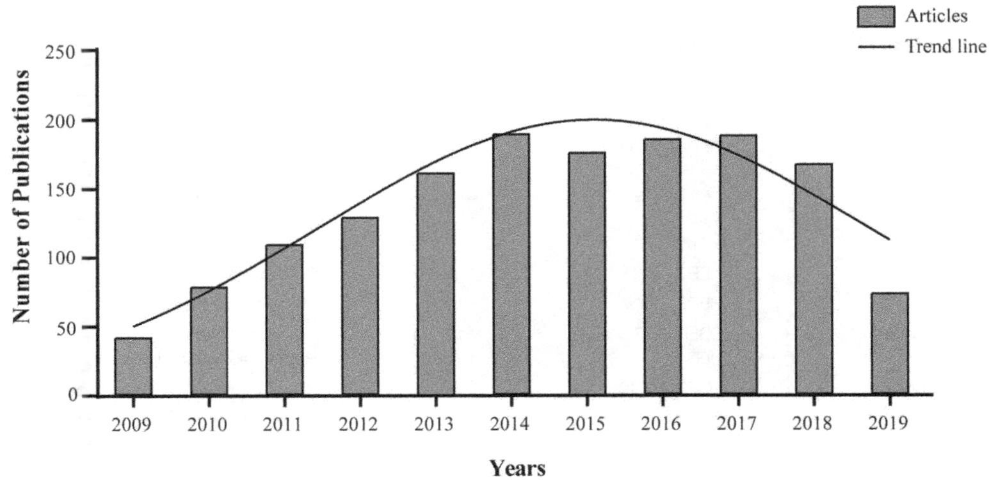

FIGURE 1 | Agents targeting the ErbB family. Search for article appearing in PUBMED database over the past 10 years using the mesh terms "Stomach Neoplasms" AND "ErbB Receptors" in the advance research builder option.

transphosphorylation. Another phase II study (http://www.clinicaltrials.gov/show/NCT01953926) is currently exploring the efficacy and safety of neratinib, an irreversible panHER inhibitor in solid tumors with activating *HER2*, *HER3* or *EGFR* mutations or with *EGFR* gene amplification. Confirmation of their efficacy could pave the way for their use in gastric cancer as well (**Table 3**).

The following novel anti-ErbB inhibitors targeting EGFR and HER2 have been approved and are currently being developed for use in patients with gastroesophageal cancer.

EGFR Inhibition

The most common approaches to the inhibition of EGFR require the use of monoclonal antibodies. Cetuximab (Erbitux®) is a chimeric monoclonal antibody (IgG1) that binds the extracellular domain of human EGFR, inducing its internalization, downregulation, and degradation. Furthermore, this antibody-receptor interaction competitively inhibits EGF binding, preventing receptor dimerization and blocking ligand-induced EGFR tyrosine kinase auto-phosphorylation and activation (85). Promising phase II data formed the basis for the phase III EXPAND trial (erbitux in combination with xeloda and cisplatin in advanced gastroesophageal cancer) in which 904 patients were randomized to receive cisplatin with capecitabine with or without cetuximab. However, a benefit in terms of progression-free (PFS) or overall survival (OS) was not observed in the cetuximab group (86).

RTOG 0436 is a randomized phase III trial comparing the efficacy of paclitaxel and cisplatin in combination with radiation therapy (daily 50.4 Gy/1.8 fractions) with or without cetuximab in patients with locally advanced esophageal cancer. The study is ongoing but currently not recruiting patients (https://clinicaltrials.gov/show/NCT00655876).

In contrast to their role in colorectal cancer, KRAS mutations have not proven to be a negative predictive biomarker of response to cetuximab in gastroesophageal cancer (87). Other biomarkers such as EGFR expression, copy number and phosporylation have also been evaluated, but sample size and the retrospective nature of the research have not led to meaningful conclusions (88, 89).

The other antibody used to inhibit EGFR is panitumumab (Vectibix®), the first fully human IgG2 monoclonal antibody targeting EGFR. Its activity in gastric cancer was studied in a randomized open-label multicenter trial on the efficacy of epirubicin, oxaliplatin, and capecitabine (EOX) with or without panitumumab in untreated advanced gastroesophageal cancer (REAL-3 study) (http://www.clinicaltrials.gov/show/NCT00824785). The results from this clinical trial did not show any benefit for the panitumumab-treated group, possibly due, in part, to reduced doses of chemotherapy administered in the combination arm, and the study was interrupted early (90).

In the ACOSOG Z4051 phase II study, patients with potentially resectable disease underwent neoadjuvant docetaxel, cisplatin, and panitumumab in combination with radiotherapy (91) (http://www.clinicaltrials.gov/show/NCT00757172). However, the activity of the multidrug combination was outweighed by the significant toxicity observed.

Nimotuzumab is a humanized therapeutic monoclonal antibody directed against EGFR. A phase II clinical trial is currently ongoing to assess the efficacy and safety of adding nimotuzumab to irinotecan after first-line treatment failure in patients with recurrent or metastatic EGFR-overexpressing gastric adenocarcinoma. In addition, as secondary aims, biomarkers for nimotuzumab efficacy in gastric cancer will be investigated (http://www.clinicaltrials.gov/show/NCT03400592).

Another phase II trial is ongoing to determine the safety and efficacy of varlitinib plus mFOLFOX6 for the treatment of gastric cancer (http://www.clinicaltrials.gov/show/NCT03130790). Varlitinib (also known as ASLAN001) is a small-molecule, adenosine triphosphate competitive inhibitor of EGFR, HER2 and HER4. EGFR inhibition by tyrosine kinase inhibitors (TKIs) such as iressa (Gefinitib®) and tarceva (Erlotinib®) (both oral

TABLE 3 | Ongoing clinical investigations of HER3 targeted agents.

Clinical trial identifier	Investigational compound	Target	Phase	Condition	Status
NCT03065387	Neratinib Palbociclib	EGFR, HER2, HER3, HER4	I	Solid tumors with EGFR mutation/amplification, HER2 mutation/amplification, HER3/4 mutation, treatment refractory and advanced or metastatic	Recruiting
CT03552406	ISU104	HER3	I	Solid Tumor	Recruiting
NCT02980341	U3-1402	HER3	I/II	Metastatic Breast Cancer	Recruiting
NCT03499626	ASLAN001	EGFR,HER2,HER3, HER4	I/II	Advanced/ Metastatic Hepatocellular Carcinoma	Recruiting
NCT01953926	Neratinib	EGFR, HER2, HER3	II	Solid tumors with somatic human epidermal growth factor receptor (EGFR, HER2, HER3) Mutations or EGFR gene amplification	Recruiting
NCT03810872	Afatinib	EGFR, HER2, HER3	II	Cancers Harboring an EGFR Mutation (Excluding Non-squamous Non- Small Cell Lung Cancer, a Registered Indication), a HER2 Mutation or a HER3 Mutation	Recruiting
NCT02501603	Afatinib	EGFR,HER2,HER3,HER4	II	Gastric Cancer, Gastroesophageal Junction Cancer	Recruiting

EGFR TKIs) has also been investigated in clinical trials on gastroesophageal cancer (92, 93).

HER2 Inhibition

On the basis of preclinical studies highlighting the significant activity of anti-HER2 therapies in both *in vitro* and *in vivo* gastric cancer models (73, 94, 95), molecular drugs targeting HER2 have been widely studied in clinical trials on gastroesophageal cancer. Trastuzumab (Herceptin®), a humanized monoclonal antibody that targets the extracellular binding domain of the HER2 receptor, was the first molecular targeted agent to be approved as standard treatment for gastric cancer (29, 96). It has been used in combination with cytotoxic chemotherapy in several clinical trials on gastric and gastroesophageal junction (GEJ) tumors (**Table 4**). The international, open-label phase III ToGA trial randomized patients with treatment-naive metastatic or locally advanced unresectable HER2-overexpressing gastric or GEJ adenocarcinoma to chemotherapy with trastuzumab or chemotherapy alone. HER2 overexpression was defined as 3+ staining by IHC or as positive FISH (29). The combination was generally well tolerated and a 2.7 month improvement in median OS was observed in the trastuzumab arm. Furthermore, response rate, time to progression and duration of response were significantly higher in the trastuzumab plus chemotherapy group.

The HELOISE trial was a randomized, multicenter, international phase IIIb study comparing the effectiveness and safety of 2 trastuzumab dosing regimens in combination with cisplatin/capecitabine in patients with metastatic gastric or GEJ cancer (http://www.clinicaltrials.gov/show/NCT01450696). This study was interrupted for futility on the basis of results from the pre-planned interim analysis confirming the standard trastuzumab dose with chemotherapy as the standard-of-care for first-line treatment.

NCT01130337 is a sponsored phase II clinical trial designed to evaluate the disease-free survival rate of a combination of capecitabine and oxaliplatin with trastuzumab administered pre-surgery in patients with resectable gastric cancer. If a complete (R0) or microscopic residual tumor (R1) resection is obtained, patients receive a further two cycles of treatment. Trastuzumab is continued for a maximum of 1 year (available online: http://clinicaltrials.gov/show/NCT01130337, results not yet posted).

Another sponsored phase II trial (TOXAG) has recently concluded proving that trastuzumab in combination with capecitabine, oxaliplatin and radiotherapy in the adjuvant setting for gastric or gastroesophageal junction adenocarcinoma is safe and tolerable (http://www.clinicaltrials.gov/show/NCT01748773).

The Her-FLOT phase II study was designed to assess the efficacy of perioperative treatment based on trastuzumab in combination with FLOT (5FU, leucovorin, docetaxel, and oxaliplatin) in patients with HER2-positive locally advanced esophagogastric adenocarcinoma. Patients were administered trastuzumab with FLOT for four cycles prior to surgical resection followed by a further four cycles of chemotherapy with trastuzumab and nine additional cycles of trastuzumab alone. The aim of the study was to determine the rate of complete pathological response (http://www.clinicaltrials.gov/show/NCT01472029, results have yet to be posted).

RTOG 1010 is an ongoing phase III trial in which patients with locally advanced HER2-overexpressing esophageal or GEJ adenocarcinoma are randomized to receive combination treatment comprising radiotherapy, paclitaxel and carboplatin

TABLE 4 | Ongoing clinical investigations of trastuzumab in gastric cancer.

Clinical trial identifier	Investigational compound	Phase	Status
NCT03680560	ACTR T Cell Product; Trastuzumab	I	Recruiting
NCT03319459	FATE-NK100; Cetuximab; Trastuzumab	I	Recruiting
NCT02805829	Trastuzumab; NK cells	I/II	Not yet recruiting
NCT02901301	Pembrolizumab; Trastuzumab; Capecitabine; Cisplatin	I/II	Recruiting
NCT01191697	Bevacizumab; Trastuzumab; Oxaliplatin; Capecitabine	II	Active, not recruiting
NCT03766607	Trastuzumab; Ramucirumab; Paclitaxel	II	Not yet recruiting
NCT02954536	Pembrolizumab; Trastuzumab; Capecitabine; Cisplatin; Oxaliplatin; 5-FU	II	Recruiting
NCT03588533	Trastuzumab; Capecitabine; Cisplatin	II	Recruiting
NCT04014075	Trastuzumab; Deruxtecan	II	Not yet recruiting
NCT02205047	Cisplatin; 5-FU; Capecitabine; Trastuzumab; Pertuzumab	II	Recruiting
NCT02678182	Capecitabine; MEDI4736; Trastuzumab; Rucaparib	II	Recruiting
NCT03556345	RC48-ADC	II	Recruiting
NCT02581462	FLOT; Herceptin; Pertuzumab	II/III	Active, not recruiting
NCT01774786	5-FU; Capecitabine; Cisplatin; Pertuzumab;Trastuzumab	III	Active, not recruiting
NCT03615326	Pembrolizumab; Cisplatin; 5-FU; Oxaliplatin; S-1; Capecitabine; Trastuzumab	III	Recruiting
NCT02578368	5-FU; Leucovorin; Oxaliplatin; Docetaxel; Trastuzumab	III	Recruiting

with or without trastuzumab prior to surgery (http://clinicaltrials.gov/show/NCT01196390, study is active but currently not recruiting).

What is emerging from these studies is that a growing number of patients are experiencing resistance to trastuzumab (97). This has aroused great interest in second- generation HER2-targeting agents such as pertuzumab (Perjeta®). Pertuzumab binds a distinct site on the HER2 receptor (extracellular domain II) and disrupts HER2 dimerization, subsequently blocking downstream signaling (98). On the basis of pre-clinical studies on GEJ and of the effectiveness of the trastuzumab and pertuzumab combination in breast cancer (99), the JACOB phase III study was designed to investigate the efficacy and safety of pertuzumab in patients with HER2-positive metastatic or locally advanced unresectable GEJ or gastric cancer receiving first-line treatment with cisplatin, fluoropyrimidine (5-fluoruracil or capecitabine) and trastuzumab (https://clinicaltrials.gov/show/NCT01774786, study is active but currently not recruiting).

Trastuzumab emtansine (TDM-1, KadCyla®) is an antibody-drug conjugate of trastuzumab and DM1 (derivative of maytansine, a macrolide isolated from plants), a powerful microtubule inhibitor In preclinical gastric cancer models, TDM-1 has demonstrated more aggressive antitumor activity than trastuzumab (100). A multicenter adaptive phase II/III of TDM-1 recruited patients with HER2-positive advanced gastric cancer in progression after first-line treatment (http://www.clinicaltrials.gov/show/NCT0164tab1939). In particular, patients with higher HER2 expression experienced a better treatment effect from TDM-1than those with lower HER2 expression (101).

Another approach to targeting HER2 is through inhibition by TKIs. Lapatinib (Tykerb® (USA)/ Tyverb® (Europe) is an oral small molecule dual TKI of EGFR and HER2 that inhibits the activation of PI3K and Ras pathways, which is activation, dependent on both receptors, leading to the downregulation of receptor tyrosine kinase phosphorylation in cancer cells. Lapatinib was evaluated in combination with standard chemotherapy in patients with HER2-positive gastric and GEJ adenocarcinomas (phase III LOGIC study, http://www.clinicaltrials.gov/show/NCT00680901). This international multicenter trial investigated whether the addition of lapatinib to a capecitabine plus oxaliplatin regimen would extend the time to progression and OS. Although the trial did not meet its primary endpoint of improved OS, some subgroups (the Asian population and patients <60 years of age) were shown to benefit.

CONCLUSIONS

Several clinical trials using ErbB receptor family targeted treatment strategies have been carried out over the past few years, with varying results. Others are currently ongoing, as extensively described in the present review. The ToGA study paved the way for the use of ErbB receptor family targeted treatments, showing that trastuzumab improves survival in HER2-overexpressing advanced gastric cancer patients. This monoclonal antibody is now acknowledged as the standard first-line treatment in this subset of patients. The role of combinations of anti-ErbB drugs and cytotoxic therapies is currently being explored in the area of advanced gastric cancer in an effort to prevent or delay drug resistance. On the other hand, drugs targeting EGFR have not repeated the encouraging results seen in early clinical trials. Similarly, lapatinib, a dual TKI of EGFR, and HER2, failed to induce a benefit in patients enrolled onto two large phase III trials. The modest efficacy of these agents may be attributable to acquired resistance or to an mismatched combination with known cytotoxic agents. Furthermore, the clinical data collected to date on molecular drugs directly targeting HER3 suggest a limited potential of these agents for the treatment of gastric cancer. However, several clinical trials are still ongoing.

It is now clear that results can only be improved by taking into account a number of important issues. First, the effects of the targeted therapy may be weakened because of differences in tumor histology (biomarkers), etiology (gastroesophageal reflux/Barret's esophagus, *H. Pylori* infection, alcohol and hot liquid intake, and smoking), and heterogeneity. Furthermore, tumor site (gastric, GEJ or esophagus) and population (Asia, America, Europe) should be considered background variables. For these reasons it is crucial to characterize tumors using established biomarkers, even though the diversity of molecular alterations acquired during malignant transformation, recurrence or metastasis makes it difficult to incorporate biomarkers into clinical trials. Finally, a better understanding of the complex interplay between growth factors and signaling pathway cross-talk would play a fundamental role in helping to identify individual patients who could benefit from ErbB receptor family targeted therapies.

CORE TIP

Despite substantial improvements in targeted therapies for advanced gastric cancer, median overall survival remains <12 months. A better understanding of the molecular pathways associated with gastric cancer carcinogenesis could lead to new and better targeted treatment options. In particular, there is increasing evidence of the important role played by ErbB family members in driving gastric cancer growth. Our paper provides an overview of published and ongoing clinical studies evaluating the antitumor potential of molecular drugs targeting EGFR and HER2.

AUTHOR CONTRIBUTIONS

CA and AT reviewed the literature and co-drafted the manuscript. SP performed the literature research. All authors read and approved the final version of the paper.

REFERENCES

1. Bray F, Ferlay J, Soerjomataram I, Siegel Rl, Torre La, Jemal A. Global cancer statistics 2018: GLOBOCAN estimates of incidence and mortality worldwide for 36 cancers in 185 countries. *CA Cancer J Clin.* (2018) 68:394–424. doi: 10.3322/caac.21492
2. Ferlay J, Steliarova-Foucher E, Lortet-Tieulent J, Rosso S, Coebergh JW, Comber H, et al. Cancer incidence and mortality patterns in Europe: estimates for 40 countries in 2012. *Eur J Cancer.* (2013) 49:1374–403. doi: 10.1016/j.ejca.2012.12.027
3. Forman D, Burley VJ. Gastric cancer: global pattern of the disease and an overview of environmental risk factors. *Best Pract Res Clin Gastroenterol.* (2006) 20:633–49. doi: 10.1016/j.bpg.2006.04.008
4. Bozzetti F, Marubini E, Bonfanti G, Miceli R, Piano C, Gennari L. Subtotal versus total gastrectomy for gastric cancer: five-year survival rates in a multicenter randomized Italian trial. Italian Gastrointestinal Tumor Study Group. *Ann Surg.* (1999) 230:170–8. doi: 10.1097/00000658-199908000-00006
5. Gouzi JL, Huguier M, Fagniez PL, Launois B, Flamant Y, Lacaine F, et al. Total versus subtotal gastrectomy for adenocarcinoma of the gastric antrum. A French prospective controlled study. *Ann Surg.* (1989) 209:162–6. doi: 10.1097/00000658-198902000-00005
6. Bennett C, Wang Y, Pan T. Endoscopic mucosal resection for early gastric cancer. *Cochrane Database Syst Rev.* (2009) 1:CD004276. doi: 10.1002/14651858.CD004276.pub3
7. Soetikno R, Kaltenbach T, Yeh R, Gotoda T. Endoscopic mucosal resection for early cancers of the upper gastrointestinal tract. *J Clin Oncol.* (2005) 23:4490–8. doi: 10.1200/JCO.2005.19.935
8. Cuschieri A, Fayers P, Fielding J, Craven J, Bancewicz J, Joypaul V, et al. Postoperative morbidity and mortality after D1 and D2 resections for gastric cancer: preliminary results of the MRC randomised controlled surgical trial. The Surgical Cooperative Group. *Lancet.* (1996) 347:995–9. doi: 10.1016/S0140-6736(96)90144-0
9. Songun I, Putter H, Kranenbarg EM, Sasako M, van de Velde CJ. Surgical treatment of gastric cancer: 15-year follow-up results of the randomised nationwide Dutch D1D2 trial. *Lancet Oncol.* (2010) 11:439–49. doi: 10.1016/S1470-2045(10)70070-X
10. Sasako M, Sano T, Yamamoto S, Kurokawa Y, Nashimoto A, Kurita A, et al. D2 lymphadenectomy alone or with para-aortic nodal dissection for gastric cancer. *N Engl J Med.* (2008) 359:453–62. doi: 10.1056/NEJMoa0707035
11. Woll E, Devries A, Eisterer W, Hejna M, Keil F, Stein H, et al. Chemotherapy in gastric cancer. *Anticancer Res.* (2008) 28:1213–9.
12. Glimelius B, Ekstrom K, Hoffman K, Graf W, Sjoden PO, Haglund U, et al. Randomized comparison between chemotherapy plus best supportive care with best supportive care in advanced gastric cancer. *Ann Oncol.* (1997) 8:163–8. doi: 10.1023/A:1008243606668
13. Wagner AD, Unverzagt S, Grothe W, Kleber G, Grothey A, Haerting J, et al. Chemotherapy for advanced gastric cancer. *Cochrane Database Syst Rev.* (2010) 3:CD004064. doi: 10.1002/14651858.CD004064.pub3
14. Van Cutsem E, Moiseyenko VM, Tjulandin S, Majlis A, Constenla M, Boni C, et al. Phase III study of docetaxel and cisplatin plus fluorouracil compared with cisplatin and fluorouracil as first-line therapy for advanced gastric cancer: a report of the V325 Study Group. *J Clin Oncol.* (2006) 24:4991–7. doi: 10.1200/JCO.2006.06.8429
15. Waters JS, Norman A, Cunningham D, Scarffe JH, Webb A, Harper P, et al. Long-term survival after epirubicin, cisplatin and fluorouracil for gastric cancer: results of a randomized trial. *Br J Cancer.* (1999) 80:269–72. doi: 10.1038/sj.bjc.6690350
16. Ajani JA, Moiseyenko VM, Tjulandin S, Majlis A, Constenla M, Boni C, et al. Clinical benefit with docetaxel plus fluorouracil and cisplatin compared with cisplatin and fluorouracil in a phase III trial of advanced gastric or gastroesophageal cancer adenocarcinoma: the V-325 Study Group. *J Clin Oncol.* (2007) 25:3205–9. doi: 10.1200/JCO.2006.10.4968
17. Cunningham D, Starling N, Rao S, Iveson T, Nicolson M, Coxon F, et al. Capecitabine and oxaliplatin for advanced esophagogastric cancer. *N Engl J Med.* (2008) 358:36–46. doi: 10.1056/NEJMoa073149
18. Al-Batran SE, Hartmann JT, Probst S, Schmalenberg H, Hollerbach S, Hofheinz R, et al. Phase III trial in metastatic gastroesophageal adenocarcinoma with fluorouracil, leucovorin plus either oxaliplatin or cisplatin: a study of the Arbeitsgemeinschaft Internistische Onkologie. *J Clin Oncol.* (2008) 26:1435–42. doi: 10.1200/JCO.2007.13.9378
19. Montagnani F, Turrisi G, Marinozzi C, Aliberti C, Fiorentini G. Effectiveness and safety of oxaliplatin compared to cisplatin for advanced, unresectable gastric cancer: a systematic review and meta-analysis. *Gastric Cancer.* (2011) 14:50–5. doi: 10.1007/s10120-011-0007-7
20. Moertel CG, Childs DS Jr, Reitemeier RJ, Colby MY Jr, Holbrook MA. Combined 5-fluorouracil and supervoltage radiation therapy of locally unresectable gastrointestinal cancer. *Lancet.* (1969) 2:865–7. doi: 10.1016/S0140-6736(69)92326-5
21. Le Chevalier T, Smith FP, Harter WK, Schein PS. Chemotherapy and combined modality therapy for locally advanced and metastatic gastric carcinoma. *Semin Oncol.* (1985) 12:46–53.
22. Macdonald JS, Smalley SR, Benedetti J, Hundahl SA, Estes NC, Stemmermann GN, et al. Chemoradiotherapy after surgery compared

with surgery alone for adenocarcinoma of the stomach or gastroesophageal junction. *N Engl J Med.* (2001) 345:725–30. doi: 10.1056/NEJMoa010187

23. Smalley SR, Benedetti JK, Haller DG, Hundahl SA, Estes NC, Ajani JA, et al. Updated analysis of SWOG-directed intergroup study 0116: a phase III trial of adjuvant radiochemotherapy vs. observation after curative gastric cancer resection. *J Clin Oncol.* (2012) 30:2327–33. doi: 10.1200/JCO.2011.36.7136
24. Stahl M, Walz MK, Stuschke M, Lehmann N, Meyer HJ, Riera-Knorrenschild J, et al. Phase III comparison of preoperative chemotherapy compared with chemoradiotherapy in patients with locally advanced adenocarcinoma of the esophagogastric junction. *J Clin Oncol.* (2009) 27:851–6. doi: 10.1200/JCO.2008.17.0506
25. Sun P, Xiang JB, Chen ZY. Meta-analysis of adjuvant chemotherapy after radical surgery for advanced gastric cancer. *Br J Surg.* (2009) 96:26–33. doi: 10.1002/bjs.6408
26. GASTRIC (Global Advanced/Adjuvant Stomach Tumor Research International Collaboration) Group, Paoletti X, Oba K, Burzykowski T, Michiels S, Ohashi Y, et al. Benefit of adjuvant chemotherapy for resectable gastric cancer: a meta-analysis. *JAMA.* (2010) 303:1729–37. doi: 10.1001/jama.2010.534
27. Cunningham D, Allum WH, Stenning SP, Thompson JN, Van de Velde CJ, Nicolson M, et al. Perioperative chemotherapy versus surgery alone for resectable gastroesophageal cancer. *N Engl J Med.* (2006) 355:11–20. doi: 10.1056/NEJMoa055531
28. Sasako M, Sakuramoto S, Katai H, Kinoshita T, Furukawa H, Yamaguchi T, et al. Five-year outcomes of a randomized phase III trial comparing adjuvant chemotherapy with S-1 versus surgery alone in stage II or III gastric cancer. *J Clin Oncol.* (2011) 29:4387–93. doi: 10.1200/JCO.2011.36.5908
29. Bang YJ, Van Cutsem E, Feyereislova A, Chung HC, Shen L, Sawaki A, et al. Trastuzumab in combination with chemotherapy versus chemotherapy alone for treatment of HER2-positive advanced gastric or gastro-oesophageal junction cancer (ToGA): a phase 3, open-label, randomised controlled trial. *Lancet.* (2010) 376:687–97. doi: 10.1016/S0140-6736(10)61121-X
30. Nagatsuma AK, Aizawa M, Kuwata T, Doi T, Ohtsu A, Fujii H, et al. Expression profiles of HER2, EGFR, MET and FGFR2 in a large cohort of patients with gastric adenocarcinoma. *Gastric Cancer.* (2015) 18:227–38. doi: 10.1007/s10120-014-0360-4
31. Yarden Y, Sliwkowski MX. Untangling the ErbB signalling network. *Nat Rev Mol Cell Biol.* (2001) 2:127–37. doi: 10.1038/35052073
32. Cohen S. The epidermal growth factor (EGF). *Cancer.* (1983) 51:1787–91. doi: 10.1002/1097-0142(19830515)51:10 < 1787::AID-CNCR2820511004 > 3.0.CO;2-A
33. Thompson DM, Gill GN. The EGF receptor: structure, regulation and potential role in malignancy. *Cancer Surv.* (1985) 4:767–88.
34. Riely GJ, Politi KA, Miller VA, Pao W. Update on epidermal growth factor receptor mutations in non-small cell lung cancer. *Clin Cancer Res.* (2006) 12:7232–41. doi: 10.1158/1078-0432.CCR-06-0658
35. Witton CJ, Reeves JR, Going JJ, Cooke TG, Bartlett JM. Expression of the HER1-4 family of receptor tyrosine kinases in breast cancer. *J Pathol.* (2003) 200:290–7. doi: 10.1002/path.1370
36. Kapitanovic S, Radosevic S, Slade N, Kapitanovic M, Andelinovic S, Ferencic Z, et al. Expression of erbB-3 protein in colorectal adenocarcinoma: correlation with poor survival. *J Cancer Res Clin Oncol.* (2000) 126:205–11.. doi: 10.1007/s004320050034
37. Wei Q, Sheng L, Shui Y, Hu Q, Nordgren H, Carlsson J. EGFR, HER2, and HER3 expression in laryngeal primary tumors and corresponding metastases. *Ann Surg Oncol.* (2008) 15:1193–201. doi: 10.1245/s10434-007 9771-3
38. Wei Q, Chen L, Sheng L, Nordgren H, Wester K, Carlsson J. EGFR, HER2 and HER3 expression in esophageal primary tumours and corresponding metastases. *Int J Oncol.* (2007) 31:493–9. doi: 10.3892/ijo.31.3.493
39. Tanner B, Hasenclever D, Stern K, Schormann W, Bezler M, Hermes M, et al. ErbB-3 predicts survival in ovarian cancer. *J Clin Oncol.* (2006) 24:4317–23. doi: 10.1200/JCO.2005.04.8397
40. Koumakpayi IH, Diallo JS, Le Page C, Lessard L, Gleave M, Begin LR, et al. Expression and nuclear localization of ErbB3 in prostate cancer. *Clin Cancer Res.* (2006) 12:2730–7. doi: 10.1158/1078-0432.CCR-05-2242
41. Reschke M, Mihic-Probst D, van der Horst EH, Knyazev P, Wild PJ, Hutterer M, et al. HER3 is a determinant for poor prognosis in melanoma. *Clin Cancer Res.* (2008) 14:5188–97. doi: 10.1158/1078-0432.CCR-08-0186
42. Yarden Y, Pines G. The ERBB network: at last, cancer therapy meets systems biology. *Nat Rev Cancer.* (2012) 12:553–63. doi: 10.1038/nrc3309
43. Seshacharyulu P, Ponnusamy MP, Haridas D, Jain M, Ganti AK, Batra SK. Targeting the EGFR signaling pathway in cancer therapy. *Expert Opin Ther Targets.* (2012) 16:15–31. doi: 10.1517/14728222.2011.648617
44. Cho HS, Mason K, Ramyar KX, Stanley AM, Gabelli SB, Denney DW Jr, et al. Structure of the extracellular region of HER2 alone and in complex with the Herceptin Fab. *Nature.* (2003) 421:756–60. doi: 10.1038/nature01392
45. Garrett TP, McKern NM, Lou M, Elleman TC, Adams TE, Lovrecz GO, et al. The crystal structure of a truncated ErbB2 ectodomain reveals an active conformation, poised to interact with other ErbB receptors. *Mol Cell.* (2003) 11:495–505. doi: 10.1016/S1097-2765(03)00048-0
46. Olayioye MA, Neve RM, Lane HA, Hynes NE. The ErbB signaling network: receptor heterodimerization in development and cancer. *EMBO J.* (2000) 19:3159–67. doi: 10.1093/emboj/19.13.3159
47. Normanno N, Bianco C, Strizzi L, Mancino M, Maiello MR, De Luca A, et al. The ErbB receptors and their ligands in cancer: an overview. *Curr Drug Targets.* (2005) 6:243–57. doi: 10.2174/1389450053765879
48. Shi F, Telesco SE, Liu Y, Radhakrishnan R, Lemmon MA. ErbB3/HER3 intracellular domain is competent to bind ATP and catalyze autophosphorylation. *Proc Natl Acad Sci USA.* (2010) 107:7692–7. doi: 10.1073/pnas.1002753107
49. Fedi P, Pierce JH, di Fiore PP, Kraus MH. Efficient coupling with phosphatidylinositol 3-kinase, but not phospholipase C gamma or GTPase-activating protein, distinguishes ErbB-3 signaling from that of other ErbB/EGFR family members. *Mol Cell Biol.* (1994) 14:492–500. doi: 10.1128/MCB.14.1.492
50. Soltoff SP, Carraway KL III, Prigent SA, Gullick WG, Cantley LC. ErbB3 is involved in activation of phosphatidylinositol 3-kinase by epidermal growth factor. *Mol Cell Biol.* (1994) 14:3550–8. doi: 10.1128/MCB.14.6.3550
51. Prigent SA, Gullick WJ. Identification of c-erbB-3 binding sites for phosphatidylinositol 3'-kinase and SHC using an EGF receptor/c-erbB-3 chimera. *EMBO J.* (1994) 13:2831–41. doi: 10.1002/j.1460-2075.1994.tb06577.x
52. Vaught DB, Stanford JC, Young C, Hicks DJ, Wheeler F, Rinehart C, et al. HER3 is required for HER2-induced preneoplastic changes to the breast epithelium and tumor formation. *Cancer Res.* (2012) 72:2672–82. doi: 10.1158/0008-5472.CAN-11-3594
53. Holbro T, Beerli RR, Maurer F, Koziczak M, Barbas CF,3rd, Hynes NE. The ErbB2/ErbB3 heterodimer functions as an oncogenic unit: ErbB2 requires ErbB3 to drive breast tumor cell proliferation. *Proc Natl Acad Sci USA.* (2003) 100:8933–8. doi: 10.1073/pnas.1537685100
54. Engelman JA, Zejnullahu K, Mitsudomi T, Song Y, Hyland C, Park JO, et al. MET amplification leads to gefitinib resistance in lung cancer by activating ERBB3 signaling. *Science.* (2007) 316:1039–43. doi: 10.1126/science.1141478
55. Choi BK, Fan X, Deng H, Zhang N, An Z. ERBB3 (HER3) is a key sensor in the regulation of ERBB-mediated signaling in both low and high ERBB2 (HER2) expressing cancer cells. *Cancer Med.* (2012) 1:28–38. doi: 10.1002/cam4.10
56. Sartor CI, Zhou H, Kozlowska E, Guttridge K, Kawata E, Caskey L, et al. Her4 mediates ligand-dependent antiproliferative and differentiation responses in human breast cancer cells. *Mol Cell Biol.* (2001) 21:4265–75. doi: 10.1128/MCB.21.13.4265-4275.2001
57. Naresh A, Long W, Vidal GA, Wimley WC, Marrero L, Sartor CI, et al. The ERBB4/HER4 intracellular domain 4ICD is a BH3-only protein promoting apoptosis of breast cancer cells. *Cancer Res.* (2006) 66:6412–20. doi: 10.1158/0008-5472.CAN-05-2368
58. Barnes NL, Khavari S, Boland GP, Cramer A, Knox WF, Bundred NJ. Absence of HER4 expression predicts recurrence of ductal carcinoma in situ of the breast. *Clin Cancer Res.* (2005) 11:2163–8. doi: 10.1158/1078-0432.CCR-04-1633
59. Kainulainen V, Sundvall M, Maatta JA, Santiestevan E, Klagsbrun M, Elenius K. A natural ErbB4 isoform that does not activate phosphoinositide 3-kinase mediates proliferation but not survival or chemotaxis. *J Biol Chem.* (2000) 275:8641–9. doi: 10.1074/jbc.275.12.8641

60. Rio C, Buxbaum JD, Peschon JJ, Corfas G. Tumor necrosis factor-alpha-converting enzyme is required for cleavage of erbB4/HER4. *J Biol Chem.* (2000) 275:10379–87. doi: 10.1074/jbc.275.14.10379
61. Ni CY, Murphy MP, Golde TE, Carpenter G. gamma -Secretase cleavage and nuclear localization of ErbB-4 receptor tyrosine kinase. *Science.* (2001) 294:2179–81. doi: 10.1126/science.1065412
62. Jones FE. HER4 intracellular domain (4ICD) activity in the developing mammary gland and breast cancer. *J Mammary Gland Biol Neoplasia.* (2008) 13:247–58. doi: 10.1007/s10911-008-9076-6
63. Zhu Y, Sullivan LL, Nair SS, Williams CC, Pandey AK, Marrero L, et al. Coregulation of estrogen receptor by ERBB4/HER4 establishes a growth-promoting autocrine signal in breast tumor cells. *Cancer Res.* (2006) 66:7991–8. doi: 10.1158/0008-5472.CAN-05-4397
64. Dulak AM, Schumacher SE, van Lieshout J, Imamura Y, Fox C, Shim B, et al. Gastrointestinal adenocarcinomas of the esophagus, stomach, and colon exhibit distinct patterns of genome instability and oncogenesis. *Cancer Res.* (2012) 72:4383–93. doi: 10.1158/0008-5472.CAN-11-3893
65. Kim MA, Lee HS, Lee HE, Jeon YK, Yang HK, Kim WH. EGFR in gastric carcinomas: prognostic significance of protein overexpression and high gene copy number. *Histopathology.* (2008) 52:738–46. doi: 10.1111/j.1365-2559.2008.03021.x
66. Kandel C, Leclair F, Bou-Hanna C, Laboisse CL, Mosnier JF. Association of HER1 amplification with poor prognosis in well differentiated gastric carcinomas. *J Clin Pathol.* (2014) 67:307–12. doi: 10.1136/jclinpath-2013-201726
67. Chen C, Yang JM, Hu TT, Xu TJ, Yan G, Hu SL, et al. Prognostic role of human epidermal growth factor receptor in gastric cancer: a systematic review and meta-analysis. *Arch Med Res.* (2013) 44:380–9. doi: 10.1016/j.arcmed.2013.07.001
68. Aydin K, Okutur SK, Bozkurt M, Turkmen I, Namal E, Pilanci K, et al. Effect of epidermal growth factor receptor status on the outcomes of patients with metastatic gastric cancer: a pilot study. *Oncol Lett.* (2014) 7:255–9. doi: 10.3892/ol.2013.1662
69. Hong L, Han Y, Yang J, Zhang H, Jin Y, Brain L, et al. Prognostic value of epidermal growth factor receptor in patients with gastric cancer: a meta-analysis. *Gene.* (2013) 529:69–72. doi: 10.1016/j.gene.2013.07.106
70. Boku N. HER2-positive gastric cancer. *Gastric Cancer.* (2014) 17:1–12. doi: 10.1007/s10120-013-0252-z
71. Gravalos C, Jimeno A. HER2 in gastric cancer: a new prognostic factor and a novel therapeutic target. *Ann Oncol.* (2008) 19:1523–9. doi: 10.1093/annonc/mdn169
72. Dang HZ, Yu Y, Jiao SC. Prognosis of HER2 over-expressing gastric cancer patients with liver metastasis. *World J Gastroenterol.* (2012) 18:2402–7. doi: 10.3748/wjg.v18.i19.2402
73. Tanner M, Hollmen M, Junttila TT, Kapanen AI, Tommola S, Soini Y, et al. Amplification of HER-2 in gastric carcinoma: association with Topoisomerase IIalpha gene amplification, intestinal type, poor prognosis and sensitivity to trastuzumab. *Ann Oncol.* (2005) 16:273–8. doi: 10.1093/annonc/mdi064
74. Janjigian YY, Werner D, Pauligk C, Steinmetz K, Kelsen DP, Jager E, et al. Prognosis of metastatic gastric and gastroesophageal junction cancer by HER2 status: a European and USA International collaborative analysis. *Ann Oncol.* (2012) 23:2656–62. doi: 10.1093/annonc/mds104
75. Gomez-Martin C, Garralda E, Echarri MJ, Ballesteros A, Arcediano A, Rodriguez-Peralto JL, et al. HER2/neu testing for anti-HER2-based therapies in patients with unresectable and/or metastatic gastric cancer. *J Clin Pathol.* (2012) 65:751–7. doi: 10.1136/jclinpath-2012-200774
76. Moelans CB, Milne AN, Morsink FH, Offerhaus GJ, van Diest PJ. Low frequency of HER2 amplification and overexpression in early onset gastric cancer. *Cell Oncol.* (2011) 34:89–95. doi: 10.1007/s13402-011-0021-0
77. He XX, Ding L, Lin Y, Shu M, Wen JM, Xue L. Protein expression of HER2, 3, 4 in gastric cancer: correlation with clinical features and survival. *J Clin Pathol.* (2015) 68:374–80. doi: 10.1136/jclinpath-2014-202657
78. Hayashi M, Inokuchi M, Takagi Y, Yamada H, Kojima K, Kumagai J, et al. High expression of HER3 is associated with a decreased survival in gastric cancer. *Clin Cancer Res.* (2008) 14:7843–9. doi: 10.1158/1078-0432.CCR-08-1064
79. Abrahao-Machado LF, Scapulatempo-Neto C. HER2 testing in gastric cancer: an update. *World J Gastroenterol.* (2016) 22:4619–25. doi: 10.3748/wjg.v22.i19.4619
80. Jacome AA, Wohnrath DR, Scapulatempo Neto C, Carneseca EC, Serrano SV, Viana LS, et al. Prognostic value of epidermal growth factor receptors in gastric cancer: a survival analysis by Weibull model incorporating long-term survivors. *Gastric Cancer.* (2014) 17:76–86. doi: 10.1007/s10120-013-0236-z
81. Atmaca A, Werner D, Pauligk C, Steinmetz K, Wirtz R, Altmannsberger HM, et al. The prognostic impact of epidermal growth factor receptor in patients with metastatic gastric cancer. *BMC Cancer.* (2012) 12:524. doi: 10.1186/1471-2407-12-524
82. Hofmann M, Stoss O, Shi D, Buttner R, van de Vijver M, Kim W, et al. Assessment of a HER2 scoring system for gastric cancer: results from a validation study. *Histopathology.* (2008) 52:797–805. doi: 10.1111/j.1365-2559.2008.03028.x
83. Albarello L, Pecciarini L, Doglioni C. HER2 testing in gastric cancer. *Adv Anat Pathol.* (2011) 18:53–9. doi: 10.1097/PAP.0b013e3182026d72
84. Tang D, Liu CY, Shen D, Fan S, Su X, Ye P, et al. Assessment and prognostic analysis of EGFR, HER2, and HER3 protein expression in surgically resected gastric adenocarcinomas. *Onco Targets Ther.* (2014) 8:7–14. doi: 10.2147/OTT.S70922
85. Martinelli E, De Palma R, Orditura M, De Vita F, Ciardiello F. Anti-epidermal growth factor receptor monoclonal antibodies in cancer therapy. *Clin Exp Immunol.* (2009) 158:1–9. doi: 10.1111/j.1365-2249.2009.03992.x
86. Lordick F, Kang YK, Chung HC, Salman P, Oh SC, Bodoky G, et al. Capecitabine and cisplatin with or without cetuximab for patients with previously untreated advanced gastric cancer (EXPAND): a randomised, open-label phase 3 trial. *Lancet Oncol.* (2013) 14:490–9. doi: 10.1016/S1470-2045(13)70102-5
87. Park SR, Kook MC, Choi IJ, Kim CG, Lee JY, Cho SJ, et al. Predictive factors for the efficacy of cetuximab plus chemotherapy as salvage therapy in metastatic gastric cancer patients. *Cancer Chemother Pharmacol.* (2010) 65:579–87. doi: 10.1007/s00280-009-1067-9
88. Luber B, Deplazes J, Keller G, Walch A, Rauser S, Eichmann M, et al. Biomarker analysis of cetuximab plus oxaliplatin/leucovorin/5-fluorouracil in first-line metastatic gastric and oesophago-gastric junction cancer: results from a phase II trial of the Arbeitsgemeinschaft Internistische Onkologie (AIO). *BMC Cancer.* (2011) 11:509. doi: 10.1186/1471-2407-11-509
89. Lordick F, Luber B, Lorenzen S, Hegewisch-Becker S, Folprecht G, Woll E, et al. Cetuximab plus oxaliplatin/leucovorin/5-fluorouracil in first-line metastatic gastric cancer: a phase II study of the Arbeitsgemeinschaft Internistische Onkologie (AIO). *Br J Cancer.* (2010) 102:500–5. doi: 10.1038/sj.bjc.6605521
90. Waddell T, Chau I, Cunningham D, Gonzalez D, Okines AF, Okines C, et al. Epirubicin, oxaliplatin, and capecitabine with or without panitumumab for patients with previously untreated advanced oesophagogastric cancer (REAL3): a randomised, open-label phase 3 trial. *Lancet Oncol.* (2013) 14:481–9. doi: 10.1016/S1470-2045(13)70096-2
91. Lockhart AC, Reed CE, Decker PA, Meyers BF, Ferguson MK, Oeltjen AR, et al. Phase II study of neoadjuvant therapy with docetaxel, cisplatin, panitumumab, and radiation therapy followed by surgery in patients with locally advanced adenocarcinoma of the distal esophagus (ACOSOG Z4051). *Ann Oncol.* (2014) 25:1039–44. doi: 10.1093/annonc/mdu091
92. Rojo F, Tabernero J, Albanell J, Van Cutsem E, Ohtsu A, Doi T, et al. Pharmacodynamic studies of gefitinib in tumor biopsy specimens from patients with advanced gastric carcinoma. *J Clin Oncol.* (2006) 24:4309–16. doi: 10.1200/JCO.2005.04.2424
93. Dragovich T, McCoy S, Fenoglio-Preiser CM, Wang J, Benedetti JK, Baker AF, et al. Phase II trial of erlotinib in gastroesophageal junction and gastric adenocarcinomas: SWOG 0127. *J Clin Oncol.* (2006) 24:4922–7. doi: 10.1200/JCO.2006.07.1316
94. Matsui Y, Inomata M, Tojigamori M, Sonoda K, Shiraishi N, Kitano S. Suppression of tumor growth in human gastric cancer with HER2 overexpression by an anti-HER2 antibody in a murine model. *Int J Oncol.* (2005) 27:681–5. doi: 10.3892/ijo.27.3.681
95. Arienti C, Zanoni M, Pignatta S, Del Rio A, Carloni S, Tebaldi M, et al. Preclinical evidence of multiple mechanisms underlying

trastuzumab resistance in gastric cancer. *Oncotarget.* (2016) 7:18424–39. doi: 10.18632/oncotarget.7575

96. Roukos DH. Targeting gastric cancer with trastuzumab: new clinical practice and innovative developments to overcome resistance. *Ann Surg Oncol.* (2010) 17:14–7. doi: 10.1245/s10434-009-0766-0
97. Shimoyama S. Unraveling trastuzumab and lapatinib inefficiency in gastric cancer: future steps (Review). *Mol Clin Oncol.* (2014) 2:175–81. doi: 10.3892/mco.2013.213
98. Agus DB, Akita RW, Fox WD, Lewis GD, Higgins B, Pisacane PI, et al. Targeting ligand-activated ErbB2 signaling inhibits breast and prostate tumor growth. *Cancer Cell.* (2002) 2:127–37. doi: 10.1016/S1535-6108(02)00097-1
99. Baselga J, Cortes J, Kim SB, Im SA, Hegg R, Im YH, et al. Pertuzumab plus trastuzumab plus docetaxel for metastatic breast cancer. *N Engl J Med.* (2012) 366:109–19. doi: 10.1056/NEJMoa1113216
100. Barok M, Tanner M, Koninki K, Isola J. Trastuzumab-DM1 is highly effective in preclinical models of HER2-positive gastric cancer. *Cancer Lett.* (2011) 306:171–9. doi: 10.1016/j.canlet.2011.03.002
101. Shah MA, Kang YK, Thuss-Patience PC, Ohtsu A, Ajani JA, Van Cutsem E, et al. Biomarker analysis of the GATSBY study of trastuzumab emtansine versus a taxane in previously treated HER2-positive advanced gastric/gastroesophageal junction cancer. *Gastric Cancer.* (2019) 22:803–16. doi: 10.1007/s10120-018-0 0923-7

18

Single Purse-String Suture for Reinforcement of Duodenal Stump During Laparoscopic Radical Gastrectomy for Gastric Cancer

Hongyong He[†], Haojie Li[†], Botian Ye and Fenglin Liu[*]

Department of General Surgery, Zhongshan Hospital, Fudan University, Shanghai, China

***Correspondence:**
Fenglin Liu
liu.fenglin@zs-hospital.sh.cn

[†]These authors have contributed equally to this work

Background: Duodenal stump leakage (DSL) is a serious surgical complication after radical gastrectomy with Roux-en-Y or BillrothII reconstruction. This study was designed to evaluate the effectiveness of laparoscopic single purse-string suture for reinforcement of duodenal stump.

Methods: A total of 183 patients harboring gastric adenocarcinoma following laparoscopic radical gastrectomy with Roux-en-Y or BillrothIIreconstruction and single purse-string suture for reinforcement of duodenal stump were retrospectively enrolled from Zhongshan Hospital of Fudan University (Shanghai, China) between January 2014 and December 2016. Operative variables and short-term complications were documented and analyzed. Clavien-Dindo classification system was used to identify surgical complications.

Results: Among 183 patients, 108 (59.02%) patients received distal gastrectomy and 75 (40.98%) received total gastrectomy. 88 (48.09%) patients underwent Roux-en-Y reconstruction and 95 (51.91%) patients underwent Billroth-II reconstruction. The mean time of laparoscopic single purse-string suture was 5.01 ± 1.33 min (range from 3.6 to 10.2 min). Postoperative early complication occurred in 26 cases of the patients. There were 4 cases of system-related complications (2.19%), including 3 cases of pulmonary infection (1.64%) and 1 cases of cardiovascular event (0.55%); and 22 cases of surgery-related complications (12.02%), including 6 cases of intra-abdominal infection (3.28%), 4 cases of pancreatic leakage (2.19%), 4 cases of wound complications (2.19%), 3 cases of gastroparesis (1.64%), 2 cases of intra-abdominal bleeding (1.09%), 2 cases of ileus (1.09%), 1 cases of lymphatic leakage (0.55%), and no duodenal stump leakage.

Conclusion: Reinforcement on duodenal stump using laparoscopic single purse-string suture during laparoscopic radical gastrectomy is simple and effective and could avoid the incidence of duodenal stump leakage to some extent.

Keywords: gastric cancer, laparoscopic radical gastrectomy, duodenal stump leakage, laparoscopic single purse-string suture, reinforcement

INTRODUCTION

Duodenal stump leakage (DSL) is serious surgical complication following radical gastrectomy with Roux-en-Y or BillrothII reconstruction (1). It is very hard to treat and is fatal in some cases (2-4). Factors associated with DSL can be divided into systemic factors and local factors (5, 6). Age, nutritional status, comorbidities were considered as systemic factors associated with DSL (5). The local factors, such as excessive vascular dissection around duodenal stump and direct thermal injury, might influence the healing of duodenal stump and result in DSL (6). In addition, DSL can also be associated with high pressure in the cavity of duodenal stump due to afferent loop obstruction or acute pancreatitis (7, 8).

Traditionally, surgeons may choose interrupted or continuous sutures to reinforce the duodenal stump in open gastrectomy (1, 8). While, it is relatively more difficult for most unexperienced surgeons to manually perform it during laparoscopic surgery as sophisticatedly as open surgery. Based on this practical problem, and the incidence of DSL is not very high, some surgeons proposed their view that duodenal stump do not need to be reinforced in laparoscopic gastrectomy. However, the consequences of DSL are very serious. It is necessary to develop a simple and effective method to reinforce the duodenal stump and release the pressure at the edge of the duodenal stump during laparoscopic surgery.

In the current study, we introduced a new and simple maneuver, single purse-string suture, for laparoscopic reinforcement of duodenal stump, which could be done by the surgeon alone easily and avoid the incidence of DSL to some extent.

METHODS

Patients

We prospectively recruited consecutive patients with gastric cancer, collected the clinicopathological data, and detailed retrospectively analyzed the clinicopathological features correlating with morbidity and mortality and their role in decreasing the incidence of complications and the death rate, and improving the effect of operation (9). Between January 2014 and December 2016, a total of 183 patients harboring gastric adenocarcinoma following laparoscopic radical gastrectomy with Roux-en-Y or Billroth II reconstruction and single purse-string suture for reinforcement of duodenal stump were retrospectively enrolled from Zhongshan Hospital of Fudan University (Shanghai, China). Excluded were patients with distant metastases, gastric stump cancer, and peritoneal dissemination. In addition, patients were excluded if they had previously been exposed to any chemotherapy, radiotherapy, targeted therapy, or intervention therapy for gastric cancer. A retrospective review of prospectively collected data was performed, and the clinicopathological features (patient's age, gender, tumor localization, co-morbidity, tumor size, history of abdominal surgery, depth of tumor invasion, lymphatic vessel invasion, distant metastases, and pathological TNM stage) and the operation results (morbidity and mortality) were analyzed. The stage of gastric cancer is classified according to the tumor-node-metastasis (TNM) staging system of the eighth UICC/AJCC manual (10). The postoperative complications are defined and graded according to the grading system of Clavien-Dindo classification (11).

Surgical Procedure

Patients were placed in a modified reverse trendelenburg position with the head slightly elevated. The primary operator stood on the left side of the patient, the first assistant was on the opposite side and the camera assistant stood between the legs of the patient.

During the port placement process, a 1–1.5 cm curved incision was made just below the umbilicus for a 10-mm trocar. After establishing pneumoperitoneum at 12 mmHg, the camera was inserted and the diagnostic laparoscopy was performed. The major operative port was placed in the left upper quadrant at the crossing of mid-clavicle line and arc of rib with a 12 mm trocar, and another trocar of 5 mm was inserted in the left lower quadrant at the crossing of mid-clavicle line and umbilical horizon. Two additional ports were placed in the right upper and right lower quadrant, both with 5 mm trocars, for the first assistant's instruments. The process of port placement could be adjusted according to the body shape of the patient and operator's preference.

Depending on the location of the tumor, the proximal free margin was at least 3 cm of esophagus for total gastrectomy and at least 5 cm for advanced tumors for distal gastrectomy. R0 resection and standard D1+/D2 lymphadenectomy was performed according to guideline of Japanese Gastric Cancer Association. Roux-en-Y and Billroth II reconstruction was performed in laparoscopic distal gastrectomy according to the size of residual stomach and operator's choice.

Laparoscopic Duodenal Stump Reinforcement

Before dissecting the duodenum, approximately 2–3 cm of dissociated duodenum stump was preserved for reinforcement. A 60 mm endoscopic linear cutter (staple height 1.5–1.8 mm) was used to cut the duodenum from left side to right side. After cutting of duodenal stump, reinforcement on duodenal stump using laparoscopic single purse-string suture was performed as follows (**Figure 1**): a. place a seromuscular purse-string suture on the duodenum wall 1.0–1.5 cm away from the duodenal stump using 3-0 single-strand absorbable suture; b. place a knot before tightening the purse-string suture; c. push the duodenal stump into the purse-string suture using laparoscopic needle holding or grasping forceps; d. tighten the knot of the purse-string suture and reinforce it with 4–5 knots.

Duodenal Stump Leakage

Duodenal stump leakage (DSL) was defined by the presence of bile in the drainage tube, which was placed near the duodenal stump during the operation; or there was regional or diffuse fluid collection near the duodenal stump and confirmed by an abdominal CT scan, which was performed in patients who represented symptoms of clinical suspects of DSL, such as severe

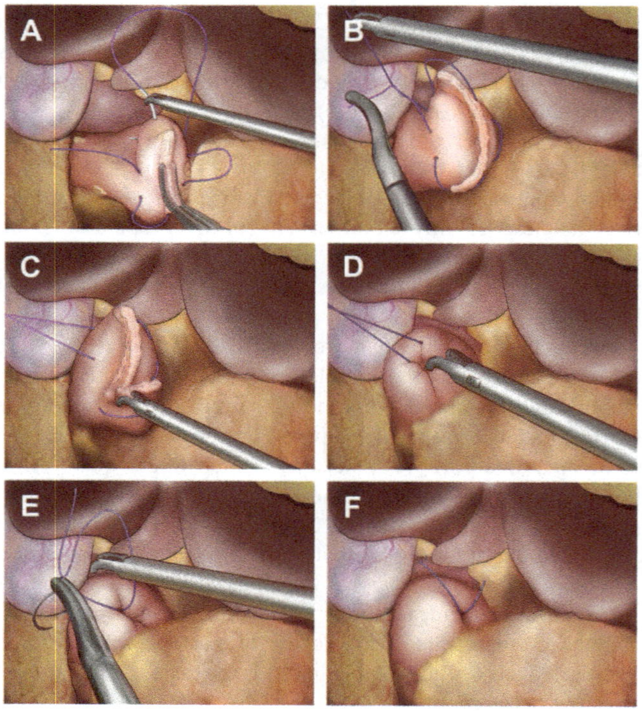

FIGURE 1 | Reinforcement on duodenal stump using laparoscopic single purse-string suture. **(A)** Place a seromuscular purse-string suture on the duodenum wall 1.0–1.5 cm away from the duodenal stump using 3–0 single-strand absorbable suture; **(B)** Place a knot before tightening the purse-string suture; **(C)** Push the duodenal stump into the purse-string suture using laparoscopic needle holding or grasping forceps; **(D)** Tighten the knot after the duodenal stump into the purse-string suture totally; **(E)** Reinforce the knots of purse-string suture with 4–5 knots; **(F)** The photo of reinforcement finished.

and abrupt abdominal pain, fever, worsening leukocytosis, and so on.

Statistical Analysis

The data were presented as mean ± standard deviation for continuous variables and as numbers and percentages for categorical variables. All analyses were performed using SPSS software (version 20.0, SPSS Inc., Chicago, IL, USA).

RESULTS

Clinicopathological Features

The clinical and pathological characteristics were summarized in **Table 1**. The mean age of the patients was 54.25 ± 9.27 ys (range from 24 to 87 ys). Most patents were male (122 of 183, 66.67%), and 66 (36.07%) patients had co-morbidity, of which, hypertension (34 of 183, 18.58%) ranked the highest. The mean preoperative blood albumin was 41.31 ± 3.88 g/L (range from 28 to 51 g/L). 9 (4.92%) patients presented with history of abdominal surgery, including cholecystectomy, appendectomy, and others. More than a half (121 of 183, 66.12%) of patients presented with

TABLE 1 | Patient demographics and clinicopathological characteristics.

Factor	No. of patients	%	Mean	SD
All patients	183	100		
Age(years)			54.25	9.27
Preoperative blood albumin, g/L			41.31	3.88
Preoperative blood creatinine, mmol/L			74.68	17.77
Gender				
Female	61	33.33		
Male	122	66.67		
Localization				
Proximal	53	28.96		
Middle	59	32.24		
Distal	71	38.80		
Co-morbidity				
Hypertension	34	18.58		
Diabetes mellitus	19	10.38		
Cardiac	13	7.10		
Tumor size (cm)			2.76	1.56
Differentiation				
Well	10	5.46		
Moderate	72	39.34		
Poorly	101	55.19		
History of abdominal surgery				
Cholecystectomy	1	0.55		
Appendectomy	5	2.73		
Others	3	1.64		
Pathological T Stage				
T1a	53	28.96		
T1b	51	27.87		
T2	39	21.31		
T3	24	13.11		
T4a	16	8.74		
T4b	0	0		
Pathological *N* Stage				
N0	123	67.21		
N1	21	11.48		
N2	25	13.66		
N3a	11	6.01		
N3b	3	1.64		
Pathological M Stage				
M0	183	100		
M1	0	0		
Pathological TNM Stage				
IA	93	50.82		
IB	28	15.30		
IIA	15	8.20		
IIB	31	16.94		
IIIA	8	4.37		
IIIB	5	2.73		
IIIC	3	1.64		
IV	0	0		

TABLE 2 | Surgical outcomes.

Outcome	No. of Patients	%	Mean	SD
All patients	183	100		
Extent of resection				
Distal gastrectomy	108	59.02		
Total gastrectomy	75	40.98		
Reconstruction				
Billroth-II	95	51.91		
Roux-en-Y	88	48.09		
Lymphadenectomy				
D1+	41	22.40		
D2	142	77.60		
Combined resection				
Gallbladder	27	14.75		
Spleen	1	0.55		
Adrenal gland	1	0.55		
Retrieved lymph node			37.83	14.35
Embedding time, minutes			5.01	1.33
Estimated blood loss, mL			136.52	86.95
Surgical time, minutes			238.02	53.07
Postoperative hospital stay, days			9.82	6.81

TABLE 3 | Morbidity and mortality.

Morbidity type/Mortality	No. of Patients	%
Morbidity	26	14.21
Surgery-related complications	22	12.02
Intra-abdominal infection	6	3.28
Pancreatic leakage	4	2.19
Wound complications	4	2.19
Gastroparesis	3	1.64
Intra-abdominal bleeding	2	1.09
Ileus	2	1.09
Lymphatic leakage	1	0.55
Duodenal stump leakage	0	0.00
System-related complications	4	2.19
Pulmonary infection	3	1.64
Cardiovascular event	1	0.55
Mortality	0	0.00
Clavien-Dindo Classification		
I	2	1.09
II	21	11.48
IIIa	2	1.09
IIIb	1	0.55

TNM stage I gastric cancer, no lymph node metastasis (123 of 183, 67.21%), and poorly differentiation (101 of 183, 55.19%).

Surgical Outcomes

Table 2 summarizes the surgical outcomes. Distal gastrectomy was performed in 108 (59.02%) patients and total gastrectomy was performed in 75 (40.98%) patients. Billroth II reconstruction was performed in 95 (51.91%) patients, Roux-en-Y reconstruction for 88 (48.09%) patients. The mean surgical time was 238.02 ± 53.07 min (range from 178 to 314 min). The procedure of laparoscopic single purse-string suture took 5.01 ± 1.33 min (range from 3.6 to 10.2 min). 37.83 ± 14.35 (range from 17 to 98) lymph nodes were retrieved from the patients enrolled in this study. There were 29 combined surgeries, including 27 cases of cholecystectomy, 1 case of splenectomy, and 1 case of adrenalectomy. Mean postoperative hospital stay was 9.82 ± 6.81 days (range from 5 to 50 days).

Morbidity and Mortality

In all, postoperative early complication occurred in 26 cases of the patients and no patient died (**Table 3**). There were 4 cases of system-related complications (2.19%), including 3 cases of pulmonary infection (1.64%) and 1 cases of cardiovascular event (0.55%); and 22 cases of surgery-related complications (12.02%), including 6 cases of intra-abdominal infection (3.28%), 4 cases of pancreatic leakage (2.19%), 4 cases of wound complications (2.19%), 3 cases of gastroparesis (1.64%), 2 cases of intra-abdominal bleeding (1.09%), 2 cases of ileus (1.09%), 1 cases of lymphatic leakage (0.55%), and no duodenal stump leakage. According to Clavien-Dindo classification, 23 patients were classified as ≤ II and 2 patients as IIIa. Only one case of intestinal obstruction recovered after reoperation, and patients with other complications were discharged successfully after conservative treatment.

Potential Mechanism

As shown in **Figure 2**, there are two potential mechanisms of the avoidance of DSL after single purse-string suture for reinforcement of duodenal stump. First, the reinforcement was performed on the relatively normal tissue in contrast to other methods, such as barbed suture and Lembert suture, which are performed on the staple-line of duodenal stump directly; Second, the field of single purse-string suture (point A) is the force-bearing point, and the staple-line of duodenal stump (weak point, point B) has been protected. Above all, the field to take the pressure of duodenum (point A) is the relatively normal tissue, and the weak point (point B) is protected and not need to take the pressure in the duodenum, especially when the afferent loop obstruction occurred, so this maneuver could avoid the incidence of DSL effectively.

Case Presentation

In Dec. 2015, a 52-year-old man with adenocarcinoma of gastric antrum was referred to our institution and had laparoscopic assisted radical distal gastrectomy with Billroth II reconstruction and single purse-string suture for reinforcement of duodenal stump. After the operation, the afferent loop obstruction occurred, and the diameter of duodenum was more than 6 cm. However, we found the duodenal stump was intact according to the image of CT scan and confirmed it during our second operation (**Figure 3**). This case showed that single purse-string suture can withstand huge pressure in the duodenum.

DISCUSSION

Duodenal stump leakage (DSL) is severe complication with a high mortality rate after radical gastrectomy with Roux-en-Y or BillrothIIreconstruction, and the incidence rate is ranging from 1.6% to 5% (1, 2). Once DSL occurred, it is very difficult to treat and the mortality rate is reported as high as 16% to 20% (8). Patient age, nutritional status, comorbidities were considered as risk system factors associated with DSL after gastrectomy (5). In addition, the surgical techniques and many other local factors, including the insufficient blood supply, the tissue vulnerability, such as local edema and scar on duodenal wall, the length of duodenal stump, and high pressure inside duodenal cavity might influence the healing of duodenal stump and result in DSL (6). So, in order to prevent DSL, reinforcement of duodenal stump is necessary and some reinforcement methods have been applied widely, including barbed suture (12), Lembert suture (13), two half-purse-string sutures (14). However, these methods require multiple stitches and knots, which is rather different for the unexperienced surgeons (12–14). This study was a retrospective, one-arm clinical trial focusing on a new maneuver, single purse-string suture, for reinforcement of duodenal stump in patients harboring gastric adenocarcinoma following laparoscopic radical gastrectomy with Roux-en-Y or BillrothIIreconstruction. The results showed that the morbidity rate was lower compared to laparoscopic assisted distal gastrectomy (morbidity rate 15.2%) in our previous CLASS-01study (15), and there was no incidence of DSL in this research, which proved that single purse-string suture is feasibility and safety.

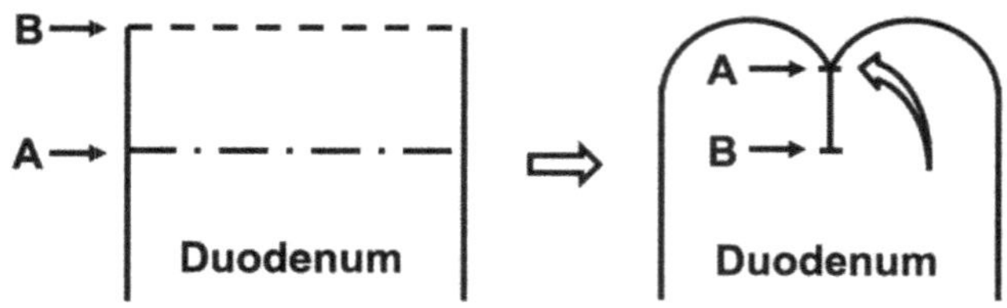

FIGURE 2 | The pattern of the reinforcement of duodenal stump with single purse-string suture. The reinforcement was performed on the relatively normal tissue, which was the field to take the pressure of duodenum (point A). The staple-line of duodenal stump was the weak point (point B), which was protected and not need to take the pressure in the duodenum after the reinforcement.

The laparoscopic duodenal stump reinforcement was thought to be relatively difficult for most even experienced surgeons to perform due to the complexity of duodenal anastomosis, the restriction of sewing angles, and the uncontrollably of knotting strength (16–18). Based on this situation, we proposed a novel reinforcement method, single purse-string suture, which is an easy and effective method to reinforce the duodenal stump, and could avoid DSL to the some extent. There are three key points about this maneuver. First, the interval of sutures is the critical point for this maneuver. The duodenal wall is vulnerable of being

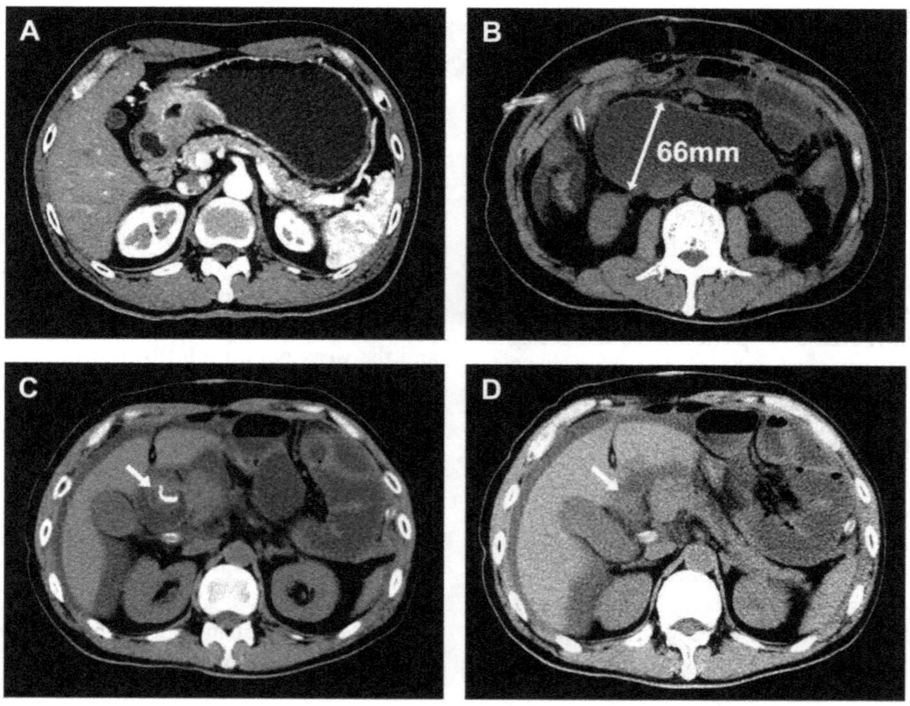

FIGURE 3 | One case of afferent loop obstruction after Billroth II reconstruction and single purse-string suture for reinforcement of duodenal stump. **(A)** Abdominal CT image of the case with adenocarcinoma of gastric antrum; **(B)** After the operation, the afferent loop obstruction occurred, and the diameter of duodenum was more than 6 cm; **(C,D)** The reinforced duodenal stump (arrows) was intact.

grasped, which could easily arouse acute local inflammation and cause local edema and tissue injuries. If the intervals of sutures are too large, the intervals may expand after local edema recedes, which may increase the risk for DSL. Therefore, we positioned our sutures with an interval of 8–10 mm, which can reinforce the duodenal stump well, and does not affect the blood supply of the duodenal stump. Second, if the length of duodenal stump is <1 cm, the single purse-string suture is not recommended. In this case, continuous suture or interrupted suture of duodenal stump is a better choice. Third, this maneuver should be performed by one operator alone. Many surgeons prefer grasping the duodenum or pushing the duodenal stump by the assistant. While, according to our experience, the kernel of controlling the knotting strength is to perform the knotting alone. The purse string suture is satisfying and trustworthy only when the direction and strength of pushing the duodenal stump are synchronous. The knotting balance could be hardly achieved by manipulation of four laparoscopic instruments.

Reinforcement suturing of the staple line after cutting the duodenum has commonly been accepted and performed for prevention of DSL in patients undergoing laparoscopic gastrectomy (1, 8). Many literatures have proved the effectiveness of reinforcement of duodenal stump in laparoscopic gastrectomy with different methods. Sang Yun Kim proved that laparoscopic reinforcement suture on staple-line of duodenal stump using barbed suture can be considered as one of prevention methods of DSL during laparoscopic gastrectomy for gastric cancer (12). Inoue et al. demonstrated the effectiveness of intracorporeal Lembert's sutures in laparoscopic distal gastrectomy receiving Roux-en-Y reconstruction while with no postoperative DSL in 223 patients (13). Ri et al. reported that duodenal stump reinforcement in laparoscopic gastrectomy with Roux-en-Y reconstruction may reduce the risk of DSL development (0.67% vs. 5.71%, $P < 0.001$) and minimize its severity (16). In addition to the reinforcement suturing of the staple line, Ojima et al. introduced a new method, reinforced stapling technique, to reinforce the reconstruction after laparoscopic gastrectomy, which is a feasible and safe procedure for gastric cancer with regard to short-term surgical outcomes (19).

There are several limitations of this study. First, this study was a retrospective analysis and the selection biases cannot be totally avoided; Second, this study was a one-arm clinical trial and there was no control group in this study, while, the result is satisfied, and the advantages of this method also can be confirmed according to previous published researches; Third, the number of patients enrolled in this study was small. The feasibility and safety of laparoscopic single purse-string suture for reinforcement of duodenal stump should be confirmed by a prospective randomized controlled multicenter clinical trial with a large sample size in the future.

In conclusion, laparoscopic single purse-string suture for reinforcement of duodenal stump showed its simplicity and efficiency, which could avoid the incidence of DSL to some extent and might improve overall outcomes of patients with gastric cancer receiving laparoscopic radical gastrectomy.

ETHICS STATEMENT

Ethical approval was granted by the Clinical Research Ethics Committee of Zhongshan Hospital of Fudan University (Shanghai, China). Signed informed consent was obtained from all patients for the acquisition and use of anonymized clinical data.

AUTHOR CONTRIBUTIONS

HH and FL: conceptualization and writing-review and editing. HH, HL, and BY: formal analysis and resources. HH: investigation and writing-original draft preparation. All the authors have approved the final manuscript.

REFERENCES

1. Zizzo M, Ugoletti L, Manzini L, Castro Ruiz C, Nita GE, Zanelli M, et al. Management of duodenal stump fistula after gastrectomy for malignant disease: a systematic review of the literature. *BMC Surgery.* (2019) 19:55. doi: 10.1186/s12893-019-0520-x
2. Cozzaglio L, Giovenzana M, Biffi R, Cobianchi L, Coniglio A, Framarini M, et al. Surgical management of duodenal stump fistula after elective gastrectomy for malignancy: an Italian retrospective multicenter study. *Gastric Cancer.* (2016) 19:273–9. doi: 10.1007/s10120-014-0445-0
3. Ali BI, Park CH, Song KY. Outcomes of non-operative treatment for duodenal stump leakage after gastrectomy in patients with gastric cancer. *J Gastric Cancer.* (2016) 16:28–33. doi: 10.5230/jgc.2016.16.1.28
4. Oh JS, Lee HG, Chun HJ, Choi BG, Lee SH, Hahn ST, et al. Percutaneous management of postoperative duodenal stump leakage with foley catheter. *Cardiovasc Interv Radiol.* (2013) 36:1344–9. doi: 10.1007/s00270-012-0518-6
5. Kim SH, Son SY, Park YS, Ahn SH, Park DJ, Kim HH. Risk factors for anastomotic leakage: a retrospective cohort study in a single gastric surgical unit. *J Gastric Cancer.* (2015) 15:167–75. doi: 10.5230/jgc.2015.15.3.167
6. Kim KH, Kim MC, Jung GJ. Risk factors for duodenal stump leakage after gastrectomy for gastric cancer and management technique of stump leakage. *Hepatogastroenterology.* (2014) 61:1446–53. doi: 10.5754/hge.14355
7. Paik HJ, Lee SH, Choi CI, Kim DH, Jeon TY, Kim DH, et al. Duodenal stump fistula after gastrectomy for gastric cancer: risk factors, prevention, and management. *Ann Surg Treat Res.* (2016) 90:157–63. doi: 10.4174/astr.2016.90.3.157
8. Aurello P, Sirimarco D, Magistri P, Petrucciani N, Berardi G, Amato S, et al. Management of duodenal stump fistula after gastrectomy for gastric cancer: Systematic review. *World J Gastroenterol.* (2015) 21:7571–6. doi: 10.3748/wjg.v21.i24.7571
9. He H, Shen Z, Wang X, Qin J, Sun Y, Qin X. Survival benefit of greater number of lymph nodes dissection for advanced node-negative gastric cancer patients following radical gastrectomy. *Jap J Clin Oncol.* (2016) 46:63–70. doi: 10.1093/jjco/hyv159
10. Amin MB, Edge SB, Greene FL, Byrd DR, Brookland RK, Washington MK, et al. *AJCC Cancer Staging Manual*(M). 8th ed. New York, NY: Springer (2016). p. 203–20.
11. Dindo D, Demartines N, Clavien PA. Classification of surgical complications: a new proposal with evaluation in a cohort

of 6336 patients and results of a survey. *Ann Surg.* (2004) 240:205–13. doi: 10.1097/01.sla.0000133083.54934.ae
12. Kim SY, Nam SH, Min JS, Kim MC. Laparoscopic reinforcement suture on staple-line of duodenal stump using barbed suture during laparoscopic gastrectomy for gastric cancer. *Ann Surg Treat Res.* (2017) 93:305–9. doi: 10.4174/astr.2017.93.6.305
13. Inoue K, Michiura T, Fukui J, Mukaide H, Ozaki T, Miki H, et al. Staple-line reinforcement of the duodenal stump with intracorporeal Lembert's sutures in laparoscopic distal gastrectomy with Roux-en-Y reconstruction for gastric cancer. *Surg Laparosc Endosc Percutan Tech.* (2016) 26:338–42. doi: 10.1097/SLE.0000000000000291
14. Shao QS, Wang YX, Ye ZY, Zhao ZK, Xu J. Application of purse-string suture for management of duodenal stump in radical gastrectomy. *Chin Med J.* (2011) 124:1018–21.
15. Hu Y, Huang C, Sun Y, Su X, Cao H, Hu J, et al. Morbidity and mortality of laparoscopic versus open D2 distal gastrectomy for advanced gastric cancer: a randomized controlled trial. *J Clin Oncol.* (2016) 34:1350–7. doi: 10.1200/JCO.2015.63.7215
16. Ri M, Hiki N, Ishizuka N, Ida S, Kumagai K, Nunobe S, et al. Duodenal stump reinforcement might reduce both incidence and severity of duodenal stump leakage after laparoscopic gastrectomy with Roux-en-Y reconstruction for gastric cancer. *Gastric Cancer.* (2019) 22:1053–9. doi: 10.1007/s10120-019-00946-8
17. Misawa K, Yoshikawa T, Ito S, Cho H, Ito Y, Ogata T. Safety and feasibility of linear stapling device with bioabsorbable polyglycolic acid sheet for duodenal closure in gastric cancer surgery: a multi-institutional phase II study. *World J Surg.* (2019) 43:192–8. doi: 10.1007/s00268-018-4748-x
18. Kim MC, Kim SY, Kim KW. Laparoscopic Reinforcement Suture (LARS) on staple line of duodenal stump using barbed suture in laparoscopic gastrectomy for gastric cancer: a prospective single arm phase II study. *J Gastric Cancer.* (2017) 17:354–62. doi: 10.5230/jgc.2017.17.e40
19. Ojima T, Nakamura M, Hayata K, Nakamori M, Yamaue H. Reinforced stapling technique for reconstruction after laparoscopic distal gastrectomy. *Surg Laparosc Endosc Percutan Tech.* (2018) 28:334–6. doi: 10.1097/SLE.0000000000000570

19

The Methods of Lymph Node Examination Make a Difference to Node Staging and Detection of N3b Node Status for Gastric Cancer

Xinhua Chen, Yuehong Chen, Yanfeng Hu, Tian Lin, Jun Luo, Tuanjie Li, Tao Li, HuiLin Huang, Yu Zhu, Tingting Li, Hao Chen, Hao Liu†, Guoxin Li*† and Jiang Yu*†*

Department of General Surgery, Nanfang Hospital, Southern Medical University, Guangzhou, China

***Correspondence:**
Hao Liu
liuhaofbi@163.com
Guoxin Li
gzliguoxin@163.com
Jiang Yu
balbc@163.com

†These authors have contributed equally to this work

Background: The number of retrieved lymph nodes (RLNs) affects the likelihood of detecting metastatic lymph nodes (MLNs) for gastric cancer (GC), but the retrieval of LNs is not satisfactory worldwide. There is no standard for LN examination.

Methods: We retrospectively analyzed 2,163 patients diagnosed with GC who underwent surgery at Nanfang Hospital between October 2004 and September 2016. According to the methods of LN examination, patients were classified into two groups: LN detection by pathologists (pathologist group) and LN examination by surgicopathologic team (surgicopathologist group). The relationship between RLNs and LN staging accuracy as well as the factors influencing the detection of MLNs were evaluated.

Results: There were 472 males in pathologist group and 467 males in surgicopathologist group. The number of RLNs and MLNs in surgicopathologist group was significantly higher than that in pathologist group (RLNs: 53.8 ± 20.9 vs. 18.8 ± 11.5, $p < 0.001$; MLNs: 5.6 ± 9.8 vs. 3.9 ± 5.7, $p < 0.001$). Notably, the detection of N3b node status was significantly improved in surgicopathologist group [83 (11.9%) vs. 34 (4.8%), $p < 0.001$]. Additionally, the detection rate of N3b status gradually increased from 0 in patients with 1-16 RLNs to 16.6% in patients with more than 49 RLNs. The MLNs detected increased gradually from 2.3 ± 3.0 in patients with 1-16 RLNs to 7.3 ± 11.7 in patients with more than 49 RLNs. Univariate and multivariate analyses indicated that LN examination by surgicopathologic team, more advanced pT, tumor size ≥5 cm and combined organ(s) resection were related to detecting more MLNs.

Conclusions: The retrieval of nodes immediately postoperatively by the surgicopathologic team could significantly improve the number of RLNs, detect more MLNs, and screen more patients with N3b node status.

Keywords: gastric cancer, lymph node, examination, node staging, N3b

INTRODUCTION

Many studies have suggested that overall survival (OS) is associated with the number of retrieved lymph nodes (RLNs) (1–3). The results based on data from the Surveillance, Epidemiology, and End Results (SEER) database showed that OS was dependent on the number of RLNs (1). For every 10 additional LNs examined, all four stage subgroups could yield superior survival, and this tendency could continue to be detected for cutoff points of up to 40 LNs. However, the number of RLNs cannot separate the impact of stage migration versus improved regional disease control to favor survival. Recently, Hayashi et al. showed that the number of RLNs < 40 could be attributed to an inferior survival for stage III gastric cancer (GC) patients who underwent total gastrectomy (2). Consistently, another large international dataset analysis, including the SEER database (n = 13,932) and the Yonsei University Gastric Cancer database (n = 11,358), also proposed that a greater number of RLNs (a minimum of 29) improves staging and OS in GC patients undergoing radical resection (3). All of these quality studies proposed a higher number of RLNs than that recommended by the 8th edition of the American Joint Committee on Cancer (AJCC) TNM staging system for GC (at least 16).

To determine why OS following operations for GC in Japan are far superior to the results obtained in Western countries, Noguchi et al. reviewed the Japanese literature and found that the meticulous histopathological evaluation of surgical specimens in Japan resulted in more accurate pathologic staging, which was one of the main reasons for the improved OS (4). Consistent with this finding, many subsequent studies also demonstrated that the number of RLNs could affect the likelihood of detecting metastatic LNs (MLNs) (5) and stage migration (6–8).

For standard D2 lymphadenectomy, which can guarantee the efficiency of locoregional disease control for resectable GC, the number of RLNs is mainly dependent on the approach of LN examination. Furthermore, the results of the retrieval of LNs in the Dutch Gastric Cancer Trial suggest that LN retrieval rather than the extent of surgical LN dissection was mainly responsible for the number of RLNs (9).

Taken together, these findings suggest that the improper approach of LN examination could result in the insufficiency of RLNs and the underestimation of LN metastasis status, which could have an undesirable impact on prognostic evaluation and the strategy formulation of adjuvant therapy. However, Sano et al. collected analytic data on 25,411 patients from 59 institutions in 15 countries, showing that the mean/median (range) number of LNs examined in Japan, Korea, selected other Asian centers and selected Western centers was 39.4/36 (1–171), 33/31 (1–129), 24.8/22 (1–103), and 29.5/27 (1–123), respectively (10).

Therefore, more standard and normative LN examination techniques are urgently needed, as well as the identification of confounding factors in nodal status assessment, to further improve the accuracy of node assessment and therefore improve survival (7, 8, 11, 12). Hence, we summarize the methods and experiences of LN examination for GC specimens at the Department of General Surgery of Nanfang Hospital by comparing the nodal yields obtained by conventional sampling by pathologists vs. immediate postoperative retrieval by the surgicopathologic team.

METHODS

Patients

In the period between October 2004 and September 2016, 2,163 consecutive patients were diagnosed with GC and underwent surgery at Nanfang Hospital, Southern Medical University. The analyses were based on the prospective GC database, which includes information on GC derived from electronic medical records that have been maintained in the Nanfang Hospital since 2004 (13). Data monitoring was performed by a specific medical recorder with ~10 years of relevant work experience. The recorded variables included demographic, clinical, pathological, and surgical characteristics. After two independent surgical oncologists reviewed the pathological reports and medical records of the patients retrospectively, patients who did not receive gastrectomy, underwent non-radical resection, had stage IV GC, underwent only D1/D1+ lymphadenectomy rather than D2/D2+ lymphadenectomy, had gastric stump cancer or had neoadjuvant chemotherapy before gastrectomy were excluded. After the above exclusion criteria were evaluated, 1,404 patients were enrolled. According to the methods of LN examination, patients were classified into two groups: conventional method for retrieving LNs by pathologists (pathologist group) and standard operating procedure (SOP) of LN examination by a specialized surgicopathologic team (surgicopathologist group) (**Figure 1**). For patients in the pathologist group, the pathologists retrieved LNs after the specimens were fixed in 10% neutral buffered formalin. For patients in surgicopathologist group, a member of the surgicopathologic team sequentially retrieved LNs postoperatively within 5 min according to the LN station and then submitted the LN specimens to the Pathology Department for further examination.

The cancer stage was determined or recoded according to the 7th edition of the AJCC TNM staging system (13). Tumor location was categorized as the upper, middle, or lower third of the stomach. The resection approach [laparoscopic gastrectomy (LG) or open gastrectomy (OG)] and reconstruction methods followed standard guidelines (14–17). The study complied with the principles set forth in the Declaration of Helsinki. The data collection protocol was approved by the Ethics Committee of Nanfang Hospital, Southern Medical University. Written informed consent was obtained from all the patients in the study.

LN Examination Approaches

Pathologist Group

LN retrieval was conventionally performed by pathologists via inspection, palpation, and/or serial sectioning of the formalin-fixed specimens.

Surgicopathologist Group

The practice of LN examination by the specialized surgicopathologic team included three parts (18): the establishment of a special team (the surgicopathologic team) to examine LNs, the development of an effective SOP for LN examination, and long-term and sustained quality control. The special team was composed of postgraduate students who were not involved in surgery but trained professionally by surgeons.

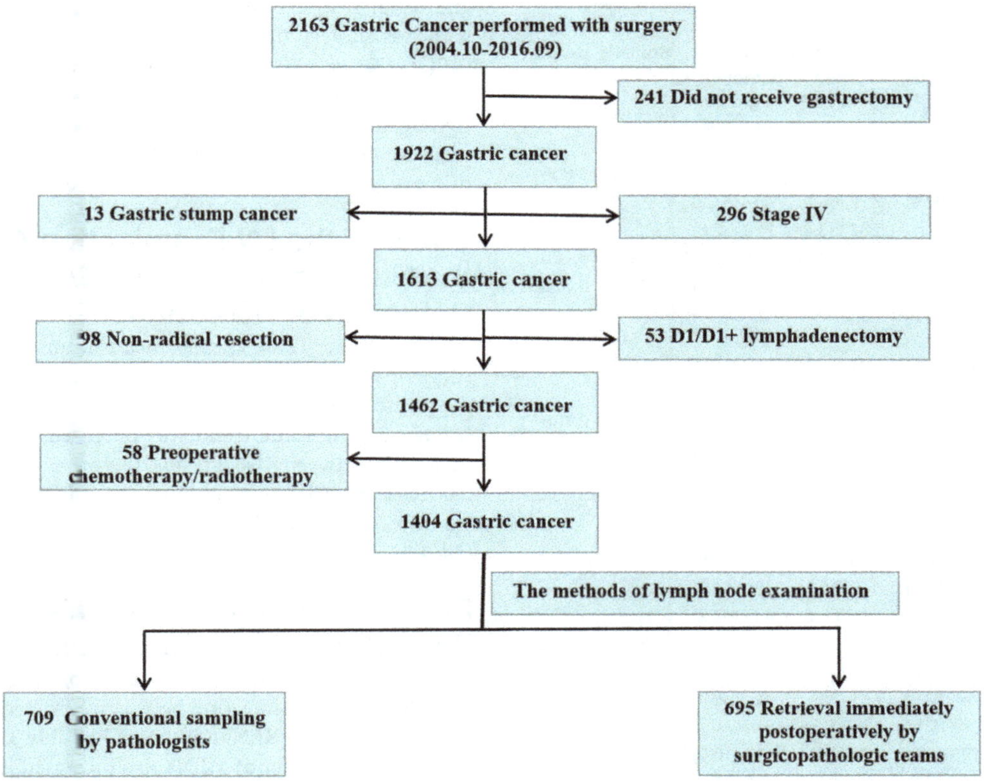

FIGURE 1 | Flow chart of the study cohort.

The SOP includes studying the anatomy of the perigastric region, learning surgical procedures to identify LN stations and specifying procedures for LN examination. The specification procedures in more detail are showed in **Appendix**. Last, quality control consisted of periodic data reporting and continuous feedback to ensure the high quality of the LN examination since personnel changes occurred often.

Statistical Analysis

Data are presented as the mean ± standard deviation (SD) for continuous variables (for variables with non-normal distributions, the medians and ranges are shown) and as numbers (%) for categorical variables. Student's t test and the Mann-Whitney U test were used to compare continuous variables, and the χ^2 test and Fisher's exact test were used to compare categorical variables as appropriate. Risk factors for the number of MLNs were evaluated by univariate analyses and multivariate analyses using a general linear regression model. $p < 0.05$ (two-tailed) was considered statistically significant. The statistical software SPSS version 17.0 for Windows (SPSS, Inc., Chicago, IL, USA) was used for all statistical analyses.

RESULTS

Patient Characteristics

The clinical and pathological characteristics of the patients are shown in **Table 1**. There were 472 males in the pathologist group and 467 males in the surgicopathologist group (p = 0.805). The mean age in the pathologist group and surgicopathologist group was 55.7 and 56.1 years (p = 0.485), with a mean body mass index of 21.6 and 22.5 kg/m^2 (p = 0.030), respectively. The clinical depth of tumor invasion (cT) was more advanced in patients in the pathologist group than in those in the surgicopathologist group [cT1/cT2/cT3/cT4: 124(17.5%)/60(8.5%)/110(15.5%)/415(58.5%) vs. 53(7.6%)/74 (10.6%)/101(14.5%)/467(67.2%), $p < 0.001$]. Similarly, pathological tumor depth (pT) was also increased in patients in the pathologist group than in those in the surgicopathologist group [pT1a/pT1b/pT2/pT3/cT4a/pT4b: 61(8.6%)/61(8.6%)/80(11.3%)/15(2.1%)/430(60.6%)/62(8.7%) vs. 71(10.2%)/88(12.7%)/69(9.9%)/111(16.0%)/309(44.5%)/ 47(67.6%), $p < 0.001$]. Nevertheless, although the clinical LN status (cN) was more advanced in the pathologist group [cN0/cTN1/cN2/cN3: 220(31.0%)/119(16.8%)/246(34.7%)/ 124(17.5%) vs. 330(47.5%)/143(20.6%)/108(15.5%)/114(16.4%), $p < 0.001$], the pathological LN status (pN) was not significantly different between the two groups [pN0/pTN1/pN2/pN3a/pN3b: 263(37.1%)/135(19.0%)/166(23.4%)/111(15.7%)/34(4.8%) vs. 328(47.2%)/92(13.2%)/86(12.4%)/106(15.3%)/83(11.9%), $p = 0.248$]. Consistent with the pT status, the patients in the pathologist group more likely underwent gastrectomy with combined organ(s) resection [60(8.5%) vs. 40(5.8%), $p = 0.049$]. Patients in the pathologist group were more inclined to undergo open surgery [345(48.7%) vs. 83(11.9%), $p < 0.001$]

TABLE 1 | Clinicopathologic characteristics of the two groups of patients.

Characteristic	Total (n = 1,404)	Pathologist group (n = 709)	Surgico-pathologist group (n = 695)	Statistic	*p-value*
Gender [n (%)]				0.061	0.805
Male	939 (66.9)	472 (66.6)	467 (67.2)		
Female	465 (33.1)	237 (33.4)	228 (32.8)		
Age, y, mean ± SD		55.7 ± 12.0	56.1 ± 11.7	−0.699	0.485
Body mass index, mean ± SD		21.6 ± 3.0	22.5 ± 8.1	−2.178	0.030
Diabetes [n (%)]				0.345	0.557
Yes	66 (4.7)	31 (4.4)	35 (5.0)		
No	1,338 (95.3)	678 (95.6)	660 (95.0)		
Tumore size [n (%)]					0.793
<5 cm	940 (67.0)	477 (67.3)	463 (66.6)		
≥5 cm	464 (33.0)	232 (32.7)	232 (33.4)		
cT-stage [n (%)]				−4.062	<0.001
cT1	177 (12.6)	124 (17.5)	53 (7.6)		
cT2	134 (9.5)	60 (8.5)	74 (10.6)		
cT3	211 (15.0)	110 (15.5)	101 (14.5)		
cT4	882 (62.8)	415 (58.5)	467 (67.2)		
pT-stage [n (%)]				−5.195	<0.001
pT1a	132 (9.4)	61 (8.6)	71 (10.2)		
pT1b	149 (10.6)	61 (8.6)	88 (12.7)		
pT2	149(10.6)	80(11.3)	69(9.9)		
pT3	126 (9.0)	15 (2.1)	111 (16.0)		
pT4a	739 (52.6)	430 (60.6)	309 (44.5)		
pT4b	109 (7.8)	62 (8.7)	47 (67.6)		
cN stage [n (%)]				−6.403	<0.001
cN0	550 (39.2)	220 (31.0)	330 (47.5)		
cN1	262 (18.7)	119 (16.8)	143 (20.6)		
cN2	354 (25.2)	246 (34.7)	108 (15.5)		
cN3	238 (17.0)	124 (17.5)	114 (16.4)		
pN stage [n (%)]				−1.155	0.248
pN0	591 (42.1)	263 (37.1)	328 (47.2)		
pN1	227 (16.2)	135 (19.0)	92 (13.2)		
pN2	252 (17.9)	166 (23.4)	86 (12.4)		
pN3a	217 (15.5)	111 (15.7)	106 (15.3)		
pN3b	117 (8.3)	34 (4.8)	83 (11.9)		
No. lesions [n (%)]				0.543	0.461
Single	1,385 (98.6)	701 (98.9)	684 (98.4)		
Multiply	19 (1.4)	8 (1.1)	11 (1.6)		
Approach [n (%)]				223.282	<0.001
Open	428 (30.5)	345 (48.7)	83 (11.9)		
Laparoscopy	976 (69.5)	364 (51.3)	612 (88.1)		
Gastrectomy [n (%)]				11.947	0.001
Distal	952 (67.8)	511 (72.1)	441 (63.5)		
Total	452 (32.2)	198 (27.9)	254 (36.5)		
Combined organ(s) resection [n(%)]				3.888	0.049
Yes	100 (7.1)	60 (8.5)	40 (5.8)		
No	1,304 (92.9)	649 (91.5)	655 (94.2)		
Surgery time [n (%)]				32.894	<0.001
<240 min	1,072 (76.4)	587 (82.8)	485 (69.8)		
≥240 min	332 (23.6)	122 (17.2)	210 (30.2)		
Blood loss [n (%)]				29.945	<0.001
<400 ml	1,268 (90.3)	610 (86.0)	658 (94.7)		
≥400 min	136 (9.7)	99 (14.0)	37 (5.3)		

and distal gastrectomy [511(72.1%) vs. 441(63.5%), $p < 0.001$], with less surgery time [surgery time ≥240 min: 122(17.2%) vs. 210(30.2%), $p < 0.001$] but more blood loss [estimated blood ≥400 ml: 99(14.0%) vs. 37(5.3%), $p < 0.001$]. There were no significant differences between the pathologist group and the surgicopathologist group in terms of tumor size, number of primary lesions, or comorbidity of diabetes.

Effect of the LN Examination Approach on the Number of RLNs and MLNs and the Detection of N3b Status

As shown in **Table 2**, the mean number of RLNs in the surgicopathologist group was significantly higher than that in the pathologist group (18.8 ± 11.5 vs. 53.8 ± 20.9, $p < 0.001$) (**Figure 2**); the same trend was observed in the mean number of MLNs between two groups (3.9 ± 5.7 vs. 5.6 ± 9.8, $p < 0.001$) (**Figure 3**). More importantly, the detection of N3b node status was significantly improved in the surgicopathologist group [34(4.8%) vs. 83(11.9%), $p < 0.001$] (**Figure 4**).

Effect of the Number of RLNs on MLNs and the Detection of N3b Status

The relationship between the number of MLNs and the number of RLNs and the association between the detection of N3b nodes and the number of RLNs are shown in **Table 3**. With the increase in RLNs, the number of MLNs also increased [1–16 RLNs vs. 17–32 RLNs vs. 33–48 RLNs vs. >49 RLNs: 2.3 ± 3.0 vs. 4.3 ± 6.1 vs. 4.6 ± 7.0 vs. 7.3 ± 11.7, $p < 0.001$] (**Figure 5**). In addition, the detection of N3b nodes was also dependent on the number of RLNs [1–16 RLNs vs. 17–32 RLNs vs. 33–48 RLNs vs. >49 RLNs: 0 vs. 25(6.9%) vs. 24(8.7%) vs. 68(13.9%), $p < 0.001$].

Factors Influencing the Detection of MLNs

As shown in **Table 4**, univariate analyses revealed that the method of LN examination, pT, tumor size, and combined organ resection were related to the number of detected MLNs. Furthermore, multivariate analyses indicated that LN examination by the specialized surgicopathologic team, more advanced pT, tumor size ≥5 cm, and combined organ(s) resection were associated with detecting a greater number of MLNs.

DISCUSSION

At most GC centers, LNs are retrieved by pathologists, especially in Western countries and in China. However, pathologists usually describe only the positive and total numbers of greater and lesser curvature LNs. By comparing the significant disparity in nodal yields between surgeons and pathologists, Bunt et al. proposed that the retrieval of LNs should be performed immediately postoperatively by surgeons (9). In their opinion, the following factors may contribute to the essential higher nodal yielding obtained by surgicopathologic teams compared with pathologists: (1) better knowledge of the locations of LNs; (2) more experienced with and dedication to the mission of retrieving more LNs (19, 20); and (3) immediate postoperative

TABLE 2 | The number of retrieved lymph nodes and metastatic lymph nodes and the dectecting of N3b status in the two groups.

Variables	Total (n = 1,404)	Pathologist group (n = 709)	Surgicopathologist group (n = 695)	Statistic	*p-value*
RLNs*, mean ± SD		18.8 ± 11.5	53.8 ± 20.9	−38.788	<0.001
MLNs#, mean ± SD		3.9 ± 5.7	5.6 ± 9.8	−3.917	<0.001
N3b status [n (%)]				−4.843	<0.001
N3b	117 (8.3)	34 (4.8)	83 (11.9)		
Non-N3b	1,287 (91.7)	675 (95.2)	612 (88.1)		

**RLNs, retrieved lymph nodes. #MLNs, metastatic lymph nodes.*

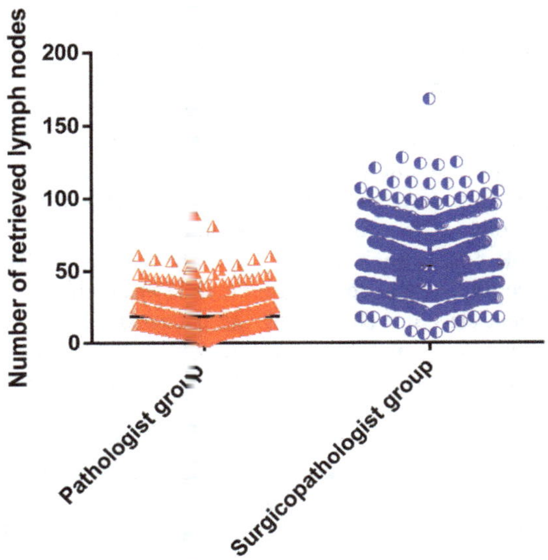

FIGURE 2 | The number of retrieved lymph nodes between the pathologist group and surgicopathologist group.

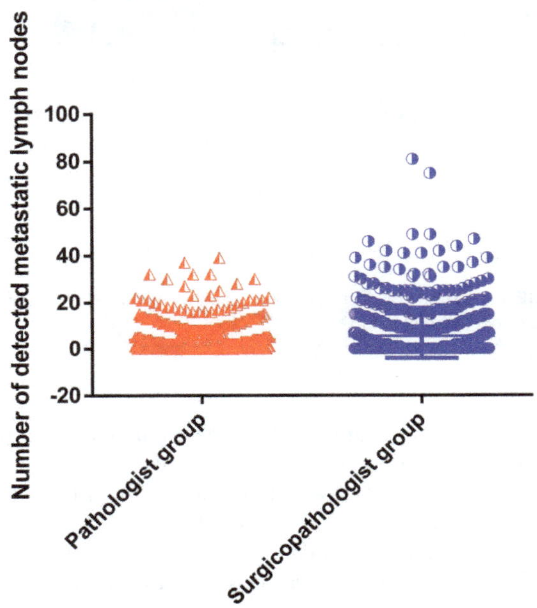

FIGURE 3 | The number of detected metastatic lymph nodes between the pathologist group and surgicopathologist group.

processing of the fresh specimen without being fixed by formalin, which facilitates the detection of LNs due to the differences in consistency from fatty tissue. LN retrieval from the operation specimen not by pathologists but by the surgicopathologic team (who have been trained with anatomical and surgical learning programs) can obtain a better three-dimensional view of the anatomical relationships. Furthermore, previous studies have demonstrated that despite some anatomical variability in the distribution of LNs, LN retrieval by the surgicopathologic team, rather than by the pathologists, could lead to more RLNs, which is helpful for standardizing the nodal status assessment (9, 21). Consistently, in our trial, the number of RLNs in the surgicopathologist group was significantly higher than that in the pathologist group (18.8 ± 11.5 vs. 53.8 ± 20.9, $p < 0.001$); the surgicopathologist group also detected a greater number of MLNs (3.9 ± 5.7 vs. 5.6 ± 9.8, $p < 0.001$). More importantly, our trial evaluated the impact of the LN examination approach and the number of RLNs on the N stage assessment, especially the N3b stage, which has not yet been investigated in other similar studies. In our study, patients in the pathologist group had more advanced cT and subsequent pT. Nevertheless, although the cN status was more advanced in the pathologist group, the pN status was not significantly different between the two groups. These results contradict the fact that the more advanced the depth of tumor invasion is, the more advanced the LN status becomes in GC (22–25). Since our trial excluded patients with preoperative chemotherapy or D1/D1+ gastrectomy, we speculated that the inconsistency between cN and pN could be attributed to the methods of LN examination. Additionally, the detection of N3b node status was significantly improved in the surgicopathologist group [34(4.8%) vs. 83(11.9%), $p < 0.001$]. Notably, the N3b status was first put forward by the 7th AJCC TNM staging system in 2014, and the 8th AJCC edition incorporated it into the TNM stage for the first time. The International Gastric Cancer Association (IGCA) Project study, which analyzed the clinical and pathological data of 25,441 patients from 15 countries and 53 institutions who underwent curative gastrectomy, demonstrated that the N3a,

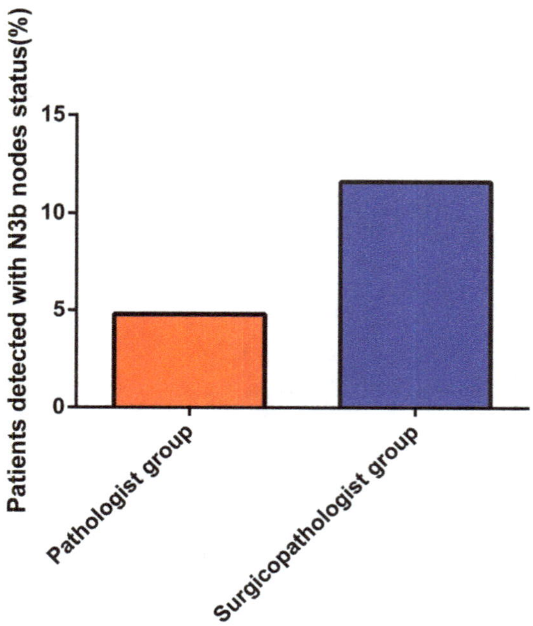

FIGURE 4 | The rate of detecting N3b status between the pathologist group and surgicopathologist group.

and N3b subgroups significantly differed in terms of the 5-year survival rate (10). On the basis of this analysis, the 8th edition AJCC attached great importance to the impact of N3b on the TNM stage. Even in early GC, the N3b node status (T1N3b) could classify patients as stage IIIB, while the T1N0, T1N1, T1N2, and T1N3a were classified as only stage IA, IB, IIA, and IIB, respectively. It showed that N3b node status could have a great impact on disease stage. Thus, the N3b subgroup should be particularly evaluated. A study based on a Chinese cohort also confirmed this phenomenon (26). In this study, N3b patients, regardless of the depth of tumor invasion, exhibited late-stage disease. Sun et al. even classified T4N3b as stage IV (27). Some fundamental research has supported the phenomenon of LN metastasis extension in clinical practice. Recently, a study conducted by Massachusetts General Hospital (MGH) showed that cancer cells from metastatic LNs can escape into the circulation and become the main source of cancer cells for distant metastasis in mouse models (28). The same conclusion was independently obtained at Medical University of Vienna using different methodologies at almost the same time (29). These findings are helpful in providing clues to the clinical significance of N3b and provide implications for facilitating a decision regarding the subsequent use of radiotherapy and chemotherapy treatment and predicting prognosis. Since all N3b patients are classified as stage IIIA or IIIB according to the 8th edition AJCC, the detection of N3b could be used to identify more high-risk stage III GC patients, which is important regarding adjuvant treatment. The positive result of the phase III trial the Adjuvant Chemotherapy Trial of S-1 for Gastric Cancer (ACTS-GC) laid the foundation of ACT for patients with stage II and III GC who had undergone D2 surgery with the regimen of a postoperative S-1 single-agent for 12 months (30). However, subgroup analysis found that the 5-year OS rate of stage IIIB GC patients was 50.2% in the group receiving S-1 after surgery and 44.1% in the group receiving surgery only (HR, 0.791; 95% CI, 0.520–1.205), indicating that there is still some room for improvement. Recently, the Japan Clinical Cancer Research Organization (JACCRO) further conducted the JACCRO GC-07 trial, showing that S-1 plus docetaxel for 6 months and followed by S-1 alone for 6 months is a better choice for stage III GC patients (31, 32). In Western patients, postoperative chemoradiotherapy should be a considered addition for these patients (33). Therefore, the improvement of detecting N3b, which could detect more stage IIIB or IIIC patients, could also make the adjuvant treatment strategy more reasonable and has great clinical significance for appraising prognosis. Overall, the upstaging caused by the N status implies a change in patient treatment (with the indication of adjuvant therapy) and adds greater clinical significance to the present study.

Importantly, surgeons can not only could retrieve more LNs but also divide LNs into stations and count sectioned LNs as a single LN at each station. The status of MLNs at each station could be vital for further investigating the regulation of LN metastasis and elucidating the metastasis model of LNs, both of which are also very important for assessing biological characteristics and making suitable treatment strategies in subsequent research. At the same time, the count of RLNs at each station could also improve quality control in the surgical treatment of GC and promote the implementation of standard D2 radical LN dissection for GC (34).

In our analysis, LN examination by the specialized surgicopathologic team, more advanced pT, tumor size ≥5 cm and combined organ resection were associated with more MLNs. Clearly, T staging, tumor size, and combined organ(s) resection represent the biological characteristics of GC that are related to LN metastasis; this has been widely proven (23, 35–37). The method of LN examination is not associated with the biological characteristics but was still related to the number of MLNs detected, which was mainly due to their impact on the number of RLNs. Given our results, the retrieval of LNs by surgeons immediately after an operation should be the preferred technique over the conventional method by pathologists.

Also, the conventional LN examination by inspection, palpation, and/or serial sectioning is prone to missing very small LNs, and small LNs can also possibly metastasize (38). Noda et al. reported that ignoring small LNs can be a major cause of staging error in GC (38). In his investigation, the mean size of metastatic LNs was 7.80 mm for a total of 23233 LNs. If all LNs with a size of 5 mm or less are ignored when fixed, then 37.8% of all MLNs would have been missed, and downstaging would occur in 14.9 and 4.2% of the cases if all LNs <6 and 4 mm, respectively, were ignored. Therefore, they proposed that all LNs 4 mm or more in size (5 mm when fresh) should be retrieved and examined. Thus, adjuvant technologies are expected to further improve the efficiency of LN examination by harvesting more LNs and

TABLE 3 | The number of metastatic lymph node and the dectecting of N3b status in the four groups with different retrieved lymph node.

RLNs*	1–16 LNs ($n = 355$)	17–32 LNs ($n = 364$)	33–48 LNs ($n = 276$)	≥49 LNs ($n = 409$)	Statistic	*p-value*
MLNs#, mean ± SD	2.3 ± 3.0	4.3 ± 6.1	4.6 ± 7.0	7.3 ± 11.7	26.414	<0.001
N3b stage [*n* (%)]					70.162	<0.001
N3b	0 (0)	25 (6.9)	24 (8.7)	68 (16.6)		
Non-N3b	355 (100)	339 (93.1)	252 (91.3)	341 (69.6)		

**RLNs, retrieved lymph nodes.* #*MLNs, metastatic lymph nodes.*

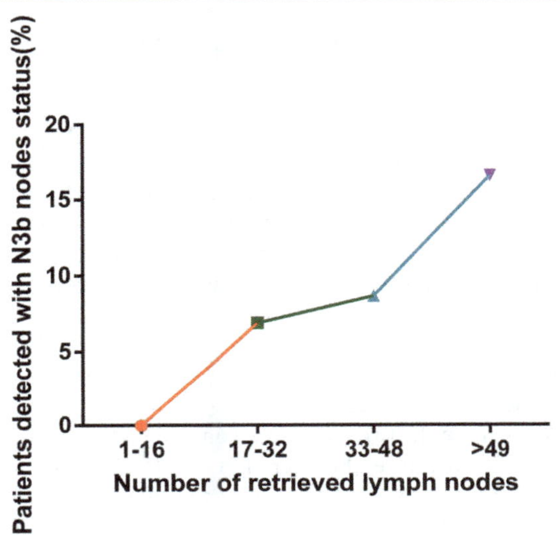

FIGURE 5 | Relationship between the number of retrieved lymph nodes and the rate of the detection of N3b status.

detecting smaller LNs on the basis of the conventional LN examination. This method includes LN-revealing solutions and lymphatic tracers.

To detect very small LNs, Koren et al. used LN-revealing solutions to prevent small LNs from being obscured by the surrounding adipose tissue (39). This method yielded LNs significantly smaller than the traditional method (mean size: 3.03 ± 3.43 vs. 6.69 ± 3.43 mm). However, this method required that the entire perigastric fat was carefully detached from the stomach and immersed for 6–12 h in ~3 times its volume of LN-revealing solution, which is a mixture composed of 65 mL of 95% ethanol, 20 mL of diethyl ether, 5 mL of glacial acetic acid and 10 mL of buffered formalin. Subsequently, the fat was washed thoroughly under running tap water and sectioned again at intervals of 2–3 mm. Thus, although this method could significantly increase the number of RLNs and decrease the size of the nodes, its operational program is tedious and time consuming, which makes it difficult to generalize in clinical practice. Subsequently, Carnoy's solution (CS) has been used as a new fat-clearing solution in LN-revealing solutions; however, it also had similar methodological limitations (40). Over decades, lymphatic tracers, including methylene blue, indocyanine green, and the intraoperative radiation technique with a gamma probe, have also been used as guidance for LN searching and dissection (41, 42). However, no ideal materials have been found due to the limitation of their staining efficiency, the relatively complicated lymphatic flow of the gastric system, radiation injury, and expense. Carbon nanoparticles (CN) are one of the most commonly used nanoparticles to trace LNs in some tumors because they are inexpensive and widely available (43–45). Recently, LN labeling with CN was applied to GC and can improve the number of RLNs and the detection of MLNs (46). To evaluate the application value of LN tracing with CN by preoperative endoscopic subserosal injection in laparoscopic radical gastrectomy, Hong et al. randomly assigned patients to a trial group and control group. The results showed that the mean number of RLNs in the trial group was significantly higher than that in the control group (35.5 ± 8.5 vs. 29.5 ± 6.5, $p < 0.05$). Regarding the LNs with and without black dye in the trial group, the rate of MLNs was significantly higher than that in LNs with black dye (17.3 vs. 4.0%, $p < 0.01$) (46). In our center, we use the method of preoperative submucosal injection of CN followed by a conventional LN examination approach in rectal cancer after neoadjuvant chemoradiotherapy. Similarly, a more precise oncologic prognostic assessment is provided by increasing the number of RLNs (21.1 vs. 8.0, $p < 0.001$) using the dye-tracing method. Furthermore, in the CN group, the mean time for LN retrieval was shorter than that in the control group (27.6 vs. 34.6 min, $p < 0.001$) (45). Li et al. conducted a prospective randomized trial to evaluate the efficiency and safety of CN for retrieving LNs in advanced GC (47). In the experimental group, 1.0 mL of CN was injected into the subserosa of the stomach at five points around the tumor about 10 min before open gastrectomy with D2 dissection. The same procedure was performed directly without any coloring material in the control arm. In line with previous studies, the mean number of RLNs was higher in the experimental group than that in the control group (38.33 vs. 28.27, $p = 0.041$). A smaller diameter of LNs was observed in the experimental arm (3.32 vs. 4.30 mm, $p = 0.023$). However, subgroup analysis showed that no additional MLNs were harvested in the experimental group. Nevertheless, the CN approach also has many potential weaknesses that limit its use, regardless of whether 0.5 mL of CN suspension is injected into the submucosal layer using a rectal speculum at 3 points around the primary tumor 1 day before surgery or whether it is injected into the subserosa of the stomach at five points around the

TABLE 4 | Univariate and multivariate analyses of factors influencing the detecting of metastatic lymph node in this cohort.

Variables	MLNs# (x ± s)	Univariate analyses		Multivariate analyses	
		Mean square	*p*	Mean square	*p*
Approach of LN examination		989.3	<0.001	848.7	<0.001
By pathologists	3.9 ± 5.7				
By surgicopathologists	5.6 ± 9.8				
Gender		90.1	0.237	0.6	0.919
Male	4.9 ± 8.5				
Female	4.4 ± 7.1				
Age		10.2	0.691	28.2	0.479
<65 years	4.7 ± 8.1				
≥65 years	4.9 ± 7.7				
Body mass index		5.0	0.782	7.9	0.707
<28 kg/m^2	4.7 ± 8.0				
≥28 kg/m^2	7.7 ± 1.3				
Diabetes		30.2	0.494	48.6	0.352
Yes	5.4 ± 8.7				
No	4.7 ± 8.0				
pT stage		1772.4	<0.001	1191.7	<0.001
pT1a	0.1 ± 0.7				
pT1b	1.2 ± 3.7				
pT2	2.0 ± 3.6				
pT3	5.3 ± 10.6				
pT4a	6.3 ± 8.6				
pT4b	8.2 ± 9.3				
No. of lesion		58.9	0.339	26.4	0.493
Single	4.8 ± 8.0				
Multiply	3.0 ± 9.6				
Tumor size [*n* (%)]		4484.7	<0.001	1472.4	<0.001
<5 cm	3.5 ± 7.1				
≥5 cm	7.3 ± 9.2				
Approach [*n* (%)]		676.7	<0.001	90.5	0.204
Open	3.7 ± 5.6				
Laparoscopy	5.2 ± 8.9				
Gastrectomy [*n* (%)]		2121.3	<0.001	61.8	0.294
Total	6.5 ± 9.1				
Distal	3.9 ± 7.3				
Combined organ(s) resection [*n* (%)]		1.1	0.897	242.3	0.038
No	4.7 ± 8.1				
Yes	4.9 ± 7.0				
Surgery time		983.2	<0.001	141.2	0.113
<240 min	4.3 ± 7.3				
≥240 min	6.3 ± 9.9				
Blood loss		0.212	0.954	3.690	0.798
<400 ml	4.8 ± 8.1				
≥400 ml	4.8 ± 7.1				

#MLNs, metastatic lymph nodes.

tumor about 10 min before surgery, both require highly technical operation, have a steep learning curve, and increase the workload for surgeons. Particularly, the injection of the CN suspension into the submucosal layer around the primary tumor is a highly technical operation, and has the risk of colliding the tumor. Furthermore, the diffusion of CN may affect the judgment of the location of the tumor and the extent of resection during surgery.

Therefore, adjuvant technology has not been widely used in the clinic as the main approach because of its inherent weaknesses. However, adjuvant technology has the potential to help detect more LNs with high efficacy, especially for small LNs, on the basis of routine LN examination relying on the operator's vision and tactile sense to detect LNs. Hence, the interdisciplinary cooperation of clinicians, basic medical researchers and chemical material researchers is expected to facilitate the development of a more accurate and effective new tracer or LN-revealing solutions.

There are also apparent limitations in our study. Although the data in our study were prospectively collected (48), our study was not prospectively designed but retrospectively analyzed. Of course, we tried our best to compensate for this limitation. For example, only standard curative D2 distal/total gastrectomy was considered, and patients with previous gastrectomy (gastric stump cancer) were excluded, as were those who underwent neoadjuvant therapy to control for other surgically-related variables. In addition, as a result of the non-prospective design, the duration of the dissection of each case was not recorded, so the assessment of the two approaches on the prospect of time was not possible. Therefore, the operation duration of each method should be taken into consideration in the design of subsequent RCTs. In addition, the size of the RLNs and MLNs in each group was not registered in our database, so we could not investigate whether the method by the specialized surgicopathologic team could retrieve smaller LNs and detect small MLNs than that by pathologists. Since ignoring small LNs can be a major cause of staging error in GC (38), the size of the RLNs and MLNs should also be recorded and analyzed in the subsequent RCTs.

CONCLUSIONS

The retrieval of LNs immediately postoperatively by the surgicopathologic team in our center could significantly improve the number of RLNs, detect more MLNs, and screen more patients with N3b node status for GC. This method could reduce stage migration and therefore has a significant impact on prognostic evaluation and the formulation of adjuvant therapy strategies.

ETHICS STATEMENT

The data collection protocol was approved by the Ethics Committee of Nanfang Hospital, Southern Medical University. Written informed consent was obtained from all the patients in the study.

AUTHOR CONTRIBUTIONS

JY, GL, and HL made substantial contributions to the conception and design, and interpretation of data. XC, YC, YH, TiaL, and JL contributed in drafting the manuscript or critically revising it for important intellectual content. XC, TuaL, TaoL, HH, YZ, TinL, and HC collected and analyzed the data. All the authors approved the final manuscript submitted. Each author participated sufficiently in the work to take public responsibility for appropriate portions of the content and agreed to be accountable for all aspects of the work in ensuring that questions related to the accuracy or integrity of any part of the work are appropriately investigated and resolved.

ACKNOWLEDGMENTS

We thank the AMERICAN JOURNAL EXPERTS(AJE) for editing a draft of this manuscript.

REFERENCES

1. Smith DD, Schwarz RR, Schwarz RE. Impact of total lymph node count on staging and survival after gastrectomy for gastric cancer: data from a large US-population database. *J Clin Oncol.* (2005) 23:7114–24. doi: 10.1200/JCO.2005.14.621
2. Hayashi S, Kanda M, Ito S, Mochizuki Y, Teramoto H, Ishigure K, et al. Number of retrieved lymph nodes is an independent prognostic factor after total gastrectomy for patients with stage III gastric cancer: propensity score matching analysis of a multi-institution dataset. *Gastric Cancer.* (2019) 22:853–63. doi: 10.1007/s10120-018-0902-2
3. Woo Y, Goldner B, Ituarte P, Lee B, Melstrom L, Son T, et al. Lymphadenectomy with optimum of 29 lymph nodes retrieved associated with improved survival in advanced gastric cancer: A 25,000-patient international database study. *J Am Coll Surg.* (2017) 224:546–55. doi: 10.1016/j.jamcollsurg.2016.12.015
4. Noguchi Y, Imada T, Matsumoto A, Coit DG, Brennan MF. Radical surgery for gastric cancer. A review of the Japanese experience. *Cancer.* (1989) 64:2053–62. doi: 10.1002/1097-0142(19891115)64:10<2053::AID-CNCR2820641014>3.0.CO;2-J
5. Axelsson CK, Mouridsen HT, Zedeler K. Axillary dissection of level I and II lymph nodes is important in breast cancer classification. The Danish Breast Cancer Cooperative Group (DBCG). *Eur J Cancer.* (1992) 28A:1415–8. doi: 10.1016/0959-8049(92)90534-9
6. Feinstein AR, Sosin DM, Wells CK. The Will Rogers phenomenon. Stage migration and new diagnostic techniques as a source of misleading statistics for survival in cancer. *N Engl J Med.* (1985) 312:1604–8. doi: 10.1056/NEJM198506203122504
7. Bunt AM, Hermans J, Smit VT, van de Velde CJ, Fleuren GJ, Bruijn JA, et al. Surgical/pathologic-stage migration confounds comparisons of gastric cancer survival rates between Japan and Western countries. *J Clin Oncol.* (1995) 13:19–25. doi: 10.1200/JCO.1995.13.1.19
8. Jessup JM. Is bigger better? *J Clin Oncol.* (1995)13:5–7. doi: 10.1200/JCO.1995.13.1.5
9. Bunt AM, Hermans J, van de Velde CJ, Sasako M, Hoefsloot FA, Fleuren G, et al. Lymph node retrieval in a randomized trial on western-type versus Japanese-type surgery in gastric cancer. *J Clin Oncol.* (1996) 14:2289–94. doi: 10.1200/JCO.1996.14.8.2289
10. Sano T, Coit DG, Kim HH, Roviello F, Kassab P, Wittekind C, et al. Proposal of a new stage grouping of gastric cancer for TNM classification: international Gastric Cancer Association staging project. *Gastric Cancer.* (2017) 20:217–25. doi: 10.1007/s10120-016-0601-9
11. Bunt AM, Hermans J, Boon MC, van de Velde CJ, Sasako M, Fleuren GJ, et al. Evaluation of the extent of lymphadenectomy in a randomized trial of Western- versus Japanese-type surgery in gastric cancer. *J Clin Oncol.* (1994) 12:417–22. doi: 10.1200/JCO.1994.12.2.417
12. Bunt TM, Bonenkamp HJ, Hermans J, van de Velde CJ, Arends JW, Fleuren G, et al. Factors influencing noncompliance and contamination in a randomized trial of "Western" (r1) versus "Japanese" (r2) type surgery in gastric cancer. *Cancer.* (1994) 73:1544–51. doi: 10.1002/1097-0142(19940315)73:6<1544::AID-CNCR2820730604>3.0.CO;2-4
13. Washington K. 7th edition of the AJCC cancer staging manual: stomach. *Ann Surg Oncol.* (2010) 17:3077–9. doi: 10.1245/s10434-010-1362-z
14. Ajani JA, D'Amico TA, Almhanna K, Bentrem DJ, Chao J, Das P, et al. Gastric cancer, Version 3.2016, NCCN clinical practice guidelines in oncology. *J Natl Compr Canc Netw.* (2016) 14:1286–312. doi: 10.6004/jnccn.2016.0137
15. Japanese Gastric Cancer Association. Japanese gastric cancer treatment guidelines 2014 (ver. 4). *Gastric Cancer.* (2017) 20:1–19. doi: 10.1007/s10120-016-0622-4
16. Smyth EC, Verheij M, Allum W, Cunningham D, Cervantes A, Arnold D. Gastric cancer: ESMO clinical practice guidelines for diagnosis, treatment and follow-up. *Ann Oncol.* (2016) 27:v38–v49. doi: 10.1093/annonc/mdw350
17. Worhunsky DJ, Ma Y, Zak Y, Poultsides GA, Norton JA, Rhoads KF, et al. Compliance with gastric cancer guidelines is associated with improved outcomes. *J Natl Compr Canc Netw.* (2015) 13:319–25. doi: 10.6004/jnccn.2015.0044
18. Zhu Y, Chen XH, Li TT, Hu YF, Li TJ, Lin T, et al. Method and experience of lymph node examination after gastrectomy with D2 lymphadenectomy for gastric cancer. *Chin J Gastrointest Surg.* (2019) 22:796–800. doi: 10.3760/cma.j.issn.1671-0274.2019.08.018
19. Kajitani T. The general rules for the gastric cancer study in surgery and pathology. Part I. Clinical classification. *Jpn J Surg.* (1981) 11:127–39. doi: 10.1007/BF02468883
20. The general rules for the gastric cancer study in surgery ad pathology. Part II. Histological classification of gastric cancer. *Jpn J Surg.* (1981) 11:140–5. doi: 10.1007/BF02468884
21. Jiang L, Yao Z, Zhang Y, Hu J, Zhao D, Zhai H, et al. Comparison of lymph node number and prognosis in gastric cancer patients with perigastric lymph nodes retrieved by surgeons and pathologists. *Chin J Cancer Res.* (2016) 28:511–8. doi: 10.21147/j.issn.1000-9604.2016.05.06
22. Ikoma N, Blum M, Chiang YJ, Estrella JS, Roy-Chowdhuri S, Fournier K, et al. Race is a risk for lymph node metastasis in patients with gastric cancer. *Ann Surg Oncol.* (2017) 24:960–5. doi: 10.1245/s10434-016-5645-x
23. Ren G, Cai R, Zhang WJ, Ou JM, Jin YN, Li WH. Prediction of risk factors for lymph node metastasis in early gastric cancer. *World J Gastroenterol.* (2013) 19:3096–107. doi: 10.3748/wjg.v19.i20.3096
24. Liang J, Liang H, Deng J, Wang X, Wang X, Wu L. Clinical study on lymph node metastasis regularity in 1456 patients with gastric cancer. *Zhonghua Wei Chang Wai Ke Za Zhi.* (2018) 21:1154–60. doi: 10.3760/cma.j.issn.1671-0274.2018.10.014
25. Chen D, Chen G, Jiang W, Fu M, Liu W, Sui J, et al. Association of the collagen signature in the tumor microenvironment with lymph node metastasis in early gastric cancer. *JAMA Surg.* (2019) 153:e185249. doi: 10.1001/jamasurg.2018.5249
26. Zhang Z, Huang JY, Wang PL, Hou WB, Yin SC, Xu HM. Should all stage N3b patients with advanced gastric cancer be considered equivalent? A 30-year single center study. *J Gastrointest Surg.* (2018) 23:1742–7. doi: 10.1007/s11605-018-3945-0
27. Sun Z, Wang ZN, Zhu Z, Xu YY, Xu Y, Huang BJ, et al. Evaluation of the seventh edition of American Joint Committee on Cancer TNM staging system for gastric cancer: results from a Chinese monoinstitutional study. *Ann Surg Oncol.* (2012) 19:1918–27. doi: 10.1245/s10434-011-2206-1
28. Pereira ER, Kedrin D, Seano G, Gautier O, Meijer E, Jones D, et al. Lymph node metastases can invade local blood vessels, exit the node, and colonize distant organs in mice. *Science.* (2018) 359:1403–7. doi: 10.1126/science.aal3622

29. Brown M, Assen FP, Leithner A, Abe J, Schachner H, Asfour G, et al. Lymph node blood vessels provide exit routes for metastatic tumor cell dissemination in mice. *Science.* (2018) 359:1408–11. doi: 10.1126/science.aa l3662
30. Sasako M, Sakuramoto S, Katai H, Kinoshita T, Furukawa H, Yamaguchi T, et al. Five-year outcomes of a randomized phase III trial comparing adjuvant chemotherapy with S-1 versus surgery alone in stage II or III gastric cancer. *J Clin Oncol.* (2011) 29:4387–93. doi: 10.1200/JCO.2011.36. 5908
31. Yoshida K, Kodera Y, Kochi M, Ichikawa W, Kakeji Y, Sano T, et al. Addition of docetaxel to oral fluoropyrimidine improves efficacy in patients with stage III gastric cancer: interim analysis of JACCRO GC-07, a randomized controlled trial. *J Clin Oncol.* (2019) 37:1296. doi: 10.1200/JCO.18.01138
32. Kodera Y, Yoshida K, Kochi M, Ichikawa W, Kakeji Y, Sano T. A randomized phase III study comparing S-1 plus docetaxel with S-1 alone as a postoperative adjuvant chemotherapy for curatively resected stage III gastric cancer (JACCRO GC-07 trial). *J Clin Oncol.* (2018) 36S.
33. Macdonald JS, Smalley SR, Benedetti J, Hundahl SA, Estes NC, Stemmermann GN, et al. Chemoradiotherapy after surgery compared with surgery alone for adenocarcinoma of the stomach or gastroesophageal junction. *N Engl J Med.* (2001) 345:725–30. doi: 10.1056/NEJMoa010187
34. Sasako M. Risk factors for surgical treatment in the Dutch Gastric Cancer Trial. *Br J Surg.* (1997) 84:1567–71. doi: 10.1111/j.1365-2168.1997.02842.x
35. Wang YW, Zhu ML, Wang RF, Xue WJ, Zhu XR, Wang LF, et al. Predictable factors for lymph node metastasis in early gastric cancer analysis of clinicopathologic factors and biological markers. *Tumour Biol.* (2016) 37:8567–78. doi: 10.1007/s13277-015-4721-3
36. Yu JW, Wu JG, Tajima Y, Li XQ, Du GY, Zheng LH, et al. Study on lymph node metastasis correlated to lymphangiogenesis, lymphatic vessel invasion, and lymph node micrometastasis in gastric cancer. *J Surg Res.* (2011) 168:188–96. doi: 10.1016/j.jss.2009.10.030
37. Huang CM, Xu M, Wang JB, Zheng CH, Li P, Xie JW, et al. Is tumor size a predictor of preoperative N staging in T2-T4a stage advanced gastric cancer? *Surg Oncol.* (2014) 23:5–10. doi: 10.1016/j.suronc.2014.01.003
38. Noda N, Sasako M, Yamaguchi N, Nakanishi Y. Ignoring small lymph nodes can be a major cause of staging error in gastric cancer. *Br J Surg.* (1998) 85:831–4. doi: 10.1046/j.1365-2168.1998.00691.x
39. Koren R, Kyzer S, Levin I, Klein B, Halpern M, Rath-Wolfson L, et al. Lymph node revealing solution: a new method for lymph node sampling: results in gastric adenocarcinoma. *Oncol Rep.* (1998) 5:341–4. doi: 10.3892/or. 5.2.341
40. Dias AR, Pereira MA, Mello ES, Zilberstein B, Cecconello I, Ribeiro JU. Carnoy's solution increases the number of examined lymph nodes following gastrectomy for adenocarcinoma: a randomized trial. *Gastric Cancer.* (2016) 19:136–42. doi: 10.1007/s10120-014-0443-2
41. Kitagawa Y, Fujii H, Mukai M, Kubota T, Ando N, Watanabe M, et al. The role of the sentinel lymph node in gastrointestinal cancer. *Surg Clin North Am.* (2000) 80:1799–809. doi: 10.1016/S0039-6109(05)70262-0
42. Wang B, Qiu NC, Zhang W, Shan CX, Jiang ZG, Liu S, et al. Sentinel node mapping for gastric cancer: a prospective multicenter trial in Japan. *J Clin Oncol.* (2013) 31:3704–10. doi: 10.1200/JCO.2013.50.3789
43. Wang Y, Deng H, Chen H, Liu H, Xue Q, Yan J, et al. The role of carbon nanoparticles in identifying lymph nodes and preserving parathyroid in total endoscopic surgery of thyroid carcinoma. *Surg Endosc.* (2015) 29:2914–20. doi: 10.1007/s00464-014-4020-x
44. Wang Y, Deng H, Chen H, Liu H, Xue Q, Yan J, et al. Preoperative submucosal injection of carbon nanoparticles improves lymph node staging accuracy in rectal cancer after neoadjuvant chemoradiotherapy. *J Am Coll Surg.* (2015) 221:923–30. doi: 10.1016/j.jamcollsurg.2015.07.455
45. Yan J, Zheng X, Liu Z, Yu J, Deng Z, Xue F, et al. A multicenter study of using carbon nanoparticles to show sentinel lymph nodes in early gastric cancer. *Surg Endosc.* (2016) 30:1294–300. doi: 10.1007/s00464-015-4358-8
46. Hong Q, Wang Y, Wang JJ, Hu CG, Fang YJ, Fan XX, et al. Application of lymph node labeling with carbon nanoparticles by preoperative endoscopic subserosal injection in laparoscopic radical gastrectomy. *Zhonghua Yi Xue Za Zhi.* (2017) 97:123–6. doi: 10.3760/cma.j.issn.0376-2491.2017. 02.009
47. Li Z, Ao S, Bu Z, Wu A, Wu X, Shan F, et al. Clinical study of harvesting lymph nodes with carbon nanoparticles in advanced gastric cancer: a prospective randomized trial. *World J Surg Oncol.* (2016) 14:88. doi: 10.1186/s12957-016-0835-3
48. Hu YF, Yu J, Zhang C, Wang YN, Cheng X, Huang F, et al. Development and implementation of a clinical data mining system for gastric cancer surgery. *Zhonghua Wei Chang Wai Ke Za Zhi.* (2010) 13:510–5. doi: 10.3760/cma.j.issn.1671-0274.2010.07.012

20

Multi-Modality Treatment for Patients with Metastatic Gastric Cancer: A Real-World Study in China

Lin Zhao [1†], Jiarui Li [1†], Chunmei Bai [1], Yongdu Nie [1] and Guole Lin [2]*

[1] *Department of Medical Oncology, Peking Union Medical College Hospital, Chinese Academy of Medical Sciences and Peking Union Medical College, Beijing, China,* [2] *Department of General Surgery, Peking Union Medical College Hospital, Chinese Academy of Medical Sciences and Peking Union Medical College, Beijing, China*

***Correspondence:**
Guole Lin
linguole@126.com

† These authors have contributed equally to this work

Introduction: People with metastatic gastric cancer (GC) have a poor prognosis. The study aims to investigate the efficacy of multi-modality treatment for patients with metastatic GC.

Methods: We retrospectively identified 267 patients with stage IV gastric cancer who were treated with systemic chemotherapy: 114 received multi-modality treatments, 153 received systematic chemotherapy alone. The survival of these two groups was compared by log rank test, the independent prognostic factors were investigated using univariate and multivariate analyses.

Results: The median survival of metastatic GC patients who received multi-modality treatment was significantly longer than those who received systematic chemotherapy alone (18.4 vs. 11.4 months, $P < 0.001$). Multivariate analysis identified tumor histologic differentiation, CA19–9 level, previous curative resection, palliative gastrectomy, and metastasectomy as independent prognostic factors for overall survival. In the multimodality treatment group, patients who received palliative gastrectomy or metastasectomy had a longer survival than those who only received intraperitoneal chemotherapy or radiotherapy (21.6 vs. 15.2 months, $P = 0.014$).

Conclusion: Multi-modality treatments offer a survival benefit for patients with metastatic GC. Future prospective studies are needed to confirm the result.

Keywords: gastric cancer, multi-modality treatment, chemotherapy, gastrectomy, metastasectomy

INTRODUCTION

Gastric cancer (GC) is the fifth most common cancers and the third leading cause of cancer death worldwide (1). Almost one million new cases of GC were diagnosed each year, and about 50% of them occurred in Eastern Asia (mainly in China) (2). Although an improvement of 5-years survival for GC was observed in the past 10 years, the prognosis of Chinese GC patients was still poor. Compared with a very high survival of GC in Korea (68·9%) and Japan (60·3%), the age-standardized 5-years relative survival was only 35.1% in China because most patients have inoperable disease at the time of initial presentation (3–5).

Gastrectomy is the only potentially curative therapy for resectable GC, but a major proportion of patients could have local or distant recurrence even after curative resection (6, 7). People with metastatic GC have a poor prognosis with a median survival time of around 4 months in the absence of systemic chemotherapy (5). For patients with metastatic diseases, it has been demonstrated in multiple trials and meta-analysis that systemic chemotherapy could extend overall survival (OS) by about 7 months more than best supportive care (8). Therefore, systemic chemotherapy is the standard treatment modality for stage IV GC patients. However, systemic chemotherapy still cannot provide significant survival benefits and the disease will progress ultimately. Although some clinical guidelines had recommendations about second- and further-line treatment regimen currently, there is still no global consensus across countries regarding the best therapeutic approach after failure of the first-line therapy (9, 10). The management of patients with metastatic GC is challenging.

Recent years, the number of options available for GC has been increasing rapidly (11). In addition to the development of new anticancer drugs, multi-modality treatments, such as palliative surgery, radiation therapy, intraperitoneal chemotherapy, and other approaches, are gaining support in the management of metastatic gastric cancer (12–18). However, despite these advances, their impact on long-term survival outcome for patients with metastatic GC remains unsatisfactory and the best form of multidisciplinary therapeutic strategy is still not established. In this real-world study, we will focus on the role of multi-modality treatment for patients with metastatic GC.

METHODS

Study Design and Participants

Between December 2011 and November 2018, a total of 267 patients with initial stage IV gastric cancer in Peking Union Medical College Hospital were included consecutively. The eligibility criteria were: (1) histologically confirmed gastric or gastroesophageal junction (GEJ) adenocarcinoma; (2) distant metastases verified by enhanced computed tomography (CT) or other approaches; (3) over 18 years old; (4) ECOG 0-2; (5) received first-line systematic treatment. Patients were divided into two groups according to treatment modality: the multi-modality treatment group comprised 114 patients and the chemotherapy only group comprised 153 patients. The multi-modality treatment group was defined as patients who received both systematic chemotherapy and other modality treatments including palliative gastrectomy and metastasectomy, intraperitoneal chemotherapy, radiotherapy, radiofrequency ablation, and transarterial chemoembolization (TACE). The chemotherapy only group was defined as patients who received systematic chemotherapy alone. This study was approved by the ethics committee of Peking Union Medical College Hospital.

Treatment

The treatment regimens of gastric cancer were mainly based on clinical guidelines of the Chinese Society of Clinical Oncology (CSCO) and the National Comprehensive Cancer Network (NCCN) (12, 19). Several cytotoxic agents are adopted to treat metastatic gastric cancer, including fluoropyrimidines (5-fluorouracil, S-1, capecitabine), platinum agents (cisplatin, oxaliplatin), taxanes (paclitaxel, docetaxel), and irinotecan. For some patients with human epidermal growth factor receptor 2 (HER2)-overexpressing tumors, trastuzumab is combined with cytotoxic chemotherapy. The method used by the hospital to test the HER2 status was immunohistochemistry and fluorescence *in situ* hybridization (FISH). Each patient's chemotherapy plan (including intraperitoneal perfusion) is individualized by senior medical oncologists in the department of medical oncology depending on the tolerance and response to different treatment regimens. All patients in this study received first-line chemotherapy. If patients had disease progression evaluated by medical oncologists and good performance status, they would consider receiving second- or further-line treatment. The palliative gastrectomy or metastasectomy were performed by surgeons from different specialties. Appropriate radiotherapy plan was determined by radiation oncologists based on the patient's general condition, irradiation field, possible normal tissue damage and so on. Radiofrequency ablation and TACE were performed by specialists from the department of radiology.

Assessment and Follow-Up

The following assessment were applied every two to three cycles typically: detailed medical history, physical examination, serum tumor marker analysis, and contrast enhanced CT of the chest, abdomen and pelvis. Additional approaches such as positron emission tomography (PET) and bone scan were undertaken depending on a clinical suspicion of recurrence or metastasis. Radiographic tumor response is quantified by using Response Evaluation Criteria in Solid Tumors (RECIST).

All patients followed up every 3 months, either in a clinical visit or by telephone. At each the out-patient review, physical examination, necessary radiological examinations (enhanced CT or occasional PET-CT), and routine laboratory examinations were performed regularly. The follow-up data were updated until January 31, 2019.

Statistical Analysis

All statistical analyses were performed using SPSS software (version 25, IBM Corp., Armonk, NY, USA). The OS is defined as the interval from the stage IV disease diagnosis to the latest follow-up or death. Continuous variables were assessed by *t*-test, and categorical variables were analyzed with Chi squared test. Related survival curves were constructed according to the Kaplan-Meier method, and a log-rank test was applied to compare these curves. The Cox proportional hazards regression model was adopted to identify the independent prognostic factors for survival, variables ($P < 0.10$) in univariate analysis were entered into multivariate analysis. A $P < 0.05$ was considered significant.

RESULTS

Patient Characteristics

The baseline characteristics of patients at diagnosis of metastatic disease are shown in **Table 1**. The average age of included patients was 56.4 years old, and 67.8% of the participants were male. At the time of stage IV disease diagnosis, the metastatic sites included peritoneum (31.8%), liver (28.1%), Krukenberg tumor (14.2%), lung (6.0%), bone (9.4%), non-regional lymph

TABLE 1 | Baseline characteristics of patients with metastatic gastric cancer.

Characteristic, *n* (%)	Total (*n* = 267)	Multimodality treatment (*n* = 114)	Chemotherapy only (*n* = 153)	*P*-value
Age (years), mean ± SD	56.4 ± 12.5	55.3 ± 11.9	57.1 ± 12.8	0.242
Sex				0.257
Male	181 (67.8)	73 (64.0)	108 (70.6)	
Female	86 (32.2)	41 (36.0)	45 (29.4)	
Differentiation				0.565
Well/median	61 (22.8)	28 (24.6)	33 (21.6)	
Poor	206 (77.2)	86 (75.4)	120 (78.4)	
HER2 status				0.520
Positive	54 (20.2)	26 (22.8)	28 (18.3)	
Negative	98 (36.7)	43 (37.7)	55 (35.9)	
Unknown	115 (43.1)	45 (39.5)	70 (45.8)	
Tumor location				0.496
Upper	79 (29.6)	29 (25.4)	50 (32.7)	
Middle	86 (32.2)	36 (31.6)	50 (32.7)	
Lower	94 (35.2)	45 (39.5)	49 (32.0)	
Diffuse	8 (3.0)	4 (3.5)	4 (2.6)	
CA19-9 level				0.184
Normal	161 (60.3)	74 (64.9)	87 (56.9)	
Elevated	106 (39.7)	40 (35.1)	66 (43.1)	
CEA level				0.062
Normal	144 (53.9)	69 (60.5)	75 (49.0)	
Elevated	123 (46.1)	45 (39.5)	78 (51.0)	
Metastatic site				
Peritoneum	85 (31.8)	43 (37.7)	42 (27.5)	0.075
Liver	75 (28.1)	27 (23.7)	48 (31.4)	0.167
Krukenberg	38 (14.2)	22 (19.3)	16 (10.5)	0.041
Lung	16 (6.0)	7 (6.1)	9 (5.9)	0.930
Bone	25 (9.4)	7 (6.1)	18 (11.8)	0.119
Non-regional lymph nodes	117 (43.8)	45 (39.5)	72 (47.1)	0.217
Other	61 (22.8)	25 (21.9)	36 (23.5)	0.925
Number of metastatic sites				0.529
1	138 (51.7)	63 (55.3)	75 (49.0)	
2	80 (30.0)	33 (28.9)	47 (30.7)	
≥3	49 (18.3)	18 (15.8)	31 (20.3)	
Curative surgery	99 (37.1)	46 (40.4)	53 (34.6)	0.339
Neoadjuvant treatment	23 (23.2)	10 (21.7)	13 (24.5)	0.257
Adjuvant treatment	85 (85.9)	39 (84.8)	46 (86.8)	0.225
Follow-up period (months), median (95%CI)	63.5 (50.4–76.5)	60.4 (48.3–72.5)	63.5 (44.7–82.3)	0.492

nodes (43.8%), and other distant metastases (22.8%). The multimodality treatment group displayed a higher proportion of Krukenberg tumors (19.3% vs. 10.5%, $P = 0.041$) than the chemotherapy only group. Curative surgery was performed in 37.1% of patients before the diagnosis of metastatic disease. Neoadjuvant treatment and adjuvant treatment were given to 23.2 and 85.9% of patients who underwent curative resection separately. The median follow-up periods of multimodality treatment group and chemotherapy only group were 60.4 (95%CI: 50.4–76.5) months and 63.5 (95%CI: 44.7–82.3) months, respectively. There was no statistical difference between the multimodality treatment group and the chemotherapy only group in age, sex, histologic differentiation, HER2 status, tumor location, tumor marker level at diagnosis, number of metastatic sites, previous curative resection, and follow-up period.

Treatment

In the first-line systematic treatment, 4.1% of them received a single drug treatment (fluoropyrimidine, taxane, or irinotecan monotherapy), 78.3% of them received a two-drug combination (fluoropyrimidine, platinum, or taxane), and 7.5% of them received a three-drug combination (**Table 2**). Only 4.9% patients received trastuzumab targeted therapy. Second-line therapy was administered in about half of patients. Among the patients that received second-line chemotherapy, the most frequent regimen type was still two-drug combination

TABLE 2 | Treatment regimens of patients with metastatic gastric cancer.

Characteristic, *n* (%)	Total (*n* = 267)	Multimodality treatment (*n* = 114)	Chemotherapy only (*n* = 153)	*P*-value
First-line treatment	267 (100)	114 (100)	153 (100)	1.000
Single-agent (fluoropyrimidine or taxane)	11 (4.1)	3 (2.6)	8 (5.2)	
Double agent combination (fluoropyrimidine, platinum, or taxane)	209 (78.3)	89 (78.1)	120 (78.4)	
Taxane + platinum + Fluoropyrimidine	20 (7.5)	10 (8.8)	10 (6.5)	0.654
Trastuzumab involved	13 (4.9)	7 (6.1)	6 (3.9)	
Others	14 (5.2)	5 (4.4)	9 (5.9)	
Second-line treatment	139 (52.1)	67 (58.8)	72 (47.1)	0.058
Single agent (fluoropyrimidine, taxane, or irinotecan)	14 (10.1)	5 (7.5)	9 (12.5)	
Double agent combination (fluoropyrimidine, platinum, taxane, or irinotecan)	102 (73.4)	49 (73.1)	53 (73.6)	
Apatinib	12 (8.6)	7 (10.4)	5 (6.9)	0.683
Trastuzumab involved	8 (5.8)	5 (7.5)	3 (4.2)	
Others	3 (2.2)	1 (1.5)	2 (2.8)	
Third-line treatment	69 (25.8)	38 (33.3)	31 (20.3)	0.016
Single agent (fluoropyrimidine, taxane, or irinotecan)	13 (18.8)	5 (13.2)	8 (25.8)	
Double agent combination (fluoropyrimidine, platinum, taxane or irinotecan)	35 (50.7)	22 (57.9)	13 (41.9)	
Apatinib	13 (18.8)	5 (13.2)	8 (25.8)	0.255
Trastuzumab involved	7 (10.1)	5 (13.2)	2 (6.5)	
Others	1 (1.4)	1 (2.6)	0 (0)	
Further-line treatment	24 (9.0)	15 (13.2)	9 (5.9)	0.040

TABLE 3 | Treatment regimens of patients received multimodality treatment.

Treatment regimens, *n* (%)	Multimodality treatment (*n* = 114)
Palliative gastrectomy	35 (30.7)
Metastasectomy	19 (16.7)
Oophorectomy	15 (78.9)
Adrenalectomy	1 (5.3)
Hepatectomy	1 (5.3)
Colectomy	1 (5.3)
Retroperitoneal lymphadenectomy	1 (5.3)
Intraperitoneal chemotherapy	37 (32.5)
Platinum	18 (48.6)
Fluoropyrimidine	15 (40.5)
Taxane	4 (10.8)
Radiotherapy	52 (45.6)
Radiofrequency ablation	6 (5.3)
TACE	6 (5.3)
Others	2 (1.8)

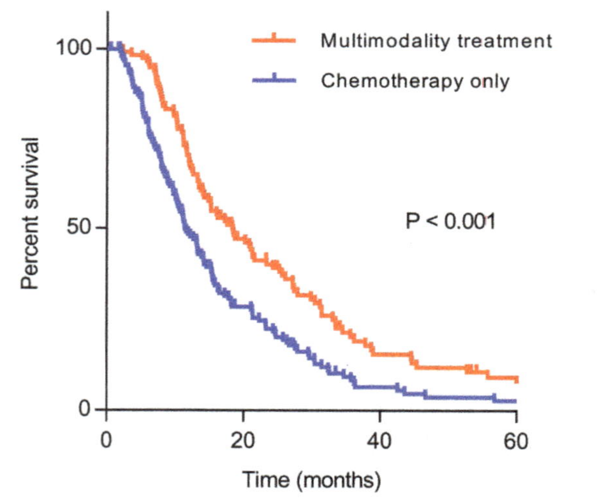

FIGURE 1 | Kaplan–Meier curve of overall survival in multimodality treatment group and chemotherapy only group.

(**Table 2**). Irinotecan or apatinib were prescribed in single agent or double agent combination regimen in second- or further-line treatment. The multimodality treatment group had a higher proportion of receiving third- (33.3 vs. 20.3%, $P = 0.016$) and further-line (13.2 vs. 5.9%, $P = 0.040$) systematic treatment than chemotherapy alone group. There was no statistical difference between these two groups in the chemotherapy regimen.

Among 114 patients who received multimodality treatment, 35 (30.7%) received palliative gastrectomy and 19 (16.7%) received metastasectomy (**Table 3**). The metastasectomy includes oophorectomy, adrenalectomy, hepatectomy, colectomy, and retroperitoneal lymphadenectomy. Fifty-two patients (45.6%) received palliative radiotherapy. In 37 patients who had peritoneal carcinomatosis and received intraperitoneal chemotherapy, fluoropyrimidine, or platinum agents were used most frequently. In addition, six patients with liver metastasis received TACE and six patients with liver metastasis received radiofrequency ablation.

TABLE 4 | Prognostic factors for OS of patients with metastatic gastric cancer on the univariate and multivariate analysis.

Characteristic	*n*	MST (m)	Univariate analysis		Multivariate analysis	
			HR (95% CI)	*P*	HR (95% CI)	*P*
Age	267	14.0	1.003 (0.993–1.014)	0.567		
Gender				0.865		
Male	181	13.4	Ref			
Female	86	15.2	1.024 (0.779–1.346)			
Location				0.305		
Upper	79	14.1	Ref			
Middle	86	13.1	1.260 (0.905–1.755)	0.171		
Lower	94	15.4	0.974 (0.702–1.353)	0.877		
Diffuse	8	14.2	1.423 (0.681–2.973)	0.348		
Differentiation				0.022		0.001
Well/median	61	21.3	Ref		Ref	
Poor	206	13.1	1.443 (1.053–1.977)		1.723 (1.231–2.410)	
CA19–9 level				<0.001		0.011
Normal	161	15.6	Ref		Ref	
Elevated	106	12.2	1.604 (1.219–2.110)		1.459 (1.089–1.956)	
CEA level				0.056		0.134
Normal	144	15.4	Ref		Ref	
Elevated	123	12.2	1.291 (0.993–1.678)		1.246 (0.935–1.660)	
Curative surgery				<0.001		<0.001
No	169	12.2	Ref		Ref	
Yes	98	18.3	0.605 (0.461–0.795)		0.588 (0.440–0.786)	
Second- and further-line chemotherapy				0.859		
No	128	11.3	Ref			
Yes	139	15.2	0.976 (0.751–1.270)			
Palliative gastrectomy				0.044		0.014
No	232	13.2	Ref		Ref	
Yes	35	18.4	0.661 (0.442–0.989)		0.590 (0.387–0.899)	
Metastasectomy				0.001		0.007
No	248	13.2	Ref		Ref	
Yes	19	35.6	0.423 (0.249–0.720)		0.468 (0.270–0.810)	
Intraperitoneal chemotherapy				0.474		
No	230	13.2	Ref			
Yes	37	17.6	0.872 (0.604–1.264)			
Radiotherapy				0.024		0.325
No	215	13.2	Ref		Ref	
Yes	52	17.6	0.682 (0.489–0.952)		0.842 (0.597–1.186)	

Survival

The median OS of patients who received multimodality treatment was prolonged significantly than patients who received systematic treatment only (18.4 vs. 11.4 months, $P < 0.001$, **Figure 1**).

Univariate analysis of clinical prognostic factors that might influence the survival was performed on all included patients. The results demonstrated that factors such as differentiation, CA19–9 level, previous curative surgery, palliative gastrectomy, metastasectomy, and radiotherapy were correlated with OS (**Table 4**). Multivariate analysis was performed by incorporating related factors with Cox regression, and the results indicated that differentiation, CA19–9 level, previous curative surgery, palliative gastrectomy, and metastasectomy were the independent prognostic factors of OS. In the multimodality treatment group, patients who received palliative surgery (gastrectomy or metastasectomy) also had a longer survival than those who received intraperitoneal chemotherapy or radiotherapy (21.6 vs. 15.2 months, $P = 0.014$, **Figure 2**).

DISCUSSION

This real-world single center study showed that median survival of patients with stage IV gastric cancer who received multimodality treatment was significantly longer compared with

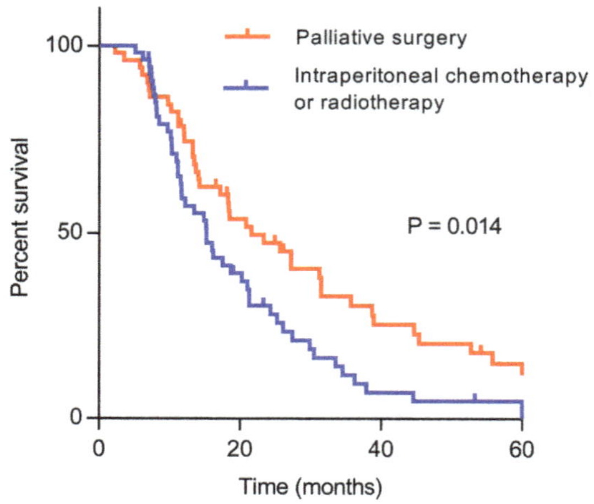

FIGURE 2 | Kaplan–Meier curve of overall survival of patients who received palliative surgery (gastrectomy or metastatectomy) and other treatments (intraperitoneal chemotherapy or radiotherapy) in multimodality treatment group.

those who received systematic therapy alone. In multivariate analysis, palliative gastrectomy, and metastasectomy were identified as independent improved survival factors, while second- and further-line chemotherapy, radiotherapy, and intraperitoneal chemotherapy were considered to be irrelevant.

Patients with stage IV GC usually have a poor prognosis and several randomized studies have provided evidence that first-line chemotherapy is more effective in terms of survival than best supportive care alone for patients with metastatic tumors (8). Therefore, patients with metastatic GC are primarily considered for systemic chemotherapy. However, treatment options after failure of standard first-line therapy are scarce and related benefit has to be weighed against treatment-related toxicities. Some randomized trials showed a survival advantage of the second- and further-line treatment over the best supportive care (20–23). However, such benefit was not seen in this real-world study even most patients still received two-drug combination regimen in the second- and further-line chemotherapy.

Surgery is not a standard treatment option for patients with stage IV GC, except for those who need alleviate symptoms such as bleeding and obstruction caused by the tumor (24). Although patients with metastases from gastric cancer are traditionally treated with systematic chemotherapy, this research and several retrospective studies indicated that gastrectomy or metastasectomy offered a more favorable survival compared with palliative chemotherapy alone by removing macroscopic lesions remaining (25–29). Even in the multimodality treatment group, patients who received surgery had a better survival than those who only received intraperitoneal chemotherapy or radiotherapy in our study. However, the clinical benefit of palliative surgery for stage IV GC is uncertain. A significant problem of these reports is selection bias. Candidates for surgical resection were more likely to have smaller disease burden and better performance status than those who received no surgical intervention. Recently, a phase III, randomized controlled trial (REGATTA trial) failed to show any survival benefit of gastrectomy in patients with advanced gastric cancer (30). Furthermore, patients undergoing gastrectomy had a significantly higher incidence of several serious adverse events related to chemotherapy in REGATTA trial. However, because of the presence of micrometastatic disease in advanced GC, it is more reasonable for advanced GC patients to receive the palliative surgery following a good response to systemic therapy. Palliative surgery in metastatic GC is a highly controversial topic, and the door to surgical resection are still not definitely closed (31). In the future, the effect of palliative resection in stage IV GC should be assessed as a component of multimodal treatment.

Peritoneal metastases are detected in about 30% of patients with advanced gastric cancer (32). Intraperitoneal chemotherapy is a reasonable strategy to approach peritoneal metastasis directly since it enables relatively high concentration of anticancer drugs to directly target cancer lesions in the peritoneum (33–35). In addition, patients with peritoneal metastasis can benefit from intraoperative chemotherapy administration combined with surgery (36). However, intraperitoneal chemotherapy in the current study yielded conflicting results and did not demonstrate a survival benefit. Similarly, the PHOENIX-GC trial failed to show statistical superiority of intraperitoneal paclitaxel in terms of overall survival (37). The possible clinical benefits of intraperitoneal chemotherapy for GC still need exploratory clinical trials.

In this research, palliative radiation therapy as a single modality in multivariate analysis also did not improve survival of metastatic GC patients. However, it is still attractive and has a well-defined role in symptomatic palliation in patients with unresectable gastric cancer, such as pain, bleeding, and obstruction (38). A population-based study demonstrated that radiation, surgery, or combination of both were associated with improved survival in advanced GC patients (39). The role of radiation therapy in stage IV GC remains controversial.

Our study has some limitations. First, this study was a retrospective design. Because of the retrospective nature, the selection bias exists inevitably and may influence the survival analysis. For example, patients with better status and less comorbidities are more likely to undergo more aggressive treatments, which may result in a better survival outcome. Second, this research was performed at a single institute. The indication for multi-modality therapy is various and dependents on the institute, the patients included in our center cannot represent the whole population of patients with stage IV GC who received multi-modality treatments. Third, as a real-world study, the heterogenous treatment schemes may be potential confounding variables that may influence the survival result although we have used the Cox regression analysis.

Up to now, it is impractical to cure stage IV GC, but the evidence is clear that using only one treatment modality cannot control this metastatic disease efficiently. Medical oncologists, surgeons, and radiologists from different disciplines should work together and offer the patients a comprehensive treatment plan to offer a chance of survival improvement. Optimal management of patients with metastatic GC is still challenging usually requires the integration of multidisciplinary therapeutic strategies either concurrently or sequentially.

CONCLUSION

In conclusion, this real-world study provided the evidence that multi-modality treatment showed a significant survival benefit for patients with metastatic gastric cancer. Palliative gastrectomy and metastasectomy were independent prognostic factors for survival. In the future, large-scale prospective randomized clinical trials are needed to determine the optimal treatment strategy for stage IV gastric cancer.

ETHICS STATEMENT

The studies involving human participants were reviewed and approved by Ethics Committee of Peking Union Medical College Hospital. Written informed consent for participation was not required for this study in accordance with the national legislation and the institutional requirements.

AUTHOR CONTRIBUTIONS

LZ, JL, CB, and GL conceived and designed the study. LZ, JL, and YN collected the data and wrote the manuscript. JL performed the statistical analyses. LZ, JL, and GL reviewed and revised the manuscript. All authors read and approved the final manuscript.

ACKNOWLEDGMENTS

We thank all patients who participated in this study.

REFERENCES

1. Ferlay J, Soerjomataram I, Dikshit R, Eser S, Mathers C, Rebelo M, et al. Cancer incidence and mortality worldwide: sources, methods and major patterns in GLOBOCAN 2012. *Int J Cancer.* (2015) 136:E359–86. doi: 10.1002/ijc.29210
2. Chen W, Zheng R, Baade PD, Zhang S, Zeng H, Bray F, et al. Cancer statistics in China, 2015. *CA Cancer J Clin.* (2016) 66:115–32. doi: 10.3322/caac.21338
3. Zeng H, Chen W, Zheng R, Zhang S, Ji JS, Zou X, et al. Changing cancer survival in China during 2003–15: a pooled analysis of 17 population-based cancer registries. *Lancet Global Health.* (2018) 6:e555–67. doi: 10.1016/S2214-109X(18)30127-X
4. Allemani C, Matsuda T, Di Carlo V, Harewood R, Matz M, Nikšić M, et al. Global surveillance of trends in cancer survival 2000–14 (CONCORD-3): analysis of individual records for 37 513 025 patients diagnosed with one of 18 cancers from 322 population-based registries in 71 countries. *Lancet.* (2018) 391:1023–75. doi: 10.1016/S0140-6736(17)33326-3
5. Van Cutsem E, Sagaert X, Topal B, Haustermans K, Prenen H. Gastric cancer. *Lancet.* (2016) 388:2654–64. doi: 10.1016/S0140-6736(16)30354-3
6. D'Angelica M, Gonen M, Brennan MF, Turnbull AD, Bains M, Karpeh MS. Patterns of initial recurrence in completely resected gastric adenocarcinoma. *Ann Surg.* (2004) 240:808–16. doi: 10.1097/01.sla.0000143245.28656.15
7. Songun I, Putter H, Kranenbarg EM, Sasako M, van de Velde CJ. Surgical treatment of gastric cancer: 15-year follow-up results of the randomised nationwide Dutch D1D2 trial. *Lancet Oncol.* (2010) 11:439–49. doi: 10.1016/S1470-2045(10)70070-X
8. Wagner AD, Syn NL, Moehler M, Grothe W, Yong WP, Tai BC, et al. Chemotherapy for advanced gastric cancer. *Cochrane Database Syst Rev.* (2017) 8:CD004064. doi: 10.1002/14651858.CD004064.pub4
9. Shen L, Shan Y-S, Hu H-M, Price TJ, Sirohi B, Yeh K-H, et al. Management of gastric cancer in Asia: resource-stratified guidelines. *Lancet Oncol.* (2013) 14:e535–47. doi: 10.1016/S1470-2045(13)70436-4
10. Muro K, Van Cutsem E, Narita Y, Pentheroudakis G, Baba E, Li J, et al. Pan-Asian adapted ESMO Clinical Practice Guidelines for the management of patients with metastatic gastric cancer: a JSMO-ESMO initiative endorsed by CSCO, KSMO, MOS, SSO, and TOS. *Ann Oncol.* (2019) 30:19–33. doi: 10.1093/annonc/mdy502
11. Sun W, Yan L. Gastric cancer: current and evolving treatment landscape. *Chin J Cancer.* (2016) 35:83. doi: 10.1186/s40880-016-0147-6
12. Wang FH, Shen L, Li J, Zhou ZW, Liang H, Zhang XT, et al. The Chinese Society of Clinical Oncology (CSCO): clinical guidelines for the diagnosis and treatment of gastric cancer. *Cancer Commun.* (2019) 39:10. doi: 10.1186/s40880-019-0349-9
13. Misleh JG, Santoro P, Strasser JF, Bennett JJ. Multidisciplinary management of gastric cancer. *Surg Oncol Clin N Am.* (2013) 22:247–64. doi: 10.1016/j.soc.2012.12.013
14. Lordick F, Siewert JR. Recent advances in multimodal treatment for gastric cancer: a review. *Gastric Cancer.* (2005) 8:78–85. doi: 10.1007/s10120-005-0321-z
15. Izuishi K, Mori H. Recent strategies for treating stage IV gastric cancer: roles of palliative gastrectomy, chemotherapy, and radiotherapy. *J Gastrointestin Liver Dis.* (2016) 25:87–94. doi: 10.15403/jgld.2014.1121.251.rv2
16. Beom SH, Choi YY, Baek SE, Li SX, Lim JS, Son T, et al. Multidisciplinary treatment for patients with stage IV gastric cancer: the role of conversion surgery following chemotherapy. *BMC Cancer.* (2018) 18:1116. doi: 10.1186/s12885-018-4998-x
17. Yang LP, Wang ZX, He MM, Jin Y, Ren C, Wang ZQ, et al. The survival benefit of palliative gastrectomy and/or metastasectomy in gastric cancer patients with synchronous metastasis: a population-based study using propensity score matching and coarsened exact matching. *J Cancer.* (2019) 10:602–10. doi: 10.7150/jca.28842
18. Desiderio J, Chao J, Melstrom L, Warner S, Tozzi F, Fong Y, et al. The 30-year experience-A meta-analysis of randomised and high-quality non-randomised studies of hyperthermic intraperitoneal chemotherapy in the treatment of gastric cancer. *Eur J Cancer.* (2017) 79:1–14. doi: 10.1016/j.ejca.2017.03.030
19. Ajani JA, D'Amico TA, Almhanna K, Bentrem DJ, Chao J, Das P, et al. Gastric cancer, version 3.2016, NCCN clinical practice guidelines in oncology. *J Natl Compr Canc Netw.* (2016) 14:1286–312. doi: 10.6004/jnccn.2016.0137
20. Kang JH, Lee SI, Lim DH, Park KW, Oh SY, Kwon HC, et al. Salvage chemotherapy for pretreated gastric cancer: a randomized phase III trial comparing chemotherapy plus best supportive care with best supportive care alone. *J Clin Oncol.* (2012) 30:1513–8. doi: 10.1200/JCO.2011.39.4585
21. Thuss-Patience PC, Kretzschmar A, Bichev D, Deist T, Hinke A, Breithaupt K, et al. Survival advantage for irinotecan versus best supportive care as second-line chemotherapy in gastric cancer–a randomised phase III study of the Arbeitsgemeinschaft Internistische Onkologie (AIO). *Eur J Cancer.* (2011) 47:2306–14. doi: 10.1016/j.ejca.2011.06.002
22. Wesolowski R, Lee C, Kim R. Is there a role for second-line chemotherapy in advanced gastric cancer? *Lancet Oncol.* (2009) 10:903–12. doi: 10.1016/S1470-2045(09)70136-6
23. Li J, Qin S, Xu J, Xiong J, Wu C, Bai Y, et al. Randomized, double-blind, placebo-controlled phase III trial of apatinib in patients with chemotherapy-refractory advanced or metastatic adenocarcinoma of the stomach or gastroesophageal junction. *J Clin Oncol.* (2016) 34:1448–54. doi: 10.1200/JCO.2015.63.5995
24. Japanese Gastric Cancer A. Japanese gastric cancer treatment guidelines 2014 (ver. 4). *Gastric Cancer.* (2017) 20:1–19. doi: 10.1007/s10120-016-0622-4

25. Markar SR, Mikhail S, Malietzis G, Athanasiou T, Mariette C, Sasako M, et al. Influence of surgical resection of hepatic metastases from gastric adenocarcinoma on long-term survival: systematic review and pooled analysis. *Ann Surg.* (2016) 263:1092–101. doi: 10.1097/SLA.0000000000001542
26. Cho JH, Lim JY, Choi AR, Choi SM, Kim JW, Choi SH, et al. Comparison of surgery plus chemotherapy and palliative chemotherapy alone for advanced gastric cancer with krukenberg tumor. *Cancer Res Treat.* (2015) 47:697–705. doi: 10.4143/crt.2013.175
27. Yan D, Du Y, Dai G, Huang L, Xu Q, Yu P. Management of synchronous krukenberg tumors from gastric cancer: a single-center experience. *J Cancer.* (2018) 9:4197–203. doi: 10.7150/jca.25593
28. Wang Y, Yu YY, Li W, Feng Y, Hou J, Ji Y, et al. A phase II trial of Xeloda and oxaliplatin (XELOX) neo-adjuvant chemotherapy followed by surgery for advanced gastric cancer patients with para-aortic lymph node metastasis. *Cancer Chemother Pharmacol.* (2014) 73:1155–61. doi: 10.1007/s00280-014-2449-1
29. Ebinger SM, Warschkow R, Tarantino I, Schmied BM, Guller U, Schiesser M. Modest overall survival improvements from 1998 to 2009 in metastatic gastric cancer patients: a population-based SEER analysis. *Gastric Cancer.* (2016) 19:723–34. doi: 10.1007/s10120-015-0541-9
30. Fujitani K, Yang H-K, Mizusawa J, Kim Y-W, Terashima M, Han S-U, et al. Gastrectomy plus chemotherapy versus chemotherapy alone for advanced gastric cancer with a single non-curable factor (REGATTA): a phase 3, randomised controlled trial. *Lancet Oncol.* (2016) 17:309–18. doi: 10.1016/S1470-2045(15)00553-7
31. D'Ugo D, Cananzi FC, Persiani R, Agnes A, Biondi A. REGATTA trial: a call for the USA and Europe. *Lancet Oncol.* (2016) 17:261–2. doi: 10.1016/S1470-2045(15)00619-1
32. Thomassen I, van Gestel YR, van Ramshorst B, Luyer MD, Bosscha K, Nienhuijs SW, et al. Peritoneal carcinomatosis of gastric origin: a population-based study on incidence, survival and risk factors. *Int J Cancer.* (2014) 134:622–8. doi: 10.1002/ijc.28373
33. Yonemura Y, Canbay E, Li Y, Coccolini F, Glehen O, Sugarbaker PH, et al. A comprehensive treatment for peritoneal metastases from gastric cancer with curative intent. *Eur J Surg Oncol.* (2016) 42:1123–31. doi: 10.1016/j.ejso.2016.03.016
34. Sugarbaker PH. Cytoreductive surgery and hyperthermic intraperitoneal chemotherapy in the management of gastrointestinal cancers with peritoneal metastases: progress toward a new standard of care. *Cancer Treat Rev.* (2016) 48:42–9. doi: 10.1016/j.ctrv.2016.06.007
35. Coccolini F, Cotte E, Glehen O, Lotti M, Poiasina E, Catena F, et al. Intraperitoneal chemotherapy in advanced gastric cancer. Meta-analysis of randomized trials. *Eur J Surg Oncol.* (2014) 40:12–26. doi: 10.1016/j.ejso.2013.10.019
36. Coccolini F, Catena F, Glehen O, Yonemura Y, Sugarbaker PH, Piso P, et al. Effect of intraperitoneal chemotherapy and peritoneal lavage in positive peritoneal cytology in gastric cancer. Systematic review and meta-analysis. *Eur J Surg Oncol.* (2016) 42:1261–7. doi: 10.1016/j.ejso.2016.03.035
37. Ishigami H, Fujiwara Y, Fukushima R, Nashimoto A, Yabusaki H, Imano M, et al. Phase III trial comparing intraperitoneal and intravenous paclitaxel plus S-1 versus cisplatin plus S-1 in patients with gastric cancer with peritoneal metastasis: PHOENIX-GC trial. *J Clin Oncol.* (2018) 36:1922–9. doi: 10.1200/JCO.2018.77.8613
38. Hazard L, O'Connor J, Scaife C. Role of radiation therapy in gastric adenocarcinoma. *World J Gastroenterol.* (2006) 12:1511–20. doi: 10.3748/wjg.v12.i10.1511
39. Gold JS, Ye S, Wang L, Zuo Z, Bei Y, Liu K. The role of surgery and radiation in advanced gastric cancer: a population-based study of Surveillance, Epidemiology, and End Results database. *PLoS ONE.* (2019) 14:e0213596. doi: 10.1371/journal.pone.0213596

21

Extracellular Matrix Characterization in Gastric Cancer Helps to Predict Prognosis and Chemotherapy Response

Zhi Yang[1†], *Feifei Xue*[2†], *Minhuan Li*[3†], *Xingya Zhu*[1†], *Xiaofeng Lu*[1], *Chao Wang*[4], *En Xu*[4], *Xingzhou Wang*[4], *Liang Zhang*[1], *Heng Yu*[1], *Chuanfu Ren*[1], *Hao Wang*[1,4], *Yizhou Wang*[1], *Jie Chen*[5*], *Wenxian Guan*[1,4*] *and Xuefeng Xia*[1,4*]

[1] *Department of General Surgery, Drum Tower Clinical Medical College of Nanjing Medical University, Nanjing, China,* [2] *Jiangsu Key Laboratory of Oral Diseases, Nanjing Medical University, Nanjing, China,* [3] *Department of Andrology, Drum Tower Clinical Medical College of Nanjing Medical University, Nanjing, China,* [4] *Department of General Surgery, Nanjing Drum Tower Hospital, The Affiliated Hospital of Nanjing University Medical School, Nanjing, China,* [5] *Department of Anesthesiology, Nanjing Drum Tower Hospital, The Affiliated Hospital of Nanjing University Medical School, Nanjing, China*

***Correspondence:**
Wenxian Guan
15850502391@163.com
Xuefeng Xia
danielxuefeng@hotmail.com
Jie Chen
jiechen028@163.com

[†]*These authors have contributed equally to this work and share first authorship*

The extracellular matrix (ECM) plays a central role in the formation of the tumor microenvironment. The deposition of the ECM is associated with poor prognosis in a variety of tumors. Aberrant ECM deposition could undermine the effect of chemotherapy and immunotherapy. However, there is no systematic analysis on the relationship between the ECM and prognosis or chemotherapy effect. In the present study, we applied the gene set variation analysis (GSVA) algorithm to score 2199 canonical pathways in 2125 cases of probe or sequencing data and identified the core matrisome as the driving factor in gastric cancer progression. We classified gastric cancer samples into three clusters according to the composition of the ECM and evaluated clinical and multi-omics characterization of ECM phenotypes. The ECM score was evaluated by GSVA score of core matrisome and a higher ECM score predicted poor prognosis of gastric cancer [Hazard Ratio (HR), 2.084; p-value $< 2 \times 10^{-16}$]. In The Cancer Genome Atlas (TCGA) cohort and KUGH, YUSH, and KUCM cohorts, we verified that patients with a low ECM score could benefit from chemotherapy. By contrast, patients with a high ECM score did not achieve satisfactory response from chemotherapy. Determining the characteristics of the ECM microenvironment might help to predict the prognosis and chemotherapy response of patients with gastric cancer, and help to resolve the enigma of chemoresistance acquisition, as well as providing inspiration to develop combination therapy.

Keywords: gastric cancer, ECM, prognostic factors, chemotherapy response, multi-omics

INTRODUCTION

Gastric cancer (GC) is the third leading cause of cancer-related death and the fifth most common cancer diagnosed worldwide (1). Surgical resection has always been the mandatory backbone treatment for resectable stage II and III GC (1). However, the significant benefit from surgical resection alone is confined to early GC, while the rate of relapse remains high for advanced GC.

Multimodal therapies, including chemotherapy, chemoradiation, and immunotherapy, have been established to prevent recurrence and have improved the survival rates of patients after surgery (1). Although the receipt of adjunctive therapies could improve prognosis for some patients with GC patients to a certain extent, variations in clinical outcome have been detected for patients who received the same treatment (2–4). Multiple molecular subtypes and ingenious prognostic models based on multi-omics data have been established for patients with resectable GC. Stomach adenocarcinoma in The Cancer Genome Atlas (TCGA) was subdivided into five molecular subtypes on the basis of molecular profiles: microsatellite instable (MSI), genomically stable (GS), Epstein–Barr virus (EBV) associated, chromosomal instability (CIN) and hypermutated-single-nucleotide variant predominant (HM-SNV) (5, 6). And the Asian Cancer Research Group (ACRG) defined four molecular subtypes, including microsatellite stable (MSS)/epithelial–mesenchymal transition (EMT), MSI, MSS/$p53^+$, and MSS/$p53^-$ (7). Oh et al. (8)identified two distinct molecular subtypes: mesenchymal phenotype(MP) and epithelial phenotype (EP). These molecular subtypes show great tumor heterogeneity, distinct clinical outcome and different response to anti-tumor therapy. Additionally, Zeng et al. (9) depicted the comprehensive landscape of tumor microenvironment characteristics and established TMEscore based on tumor immune infiltration patterns to predict immunotherapy response in gastric cancer. Zhang et al. (10) characterized m^6A modification patterns in gastric cancer and constructed m6Ascore based on 21 m^6A regulators, which could also discriminate distinct TME and do well in predicting benefits from immunotherapy for patients with gastric cancer. Cheong et al. (11) developed and validated a model with four classifier genes (GZMB, WARS, SFRP4, and CDX1) for predicting adjuvant chemotherapy response in patients with resectable, stage II–III gastric cancer. Benefited from these classification and scoring system, the tumor heterogeneity could be defined, evaluated and precisely targeted.

The extracellular matrix (ECM) regulates tissue development and homeostasis (12). It consists of biochemically and biomechanically distinct macromolecules, including glycoproteins, collagens, and proteoglycans, which assemble into a three-dimensional supramolecular network that regulates cell growth, survival, motility, and differentiation (13). As a major component of the tumor microenvironment, the ECM could affect the hallmarks of cancer and is involved in all the cellular processes contributing to cancer initiation, progression, and dissemination (14, 15). Researchers found that increased ECM stiffness is required for the transformation of normal cells into tumor through YAP/TAZ mechanotransduction (16), and could also drive EMT, invasion and metastasis *via* TWIST1-G3BP2 mechanotransduction (17). In gastric cancer, the stiffness of the ECM could induce hypomethylation of the promoter region of mechanosensitive Yes-associated protein (YAP) and activate the oncogenic activity of YAP (18). Clinical observations also confirmed that an increased ECM content correlates with more aggressive tumors and poorer prognosis (Socovich and Naba 2019). Intriguingly, in pancreatic ductal adenocarcinoma, decreasing ECM with an anti–lysyl oxidase like-2 (anti-LOXL2) antibody in syngeneic orthotopic PDA mouse models accelerated tumor growth, resulting in diminished overall survival, which suggested a protective role of ECM (20). In addition, tumor ECM is also an affecting factor of cancer therapy. A pan-cancer analysis showed that ECM deposition induced by TGF-β signalling could predict failure of PD-1 blockade (21). On the contrary, inhibiting ECM deposition could soften metastases of colorectal cancer and increase the anti-angiogenic effects of bevacizumab (22). However, until recently, we were not aware of the whole picture of the complexity of the tumor ECM, nor had we determined, to what extent, the ECM is involved in cancer progression. Rapidly developing high throughput sequencing and bioinformatic technologies are of great help to precisely characterize the ECM composition in tumor microenvironments. In this study, we are going to characterize the landscape of ECM in gastric cancer and discuss its clinical implications.

MATERIALS AND METHODS

Gene Expression Data Gathering and Processing

We searched in The Cancer Genome Atlas (TCGA) database and Gene-Expression Omnibus (GEO) for open source gene-expression data with full clinical annotation of gastric cancer. Only those with a sample size greater than 50 and available survival information were included for further analysis. In total, 2125 gastric cancer samples were integrated, including 7 cohorts from the GEO database (https://www.ncbi.nlm.nih.gov/; geo accession numbers: GSE13861 [Yonsei University Severance Hospital (YUSH) cohort], GSE15459, GSE26253, GSE26942, GSE29272, GSE66229, GSE84437 [Asian Cancer Research Group (ACRG) cohort] and TCGA-STAD cohort (**Supplementary Table S1**). The GSE26942 cohort was merged with GSE26899 for the Korea University Guro Hospital (KUGH) cohort and with GSE26901 for the Kosin University College of Medicine (KUCM) cohort. In brief, primary microarray data sets downloaded from GEO were analyzed with background adjustment and normalized using the microarray data package in the R language environment (23). For the TCGA-STAD cohort, latest RNA-sequencing data (HTSeq-FPKM) were retrieved through the R package TCGAbiolinks 2.16.4, which was further transformed into transcripts per kilobase million (TPM) to make it more comparable with the microarray data. All the gene expression data sets were transformed into a log2 base before further analysis. To merge multiple gene expression data sets, a batch normalization algorithm was employed to remove batch effects using the R package sva 3.36.0.

Clinical and Genomic Data Collection

Up to date clinical information for the TCGA-STAD cohort was downloaded and prepared using the R package TCGAbiolinks

2.16.4 and that of other cohorts was directly downloaded as attached files from GEO database or from the **Supplementary Materials** in the related literature. Multi-omics data of the TCGA-STAD cohort, including somatic mutation, copy number variation (CNV), and DNA methylation (Illumina Human Methylation 450K), were obtained from UCSC Xena (https://xenabrowser.net/). All the multi-omics data analysis was limited to samples with available mRNA data; therefore, we analyzed 366 samples for somatic mutation, 374 samples for CNVs, and 336 samples for DNA methylation.

Gene Set Variation Analysis

We downloaded 2922 canonical pathways gene sets integrated from authoritative pathway databases, including the BioCarta pathway database, the Kyoto Encyclopedia of Genes and Genomes (KEGG) pathway database, the PID pathway database, the Reactome pathway database, and the WikiPathways pathway database, from the Molecular Signatures Database (MSigDB, https://www.gsea-msigdb.org/gsea/index.jsp) (24). The normalized GSVA score of each canonical pathway gene set was measured for each gastric cancer sample using the GSVA algorithm in the R package GSVA 1.36.2 (25). The ECM score was measured as the GSVA score of the core matrisome gene set downloaded from MatrisomeDB (http://www.pepchem.org/matrisomedb), an updated version with slight changes (26).

Gene Set Enrichment Analysis

The GSEA algorithm was used to analyze the enriched biological processes between different groups. In brief, the differential genes between two groups were measured with the R package limma 3.44.3, and were subsequently pre-ranked by log2 fold-change and submitted to the R package clusterProfiler 3.16.1 to run the GSEA. Results with a p-value < 0.05 and a q-value < 0.05 were considered statistically significant.

Consensus Clustering for the Extracellular Matrix Composition

To identify different ECM composition patterns and classify patients into distinct groups for further analysis, Unsupervised clustering analysis (based on the Euclidean distance and Ward's linkage) was carried out based on the expression of 274 kinds of ECM in the merged data set and the ACRG cohort. The R package ConsensuClusterPlus 1.52.0 was used to perform the clustering procedure and to determine the optimal number of clusters, which was repeated 1000 times to guarantee the stability of classification.

Estimation Tumor Microenvironment Cell Infiltration

To explore the immune cell infiltration composition of different ECM clusters, the CIBERSORT algorithm was used to analyze the proportions of 22 types of immune cells in each sample of the ACRG cohort using the R package CIBERSORT (27). CIBERSORT employed a deconvolution algorithm, along with support vector regression, to work on 547 specific immune cell-related genes and deconstructed 22 main types of immune cells, including $CD8^+$ T cells, regulatory T cells (Tregs), M0 macrophages, M1 macrophages, and M2 macrophages. 1,000 permutations were performed to achieve robust quantification of the relative abundance of each infiltrated immune cell.

Gene Silencing by Small Interfering RNA Transfection

AGS and Hs746T cells were seeded in 6-well plates at 2×10^5 cell per well overnight, and then treated with 2 μg of negative control small interfering RNA (siRNA), FBN1-siRNA (targeting FBN1 encoding fibrillin 1) and LAMC1-siRNA (targeting LAMC1 encoding laminin subunit gamma 1) constructed by Shanghai GenePharma Company (Shanghai, China) along with 5 μL siRNA interferin reagent (Polyplus, New York, NY, USA). After incubation at 37°C with 5% CO_2 for 48 h, the efficiency of gene silencing was determined using qRT-PCR.

Apoptosis Assay

For the apoptosis assay, cells were seeded into a six-well plate and subjected to different treatments. The cell apoptosis assay was operated according to the manual of the fluorescein isothiocyanate (FITC) Annexin V Apoptosis Detection Kit (BD Biosciences, San Jose, CA, USA). The results were analyzed using FlowJo 10 software (FlowJo, Ashland, OR, USA).

Transwell Invasion Assay

For the Transwell invasion assay, 5×10^4 cells in a volume of 200 μL of serum-free medium were added into a Transwell chamber containing a polycarbonate membrane with 8.0 μm pores (353097; BD Falcon) and covered with a layer of Matrigel matrix (56234; Corning Inc., Corning, NY, USA). The chamber was then placed in a 24-well plate containing 600 μL of medium with 10% fetal bovine serum and incubated at 37°C with 5% CO_2. After 24 h of incubation, non-migrated cells were wiped away and the remaining cells that had migrated through the bottom of the chamber were fixed in 4% paraformaldehyde followed by crystal violet staining and counting under a microscope.

Statistical Analysis

Unpaired Student t tests and Wilcoxon rank-sum tests were used to evaluate the statistical significance of normally distributed and non-normally distributed variables, respectively, when comparing two groups. Kruskal-Wallis tests and One-way analysis of variance (ANOVA) was used to conduct difference comparisons of more than two groups (28). Spearman and distance correlational analyses were conducted using the R package Hmisc 4.4.1. Objects with a Spearman correlation coefficient greater than 0.5 were deemed strongly correlated (29). The hazard ratios (HR) of all prognostic factors was calculated using a univariate Cox proportional hazards regression model. The "surv_cutpoint" function of the R package survminer 0.4.8 was used to estimate the best cut off point for prognostic factors according to their relationship with the patients' survival probability with the maximum rank statistic. For the ECM score, patients were then divided into ECM score low and ECM high groups according to the best cut off point. Then, survival curves were drawn using the Kaplan–Meier method. The statistical significance of the difference in survival probability was estimated using the log-rank test. The R package forestplot 1.10 was used to show the univariate prognosis analyses of different groups of prognostic factors. The visualization of ECM clusters was facilitated by the R package umap 0.2.6., to perform dimensionality reduction. The networks of canonical signaling pathways were constructed using the software Cytoscape 3.7.2 and the hub pathway was estimated by the Cytoscape plug-in CytoHubba. The R package ComplexHeatmap 2.4.3 generated all the heat maps. A Waterfall Chart was used to exhibit the overview of gene mutation landscape, which was generated the R package maftools 2.4.12. The statistical difference of CNVs between the ECM low and ECM high group was determined using the R package cnvaq 0.1.3. Then, the IGV 2.8.2 software was employed to visualize the CNV landscape of the two groups.

All the above analyses were performed using the R 4.0.0 software. All the statistical analyses were two-sided and a p-value < 0.05 was considered statistically significant.

RESULTS

Identification of the Core Matrisome as the Major Factor Involved in Gastric Cancer Progression

In total, eight eligible GC cohorts (GSE13861, GSE15459, GSE26253, GSE26942, GSE29272, ACRG/GSE66229, GSE84437, and TCGA-STAD) were used in our study. Six cohorts with microarray data (GSE13861, GSE15459, GSE26942, GSE29272, ACRG/GSE66229, and GSE84437) were merged into a meta-cohort (n = 1323). GSE26253 was not merged because of its limited number of gene probes and the sequence data of TCGA-STAD cohort was dismissed because it was being incompatible with the microarray data for technical reasons. Then, we calculated the GSVA score of 2199 canonical pathways for all the cohorts engaged in our study. First, the hazard ratio (HR) of the canonical pathways for overall survival (OS) of patients with gastric cancer were calculated in the meta-cohort (**Figure 1A**). The Wnt signaling pathway, the common pathway of fibrin clot formation, and autophagy were among the top risk pathways, and the caspase pathway, tumor necrosis factor receptor 1 (TNFR1) pathway, and Fas signaling pathway were among the top favorable pathways (**Supplementary Figure S1B**).

Then, we computed the HR of all the canonical pathways for four cohorts with more than 300 tumor samples (TCGA-STAD, ACRG/GSE66229, GSE84437, and meta-cohort; GSE26253 was not engaged because of its limited number gene probes). The intersection of those pathways, 147 in total, were considered to correlate stably with patients' prognosis (**Figure 1B** and **Supplementary Table S2**). These 147 common pathways were further used to perform unsupervised hierarchical clustering for 1323 tumor samples in the meta-cohort. The result showed that these samples could be divided into three distinct subclusters, which displayed significant differences in survival (log-rank test, p-value < 0.001; **Figure 1D**).

To depict the biological processes that characterized the three pathway clusters, we performed GSEA for each cluster against the whole meta-cohort. The results showed that the top 10 gene ontology (GO) biological processes enriched in pathway cluster A primarily correlated with extracellular matrix organization and those of pathway cluster C were primarily correlated with mitosis and DNA replication (**Supplementary Figures S1C, D**), suggesting the importance of these pathways in gastric cancer progression. No pathway was enriched in pathway cluster B, implying it was intermediate between pathway cluster A and C.

To identify the core pathway involved in the OS of patients with gastric cancer, we calculated the Spearman correlation coefficient among the 147 common pathways in the four cohorts that had more than 300 tumor samples (**Supplementary Table S3**). Only those pathways with absolute value of the Spearman correlation coefficient greater than 0.5 were considered strongly correlated. The connectivity of each pathway in the correlation network was estimated for the four cohorts. Then, we constructed the clustering network of prognostic pathways for the meta cohort according to the intersection of these gene sets (**Figure 1C**). It showed that the most enriched pathways were extracellular matrix remodeling related pathways and glycosaminoglycan metabolism related pathways with higher degree and more closely related to prognosis followed by apoptosis related pathways. Moreover, the top 10 pathways ranked by degree for each cohort were estimated (**Supplementary Figures S1E–H**). The top four pathways with highest mean degree among the four cohorts were the core matrisome, ECM glycoproteins, ECM proteoglycans, and elastic fiber formation, all of which were included in the top 10 pathways in each of the four chosen cohorts, again indicating the key role of the ECM in gastric cancer progression.

Considering the striking performance of the ECM among all the prognostic pathways, we extracted the gene set of "core matrisome" from MatrisomeDB, consisting of all the ECM-related genes, including those encoding 195 ECM glycoproteins, 44 ECM collagens, and 35 proteoglycans (**Supplementary Table S4**). These ECM-related genes were then used to cluster the meta-cohort into three groups named ECM cluster A, ECM cluster B, and ECM cluster C (**Figure 1F**); the ECM clustering shared great similarity with the pathway clusters (**Supplementary Table S5**; Kappa value = 0.69, p-value < 0.0001). As expected, the three ECM clusters displayed significant differences in survival (**Figure 1E**; log-rank test, p-value < 0.001). In summary, this evidence strongly supported the core matrisome as the major pathway in gastric cancer progression.

Clinical and Different Biological Progress Traits of ECM Phenotypes in ACRG Cohort

To explore the clinical and transcriptomic characterization of ECM phenotypes, we chose the ACRG cohort for further study. Similarly, we clustered the 300 samples into three pathway clusters with 147 common prognostic pathways and three ECM clusters with 274 ECM genes (**Figures 2A, B** and **Supplementary Figures S2A–E**). There was high consistency between the pathway clusters and the ECM clusters (**Supplementary Table S6**; kappa value = 0.68, p-value < 0.0001), and different ECM clusters showed great differences in OS and relapse free survival (RFS) (**Figure 2C**, log-rank test, p-value = 7.4×10^{-7}; **Supplementary Figure S2H**, log-rank test, p-value = 7×10^{-7}). The most enriched biological processes still

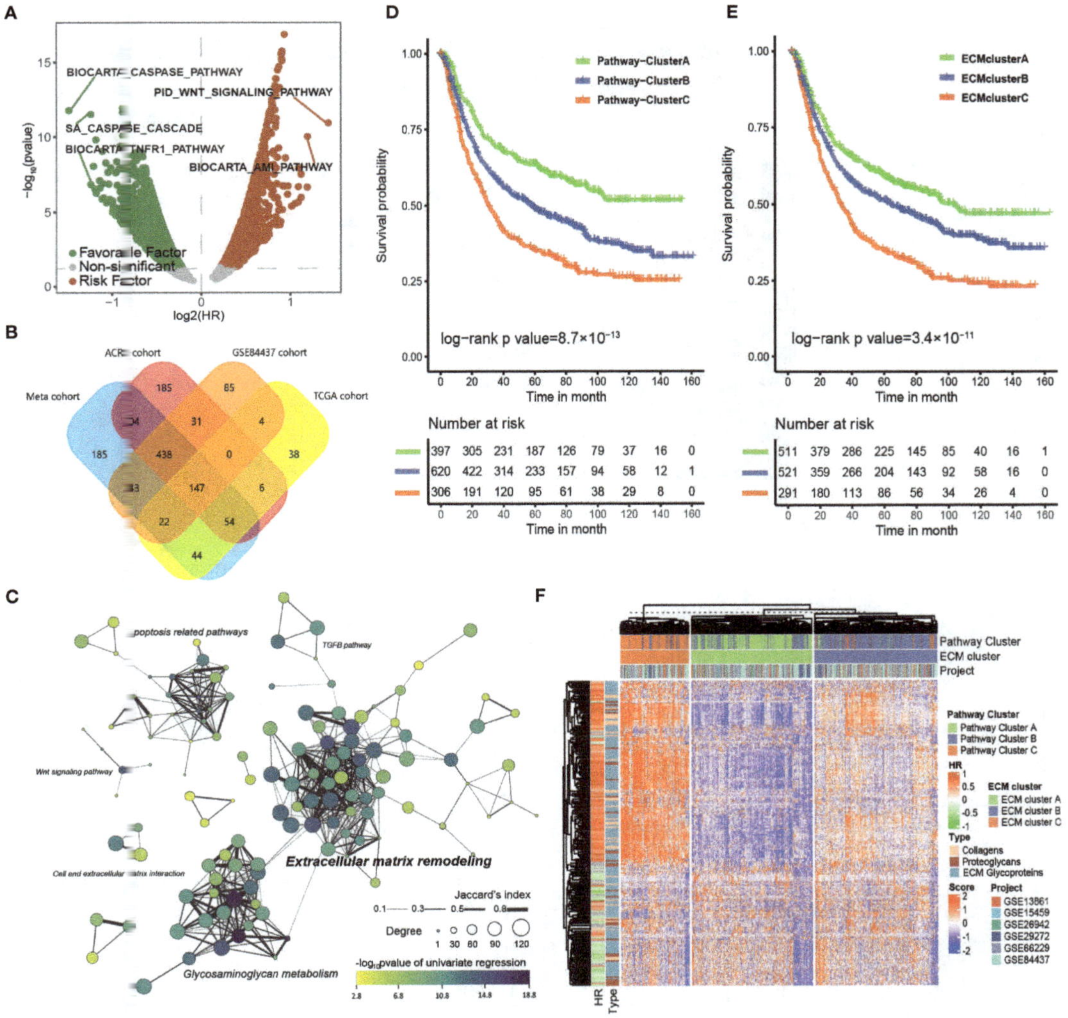

FIGURE 1 | The core matrisome is major pathway involved in gastric cancer progression. **(A)** Volcano plot of prognostic pathways. The x-axis shows the log2 transformed hazard ratio and the y-axis shows −log10 transformed log rank p-values. Red dots indicate risk pathways; green dots indicate favorable pathways; and Grey dots indicate non-prognostic pathways. **(B)** Venn plot of the prognostic pathways in the TCGA-STAD cohort, ACRG cohort, GSE84437 cohort, and the meta-cohort. **(C)** Network of prognostic pathways in the meta-cohort. Each dot represents a prognostic pathway in gastric cancer. A line connecting two pathways means the Jaccard's index between gene sets of the two pathways. The size of the dot represents the degree of the pathway in correlation network of these pathways. The color filling the dot shows the −log10 transformed p-value of univariate cox regression for the GSVA score of the corresponding gene set. **(D)** Kaplan–Meier curves for the overall survival of 1323 patients in the meta-cohort with 3 distinct pathway clusters. The sample size of pathway clusters A, B, and C were n = 397, n = 620, and n = 306, respectively. Log-rank test, p -value = 8.7×10^{-13}. **(E)** Kaplan–Meier curves for overall survival of 1323 patients in the meta-cohort with 3 distinct ECM clusters. The sample size of ECM clusters A, B, and C were n = 511, n = 521, and n = 291, respectively. Log-rank test, p-value = 3.4×10^{-11}. **(F)** Heat map showing the unsupervised clustering of 274 types of ECM for 1323 patients in the meta-cohort. The ECM clustering resembled the pathway clustering to a great extent. The hazard ratio and subtypes of ECM in the meta cohort are also shown in annotation on the right.

shared great similarity with those in the meta-cohort (**Supplementary Figures S2F, G**).

The GSVA score of the "core matrisome" was used as the ECM score for the gene set that consisted of all the ECM genes and could reflect the ECM deposition status. We also tried to shorten this list to obtain a more precise list of ECM-related genes by taking the intersection of differential genes between ECM score high and the ECM score low group in the above four cohorts (**Supplementary Table S7**). However, the shortened gene list was less competent in predicting prognosis. The three ECM clusters had distinct ECM scores (**Supplementary Figure S2I**). As expected, the ECM score could predict OS (**Figure 2D**; HR = 2.19, log-rank test, p-value = 2.8×10^{-6}) and RFS (**Supplementary Figure S2J**; HR = 2.47, log-rank test, p-value = 5.6×10^{-7}). Tumors at stage III/IV had higher ECM scores than those of tumors at stage I/II (**Figure 2E**). Molecular subtypes analysis showed that most of ECM cluster C overlapped with the EMT subtype and none of ECM cluster A belonged to

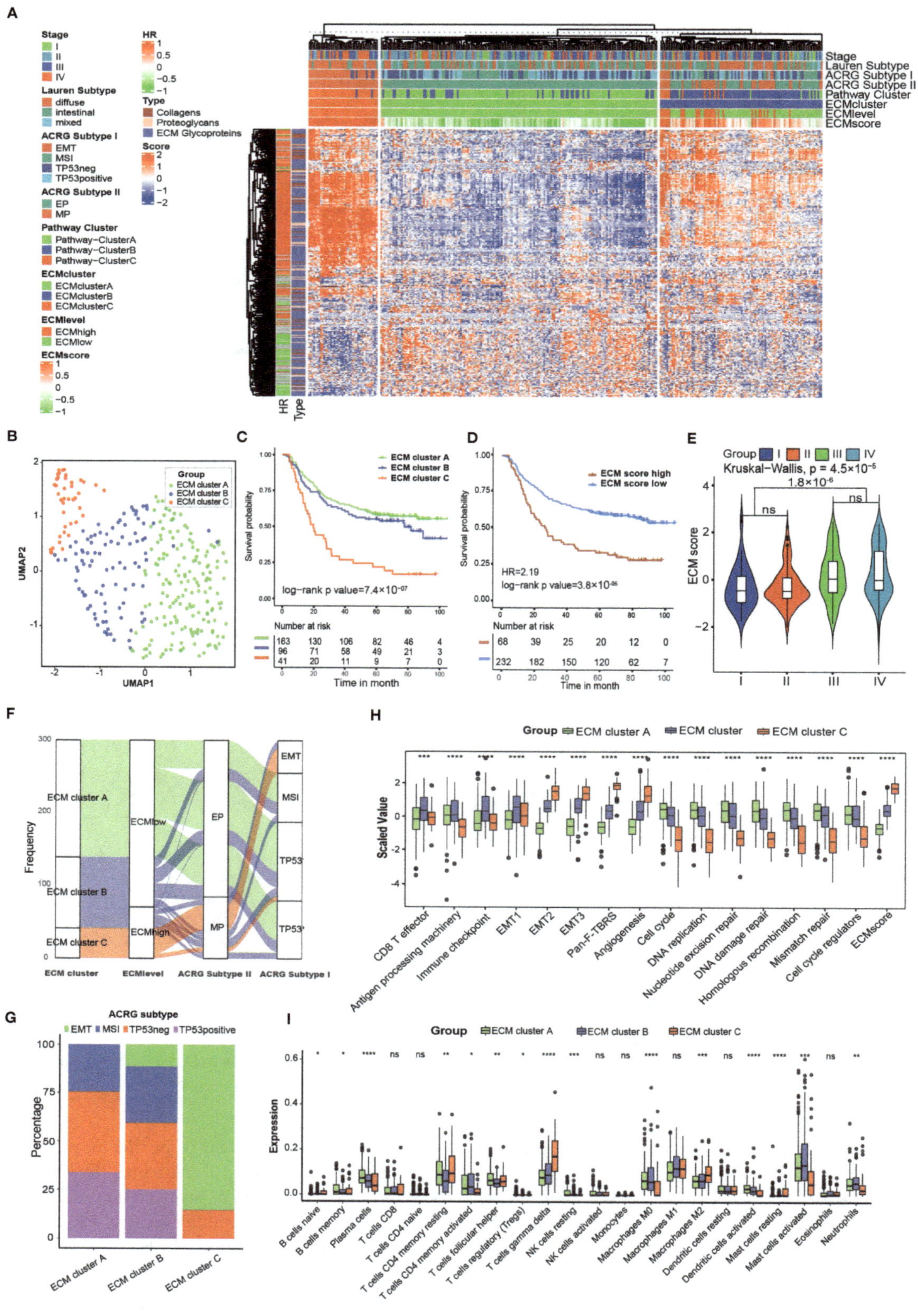

FIGURE 2 | Continued

FIGURE 2 | Clinical and transcriptome characteristics of ECM clusters in the ACRG cohort. **(A)** Heat map showing unsupervised clustering of 274 types of ECM for 300 patients in the ACRG cohort. Tumor stage, Lauren subtype, ACRG subtype I, ACRG subtype II, Pathway cluster, ECM level, and ECM score are shown as patient annotation. The hazard ratio and subtypes of ECM in the ACRG cohort are also shown in the ECM annotation. **(B)** A UMAP plot of 300 patients by dimensionality reduction of 274 types of ECM showing 3 distinct ECM clusters. **(C)** Kaplan–Meier curves for overall survival of 300 patients in the ACRG cohort with 3 distinct ECM clusters. The sample size of ECM clusters A, B, and C were n = 163, n =9 6, and n = 41, respectively. Log-rank test, p-value =7.4×10^{-7}. **(D)** Kaplan–Meier curves for the ECM score by the best cut off value in the ACRG cohort. The numbers of patients in the ECM score high and ECM score low groups were n = 68 and n = 232, respectively. Log-rank test, p-value = 3.8×10^{-6}. **(E)** Violin plot showing that the ECM scores are different among different tumor stages. Kruskal–Wallis test, p-value = 4.5×10^{-5}. The ECM score of stage I and II is lower than that in stage III and IV, Student's t test, p-value = 1.8×10^{-6}. **(F)** Alluvial diagram showing the different ECM clusters in the different ECM levels, ACRG subtype I, and ACRG subtype II. **(G)** Stacked bar chart showing the proportion of ACRG subtypes in the different ECM clusters. **(H, I)** Different biological status and immune cell infiltration patterns of ECM clusters. The top and bottom of the boxes represent the interquartile range of the values. The thick lines in the middle of the boxes represent the median values. The black dots show the outliers. The statistical differences among different ECM clusters were evaluated using the Kruskal–Wallis test. Statistical p-value (*P < 0.05; **P < 0.01; ***P < 0.001, ****P < 0.0001). ns, not significant.

the EMT subtype. Additionally, a higher ECM score was highly associated with a mesenchymal phenotype and diffuse type of Lauren class (**Figures 2F, G** and **Supplementary Figure S2K**) (8). Activation of the EMT program could permit tumors to enter the cancer stem cell (CSC) state, which is resistant to most conventional therapeutics and the major reason for failure of eradicating carcinoma (30, 31). Thus, we deduced that ECM deposition constructed the niche for CSC, which could hinder the efficacy of multiple therapeutics.

The core matrisome turned out to be the major factor in gastric cancer progression; therefore, we characterized the ECM phenotypes with relevant biological processes involved in cancer progression (**Supplementary Table S8**) (32). The results showed that almost all chosen biological processes exhibited significant differences among the three ECM clusters (**Figure 2H**). The ECM score correlated positively with EMT-related processes and negatively with processes involved in DNA replication and DNA repair, which happened to be the feature of CSCs (**Supplementary Figure S2A** and **Supplementary Table S9**). We also analyzed the expression of transforming growth factor beta (TGFβ)-EMT pathway-related genes (*VIM, COL4A1, PDGFRA, SMAD9, TGFB2, TWIST1, ZEB2, CDH1*), DNA damage repair-related genes (*BRCA1, BRCA2, MLH1, MSH2, MGMT, APEX1, FEN1*), and immune checkpoint-related genes (*CD80, CD86, CTLA4, HAVCR2, IDO1, LAG3, PD1, PDL1, TIGIT, TNFRSF9*) in the ECM clusters of the ACRG cohort. The results were consistent with the related biological processes (**Supplementary Figures S3C–E**).

Additionally, the results indicated that different ECM phenotypes showed different immunocompetences. Therefore, we analyzed the immune infiltration pattern of the ECM phenotypes. ECM cluster C showed highest level of M2 and T gamma delta cells, which were identified risk factors for the OS of patients with gastric cancer, and lowest level of activated dendritic cells, M0 macrophages, activated mast cells, and neutrophils, which were identified as favorable factors for the OS of patients with gastric cancer (**Figure 2I**) (9).

Clinical and Multi-Omics Traits of ECM Phenotypes in the TCGA Cohort

Benefitting from multi-omics data, the TCGA cohort contains data related to constructed comprehensive molecular subtypes for gastric cancer, including genome stable (GS), microsatellite instability (MSI), EBV infection, and chromosomal instability (CIN). A higher ECM score was associated with the GS subtype and unfavorable prognosis, whereas a lower ECM score was associated with the EBV or MSI subtypes and favorable prognosis (**Figure 3A**, log-rank test, p-value = 0.0046; **Figure 3B**).

Gene instability, evaluated using the tumor mutation burden (TMB), would result in more neo-antigens, increasing the opportunity for immune recognition and clearance (33, 34). Besides, chemotherapeutic drugs function through damaging DNA integrity of rapidly cycling cancer cells (35). Thus, evaluation of the gene mutation load is very important for the precise administration of medication. First, we found that the high ECM score group had a lower TMB than the low ECM score group in the TCGA cohort (**Figure 3C**; Wilcoxon rank sum test, p-value = 2.9×10^{-7}). In addition, the TMB correlated negatively with the ECM score (**Figure 3D**; Spearman correlation, r = −0.38, p-value = $6.4{\times}10^{-14}$). Subgroup analysis showed that the correlation between ECM score and TMB differed in different molecular subtypes (**Supplementary Figures S4A–E**), which was highest in GS group (Spearman correlation, r = −0.5, p-value = 0.0014) and insignificant in MSI group (p>0.05). Furthermore, the low ECM score group presented a more extensive TMB than the high ECM score group for the levels of individual altered genes in the top 30 most frequently mutated genes (**Figure 3E**). According to **Figure 2H**, the ECM score correlated negatively with DNA replication, which might explain why a higher ECM score was associated with a lower TMB. Similarly, the high ECM score group tended to have less gain or loss in copy number and more wild-type genes (**Figure 3F**). In addition, the total CNV was also correlated negatively with the ECM score (**Figure 3G**; Spearman correlation, r= −0.39, p-value = $8.1{\times}10^{-15}$), and the results in different molecular subtypes were about the same (**Supplementary Figures S4F–J**).

Epigenetic abnormalities are widespread among all tumor types, which also play an important role in drug resistance and immune surveillance (36–38). Therefore, we examined the association of the ECM score with DNA methylation. Interestingly, the high ECM score group had a lower level of DNA methylation in all DNA parts except for 3' untranslated region, and the CpG island and CpG shore, which are associated with inhibiting gene expression, were enriched in the low ECM score group (**Figure 3H** and **Supplementary Figures S4K–L**). Furthermore, we compared the CpG island abundance between the high ECM score and the low ECM score group. GSEA enrichment results showed that, in the high ECM score group, the most hypomethylated biological processes were synapse development and cell differentiation, which may lead to EMT

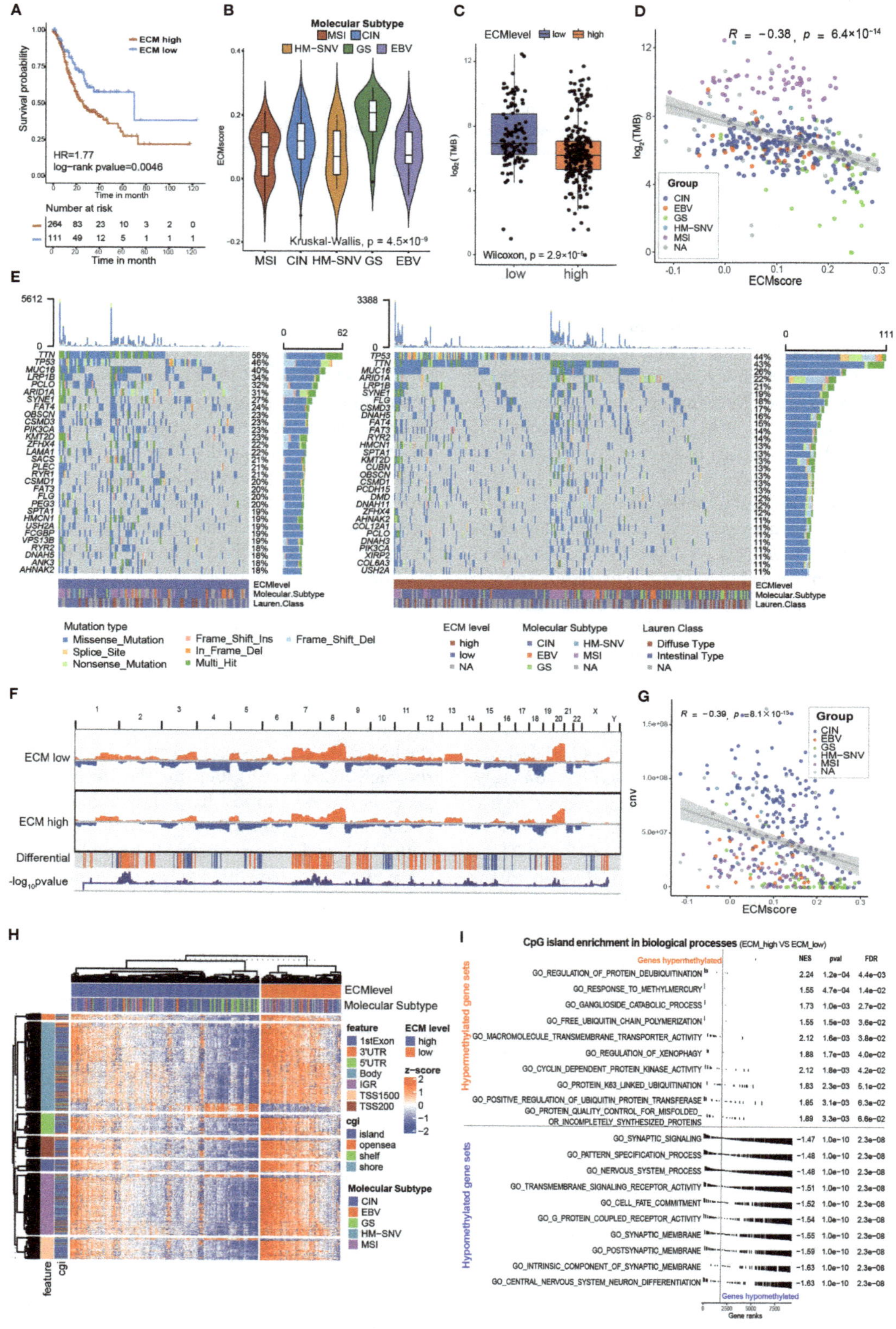

FIGURE 3 | Continued

FIGURE 3 | Characteristics of the ECM pattern in TCGA-STAD molecular subtypes and multi-omics level. **(A)** Kaplan–Meier curves for the ECM score by best cut off value in the TCGA-STAD cohort. The numbers of patients in the ECM score high and ECM score low groups were n = 264 and n = 111, respectively. Log-rank test, p-value = 0.0046. **(B)** Violin plot showing that the ECM scores are different among different molecular subtypes in the TCGA-STAD cohort. Kruskal–Wallis test, p-value = 4.5×10^{-9}. MSI (n = 61), CIN (n = 207), HM-SNV (n = 7), GS (n = 45), EBV (n = 27). **(C)** Difference in the TMB between the ECM high and ECM low groups. The scattered dots indicate the TMB of each sample. The top and bottom of the boxes represent the interquartile range of the values. The thick lines in the middle of the boxes represent the median value. Wilcoxon rank sum test, p-value = 2.9×10^{-7}. **(D)** Scatter plot depicting the correlation between the ECM score and the TMB. Spearman correlation analysis, R = −0.38, p-value = 6.4×10^{-14}. The color of the dots represents the molecular subtypes annotated by the legend. **(E)** An Oncoprint showing the gene mutation map of the ECM high (right, red) and ECM low (left, blue) groups. Each column represents a patient and the barplot in the right of each group indicates the gene mutation frequency of each gene in the corresponding group. The barplot on the top shows the TMB. The gene mutation types are annotated in the legend. Molecular subtypes and Lauren subtypes are also shown as patient annotation. **(F)** CNV pattern of the ECM high and ECM low groups. The length of the plot represents the whole genome and each vertical line represents a gene; red for gain of copy number and blue for loss of copy number. The penultimate line mark the genes with differential copy number between the two groups; a red stripe for higher and a blue stripe for lower copy number in the ECM high group. The last line indicates the −log10 transformed chi-squared test p-value of the copy number difference. **(G)** Scatter plot depicting the correlation between the ECM score and CNV. Spearman correlation analysis, R = −0.39, P = 8.1×10^{-15}. The color of the dots represents the molecular subtypes annotated by the legend. **(H)** Heat map exhibiting the DNA methylation pattern of the ECM high and ECM low groups. The locations of each DNA methylation site are indicated in the left annotation. The molecular subtype is shown as patient annotation. **(I)** GSEA enrichment of CpG islands in biological processes between ECM high group and ECM low groups. The upper part shows the top10 hypermethylated biological processes and the lower part shows the top10 hypomethylated biological processes. The enrichment plot, normalized enrichment score (NES), p value and false discovery rate (FDR) are shown in the right.

and cell stemness, and the most hypermethylated biological processes were less significant to be mentioned (**Figure 3I**). Global hypomethylation is an important feature of naïve pluripotent cells and complex regulation of the epigenome also promotes CSCs formation (39, 40). Therefore, we speculated that ECM deposition might promote CSC formation through an epigenetic mechanism.

The ECM Score Predicts Chemotherapeutic Benefits

Upon dividing the specific data sets by the best cutoff value of the ECM score, significant differences in OS were observed between the low and high ECM score groups for all gastric cancer data sets except GSE29272 (HR, 1.43; 95% CI, 0.99–2.07) (**Figure 4A** and **Supplementary Table S10**). Meanwhile, the prognostic value of the ECM score was also validated in five other independent data sets (GSE13861: HR, 3,21; 95% CI, 1.47–7.0; GSE15459: HR, 2.69; 95% CI, 1.57–4.6; GSE26253: HR, 2.19; 95% CI, 1.62-2.97; GSE26942: HR, 2.67; 95% CI, 1.75–4.08; GSE84437: HR, 2.15; 95% CI, 1.52–3.04; **Supplementary Figures S5C–G**). Moreover, the ECM score could also predict poor prognosis in each stage of gastric cancer (stage I: HR, 3.48; 95% CI, 1.91–6.34; stage II: HR, 2.16; 95% CI, 1.54–3.04; stage III: HR, 1.71; 95% CI, 1.40–2.09; and stage IV: HR, 2.03; 95% CI, 1.55–2.68). These results suggested that the ECM score could be prognostic factor that is independent of tumor stage in gastric cancer (**Supplementary Figures S5A, B**).

Next, we investigated the performance of the ECM score in pan-cancer. We evaluated the predictive value of the ECM score for 14 types of solid tumors in the TCGA cancer cohort, comprising 6251 samples in total (**Supplementary Table S11**). The results showed that the ECM score was a risk factors for eight types of cancer in the TCGA cohorts, including thyroid cancer, brain lower grade glioma, skin cutaneous melanoma, uterine corpus endometrial carcinoma, ovarian serous cystadenocarcinoma, glioblastoma, kidney renal clear cell carcinoma, and lung squamous cell carcinoma, but was irrelevant to other types of cancer, which indicated the biological heterogeneity of the ECM among distinct cancer types (**Figure 4B**).

Chemotherapy is a crucial treatment to supplement surgery in patients with gastric cancer. However, currently, there is no biomarker that can effectively predict a patient's chemotherapy response and even guide the choice of chemotherapeutic regimens. Our results demonstrated that a higher ECM score was associated with the EMT molecular subtype in the ACRG cohort and with the GS molecular subtype in the TCGA-STAD cohort, which were tolerant to chemotherapy. To explore the capacity of the ECM score to predict the chemotherapy response, we first evaluated the best cut off value of the ECM score for patients in the TCGA-STAD cohort who had received chemotherapy according to their prognosis, which could divide the TCGA-STAD cohort into ECM low and ECM high groups. Combined with the chemotherapeutic history, the best cut off value further stratified the TCGA-STAD cohort into Chemo$^+$/ECM high, Chemo$^-$/ECM high, Chemo$^+$/ECM low, Chemo$^-$/ECM score low groups. Interestingly, survival analysis indicated that patients with a low ECM score could benefit from chemotherapy (**Figure 4C**; log-rank test, p-value = 0.019), while there was no significant difference between the chemotherapy and non-chemotherapy group even when the sample size was larger (**Figure 4D**; log-rank test, p-value > 0.05). Besides, more patients with a low ECM score showed a complete response to chemotherapy and less progressive disease compared with patients with a high ECM score (**Supplementary Figure S5H**). To further verify this result, stage II, III, or IV gastric cancer without distant metastasis (n = 180) in three cohorts [GSE26899 for the KUGH cohort, GSE26901 for the KUCM cohort, and GSE13861 for the YUSH cohort; (**Supplementary Table S12**)] with complete chemotherapy information were integrated for survival analysis (log-rank test, p-value = 6.5×10^{-6}) Likewise, patients with a low ECM score could achieve a satisfactory chemotherapy response (**Figure 4E**; log-rank p-value = 0.00019), while patients with a high ECM score could not (**Figure 4F**; log-rank test, p-value > 0.05). Our results strongly supported the view that the ECM score could predict poor prognosis and the response to chemotherapy.

In Vitro Study Indicated That the ECM Could Influence the Invasion and Chemoresistance of Gastric Cancer Cells

To further verify our analysis, we chose two representative ECM genes for the *in vitro* experiment. Firstly, we conducted Spearman correlation analysis for two ECM genes according to their expression levels in the TCGA-STAD, ACRG/GSE66229,

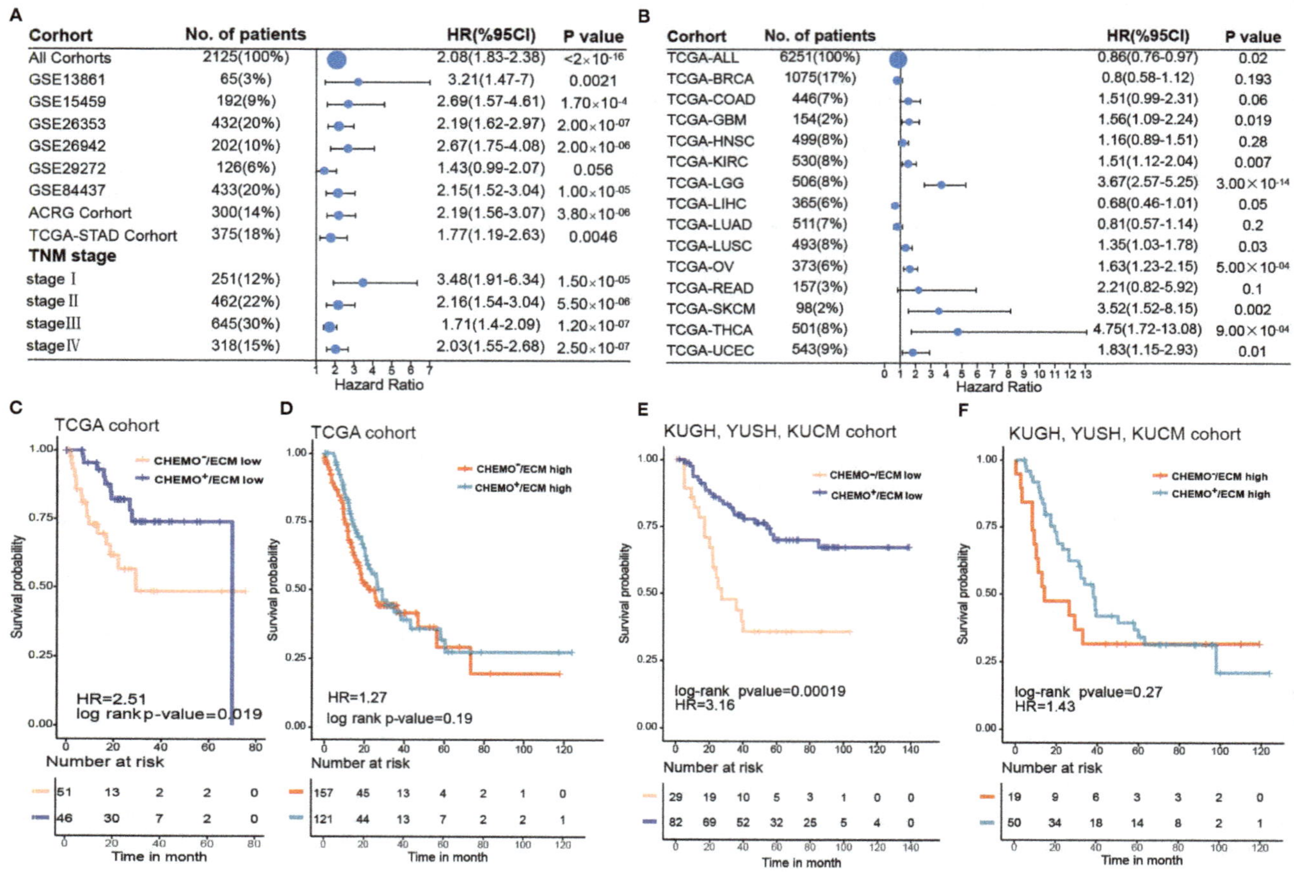

FIGURE 4 | ECM score is a prognostic biomarker and could predict chemotherapy response. **(A)** Forest plot showing the difference in prognosis between ECM high and low groups in independent gastric cancer cohorts and different tumor stages. The horizontal coordinates represent the hazard ratio of the ECM high group relative to the ECM low group and the horizontal line represents the 95% confident interval of the hazard ratio. The size of the dot indicates the sample size of the independent group. **(B)** Forest plot showing the difference in prognosis between the ECM high and low groups in 14 types of solid tumors from the TCGA datasets. The horizontal coordinates represent the hazard ratio of the ECM high group relative to the ECM low group and the horizontal line represents the 95% confident interval of hazard ratio. The size of the dot indicates the sample size of the independent group. **(C)** Kaplan–Meier curves for overall survival of the ECM high group in the TCGA-STAD cohort grouped by chemotherapeutic history. $CHEMO^-$/ECM high, n = 157; $CHEMO^+$/ECM high, n = 121. Log-rank test, p-value = 0.19. **(D)** Kaplan–Meier curves for overall survival of the ECM low group in the TCGA-STAD cohort grouped by chemotherapeutic history. $CHEMO^-$/ECM low, n = 51; $CHEMO^+$/ECM low, n = 46. Log-rank test, p-value = 0.019. **(E)** Kaplan–Meier curves for overall survival of the ECM high group in the KUGH, YUSH, and KUCM cohorts grouped by chemotherapeutic history. $CHEMO^-$/ECM high, n = 19; $CHEMO^+$/ECM high, n = 50. Log-rank test, p-value = 0.27. **(F)** Kaplan–Meier curves for overall survival of the ECM low group in the KUGH, YUSH, KUCM cohort grouped by chemotherapeutic history. $CHEMO^-$/ECM low, n = 29; $CHEMO^+$/ECM low, n = 82. Log-rank test, p-value = 0.00019.

GSE84437, and the meta-cohort and submitted the correlation networks to Cytoscape to find a hub gene for ECM deposition (**Supplementary Figures S6A–E** and **Supplementary Table S13**). *FBN1* was identified as the only common top 10 hub gene among all the cohorts. Fibrillin 1 serves as scaffold for elastic fibers and as a reservoir for growth factors like TGFβ (**Figure 5A**) (41, 42). Then, we performed univariate Cox regression for all the ECM genes in the meta-cohort and identified *LAMC1*, which encodes laminin subunit gamma 1, an essential component of the basement membrane that is involved in multiple types of cancer progression (43–46), as the risk factor with the lowest p-value (**Figure 5B**). Both genes correlated significantly with poor prognosis in the meta-cohort (**Figures 5C, D**; *LAMC1*: HR = 1.71, log-rank test, p-value < 0.0001; *FBN1*: HR = 1.74, log-rank test, p-value < 0.0001). After knocking down the expression of *LAMC1* and *FBN1* separately in Hs746T cells, a metastatic and mesenchymal like cell line, the invasiveness of Hs746T cells was compromised significantly. Similar but less conspicuous results were when the experiment was repeated in AGS cells, a primary and epithelial like cell line (**Figures 5E, F**). We speculated that relative lower expression of the targeted genes in AGS cells accounted for the less significant influence of treatment. However, it is plausible to claim that the ECM could have impact on the EMT phenotype. To check whether the ECM could influence the chemotherapeutic response, we treated Hs746T and AGS cells with 10 μM 5 fluorouracil (5FU), a first-line chemotherapy drug, (1) combined

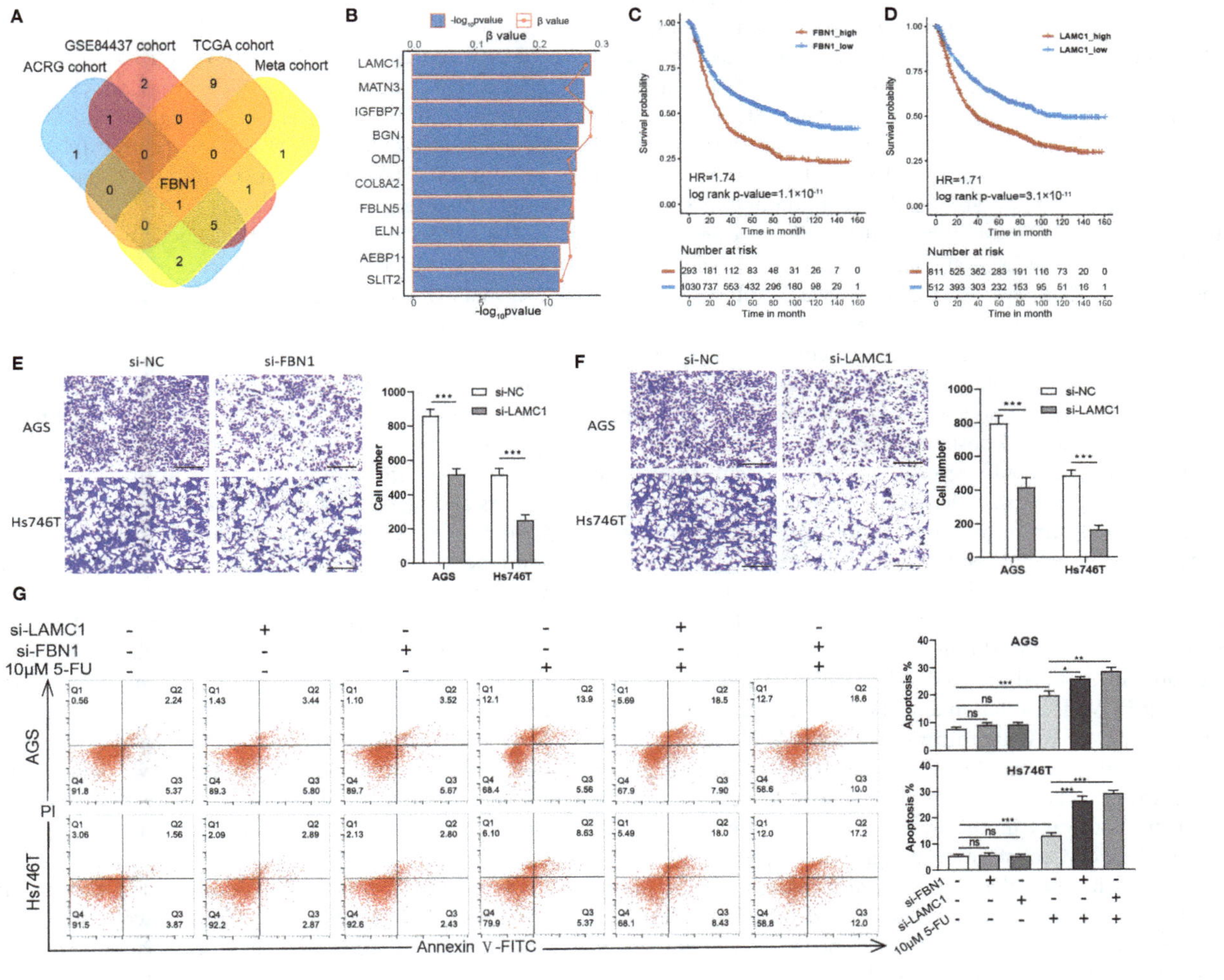

FIGURE 5 | ECM could influence the invasion and drug tolerance of gastric cancer cells. **(A)** A Venn diagram showing the intersection of top 10 hub ECM genes of four cohorts (TCGA-STAD, ACRG, GSE84437 and meta-cohort). *FBN1* is the only common hub ECM gene in the four cohorts. **(B)** Univariate Cox regression results of all ECM in the meta cohort. The top 10 ECM genes with the lowest p values are shown. The horizontal bars shows the $-\log_{10}$ p-value of the univariate Cox regression and the horizontal coordinates of the dots show the β value of univariate Cox regression. **(C, D)** Kaplan–Meier curves for *FBN1* and *LAMC1* by best cut off value in the meta cohort. *FBN1*: HR, 1.74, Log-rank p-value = 1.1×10^{-11}. *LAMC1*: HR, 1.71, Log-rank p-value = 3.1×10^{-11}. **(E, F)** Transwell invasion assay performed in AGS and Hs746T cells transfected with control siRNA, *FBN1* siRNA, or *LAMC1* siRNA. **(G)** Apoptosis was determined using fluorescence activated cell sorting (FACS) analysis by Annexin V-FITC and propidium iodide (PI) co-staining (left panel), and Annexin V^+ cell populations were defined as apoptotic (right panel). Statistical p-value (*P < 0.05; **P < 0.01; ***P < 0.001; ns, not significant).

with *LAMC1* or *FBN1* knockdown for 48 h. Knocking down *LAMC1* or *FBN1* did not influence the survival of Hs746T or AGS cells. However, knocking down *LAMC1* or *FBN1*, or both could sensitize Hs746T cells to 5-FU; the same phenomenon was observed in AGS cells but with less significance. In addition, the mesenchymal-like Hs746T cell line was more tolerant to 5-FU than the epithelial-like AGS cell line (**Figure 5G**).

DISCUSSION

Growing evidence suggests that the ECM is an indispensable but enigmatic component of the tumor microenvironment (13, 15). Aberrant constitution of the ECM is involved in all the cellular processes throughout cancer initiation, progression, and dissemination, and, in most cases, correlated with more aggressive tumors and poorer prognosis (19). In breast cancer, researchers found that decellularized ECM from tumor-bearing and obese mammary glands drives triple-negative breast cancer (TNBC) cell invasion, and collagen VI was found to be the driver protein by proteomic analysis (47). In colon cancer, Romero-López et al. (48) extracted and compared ECM from normal human colon and colon tumor that had metastasized to liver and even seeded tumor cells in these ECM. The results showed that cells seeded in tumor ECM had higher levels of free NADH along with glycolytic rate and more capable of inducing tumor-like vasculature compared with those seeded in normal ECM. Contradictorily, in pancreatic ductal adenocarcinoma, decreasing ECM with an anti-LOXL2 antibody *in vivo* boosted tumor growth and diminished overall survival, suggesting a protective role of ECM (20). Also, in melanoma, there is evidence that aging fibroblasts were less capable of secreting ECM, especially HAPLN1, resulting in a more aligned ECM that promoted metastasis of melanoma cells (49). Hence, it seems that the ECM also share heterogeneity among different tumor types and the interplay between ECM and tumor cells is still intricate.

Additionally, the ECM is also an interference factor during anti-tumor therapy. Excessive ECM deposition and stiffening in solid tumors could also induce physical and biological barriers for chemotherapy, a major problem faced by current cancer research. For example, ECM deposition in liver metastasis of colorectal tumor could enhance angiogenesis and anti-angiogenic therapy resistance, while inhibiting ECM deposition with drugs targeting the renin-angiotensin system could reverse resistance to anti-angiogenic bevacizumab (22). Also, decreasing ECM stiffness with lysyl oxidase (LOX) inhibitors increased drug penetration and overcame chemotherapy resistance in triple negative breast cancer (50). However, to date, the clinical and multi-omics characterization of the ECM in gastric cancer and the potential of the ECM to predict prognosis and chemotherapy response had not yet been systematically explored, neither did any clinical trials investigate the role of ECM deposition in anti-tumor therapy resistance.

Exploiting GSVA algorithms, we scored all the gene set canonical pathways and ECM was identified as core factor in gastric cancer progression with highest degree among all prognostic pathways in the overlap of four cohort. Then, we resolved the ECM constitution pattern and depicted the overall landscape of the clinical and multi-omics characterization of the ECM in gastric cancer. Integrated analysis detected that the ECM score performed well to predict the prognosis and chemotherapy response in gastric cancer. The ECM score was a robust risk factor in different stage of gastric cancer and in different cohorts. It was verified in both the TCGA-STAD cohort and the KUGH, YUSH, and KUCM cohorts that chemotherapy showed a poor effect in patients with gastric cancer with a high ECM score, the result of which might be instructional for precision medicine.

In the ACRG cohort, the ECM score was exclusively high in patients with the EMT molecular subtype. Previous studies had identified EMT or a mesenchymal phenotype as predicators for poor prognosis and resistance to anti-cancer drug therapy in multiple cancer types (8, 30, 51–53). The EMT-like change could also enable cancer cells to acquire a cancer stem cell phenotype, which has received unanimous acceptance as the backbone of drug resistance (30). Counterintuitively, our results showed that cancers with a higher ECM score showed a remarkably low level of proliferation activity, which might be ascribed to the dominant state of CSCs. There is considerable evidence demonstrating that ECM remodeling could be the upstream signal that regulates the EMT or CSCs phenotype through a mechanochemical pathway in cancer cells (15, 54–56).

In the TCGA-STAD cohort, the ECM score was exclusively high in patients of the GS molecular subtype. The GS molecular subtype is characterized by a low TMB. Most chemotherapy imposes DNA damage on rapidly proliferating cancer cells that lack adequate DNA repair (35). Hence, we deduced that gene stability and relatively slow DNA replication could restrain the effectiveness of chemotherapeutic drugs, which happened to be the feature of those cancers with a high ECM score. Our results demonstrated that the ECM score was closely related to the TMB as well as CNV, further explaining its capacity to predict drug response.

The role of non-genetic or epigenetic mechanisms to regulate drug resistance is vital but poorly understood. Aberrant epigenetic regulation is common among all tumor types and has long been considered as a regulator of drug resistance, and several epigenetic therapies have been involved in preclinical trials (57–60). Our data indicated that ECM deposition in gastric cancer might alter epigenetic states, thus influencing the drug response. Determining the interconnection between ECM remodeling and epigenetic alteration would deepen our understanding of drug-tolerant cancer.

Increased use of immunotherapy has revealed the presence of immune tolerance (61–64). It is not surprising that in accordance with our results, the tumor-associated ECM could also have immune modulatory effects and could regulate the migration and localization of immune cells (65, 66). Actually, combined treatment targeting both the immune and stroma microenvironment could lead to remarkable therapeutic effects (67, 68). Finally, we chose two representative ECM genes, *LAMC1* and *FBN1*, to further verify our findings. Knocking down these two genes impaired the invasion ability of cancer cells and sensitized cancer cells to chemotherapeutic drugs, which, to some extent, corroborated our analyses.

In short, in the current study, gene expression analysis identified ECM as the driving factor involved in gastric cancer progression. Hence, we systematically discussed the landscape of clinical, biological, and multi-omics characterization of the ECM constitution pattern in gastric cancer and found a higher ECM score is tightly associated with an epithelial to mesenchyme transition (EMT) phenotype, a gene stable (GS) molecular subtype, markedly lower somatic mutation rates, and a lower level of DNA methylation. In addition, the ECM score was identified as robust prognostic biomarker and predictive factor for the response to chemotherapy resistance, which was further verified experimentally. Our findings imply that ECM may foster chemotherapy resistance in gastric cancer genetically and epigenetically. Further investigation would help to solve the enigma of chemoresistance acquisition. The establishment of ECM score could also help to design personalized and precise chemotherapy and provide inspiration to develop combination therapy. Nevertheless, our study has some limitations as well. Detailed information regarding the treatment history of the enrolled patients with gastric cancer was inadequate, such as the prescription and duration of the chemotherapy, and the receipt of any other treatment, which would interfere with the precise identification of the best cut off point. Further treatment information gathering would help to refine the prediction model. Additionally, tumor heterogeneity is the main cause of chemotherapy tolerance, which means that sequencing of mixed tumor tissues might inevitably lead to bias. Standardized and sub-regional sample collection and, if conditional, single cell sequencing, would ensure an in-depth exploration of the role of the ECM in chemoresistance.

AUTHOR CONTRIBUTIONS

Conception and design of the study: XX, JC, and WG. Data collection and preprocessing: ML and XZ. Analysis and interpretation of data: ZY and FX. Manuscript writing: ZY, ML, and XZ. Study selection, *in vitro* experiment and statistical expertise: CW, EX, XW, LZ, HY, CR, HW, and YW. All authors contributed to the article and approved the submitted version.

REFERENCES

1. Smyth EC, Nilsson M, Grabsch HI, van Grieken NC, Lordick F. Gastric Cancer. *Lancet* (2020) 396:635–48. doi: 10.1016/S0140-6736(20)31288-5
2. Kang YK, Boku N, Satoh T, Ryu MH, Chao Y, Kato K, et al. Nivolumab in Patients With Advanced Gastric or Gastro-Oesophageal Junction Cancer Refractory to, or Intolerant of, at Least Two Previous Chemotherapy Regimens (ONO-4538-12, ATTRACTION-2): A Randomised, Double-Blind, Placebo-Controlled, Phase 3 Trial. *Lancet* (2017) 390:2461–71. doi: 10.1016/S0140-6736(17)31827-5
3. Noh SH, Park SR, Yang HK, Chung HC, Chung IJ, Kim SW, et al. Adjuvant Capecitabine Plus Oxaliplatin for Gastric Cancer After D2 Gastrectomy (CLASSIC): 5-Year Follow-Up of an Open-Label, Randomised Phase 3 Trial. *Lancet Oncol* (2014) 15:1389–96. doi: 10.1016/S1470-2045(14)70473-5
4. Jiang Y, Li T, Liang X, Hu Y, Huang L, Liao Z, et al. Association of Adjuvant Chemotherapy With Survival in Patients With Stage II or III Gastric Cancer. *JAMA Surg* (2017) 152:e171087. doi: 10.1001/jamasurg.2017.1087
5. Liu Y, Sethi NS, Hinoue T, Schneider BG, Cherniack AD, Sanchez-Vega F, et al. Comparative Molecular Analysis of Gastrointestinal Adenocarcinomas. *Cancer Cell* (2018) 33:721–35.e8. doi: 10.1016/j.ccell.2018.03.010
6. Bass AJ, Thorsson V, Shmulevich I, Reynolds SM, Miller M, Bernard B, et al. Comprehensive Molecular Characterization of Gastric Adenocarcinoma. *Nature* (2014) 513:202–9. doi: 10.1038/nature13480
7. Cristescu R, Lee J, Nebozhyn M, Kim K-M, Ting JC, Wong SS, et al. Molecular Analysis of Gastric Cancer Identifies Subtypes Associated With Distinct Clinical Outcomes. *Nat Med* (2015) 21:449–56. doi: 10.1038/nm.3850
8. Oh SC, Sohn BH, Cheong J-H, Kim S-B, Lee JE, Park KC, et al. Clinical and Genomic Landscape of Gastric Cancer With a Mesenchymal Phenotype. *Nat Commun* (2018) 9:1777. doi: 10.1038/s41467-018-04179-8
9. Zeng D, Li M, Zhou R, Zhang J, Sun H, Shi M, et al. Tumor Microenvironment Characterization in Gastric Cancer Identifies Prognostic and Immunotherapeutically Relevant Gene Signatures. *Cancer Immunol Res* (2019) 7:737–50. doi: 10.1158/2326-6066.CIR-18-0436
10. Zhang B, Wu Q, Li B, Wang D, Wang L, Zhou YL. M6a Regulator-Mediated Methylation Modification Patterns and Tumor Microenvironment Infiltration Characterization in Gastric Cancer. *Mol Cancer* (2020) 19:53. doi: 10.1186/s12943-020-01170-0
11. Cheong J-H, Yang H-K, Kim H, Kim WH, Kim Y-W, Kook M-C, et al. Predictive Test for Chemotherapy Response in Resectable Gastric Cancer: A Multi-Cohort, Retrospective Analysis. *Lancet Oncol* (2018) 19:629–38. doi: 10.1016/S1470-2045(18)30108-6
12. Mammoto T, Ingber DE. Mechanical Control of Tissue and Organ Development. *Development* (2010) 137:1407–20. doi: 10.1242/dev.024166
13. Hynes RO. The Extracellular Matrix: Not Just Pretty Fibrils. *Science* (2009) 326:1216–9. doi: 10.1126/science.1176009
14. Hanahan D, Weinberg RA. Hallmarks of Cancer: The Next Generation. *Cell* (2011) 144:646–74. doi: 10.1016/j.cell.2011.02.013
15. Pickup MW, Mouw JK, Weaver VM. The Extracellular Matrix Modulates the Hallmarks of Cancer. *EMBO Rep* (2014) 15:1243–53. doi: 10.15252/embr.201439246
16. Panciera T, Citron A, Di Biagio D, Battilana G, Gandin A, Giulitti S, et al. Reprogramming Normal Cells Into Tumour Precursors Requires ECM Stiffness and Oncogene-Mediated Changes of Cell Mechanical Properties. *Nat Mater* (2020) 19:797–806. doi: 10.1038/s41563-020-0615-x
17. Wei SC, Fattet L, Tsai JH, Guo Y, Pai VH, Majeski HE, et al. Matrix Stiffness Drives Epithelial-Mesenchymal Transition and Tumour Metastasis Through a TWIST1-G3BP2 Mechanotransduction Pathway. *Nat Cell Biol* (2015) 17:678–88. doi: 10.1038/ncb3157
18. Jang M, An J, Oh SW, Lim JY, Kim J, Choi JK, et al. Matrix Stiffness Epigenetically Regulates the Oncogenic Activation of the Yes-Associated Protein in Gastric Cancer. *Nat BioMed Eng* (2021) 5:114–23. doi: 10.1038/s41551-020-00657-x
19. Socovich AM, Naba A. The Cancer Matrisome: From Comprehensive Characterization to Biomarker Discovery. *Semin Cell Dev Biol* (2019) 89:157–66. doi: 10.1016/j.semcdb.2018.06.005
20. Jiang H, Torphy RJ, Steiger K, Hongo H, Ritchie AJ, Kriegsmann M, et al. Pancreatic Ductal Adenocarcinoma Progression Is Restrained by Stromal Matrix. *J Clin Invest* (2020) 130:4704–9. doi: 10.1172/JCI136760
21. Chakravarthy A, Khan L, Bensler NP, Bose P. Carvalho DD De. TGF-β-Associated Extracellular Matrix Genes Link Cancer-Associated Fibroblasts to Immune Evasion and Immunotherapy Failure. *Nat Commun* (2018) 9:4692. doi: 10.1038/s41467-018-06654-8
22. Shen Y, Wang X, Lu J, Salfenmoser M, Wirsik NM, Schleussner N, et al. Reduction of Liver Metastasis Stiffness Improves Response to Bevacizumab in Metastatic Colorectal Cancer. *Cancer Cell* (2020) 37:800–17.e7. doi: 10.1016/j.ccell.2020.05.005
23. Bolstad BM, Irizarry RA, Astrand M. Speed TP. A Comparison of Normalization Methods for High Density Oligonucleotide Array Data Based on Variance and Bias. *Bioinformatics* (2003) 19:185–93. doi: 10.1093/bioinformatics/19.2.185
24. Liberzon A, Birger C, Thorvaldsdottir H, Ghandi M, Mesirov JP, Tamayo P. The Molecular Signatures Database (MSigDB) Hallmark Gene Set Collection. *Cell Syst* (2015) 1:417–25. doi: 10.1016/j.cels.2015.12.004
25. Hanzelmann S, Castelo R, Guinney J. GSVA: Gene Set Variation Analysis for Microarray and RNA-Seq Data. *BMC Bioinf* (2013) 14:7. doi: 10.1186/1471-2105-14-7
26. Shao X, Taha IN, Clauser KR, Gao YT, Naba A. MatrisomeDB: The ECM-Protein Knowledge Database. *Nucleic Acids Res* (2020) 48:D1136–44. doi: 10.1093/nar/gkz849
27. Newman AM, Liu CL, Green MR, Gentles AJ, Feng W, Xu Y, et al. Robust Enumeration of Cell Subsets From Tissue Expression Profiles. *Nat Methods* (2015) 12:453–7. doi: 10.1038/nmeth.3337
28. Hazra A, Gogtay N. Biostatistics Series Module 3: Comparing Groups: Numerical Variables. *Indian J Dermatol* (2016) 61:251–60. doi: 10.4103/0019-5154.182416
29. Cohen J. *Statistical Power Analysis for the Behavioral Sciences*. Hoboken: Taylor and Francis (2013).
30. Shibue T, Weinberg RA. EMT, CSCs, and Drug Resistance: The Mechanistic Link and Clinical Implications. *Nat Rev Clin Oncol* (2017) 14:611–29. doi: 10.1038/nrclinonc.2017.44
31. Holohan C, van Schaeybroeck S, Longley DB, Johnston PG. Cancer Drug Resistance: An Evolving Paradigm. *Nat Rev Cancer* (2013) 13:714–26. doi: 10.1038/nrc3599
32. Mariathasan S, Turley SJ, Nickles D, Castiglioni A, Yuen K, Wang Y, et al. Tgfβ Attenuates Tumour Response to PD-L1 Blockade by Contributing to Exclusion of T Cells. *Nature* (2018) 554:544–8. doi: 10.1038/nature25501
33. Klein O, Kee D, Markman B, Carlino MS, Underhill C, Palmer J, et al. Evaluation of TMB as a Predictive Biomarker in Patients With Solid Cancers

Treated With Anti-PD-1/CTLA-4 Combination Immunotherapy. *Cancer Cell* (2021) 39:592–3. doi: 10.1016/j.ccell.2021.04.005

34. Samstein RM, Lee C-H, Shoushtari AN, Hellmann MD, Shen R, Janjigian YY, et al. Tumor Mutational Load Predicts Survival After Immunotherapy Across Multiple Cancer Types. *Nat Genet* (2019) 51:202–6. doi: 10.1038/s41588-018-0312-8
35. Bouwman P, Jonkers J. The Effects of Deregulated DNA Damage Signalling on Cancer Chemotherapy Response and Resistance. *Nat Rev Cancer* (2012) 12:587–98. doi: 10.1038/nrc3342
36. Morel D, Jeffery D, Aspeslagh S, Almouzni G, Postel-Vinay S. Combining Epigenetic Drugs With Other Therapies for Solid Tumours - Past Lessons and Future Promise. *Nat Rev Clin Oncol* (2020) 17:91–107. doi: 10.1038/s41571-019-0267-4
37. Brown R, Curry E, Magnani L, Wilhelm-Benartzi CS, Borley J. Poised Epigenetic States and Acquired Drug Resistance in Cancer. *Nat Rev Cancer* (2014) 14:747–53. doi: 10.1038/nrc3819
38. Jones PA, Ohtani H, Chakravarthy A, de Carvalho DD. Epigenetic Therapy in Immune-Oncology. *Nat Rev Cancer* (2019) 19:151–61. doi: 10.1038/s41568-019-0109-9
39. Leitch HG, Surani MA, Hajkova P. DNA (De)Methylation: The Passive Route to Naïvety? *Trends Genet* (2016) 32:592–5. doi: 10.1016/j.tig.2016.08.005
40. Wainwright EN, Scaffidi P. Epigenetics and Cancer Stem Cells: Unleashing, Hijacking, and Restricting Cellular Plasticity. *Trends Cancer* (2017) 3:372–86. doi: 10.1016/j.trecan.2017.04.004
41. Zilberberg L, Todorovic V, Dabovic B, Horiguchi M, Couroussé T, Sakai LY, et al. Specificity of Latent TGF-β Binding Protein (LTBP) Incorporation Into Matrix: Role of Fibrillins and Fibronectin. *J Cell Physiol* (2012) 227:3828–36. doi: 10.1002/jcp.24094
42. Godwin AR, Singh M, Lockhart-Cairns MP, Alanazi YF, Cain SA, Baldock C. The Role of Fibrillin and Microfibril Binding Proteins in Elastin and Elastic Fibre Assembly. *Matrix Biol* (2019) 84:17–30. doi: 10.1016/j.matbio.2019.06.006
43. Han Z-R, Jiang X-L, Fan W-C. LAMC1 s Related to the Poor Prognosis of Patients With Gastric Cancer and Facilitates Cancer Cell Malignancies. *Neoplasma* (2021) 8(4):711–8. doi: 10.4149/neo_2021_201117N1239
44. Liu J, Liu D, Yang Z, Yang Z. High LAMC1 Expression in Glioma s Associated With Poor Prognosis. *Onco Targets Ther* (2019) 12:4253–60. doi: 10.2147/OTT.S205333
45. Ye G, Qin Y, Wang S, Pan D, Xu S, Wu C, et al. Lamc1 Promotes the Warburg Effect in Hepatocellular Carcinoma Cells by Regulating PKM2 Expression Through AKT Pathway. *Cancer Biol Ther* (2019) 20:711–9. doi: 10.1080/15384047.2018.1564558
46. Kashima H, Wu R-C, Wang Y, Sinno AK, Miyamoto T, Shiozawa T, et al. Laminin C1 Expression by Uterine Carcinoma Cells s Associated With Tumor Progression. *Gynecol Oncol* (2015) 139:338–44. doi: 10.1016/j.ygyno.2015.08.025
47. Wishart AL, Conner SJ, Guarin JR, Fatherree JP, Peng Y, McGinn RA, et al. Decellularized Extracellular Matrix Scaffolds Identify Full-Length Collagen VI as a Driver of Breast Cancer Cell Invasion in Obesity and Metastasis. *Sci Adv* (2020) 6(43):eabc3175. doi: 10.1126/sciadv.abc3175
48. Romero-López M, Trinh AL, Sobrino A, Hatch MM, Keating MT, Fimbres C, et al. Recapitulating the Human Tumor Microenvironment: Colon Tumor-Derived Extracellular Matrix Promotes Angiogenesis and Tumor Cell Growth. *Biomaterials* (2017) 116:118–29. doi: 10.1016/j.biomaterials.2016.11.034
49. Kaur A, Ecker BL, Douglass SM, Kugel CH, Webster MR, Almeida FV, et al. Remodeling of the Collagen Matrix in Aging Skin Promotes Melanoma Metastasis and Affects Immune Cell Motility. *Cancer Discov* (2019) 9:64–81. doi: 10.1158/2159-8290.CD-18-0193
50. Saatci O, Kaymak A, Raza U, Ersan PG, Akbulut O, Banister CE, et al. Targeting Lysyl Oxidase (LOX) Overcomes Chemotherapy Resistance in Triple Negative Breast Cancer. *Nat Commun* (2020) 11:2416. doi: 10.1038/s41467-020-16199-4
51. Byers LA, Diao L, Wang J, Saintigny P, Girard L, Peyton M, et al. An Epithelial-Mesenchymal Transition Gene Signature Predicts Resistance to EGFR and PI3K Inhibitors and Identifies Axl as a Therapeutic Target for Overcoming EGFR Inhibitor Resistance. *Clin Cancer Res* (2013) 19:279–90. doi: 10.1158/1078-0432.ccr-12-1558
52. Farmer P, Bonnefoi H, Anderle P, Cameron D, Wirapati P, Wirapati P, et al. A Stroma-Related Gene Signature Predicts Resistance to Neoadjuvant Chemotherapy in Breast Cancer. *Nat Med* (2009) 15:68–74. doi: 10.1038/nm.1908
53. Zheng X, Carstens JL, Kim J, Scheible M, Kaye J, Sugimoto H, et al. Epithelial-To-Mesenchymal Transition Is Dispensable for Metastasis But Induces Chemoresistance in Pancreatic Cancer. *Nature* (2015) 527:525–30. doi: 10.1038/nature16064
54. Plotnikov SV, Pasapera AM, Sabass B, Waterman CM. Force Fluctuations Within Focal Adhesions Mediate ECM-Rigidity Sensing to Guide Directed Cell Migration. *Cell* (2012) 151:1513–27. doi: 10.1016/j.cell.2012.11.034
55. Vogel V. Unraveling the Mechanobiology of Extracellular Matrix. *Annu Rev Physiol* (2018) 80:353–87. doi: 10.1146/annurev-physiol-021317-121312
56. Kesh K, Gupta VK, Durden B, Garrido V, Mateo-Victoriano B, Lavania SP, et al. Therapy Resistance, Cancer Stem Cells and ECM in Cancer: The Matrix Reloaded. *Cancers (Basel)* (2020) 12(10):3067. doi: 10.3390/cancers12103067
57. Baylin SB, Jones PA. A Decade of Exploring the Cancer Epigenome - Biological and Translational Implications. *Nat Rev Cancer* (2011) 11:726–34. doi: 10.1038/nrc3130
58. Glasspool RM, Teodoridis JM, Brown R. Epigenetics as a Mechanism Driving Polygenic Clinical Drug Resistance. *Br J Cancer* (2006) 94:1087–92. doi: 10.1038/sj.bjc.6603024
59. Easwaran H, Tsai H-C, Baylin SB. Cancer Epigenetics: Tumor Heterogeneity, Plasticity of Stem-Like States, and Drug Resistance. *Mol Cell* (2014) 54:716–27. doi: 10.1016/j.molcel.2014.05.015
60. Zhang Y-W, Zheng Y, Wang J-Z, Lu X-X, Wang Z, Chen L-B, et al. Integrated Analysis of DNA Methylation and mRNA Expression Profiling Reveals Candidate Genes Associated With Cisplatin Resistance in Non-Small Cell Lung Cancer. *Epigenetics* (2014) 9:896–909. doi: 10.4161/epi.28601
61. Sharma P, Hu-Lieskovan S, Wargo JA, Ribas A. Primary, Adaptive, and Acquired Resistance to Cancer Immunotherapy. *Cell* (2017) 168:707–23. doi: 10.1016/j.cell.2017.01.017
62. Lovly CM, Shaw AT. Molecular Pathways: Resistance to Kinase Inhibitors and Implications for Therapeutic Strategies. *Clin Cancer Res* (2014) 20:2249–56. doi: 10.1158/1078-0432.CCR-13-1610
63. Kalbasi A, Ribas A. Tumour-Intrinsic Resistance to Immune Checkpoint Blockade. *Nat Rev Immunol* (2020) 20:25–39. doi: 10.1038/s41577-019-0218-4
64. Aldea M, Andre F, Marabelle A, Dogan S, Barlesi F, Soria J-C. Overcoming Resistance to Tumor-Targeted and Immune-Targeted Therapies. *Cancer Discov* (2021) 11:874–99. doi: 10.1158/2159-8290.cd-20-1638
65. Salmon H, Franciszkiewicz K, Damotte D, Dieu-Nosjean M-C, Validire P, Trautmann A, et al. Matrix Architecture Defines the Preferential Localization and Migration of T Cells Into the Stroma of Human Lung Tumors. *J Clin Invest* (2012) 122:899–910. doi: 10.1172/JCI45817
66. Gajewski TF, Schreiber H, Fu Y-X. Innate and Adaptive Immune Cells in the Tumor Microenvironment. *Nat Immunol* (2013) 14:1014–22. doi: 10.1038/ni.2703
67. Ravi R, Noonan KA, Pham V, Bedi R, Zhavoronkov A, Ozerov IV, et al. Bifunctional Immune Checkpoint-Targeted Antibody-Ligand Traps That Simultaneously Disable Tgfβ Enhance the Efficacy of Cancer Immunotherapy. *Nat Commun* (2018) 9:741. doi: 10.1038/s41467-017-02696-6
68. Lan Y, Zhang D, Xu C, Hance KW, Marelli B, Qi J, et al. Enhanced Preclinical Antitumor Activity of M7824, a Bifunctional Fusion Protein Simultaneously Targeting PD-L1 and TGF-β. *Sci Transl Med* (2018) 10(424):eaan5488. doi: 10.1126/scitranslmed.aan5488

22

Perineural Invasion and Postoperative Adjuvant Chemotherapy Efficacy in Patients with Gastric Cancer

Qing Tao [1†], Wen Zhu [1†], Xiaohui Zhao [2], Mei Li [2], Yongqian Shu [3], Deqiang Wang [1] and Xiaoqin Li [1*]*

[1] Department of Medical Oncology, Affiliated Hospital of Jiangsu University, Zhenjiang, China, [2] Department of Pathology, Affiliated Hospital of Jiangsu University, Zhenjiang, China, [3] Department of Medical Oncology, Jiangsu Province Hospital, Nanjing, China

Correspondence:
Deqiang Wang
deqiang_wang@aliyun.com
Xiaoqin Li
1000011452@ujs.edu.cn

†These authors have contributed equally to this work

Purpose: There is currently a lack of validated predictors for adjuvant chemotherapy efficacy in patients with gastric cancer (GC). Perineural invasion (PNI) is the process of neoplastic invasion of the nerves, accompanied by tumor microenvironment (TME) changes. TME can determine treatment outcome while the impact of PNI on chemotherapy efficacy remains unknown in GC. We investigated the association between PNI and the efficacy of postoperative adjuvant chemotherapy in patients with resected GC.

Methods: Patients who underwent radical resection of stage IB-III GC with or without fluoropyrimidine (FU)-based adjuvant chemotherapy were retrospectively selected from two separate patient cohorts. PNI was confirmed with S100 immunohistochemistry (IHC). Tumor hypoxia and activity of selected pathways were quantified by mRNA-based signature scoring based on publicly available data. A hypoxia biomarker, ERO1A, and a FU resistance biomarker, thymidylate synthase (TS), were assessed by IHC, respectively.

Results: Two cohorts included 223 and 599 patients, respectively. Adjuvant chemotherapy significantly improved overall survival (OS) and disease-free survival (DFS) in PNI-positive but not in PNI-negative patients, which was not impacted by stages. Multivariate models showed that adjuvant chemotherapy was an independent predictor for OS and DFS in PNI-positive patients in both cohorts. For TME, PNI-negative tumors were more hypoxic than were PNI-positive tumors, and displayed relative up-regulation of signaling along the pathways that are important in FU metabolism or resistance. Expressions of ERO1A and TS significantly decreased in PNI-positive compared to PNI-negative tumors.

Conclusions: PNI might help predict adjuvant chemotherapy benefit in patients with resected GC. Validation in prospective studies is required. Novel treatment strategies need to be developed in PNI-negative patients.

Keywords: perineural invasion, gastric cancer, adjuvant chemotherapy, tumor microenvironment, hypoxia, thymidylate synthase

INTRODUCTION

China is the world leader in gastric cancer (GC) incidence (1). Currently, radical resection is the main curative method for GC. In East Asia, D2 radical gastrectomy is currently the standard procedure recommended for resectable GC (2). However, surgery alone is insufficient to remove GC and many patients remain at risk of local recurrence and distant metastasis. Randomized phase III clinical trials have demonstrated that fluoropyrimidine (FU)-based adjuvant chemotherapy, following radical gastrectomy, could significantly prolong survival of patients with GC compared to surgery alone (3, 4). Nevertheless, studies have shown that 30–40% of patients treated with surgery and adjuvant chemotherapy relapse within 5 years (3, 4), illustrating variability in response to adjuvant chemotherapy among patients and the need for predictive markers for the efficacy of adjuvant chemotherapy.

Perineural invasion (PNI) is the process of neoplastic invasion of the nerves. PNI is an important marker of local tumor progression, indicative of prognosis in many types of tumors (5, 6). PNI is common in GC; however, the relationship between PNI occurrence and GC prognosis is controversial. A meta-analysis (7) has reported that PNI occurrence affects disease-free survival (DFS) and overall survival (OS) in patients with resected GC. Nevertheless, the strength of evidence upon which this conclusion has been made is weak, as few studies have reported PNI-specific results; in addition, there was high heterogeneity between the studies included in pooled results. In particular, six studies included in this meta-analysis, which involved over 15,000 patients, did not support the independent prognostic role of PNI (7). Of note, the results from these studies were consistent with findings presented in two recent reports (8, 9).

While several studies have investigated the prognostic role of PNI, few studies have investigated the association between PNI and efficacy of adjuvant chemotherapy. In stage II colorectal cancer, Huh (10) found that adjuvant chemotherapy significantly improved 5-year DFS in PNI-positive but not in PNI-negative patients. This finding has been recently confirmed by Cienfuegos et al. (11). Moreover, Suzuki et al. (12) reported similar results in patients with stage III colorectal cancer. Finally, in a recent study, Song et al. (13) revealed that among patients with locally advanced rectal cancer treated with preoperative chemoradiotherapy and radical surgery, PNI-positive patients were more likely than PNI-negative patients to benefit from postoperative adjuvant chemotherapy when distant failure rate was the primary outcome of interest. These results suggest a role of PNI in predicting adjuvant chemotherapy efficacy in colorectal cancer. However, such a role of PNI in GC remains unknown.

The rationality of the potential association between PNI and treatment efficacy is strengthened by progress in understanding molecular mechanisms of PNI. Recent studies emphasize the interactions between perineural microenvironment (PME) and tumor cells (6). PME is composed of neural cells, supporting cells, extracellular matrix, blood vessels, and inflammatory and immune components. Nerve cells and tumor cells can interact directly or through complex signal transduction among various signaling molecules and their receptors. PNI occurs through changes in nerve cells, tumor cells, supporting cells and even the entire PME. Finally, PME evolves into tumor microenvironment (TME). Of note, clinical relevance of TME has been reported in various malignancies (14, 15). Particularly, TME evaluation has been validated as a robust predictor for the efficacy of immunotherapy and adjuvant chemotherapy in GC (16, 17). These findings indicate that PNI may impact treatment efficacy based on TME changes.

In this study, we used two independent patient cohorts to investigate the prognostic and predictive value of PNI in patients with resected GC. We also explored the potential mechanism underlying the clinical significance of PNI, which has not been previously reported, using public RNA sequencing data and a validation protocol for our samples.

MATERIALS AND METHODS

Patients

This study involved two patient cohorts. The Jiangsu Province Hospital (JPH) cohort included 223 patients with GC, diagnosed between 2011 and 2013 at the JPH, Nanjing. The Affiliated Hospital of Jiangsu University (AHJU) cohort included 599 patients with GC, admitted to the AHJU in Zhenjiang city between 2011 and 2016 and screened from a prospective GC database (18).

All patients met the following inclusion criteria: (1) age $\geq$18 and $\leq$75 years; (2) history of D2 radical gastrectomy with R0 resection; (3) pathologically-confirmed diagnosis of stage IB-III gastric adenocarcinoma; and (4) FU-based adjuvant chemotherapy or observation during post-surgical follow-up. FU-based adjuvant chemotherapy involved 5-fluorouracil, capecitabine, or S-1 (tegafur-gimeracil-oteracil potassium capsules). Patients were excluded from the study for the following: insufficient clinicopathological data or prior history of radiation therapy, other chemotherapies, or biologic targeted therapies, including neoadjuvant therapy. Clinical and clinicopathologic classification and stage of GC were determined according to the American Joint Committee on Cancer (AJCC) criteria. The hospital's ethics committee approved the research protocol, and all patients signed informed consent.

PNI Detection

Paraffin-embedded tissue sections of surgical specimens were used to assess PNI, which was defined according to previously reported criteria (5). S100 protein immunohistochemistry (IHC) staining, which is specific for nerves in gastric tissues, was used to assist in the detection of the nerves (19). Hematoxylin and eosin (HE) staining was used to confirm the nerve structure. For each specimen, three independent representative tissue sections were prepared, and the specimens were classified as PNI-positive when PNI was observed in any of the three sections.

IHC Analysis

Antibodies (Abcam, UK) of S100 (ab52642), thymidylate synthetase (TS, *TYMS*; ab108995) and ERO1A (ab177156) were used for IHC staining with the streptavidin-perosidase method based on a 2-step protocol (20). Positive S100 expression was

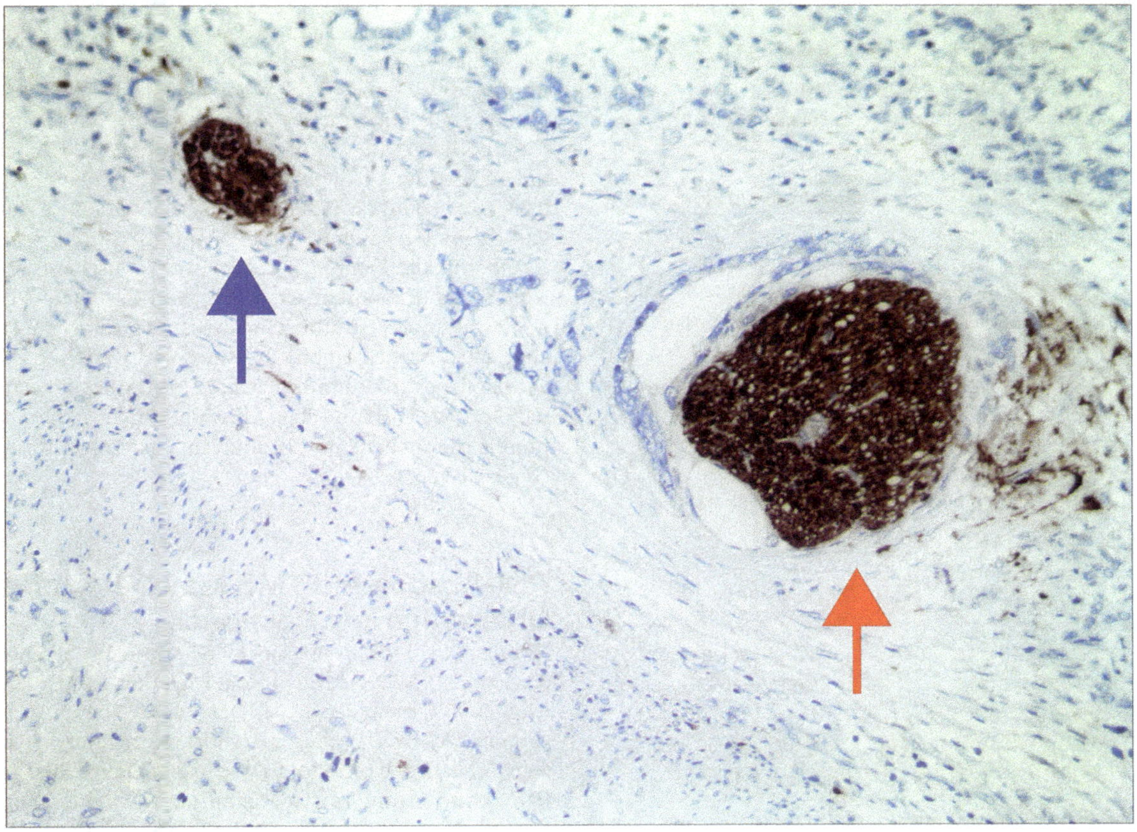

FIGURE 1 | Representative micrographs of nerves invaded (red arrow) and uninvaded (blue arrow) by tumors at 200× magnification.

defined as the presence of nerve staining irrespective of their proportion or intensity, however, S100 staining was generally strong in our samples. Positive TS expression was defined as the presence of nuclear and/or cytoplasm staining of tumor cells irrespective of their proportion or intensity. Positive ERO1A expression had been defined by Seol et al. (21).

Microarray Data

GC mRNA abundance data from the Asian Cancer Research Group (ACRG) are freely available and were downloaded from the NCBI Gene Expression Omnibus (GEO; GSE62254) and processed as previously described (16). Corresponding PNI data (**Table S1**) were obtained from the supplementary materials in published literature (22).

Signature Scoring

Tumor hypoxia were quantified through mRNA-based scoring, using R package known as the *Parametric Gene Set Enrichment Analysis* (PGSEA; http://www.bioconductor.org/), which is based on well-established signatures developed by others, as described elsewhere (23–27). The activities of the selected pathways were also quantified by the same method based on gene sets developed by The Kyoto Encyclopedia of Genes and Genomes (KEGG).

Statistical Analysis

Overall survival (OS) was defined as the time period from the date of operation to the end of follow-up or cancer-related death. Disease-free survival (DFS) was defined as the time period from the date of operation to the date of recurrence, metastasis, or end of follow-up. A two-sided χ^2 test, Student's *t*-test, or Mann–Whitney *U*-test, as required, were used to compare the groups of enumeration data. Correlation coefficient was computed by Spearman correlation analysis. Survival analysis was performed using the Kaplan–Meier method plus the Log-rank test. Prognostic factors were determined using univariate and multivariate Cox proportional hazards models. Hazard ratios (HR), along with their 95% confidence intervals (CIs), were calculated. Two-sided $p < 0.05$ was considered statistically significant. We used R (version 3.6.1) and R Bioconductor packages for all analyses.

RESULTS

Patient Characteristics

Typical micrograph of PNI is presented in **Figure 1**. The incidence of PNI was 33.6 and 56.3% in the JPH and AHJU cohort, respectively (**Table 1**). In both cohorts, PNI was more frequent in tumors with lymphovascular invasion and TNM stage

TABLE 1 | Patient characteristics according to status of perineural invasion.

Characteristic	JPH cohort: No (%)			AHJU cohort: No (%)		
	PNI- 148 (66.4)	PNI+ 75 (33.6)	*P*-value	PNI- 262 (43.7)	PNI+ 337 (56.3)	*P*-value
Age (years)						
<65	106 (65.4)	56 (34.6)	0.630	159 (46.0)	187 (54.0)	0.201
≥65	42 (68.9)	19 (31.1)		103 (40.7)	150 (59.3)	
Sex						
Female	46 (73.0)	17 (27.0)	0.187	74 (48.1)	80 (51.9)	0.211
Male	102 (63.8)	58 (36.3)		188 (42.2)	257 (57.8)	
Tumor location						
Non-cardia	96 (66.7)	48 (33.3)	0.898	141 (52.0)	130 (48.0)	<0.001
Cardia	52 (65.8)	27 (34.2)		121 (36.9)	207 (63.1)	
Histology grade						
I/II	73 (64.0)	41 (36.0)	0.451	168 (49.7)	170 (50.3)	0.001
III	75 (68.8)	34 (31.2)		94 (36.0)	167 (64.0)	
Lymphovascular invasion						
Negative	117 (70.9)	48 (29.1)	0.015	201 (50.1)	200 (49.9)	<0.001
Positive	31 (53.4)	27 (46.6)		61 (30.8)	137 (69.2)	
TNM stage						
IB/II	61 (77.2)	18 (22.8)	0.011	151 (63.4)	87 (36.6)	<0.001
III	87 (60.4)	57 (39.6)		111 (30.7)	250 (69.3)	
Adjuvant chemotherapy						
Untreated	15 (60.0)	10 (40.0)	0.474	76 (40.0)	114 (60.0)	0.209
Treated	133 (67.2)	65 (32.8)		186 (45.5)	223 (54.5)	

JPH, Jiangsu Province Hospital; AHJU, Affiliated Hospital of Jiangsu University.

III ($p < 0.05$). In the AHJU cohort, PNI was also more frequent in cardia tumors and tumors with histologic grade III ($p < 0.05$). Significant heterogeneity was observed for the clinicopathologic characteristics of patients between the JPH and AHJU cohorts, verifying that they were independent.

Association of PNI With Patient Prognosis

In the JPH cohort, PNI was not associated with OS or DFS ($p > 0.05$; **Figures 2A,B**). In the AHJU cohort, PNI was associated with poor OS ($p = 0.045$; **Figure 2C**) but it was not associated with DFS ($p > 0.05$; **Figure 2D**). However, multivariate analyses showed that PNI was not an independent predictor of OS (HR = 0.82, 95% CI: 0.58–1.15, $p = 0.243$; **Figure 2E**). Finally, PNI did not correlate with OS and DFS in a combined cohort including all patients ($p > 0.05$; **Figure S1**).

Association Between PNI and Chemotherapy Benefit

In the JPH cohort, FU-based adjuvant chemotherapy did not impact OS or DFS among patients with PNI-negative tumors ($p > 0.05$; **Figures 3A,B**). In contrast, adjuvant chemotherapy improved OS and DFS among patients with PNI-positive tumors ($p < 0.05$; **Figures 3C,D**). The multivariate models indicated that adjuvant chemotherapy was an independent predictor for both OS (HR = 0.38, 95% CI: 0.17–0.88, $p = 0.023$) and DFS (HR = 0.33, 95% CI: 0.15–0.74, $p = 0.008$) among patients with PNI-positive tumors (**Figure 3E**).

Similarly, in the AHJU cohort, adjuvant chemotherapy improved OS and DFS among patients with PNI-positive tumors but not among patients with PNI-negative tumors (**Figures 4A–D**). Moreover, adjuvant chemotherapy independently predicted OS (HR = 0.57, 95% CI: 0.38–0.85, $p = 0.006$) and DFS (HR = 0.63, 95% CI: 0.44–0.90, $p = 0.011$) among patients with PNI-positive tumors (**Figure 4E**). Results for the combined cohort were consistent with findings from separate cohort analyses (**Figure S2**).

Furthermore, stratified analyses according to stages were conducted in the combined cohort, and we found that patients with PNI-positive tumors benefited from adjuvant chemotherapy in both stage IB/II and stage III while patients with PNI-negative tumors cannot benefit from adjuvant chemotherapy in any stages (**Figure S3**).

PNI-Associated TME May Determine Chemotherapy Response

Hypoxia in TME is a critical determinant of chemotherapy efficacy (28). We quantified tumor hypoxia in ACRG (**Table S2**), using well-established mRNA-based hypoxia signatures (**Figure 5A**). PNI-negative tumors were more hypoxic than were PNI-positive tumors ($p < 0.05$; **Figure 5B**). In contrast, PNI-positive tumors had significantly higher Yang hypoxia signature scores ($p < 0.05$; **Figure 5B**), which predicted favorable therapy response in patients with bladder cancer (27).

In order to verify the hypoxia difference between PNI-positive and PNI-negative tumors, we detected the protein expression of ERO1A, a novel endogenous marker of hypoxia in cancer (29), in 49 GC tissues of the AHJU cohort (**Figure 5C**). The ERO1A-positive rate was significantly lower in PNI-positive tumors than in PNI-negative tumors ($p = 0.015$; **Figure 5D**).

Hypoxia renders tumors resistant to chemotherapy by affecting signaling crucial for therapy response (28). As a result, we chose to observe the KEGG pathways, which could impact FU metabolism or sensitivity, including entries of pyrimidine metabolism, one carbon pool by folate, and antifolate resistance. We conducted signature scoring for these pathways in ACRG (**Figure 6A**; **Table S3**). These pathway scores significantly correlated with hypoxia scores ($p < 0.05$; **Figure 6B**). Then, we found that PNI-positive tumors obtained significantly lower scores for the pathways of interest than did PNI-negative tumors ($p < 0.05$; **Figure 6C**).

We next analyzed the relationship between PNI and *TYMS* mRNA expression, a biomarker of FU resistance and a key enzyme in all of the abovementioned pathways (30). We revealed that *TYMS* mRNA significantly correlated with hypoxia scores (**Figure 6B**) and reduced in PNI-positive compared to PNI-negative tumors ($p < 0.001$; **Figure 6C**). Furthermore, protein expression of TS, encoding by *TYMS*, was assessed by using IHC in the AHJU cohort (**Figure 6D**). The TS-positive rate was also significantly lower in PNI-positive tumors than in PNI-negative tumors ($p = 0.013$; **Figure 6E**).

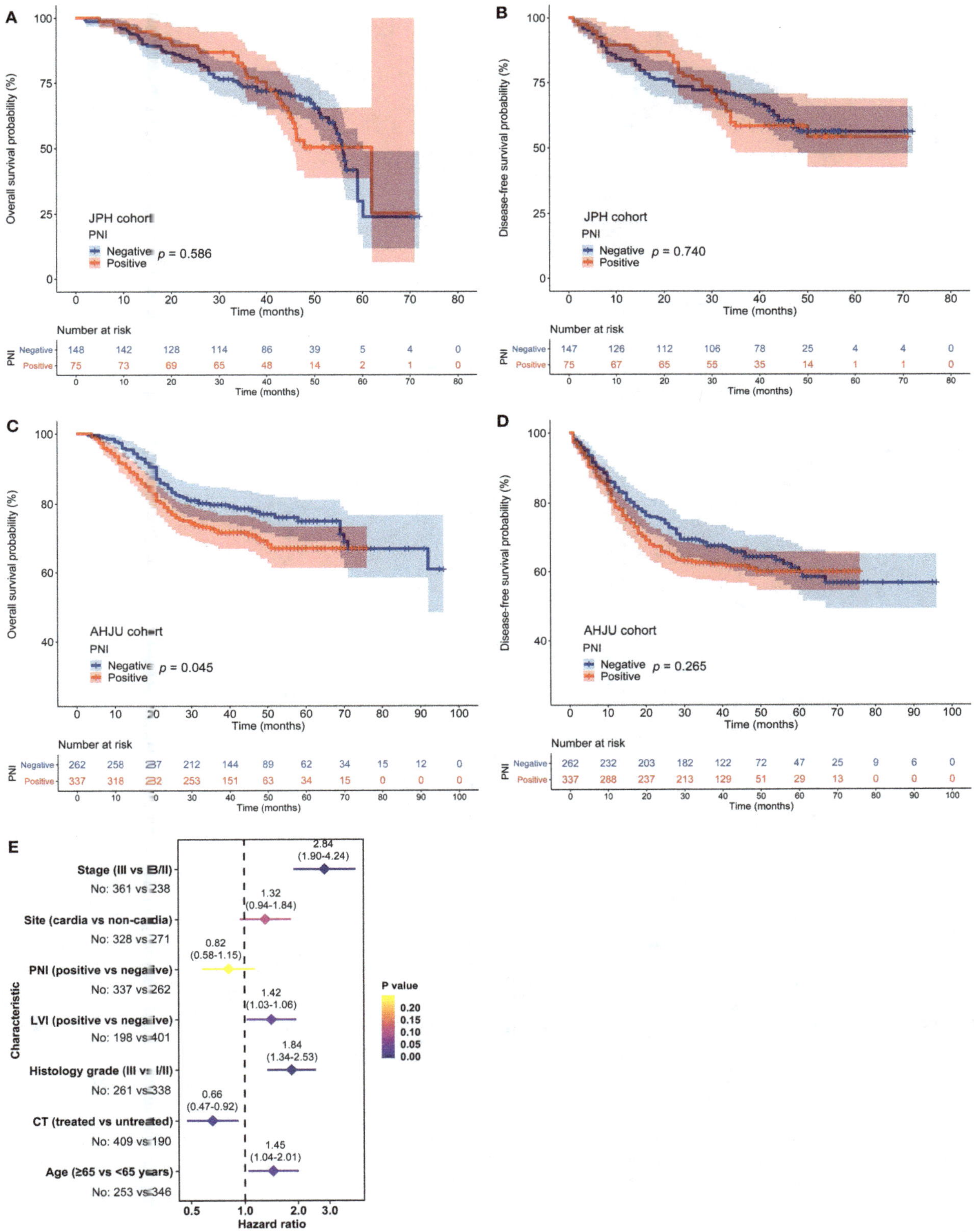

FIGURE 2 | Impact of perineural invasion (PNI) on patient survival. **(A–D)** Overall survival (OS) and disease-free survival in patients with resected gastric cancer according to PNI status. **(E)** Multivariate analyses of variables associated with OS, selected for their prognostic significance established in univariate analysis. LVI, lymphovascular invasion; CT, chemotherapy.

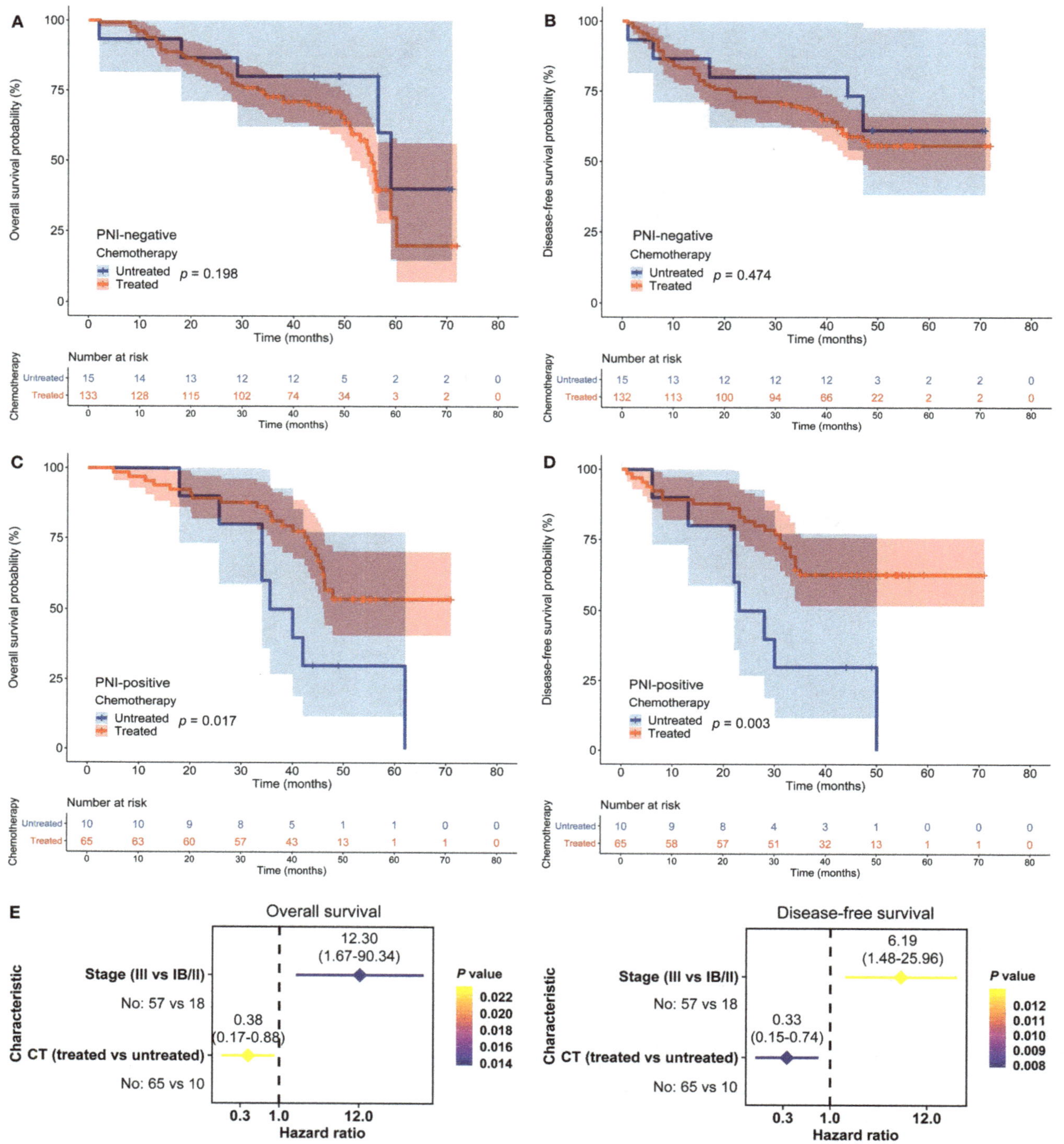

FIGURE 3 | Impact of perineural invasion (PNI) on the efficacy of adjuvant chemotherapy in the Jiangsu Province Hospital cohort. **(A–D)** Overall survival (OS) and disease-free survival (DFS) in patients with resected gastric cancer according to PNI and treatment status. **(E)** Multivariate analyses of variables associated with OS and DFS, selected for their prognostic significance established in univariate analysis. CT, chemotherapy.

DISCUSSION

Previous studies have shown significant genetic and biological heterogeneity among patients with GC, suggesting that prognostic or predictive markers are required to improve patient outcomes. Progress in understanding molecular mechanisms of GC has contributed to the development of novel biomarkers (22, 31), which often involve complex equipment and procedures,

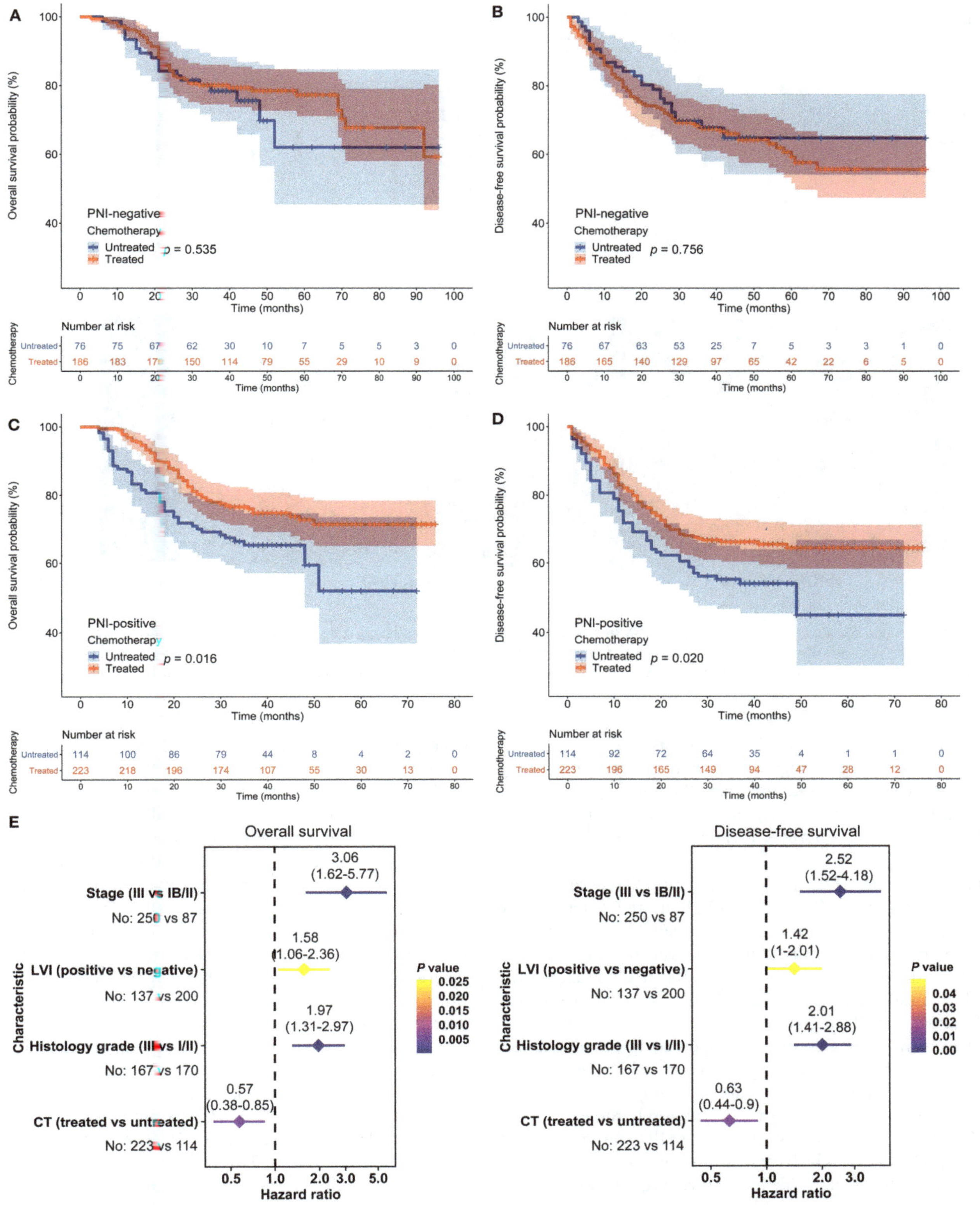

FIGURE 4 | Impact of perineural invasion (PNI) on the efficacy of adjuvant chemotherapy in the Affiliated Hospital of Jiangsu University cohort. **(A–D)** Overall survival (OS) and disease-free survival (DFS) in patients with resected gastric cancer according to PNI and treatment status. **(E)** Multivariate analyses of variables associated with OS and DFS, selected for their prognostic significance established in univariate analysis. LVI, lymphovascular invasion; CT, chemotherapy.

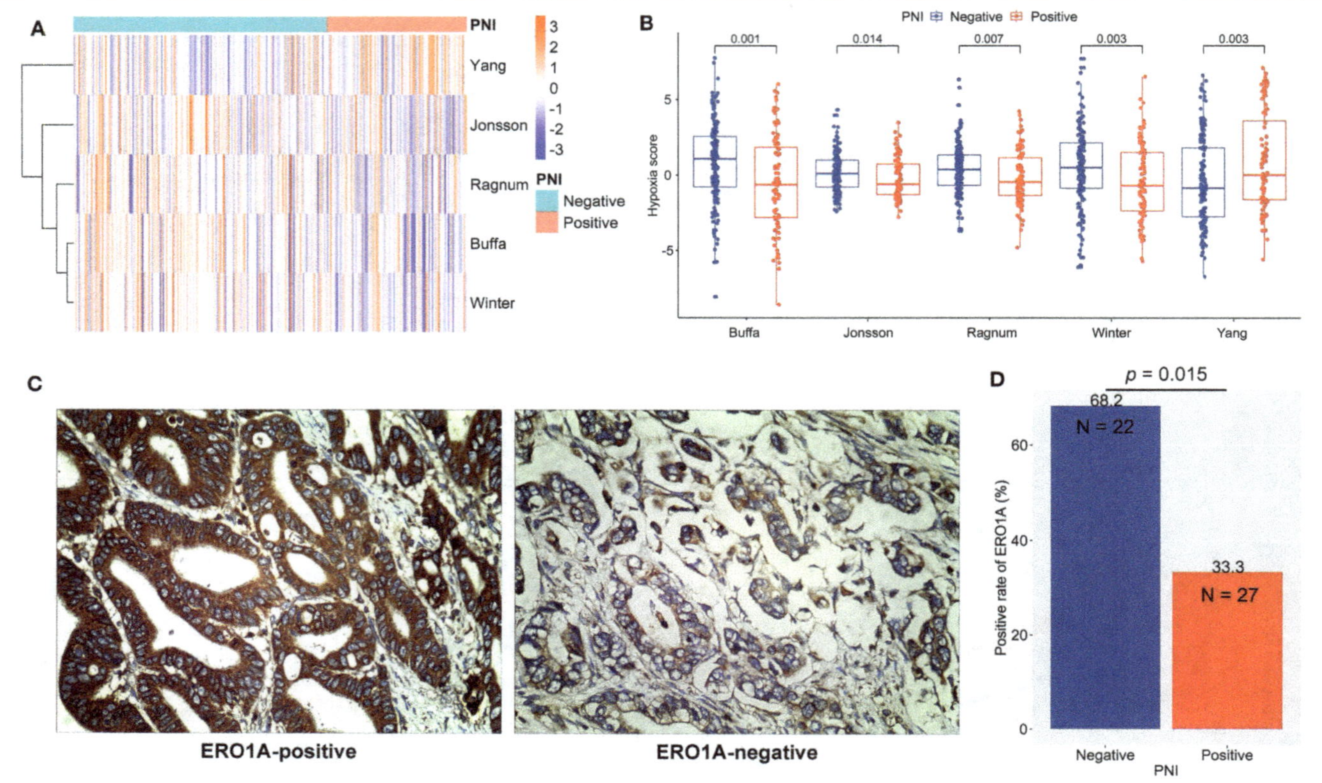

FIGURE 5 | Tumor hypoxia and perineural invasion (PNI). **(A,B)** Differences in hypoxia scores (signature authors are shown) in ACRG between PNI-positive and PNI-negative GC: A clustered heat map **(A)** and direct comparisons **(B)**. **(C)** Typical micrographs of ERO1A-negative and ERO1A-positive tumors, at 400× magnification. **(D)** Different positive rates of ERO1A between PNI-positive and PNI-negative GC. ACRG, Asian Cancer Research Group; GC: gastric cancer.

as well as time and additional cost. In this study, we showed that an established pathological characteristic, PNI, might help predict the efficacy of adjuvant chemotherapy in patients with resected GC. This finding may help improve patient selection and, consequently, improve therapy outcomes in patients with GC.

Previous studies have reported frequency of PNI occurrence in GC in the range from 6.8 to 75.6% (7), indicating heterogeneity of this patient population as well as variability in accuracy of detection methods, and differences in assessment criteria, among others. In the present study, we used S100 IHC to detect PNI, which is considered a classic approach (19). Moreover, we defined PNI according to Liebig et al's. proposal (5) that incorporated many recognized features of PNI. Adoption of these methods can help decrease the false negative/positive rate in PNI detection.

In our study, both the cardia GC proportion (54.8 vs. 35.4%) and the PNI incidence of this subgroup (63.1 vs. 34.2%) were significantly higher in the AHJU cohort than that in the JPH cohort, which may contribute to the large gap observed for the PNI incidences between these two cohorts. The AHJU cohort and the JPH cohort were heterogeneous, patients in AHJU mainly came from local cities such as Yangzhong city which is well-known for high incidences of gastrointestinal cancers (32), while many patients in JPH came from peripheral provinces and cities because JPH is a regional medical center.

The PME, also known as the perineural niche, is crucial to the pathogenesis of PNI (6, 33). Especially, tumor cells may have passion for PME. First, new tumor cells might prefer to penetrate the soft perineurium rather than the dense desmoplastic microenvironment of the primary tumor. Second, the nutrient-rich perineural space, characterized by extensive vascular and lymphatic supply, might trigger migration of tumor cells growing in a hypoxic and nutrient-deprived microenvironment. These theories suggest that PNI can effectively relieve tumor hypoxia, which is consistent with our finding that PNI-positive tumors were less hypoxic than were PNI-negative tumors.

We further found that in PNI-negative tumors, pathways that are important for FU metabolism or resistance, which could response to hypoxia (34, 35), were upregulated. Finally, in the present study *TYMS* mRNA and TS protein, a target for FU and biomarker of FU resistance (30), were overexpressed in PNI-negative relative to PNI-positive tumors. Recently, in a cohort of 285 GC patients, Pereira (36) found that high TS expression independently predicted poor DFS in stage III GC patients who received 5-FU-based adjuvant chemotherapy. These findings might explain the role of PNI in predicting the efficacy of adjuvant chemotherapy.

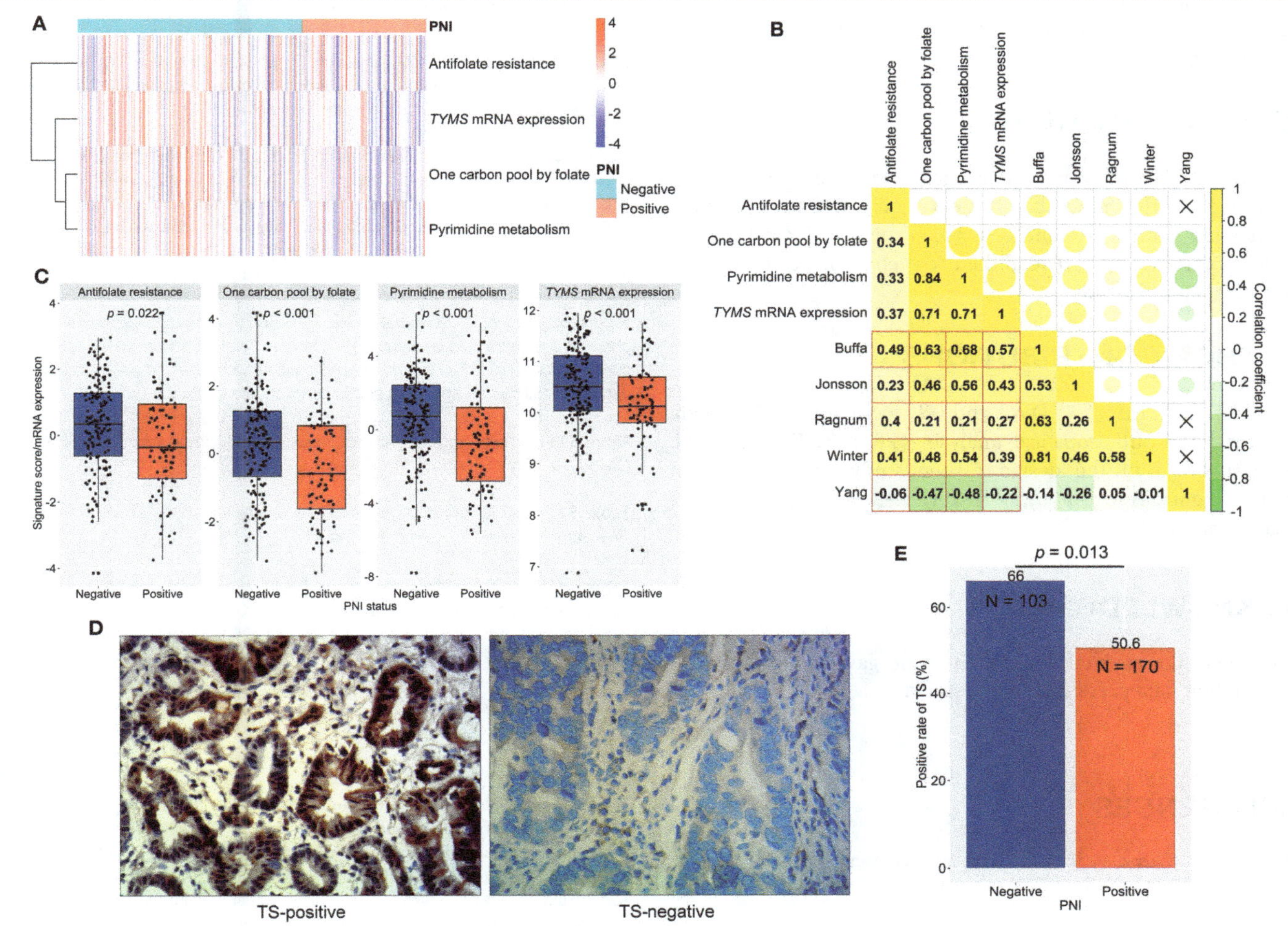

FIGURE 6 | Signaling scores, thymidylate synthetase (TS, *TYMS*) expression, and perineural invasion (PNI). **(A)** A clustered heat map for signaling scores and *TYMS* expression in ACRG. **(B)** The correlations between hypoxia scores (signature authors are shown) and signaling scores (Spearman correlation coefficients were shown and a fork mark indicated non-significant correlation). **(C)** Differences in signaling scores and *TYMS* expression between PNI-positive and PNI-negative GC. **(D)** Typical micrographs of TS-negative and TS-positive tumors, at 400× magnification. **(E)** Different positive rates of TS between PNI-positive and PNI-negative GC. GC, gastric cancer; ACRG, Asian Cancer Research Group.

Nevertheless, in the present study, PNI was not prognostic in resected GC. Considering the benefits of chemotherapy that were observed among patients with PNI-positive tumors but not among patients with PNI-negative tumors, a potential explanation may be that the adverse impact of PNI on survival could be reversed by adjuvant chemotherapy, which has been reported in patients with colorectal cancer (11, 12). Similarly, the prognostic effect of microsatellite instability (MSI), a potential biomarker for the efficacy of adjuvant chemotherapy in GC, could be attenuated by adjuvant chemotherapy (37). In terms of previous reports about the significant effects of PNI on prognosis (7), we cautioned that some early studies might have been affected by a lack of effective adjuvant therapies among patients with PNI-positive tumors.

This study has some limitations. First, this was a retrospective study, in which patients were not randomly selected. Prospective validation studies are warranted. However, our results were consistent for two independent cohorts, indicating robustness of our findings. Second, PNI might have existed in tumor tissues that were not sampled for testing in this study. Although we used three independent tissue sections to confirm PNI, some false PNI-negative results might have affected our findings. In addition, ethnic differences in the prognostic role of PNI in GC have been reported (7), suggesting the present results need to be verified in non-Chinese populations. Furthermore, data on some clinicopathological features, such as Lauren histotype, were not available in our study.

In conclusion, we revealed that PNI might be an independent predictor for adjuvant chemotherapy efficacy in patients with resected GC; however, its prognostic role remains conflicting. If validated by prospective studies, PNI might become a convenient marker to improve patient selection for adjuvant chemotherapy. Finally, novel treatment strategies need to be developed in PNI-negative patients.

ETHICS STATEMENT

The studies involving human participants were reviewed and approved by the ethics committees from Affiliated Hospital of Jiangsu University and Jiangsu Province Hospital. The patients/participants provided their written informed consent to participate in this study.

AUTHOR CONTRIBUTIONS

QT, WZ, XZ, ML, YS, DW, and XL were involved in data interpretation and statistical analysis. QT, WZ, DW, and XL were involved in the design of the study and preparation of the manuscript. All authors reviewed and approved the final manuscript.

ACKNOWLEDGMENTS

We would like to thank the patients who gave their consent to having their data presented in this study.

SUPPLEMENTARY MATERIAL

Figure S1 | Impact of perineural invasion (PNI) on patient survival in a combined patient cohort. **(A,B)** Overall survival and disease-free survival among patients with resected gastric cancer according to the PNI status.

Figure S2 | Impact of perineural invasion (PNI) on the efficacy of adjuvant chemotherapy in a combined patient cohort. **(A-D)** Overall survival (OS) and disease-free survival (DFS) among patients with resected gastric cancer according to PNI and treatment status. **(E)** Multivariate analyses of variables associated with OS and DFS, selected for their prognostic significance established in univariate analysis. LVI, lymphovascular invasion; CT, chemotherapy.

Figure S3 | Impact of perineural invasion (PNI) on the efficacy of adjuvant chemotherapy stratified by stages in a combined patient cohort. **(A–D)** Overall survival and disease-free survival among patients with resected gastric cancer according to PNI and treatment status stratified by stages.

Table S1 | Perineural invasion data of gastric cancer samples from the Asian Cancer Research Group.

Table S2 | Hypoxia scores of gastric cancer samples from the Asian Cancer Research Group.

Table S3 | Selected pathway scores and *TYMS* mRNA expression of gastric cancer samples from the Asian Cancer Research Group.

REFERENCES

1. Chen W, Zheng R, Baade PD, Zhang S, Zeng H, Bray F, et al. Cancer statistics in China, (2015). *CA Cancer J Clinh.* (2016) 66:115–32. doi: 10.3322/caac.21338
2. Schmidt B, Yoon SS. D1 versus D2 lymphadenectomy for gastric cancer. *J Surg Oncol.* (2013) 107:259–64. doi: 10.1002/jso.23127
3. Cai Z, Yin Y, Yin Y, Shen C, Wang J, Yin X, et al. Comparative effectiveness of adjuvant treatments for resected gastric cancer: a network meta-analysis. *Gastric Cancer.* (2018) 21:1031–40. doi: 10.1007/s10120-018-0831-0
4. Cai Z, Yin Y, Shen C, Wang J, Yin X, Chen Z, et al. Comparative effectiveness of preoperative, postoperative and perioperative treatments for resectable gastric cancer: a network meta-analysis of the literature from the past 20 years. *Surg Oncol.* (2018) 27:563–74. doi: 10.1016/j.suronc.2018.07.011
5. Liebig C, Ayala G, Wilks JA, Berger DH, Albo D. Perineural invasion in cancer: a review of the literature. *Cancer.* (2009) 115:3379–91. doi: 10.1002/cncr.24396
6. Chen SH, Zhang BY, Zhou B, Zhu CZ, Sun LQ, Feng YJ. Perineural invasion of cancer: a complex crosstalk between cells and molecules in the perineural niche. *Am J Cancer Res.* (2019) 9:1–21.
7. Deng J, You Q, Gao Y, Yu Q, Zhao P, Zheng Y, et al. Prognostic value of perineural invasion in gastric cancer: a systematic review and meta-analysis. *PLoS ONE.* (2014) 9:e88907. doi: 10.1371/journal.pone.0088907
8. España-Ferrufino A, Lino-Silva LS, Salcedo-Hernández RA. Extramural perineural invasion in pT3 and pT4 gastric carcinomas. *J Pathol Transl Med.* (2018) 52:79–84. doi: 10.4132/jptm.2017.11.01
9. de Franco L, Marrelli D, Voglino C, Vindigni C, Ferrara F, Di Mare G, et al. Prognostic value of perineural invasion in resected gastric cancer patients according to lauren histotype. *Pathol Oncol Res.* (2018) 24:393–400. doi: 10.1007/s12253-017-0257-8
10. Huh JW, Kim HR, Kim YJ. Prognostic value of perineural invasion in patients with stage II colorectal cancer. *Ann Surg Oncol.* (2010) 17:2066–72. doi: 10.1245/s10434-010-0982-7
11. Cienfuegos JA, Martínez P, Baixauli J, Beorlegui C, Rosenstone S, Sola JJ, et al. Perineural invasion is a major prognostic and predictive factor of response to adjuvant chemotherapy in stage I-II colon cancer. *Ann Surg Oncol.* (2017) 24:1077–84. doi: 10.1245/s10434-016-5561-0
12. Suzuki T, Suwa K, Ogawa M, Eto K, Kawahara H, Fujita T, et al. Adjuvant chemotherapy for the perineural invasion of colorectal cancer. *J Surg Res.* (2015) 199:84–9. doi: 10.1016/j.jss.2015.03.101
13. Song JH, Yu M, Kang KM, Lee JH, Kim SH, Nam TK, et al. Significance of perineural and lymphovascular invasion in locally advanced rectal cancer treated by preoperative chemoradiotherapy and radical surgery: can perineural invasion be an indication of adjuvant chemotherapy. *Radiother Oncol.* (2019) 133:125–31. doi: 10.1016/j.radonc.2019.01.002
14. Turley SJ, Cremasco V, Astarita JL. Immunological hallmarks of stromal cells in the tumour microenvironment. *Nat Rev Immunol.* (2015) 15:669–82. doi: 10.1038/nri3902
15. Fridman WH, Zitvogel L, Sautès-Fridman C, Kroemer G. The immune contexture in cancer prognosis and treatment. *Nat Rev Clin Oncol.* (2017) 14:717–34. doi: 10.1038/nrclinonc.2017.101
16. Zeng D, Li M, Zhou R, Zhang J, Sun H, Shi M, et al. Tumor microenvironment characterization in gastric cancer identifies prognostic and immunotherapeutically relevant gene signatures. *Cancer Immunol Res.* (2019) 7:canimm.0436. doi: 10.1158/2326-6066.CIR-18-0436
17. Jiang Y, Zhang Q, Hu Y, Li T, Yu J, Zhao L, et al. ImmunoScore signature: a prognostic and predictive tool in gastric cancer. *Ann Surg.* (2018) 267:504–13. doi: 10.1097/SLA.0000000000002116
18. Zhao X, Dai D, Li X, Shen B, Chen X, Shu Y, et al. A polymorphism within the mismatch repair gene predicts prognosis and adjuvant chemotherapy benefit in gastric cancer. *Gastric Cancer.* (2019) 22:1121–9. doi: 10.1007/s10120-019-00962-8
19. Kurtz KA, Hoffman HT, Zimmerman MB, Robinson RA. Perineural and vascular invasion in oral cavity squamous carcinoma: increased incidence on re-review of slides and by using immunohistochemical enhancement. *Arch Pathol Lab Med.* (2005) 129:354–9. doi: 10.1043/1543-2165(2005)129<354:PAVIIO>2.0.CO;2

20. Wang D, Li X, Shen B, Chen X, Shu Y. Histone chaperone CHAF1A impacts the outcome of fluoropyrimidines-based adjuvant therapy in gastric cancer by regulating the expression of thymidylate synthetase. *Gene.* (2019) 716:144034. doi: 10.1016/j.gene.2019.144034
21. Seol SY, Kim C, Lim JY, Yoon SO, Hong SW, Kim JW, et al. Overexpression of endoplasmic reticulum oxidoreductin 1-α (ERO1L) is associated with poor prognosis of gastric cancer. *Cancer Res Treat.* (2016) 48:1196–209. doi: 10.4143/crt.2015.189
22. Cristescu R, Lee J, Nebozhyn M, Kim KM, Ting JC, Wong SS, et al. Molecular analysis of gastric cancer identifies subtypes associated with distinct clinical outcomes *Nat Med.* (2015) 21:449–56. doi: 10.1038/nm.3850
23. Buffa FM, Harris AL, West CM, Miller CJ. Large meta-analysis of multiple cancers reveals a common, compact and highly prognostic hypoxia metagene. *Br J Cancer.* (2010) 102:428–35. doi: 10.1038/sj.bjc.6605450
24. Jonsson M, Ragnum HB, Julin CH, Yeramian A, Clancy T, Frikstad KM, et al. Hypoxia-independent gene expression signature associated with radiosensitisation of prostate cancer cell lines by histone deacetylase inhibition. *Br J Cancer.* (2016) 115:929–39. doi: 10.1038/bjc.2016.278
25. Ragnum HB, Vlatkovic L, Lie AK, Axcrona K, Julin CH, Frikstad KM, et al. The tumour hypoxia marker pimonidazole reflects a transcriptional programme associated with aggressive prostate cancer. *Br J Cancer.* (2015) 112:382–90. doi: 10.1038/bjc.2014.604
26. Winter SC, Buffa FM, Silva P, Miller C, Valentine HR, Turley H, et al. Relation of a hypoxia metagene derived from head and neck cancer to prognosis of multiple cancers. *Cancer Res.* (2007) 67:3441–9. doi: 10.1158/0008-5472.CAN-06-3322
27. Yang L, Taylor J, Eustace A, Irlam JJ, Denley H, Hoskin PJ, et al. A gene signature for selecting benefit from hypoxia modification of radiotherapy for high-risk bladder cancer patients. *Clin Cancer Res.* (2017) 23:4761–8. doi: 10.1158/1078-0432.CCR-17-0038
28. Wilson WR, Hay MP. Targeting hypoxia in cancer therapy. *Nat Rev Cancer.* (2011) 11:393–410. doi: 10.1038/nrc3064
29. Takei N, Yoneda A, Kosaka M, Sakai-Sawada K, Tamura Y. ERO1α is a novel endogenous marker of hypoxia in human cancer cell lines. *BMC Cancer.* (2019) 19:510. doi: 10.1186/s12885-019-5727-9
30. Wilson PM, Danenberg PV, Johnston PG, Lenz HJ, Ladner RD. Standing the test of time: targeting thymidylate biosynthesis in cancer therapy. *Nat Rev Clin Oncol.* (2014) 11:282–98. doi: 10.1038/nrclinonc.2014.51
31. Sohn BH, Hwang JE, Jang HJ, Lee HS, Oh SC, Shim JJ, et al. Clinical significance of four molecular subtypes of gastric cancer identified by the cancer genome atlas project. *Clin Cancer Res.* (2017) 23:4441–9. doi: 10.1158/1078-0432.CCR-16-2211
32. Shao Y, Hua Z, Zhao L, Shen Y, Guo X, Niu C, et al. Time trends of gastrointestinal cancers incidence and mortality in Yangzhong From 1991 to 2015: an updated age-period-cohort analysis. *Front Oncol.* (2018) 8:638. doi: 10.3389/fonc.2018.00638
33. Abiatari I, DeOliveira T, Kerkadze V, Schwager C, Esposito I, Giese NA, et al. Consensus transcriptome signature of perineural invasion in pancreatic carcinoma. *Mol Cancer Ther.* (2009) 8:1494–504. doi: 10.1158/1535-7163.MCT-08-0755
34. Shukla SK, Purohit V, Mehla K, Gunda V, Chaika NV, Vernucci E, et al. MUC1 and HIF-1alpha signaling crosstalk induces anabolic glucose metabolism to impart gemcitabine resistance to pancreatic cancer. *Cancer Cell.* (2017) 32:71–87.e7. doi: 10.1016/j.ccell.2017.06.004
35. Tampellini M, Bironzo P, Di Maio M, Scagliotti GV. Thymidine phosphorylase: the unforeseen driver in colorectal cancer treatment. *Future Oncol.* (2018) 14:1223–31. doi: 10.2217/fon-2017-0627
36. Pereira MA, Ramos M, Dias AR, Faraj SF, Cirqueira C, de Mello ES, et al. Immunohistochemical expression of thymidylate synthase and prognosis in gastric cancer patients submitted to fluoropyrimidine-based chemotherapy. *Chin J Cancer Res.* (2018) 30:526–36. doi: 10.21147/j.issn.1000-9604.2018.05.06
37. Kim SY, Choi YY, An JY, Shin HB, Jo A, Choi H, et al. The benefit of microsatellite instability is attenuated by chemotherapy in stage II and stage III gastric cancer: results from a large cohort with subgroup analyses. *Int J Cancer.* (2015) 137:819–25. doi: 10.1002/ijc.29449

Permissions

All chapters in this book were first published by Frontiers; hereby published with permission under the Creative Commons Attribution License or equivalent. Every chapter published in this book has been scrutinized by our experts. Their significance has been extensively debated. The topics covered herein carry significant findings which will fuel the growth of the discipline. They may even be implemented as practical applications or may be referred to as a beginning point for another development.

The contributors of this book come from diverse backgrounds, making this book a truly international effort. This book will bring forth new frontiers with its revolutionizing research information and detailed analysis of the nascent developments around the world.

We would like to thank all the contributing authors for lending their expertise to make the book truly unique. They have played a crucial role in the development of this book. Without their invaluable contributions this book wouldn't have been possible. They have made vital efforts to compile up to date information on the varied aspects of this subject to make this book a valuable addition to the collection of many professionals and students.

This book was conceptualized with the vision of imparting up-to-date information and advanced data in this field. To ensure the same, a matchless editorial board was set up. Every individual on the board went through rigorous rounds of assessment to prove their worth. After which they invested a large part of their time researching and compiling the most relevant data for our readers.

The editorial board has been involved in producing this book since its inception. They have spent rigorous hours researching and exploring the diverse topics which have resulted in the successful publishing of this book. They have passed on their knowledge of decades through this book. To expedite this challenging task, the publisher supported the team at every step. A small team of assistant editors was also appointed to further simplify the editing procedure and attain best results for the readers.

Apart from the editorial board, the designing team has also invested a significant amount of their time in understanding the subject and creating the most relevant covers. They scrutinized every image to scout for the most suitable representation of the subject and create an appropriate cover for the book.

The publishing team has been an ardent support to the editorial, designing and production team. Their endless efforts to recruit the best for this project, has resulted in the accomplishment of this book. They are a veteran in the field of academics and their pool of knowledge is as vast as their experience in printing. Their expertise and guidance has proved useful at every step. Their uncompromising quality standards have made this book an exceptional effort. Their encouragement from time to time has been an inspiration for everyone.

The publisher and the editorial board hope that this book will prove to be a valuable piece of knowledge for researchers, students, practitioners and scholars across the globe.

List of Contributors

Juan Wang, Quan Wang and Gang Ji
Department of Digestive Surgery, Xi Jing Hospital, The Fourth Military Medical University, Xi'an, China

Min Yang
Emergency Department, Huangpu Branch of the Ninth People's Hospital Affiliated to the Medical College of Shanghai Jiaotong University, Shanghai, China

Yunhe Gao, Bo Wei, Aizhen Cai, Jiyang Li and Lin Chen
Department of General Surgery, Chinese PLA General Hospital, Beijing, China
General Surgery Institute, Chinese PLA General Hospital, Beijing, China

Hongqing Xi, Jianxin Cui, Kecheng Zhang, Hua Li and Zhi Qiao
Department of General Surgery, Chinese PLA General Hospital, Beijing, China

Weishen Shen
Department of General Surgery, Chinese PLA General Hospital, Beijing, China
Nanjing General Hospital of Nanjing Military Command, Nanjing, China

Rafael Rosell
Catalan Institute of Oncology, Germans Trias i Pujol Health Science Institute and Hospital, Barcelona, Spain

Joseph Chao
Department of Medical Oncology and Therapeutics Research, City of Hope Comprehensive Cancer Center, Duarte, CA, United States

Tianhui Chen
Department of Cancer Prevention, Institute of Cancer and Basic Medicine (ICBM), Zhejiang Provincial Office for Cancer Prevention and Control, Cancer Hospital of the University of CAS, Chinese Academy of Sciences (CAS), Hangzhou, China

Samuel Klempner
The Angeles Clinic and Research Institute, Los Angeles, CA, United States
Samuel Oschin Comprehensive Cancer Institute, Cedars-Sinai Medical Center, Los Angeles, CA, United States

Chang Min Lee
Department of Surgery, Korea University College of Medicine, Seoul, South Korea
Department of Surgery, Korea University Medical Center Ansan Hospital, Ansan, South Korea

San Lee and Danbi Lee
Department of Surgery, Korea University Medical Center Ansan Hospital, Ansan, South Korea

Sungsoo Park
Department of Surgery, Korea University College of Medicine, Seoul, South Korea
Department of Surgery, Korea University Medical Center Anam Hospital, Seoul, South Korea

Zepang Sun, Hao Liu, Weicai Huang, Zhen Han, Hao Chen, Mingli Zhao, Yanfeng Hu, Yuming Jiang and Guoxin Li
Department of General Surgery, Nanfang Hospital, Southern Medical University, Guangzhou, China

Tian Lin and Jiang Yu
Department of General Surgery, Nanfang Hospital, Southern Medical University, Guangzhou, China

Chaogang Yang, Shuyi Wang and Bin Xiong
Department of Gastrointestinal Surgery, Zhongnan Hospital of Wuhan University, Wuhan, China
Hubei Key Laboratory of Tumor Biological Behaviors, Wuhan, China
Hubei Cancer Clinical Study Center, Wuhan, China

Fangfang Chen
Hubei Key Laboratory of Tumor Biological Behaviors, Wuhan, China
Hubei Cancer Clinical Study Center, Wuhan, China
Department of Breast and Thyroid Surgery, Zhongnan Hospital of Wuhan University, Wuhan, China

Shuchun Li and Lu Zang
Department of Surgery, Ruijin Hospital, Shanghai Jiaotong University School of Medicine, Shanghai, China
Shanghai Minimally Invasive Surgery Center, Shanghai, China

Chang In Choi
Department of Surgery, Biomedical Research Institute, Pusan National University College of Medicine, Busan, South Korea

Ji Ho Park
Department of Surgery, Gyeongsang National University School of Medicine, Jinju, South Korea

Ye Seob Jee
Department of Surgery, Dankook University College of Medicine, Cheonan, South Korea

Han Hong Lee
Department of Surgery, College of Medicine, The Catholic University of Korea, Seoul, South Korea

Oh Jeong
Department of Surgery, Chonnam National University Medical School, Gwangju, South Korea

Zai Luo, Zeyin Rong and Chen Huang
Department of General Surgery, Shanghai General Hospital, School of Medicine, Shanghai Jiao Tong University, Shanghai, China

Won Jun Kim and Liang An
Korea University Medical Center, College of Medicine, Seoul, South Korea

Jong-Han Kim
Department of Surgery, Korea University Medical Center, Guro Hospital, Seoul, South Korea

Tom van den Ende, Frank A. Abe Nijenhuis, Héctor G. van den Boorn, Emil ter Veer, Martijn G. H. van Oijen and Hanneke W. M. van Laarhoven
Department of Medical Oncology, Cancer Center Amsterdam, Amsterdam University Medical Centers (UMC), University of Amsterdam, Amsterdam, Netherlands

Maarten C. C. M. Hulshof
Department of Radiotherapy, Cancer Center Amsterdam, Amsterdam University Medical Centers (UMC), University of Amsterdam, Amsterdam, Netherlands

Suzanne S. Gisbertz
Department of Surgery, Cancer Center Amsterdam, Amsterdam University Medical Centers (UMC), University of Amsterdam, Amsterdam, Netherlands

Mengdi Yang, Zhiyuan Jiang, Guangyu Yao, Zhiyu Wang, Jing Sun and Hui Zhao
Department of Internal Oncology, Shanghai Jiao Tong University Affiliated Sixth People's Hospital, Shanghai, China

Huanlong Qin
Department of Gastrointestinal Surgery, Shanghai Tenth People's Hospital Affiliated with Tongji University, Shanghai, China

Liangliang An, Haidong Cheng and Mingxing Hou
Department of General Surgery, Affiliated Hospital of Inner Mongolia Medical University, Hohhot, China

Sharen Gaowa
Department of Pathology, College of Basic Medicine, Inner Mongolia Medical University, Hohhot, China

Fei Zhang, Xuanzhang Huang, Peng Gao, Zhexu Guo, Jinxin Shi, Zhonghua Wu and Zhenning Wang
Key Laboratory of Precision Diagnosis and Treatment of Gastrointestinal Tumors, Ministry of Education, Department of Surgical Oncology and General Surgery, The First Affiliated Hospital of China Medical University, Shenyang, China

Cen Zhou and Yongxi Song
Department of Surgical Oncology and General Surgery, Key Laboratory of Precision Diagnosis and Treatment of Gastrointestinal Tumors, Ministry of Education, The First Affiliated Hospital of China Medical University, Shenyang, China

Yunshu Su
Department of Thoracic Surgery, Renmin Hospital of Wuhan University, Wuhan, China

Jinqi Huang
Division of Cardiothoracic Surgery, Central Hospital of EnShi Tujia and Miao Autonomous Prefecture, EnShi Clinical College of Wuhan University, EnShi, China

Jichang Hu
Department of Pathology, Renmin Hospital of Wuhan University, Wuhan, China

Xi Zhong and Jie Sun
Department of Surgical Oncology and General Surgery, Key Laboratory of Precision Diagnosis and Treatment of Gastrointestinal Tumors, Ministry of Education, The First Affiliated Hospital of China Medical University, Shenyang, China

Xiaoyong Shen
Department of Radiology, First Affiliated Hospital, Zhejiang University School of Medicine, Hangzhou, China

Fan Yang, Modan Yang, Jianyong Zhuo, Jianguo Wang, Di Lu, Zhikun Liu, Shu-sen Zheng and Xiao Xu
Department of Hepatobiliary and Pancreatic Surgery, First Affiliated Hospital, Zhejiang University School of Medicine, Hangzhou, China

Pengfei Yang
Sir Run Run Shaw Hospital, Zhejiang University School of Medicine, Hangzhou, China
Institute of Translational Medicine, Zhejiang University, Hangzhou, China
College of Biomedical Engineering & Instrument Science, Zhejiang University, Hangzhou, China

Lei Xu
Sir Run Run Shaw Hospital, Zhejiang University School of Medicine, Hangzhou, China
Institute of Translational Medicine, Zhejiang University, Hangzhou, China

Tianye Niu
Sir Run Run Shaw Hospital, Zhejiang University School of Medicine, Hangzhou, China
Institute of Translational Medicine, Zhejiang University, Hangzhou, China
Nuclear & Radiological Engineering and Medical Physics Programs, Woodruff School of Mechanical Engineering, Georgia Institute of Technology, Atlanta, GA, United States

Chiara Arienti, Sara Pignatta and Anna Tesei
Biosciences Laboratory, Istituto Scientifico Romagnolo per lo Studio e la Cura dei Tumori (IRST) IRCCS, Meldola, Italy

Hongyong He, Haojie Li, Botian Ye and Fenglin Liu
Department of General Surgery, Zhongshan Hospital, Fudan University, Shanghai, China

Xinhua Chen, Yuehong Chen, Jun Luo, Tuanjie Li, Tao Li, HuiLin Huang, Yu Zhu and Tingting Li
Department of General Surgery, Nanfang Hospital, Southern Medical University, Guangzhou, China

Lin Zhao, Jiarui Li, Chunmei Bai and Yongdu Nie
Department of Medical Oncology, Peking Union Medical College Hospital, Chinese Academy of Medical Sciences and Peking Union Medical College, Beijing, China

Guole Lin
Department of General Surgery, Peking Union Medical College Hospital, Chinese Academy of Medical Sciences and Peking Union Medical College, Beijing, China

Zhi Yang, Xingya Zhu, Xiaofeng Lu, Liang Zhang, Heng Yu, Chuanfu Ren and Yizhou Wang
Department of General Surgery, Drum Tower Clinical Medical College of Nanjing Medical University, Nanjing, China

Feifei Xue
Jiangsu Key Laboratory of Oral Diseases, Nanjing Medical University, Nanjing, China

Minhuan Li
Department of Andrology, Drum Tower Clinical Medical College of Nanjing Medical University, Nanjing, China

Chao Wang, En Xu and Xingzhou Wang
Department of General Surgery, Nanjing Drum Tower Hospital, The Affiliated Hospital of Nanjing University Medical School, Nanjing, China

Hao Wang, Wenxian Guan and Xuefeng Xia
Department of General Surgery, Drum Tower Clinical Medical College of Nanjing Medical University, Nanjing, China
Department of General Surgery, Nanjing Drum Tower Hospital, The Affiliated Hospital of Nanjing University Medical School, Nanjing, China

Jie Chen
Department of Anesthesiology, Nanjing Drum Tower Hospital, The Affiliated Hospital of Nanjing University Medical School, Nanjing, China

Qing Tao, Wen Zhu, Deqiang Wang and Xiaoqin Li
Department of Medical Oncology, Affiliated Hospital of Jiangsu University, Zhenjiang, China

Xiaohui Zhao and Mei Li
Department of Pathology, Affiliated Hospital of Jiangsu University, Zhenjiang, China

Yongqian Shu
Department of Medical Oncology, Jiangsu Province Hospital, Nanjing, China

Index